PEDIATRIC AND
ADOLESCENT
HYPERTENSION

PEDIATRIC AND ADOLESCENT HYPERTENSION

EDITED BY

JENNIFER M. H. LOGGIE MD

CHILDREN'S HOSPITAL
MEDICAL CENTER
CINCINNATI, OHIO

BOSTON

BLACKWELL SCIENTIFIC PUBLICATIONS

OXFORD LONDON EDINBURGH
MELBOURNE PARIS BERLIN VIENNA

© 1992 by
Blackwell Scientific Publications, Inc.
Editorial offices:
3 Cambridge Center, Cambridge
  Massachusetts 02142, USA
Osney Mead, Oxford OX2 0EL, England
25 John Street, London WC1N 2BL
  England
23 Ainslie Place, Edinburgh EH3 6AJ
  Scotland
54 University Street, Carlton
  Victoria 3053, Australia

Other editorial offices:
Arnette SA
  2 rue Casimir-Delavigne
  75006 Paris
  France

Blackwell Wissenschaft
  Meinekestrasse 4
  D-1000 Berlin 15
  Germany

Blackwell MZV
  Feldgasse 13
  A-1238 Wien
  Austria

First published 1992

Set by Setrite Typesetters Ltd, Hong Kong
Printed and bound in the United States of
America by BookCrafters, Chelsea, Michigan

92 93 94 95 5 4 3 2 1

DISTRIBUTORS

USA
  Blackwell Scientific Publications, Inc.
  3 Cambridge Center
  Cambridge, MA 02142
  (*Orders*: Tel: 800 759−6102)

Canada
  Times Mirror Professional Publishing, Ltd
  5240 Finch Avenue East
  Scarborough, Ontario M1S 5A2
  (*Orders*: Tel: 416 298−1588)

Australia
  Blackwell Scientific Publications
  (Australia) Pty Ltd
  54 University Street
  Carlton, Victoria 3053
  (*Orders*: Tel: 03 347 0300)

Outside North America and Australia
  Marston Book Services Ltd
  PO Box 87
  Oxford OX2 0DT
  (*Orders*: Tel: 0865 791155
           Fax: 0865 791927
           Telex: 837515)

Library of Congress
Cataloging-in-Publication Data

Pediatric and adolescent hypertension
edited by Jennifer M. H. Loggie.
     p.   cm.
  Includes bibliographical references
  and index.
  ISBN 0−86542−097−1
  1. Hypertension in children.
  2. Hypertension in adolescence.
  I. Loggie, Jennifer M. H., 1936−
DNLM: 1 Hypertension − in adolescence.
  2. Hypertension − in infancy & childhood.
WG 340 J98
RJ426.H9J872 1992
618.92' 132 − dc20

Contents

List of Contributors

GERALD S. ARBUS MD, FRCP (C)
*Associate Professor of Pediatrics, Chief, Division of
Nephrology, The Hospital for Sick Children; Associate
Professor, Department of Pediatrics, Faculty of Medicine,
University of Toronto, Toronto, Ontario, Canada M5G IX8*

MICHAEL D. BAILIE MD, PhD
*Professor and Chairman of Pediatrics, Director, University
of Illinois, College of Medicine at Peoria, Illinois Drive,
Peoria, IL 61656*

WILLIAM S. BALL JR MD
*Associate Professor of Radiology and Pediatrics;
Chief, Section of Vascular Interventional Radiology,
Children's Hospital Medical Center; University of
Cincinnati College of Medicine, Cincinnati, OH 45229*

WILL R. BLACKBURN MD
*Professor of Pediatrics, Director, Pediatric—Perinatal
Pathology, Department of Pathology, University of South
Alabama, College of Medicine, 2451 Fillingim St, Mobile,
AL 36617*

FRANK G. BOINEAU MD
*Professor of Pediatrics and Head, Pediatric Nephrology,
Division of Nephrology, Tulane University Medical Center,
5534 Hutchinson Bldg, New Orleans, LA 70112*

JANE E. BRAZY MD
*Associate Professor of Pediatrics; Director, Wisconsin
Perinatal Center; University of Wisconsin/Meriter
Hospital, Madison General, 202 South Park St, Madison,
WI 53715*

RUSSELL W. CHESNEY MD
*Division of Pediatric Nephrology, Department of Pediatrics,
University of Tennessee, Memphis, College of Medicine; Le
Bonheur Children's Medical Center, Memphis, TN 38103*

JAMES L. CHRISTIANSEN MD
*Assistant Professor, Pediatric Cardiology, Department of
Pediatrics, The University of Iowa Hospitals and Clinics,
The University of Iowa, Iowa City, Iowa 52242*

JOSÉ C. CORTEZ MD
*Resident, Division of Urology, Department of Surgery,
University of Cincinnati College of Medicine; 231 Bethesda
Av., Cincinnati, OH 45267*

CHRISTOPHER CRAWFORD
*Academic Research Specialist, Division of Pediatric
Endocrinology, Department of Pediatrics, New York
Hospital—Cornell Medical Center, New York, NY 10021*

STEPHEN R. DANIELS MD, PhD
*Associate Professor of Pediatrics; Assistant Professor of
Environmental Health, University of Cincinnati College of
Medicine; Cardiologist, Children's Hospital Medical Center,
Elland & Bethesda Aves, Cincinnati, OH 45229*

DARRYL C. DE VIVO MD
*Sidney Carter Professor of Neurology, Professor of
Pediatrics, Director of Pediatric Neurology, College of
Physicians and Surgeons of Columbia University;
Departments of Neurology and Pediatrics, Division of
Pediatric Neurology, Neurological Institute, 710 West
168th St, New York, NY 10032*

HARRIET P. DUSTAN MD
*Emeritus Professor of Medicine, University of Alabama,
School of Medicine, Birmingham, AL 35294. Present
address: 28 Hagan Drive, Essex, VT 05452*

ZEINAB M. ELKWIRY MB, ChB, MS, MPH
2505 Clover Glen, Edmond, OK 73013

and Hypertension, The Medical College of Pennsylvania, 3300 Henry Ave, Philadelphia, PA 19129

MICHELLE FARINE MD, FRCP (C)

Staff Pediatrician, Hospital for Sick Children; Assistant Professor, Department of Pediatrics, Faculty of Medicine, University of Toronto, Toronto, Ontario, Canada M59 IX8

ROBIN A. FELDER PhD

Assistant Professor of Pathology; Associate Director, Clinical Chemistry and Toxicology, University of Virginia Medical Center, Charlottesville, VA 22908

DAVID E. FIXLER MD

Director of Cardiology, University of Texas Health Science Center at Dallas, Southwestern Medical School, 5323 Harry Hines Blvd, Dallas, TX 75235−9063

LARRY E. FLEISCHMANN MD

Professor of Pediatrics; Director, Division of Pediatric Nephrology, Children's Hospital of Michigan, 3901 Beaubien Blvd, Detroit, MI 48201

AARON L. FREIDMAN MD

Professor of Pediatrics, Division of Pediatric Nephrology, Department of Pediatrics, University of Wisconsin Center for the Health Sciences, Madison, WI 53705

WILLIAM J. FRY MD

Catherine McAuley Health Center, Head, Department of General Surgery, St. Joseph Mercy Hospital, PO Box 995, Ann Arbor, MI 48106

ALAN B. GRUSKIN MD

Professor and Chairman, Department of Pediatrics; Pediatrician-in-Chief, Children's Hospital of Michigan, 3901 Beaubien Blvd, Detroit, MI 48201

JONATHAN D. HEILICZER MD

Director, Section of Pediatric Nephrology; Assistant Professor of Pediatrics, Rush Medical College, Chicago, IL 60612

ARNO R. HOHN MD

Professor of Pediatrics, Head, Division of Pediatric Cardiology, University of Southern California, Children's Heart Center, Children's Hospital of Los Angeles, 4650 Sunset Blvd, Los Angeles, CA 90027

JULIE R. INGELFINGER MD

Associate Professor of Pediatrics, Harvard Medical School, Co-chief, Pediatric Nephrology Unit, Massachusetts General Hospital, Bartlett Hall Extension #4, Fruit Street, Boston, MA 02114

PEDRO A. JOSE MD, PhD

Professor of Pediatrics; Director, Pediatric Nephrology, Georgetown University Medical Center, Washington, DC 20007−2197

ALLEN P. KILLAM MD

Professor, Department of Obstetrics and Gynecology, Director, Division of Perinatology, Box 3122, Duke University Medical Center, Durham, NC 27710

GARY R. LERNER MD

Assistant Professor of Clinical Pediatrics; Medical Director, Hemodialysis Unit, Children's Hospital of Los Angeles, University of Southern California School of Medicine, 4650 Sunset Blvd, Los Angeles, CA 90027

JOHN E. LEWY MD

Reily Professor and Chairman, Department of Pediatrics, Tulane University School of Medicine, Tulane University Medical Center, 1430 Tulane Ave, New Orleans, LA 70112

JENNIFER M. H. LOGGIE MD

Professor of Pediatrics, Department of Pediatrics, University of Cincinnati College of Medicine; Director, Division of Clinical Pharmacology, Children's Hospital Medical Center, Elland & Bethesda Aves, Cincinnati, OH 45229

BARRY MARCUS MD

Assistant Professor of Clinical Pediatrics, Division of Cardiology, University of Southern California, Children's Heart Center, Children's Hospital of Los Angeles, 4650 Sunset Blvd, Los Angeles, CA 90027

GERARD R. MARTIN MD

Clinical Assistant Professor of Child Health and Development; Director of Pediatric Echocardiography, George Washington University, Washington, DC 20010

WALLACE W. McCRORY MD

Professor of Pediatrics, Director, Division of Pediatric Nephrology, New York Hospital−Cornell University Medical Center, New York, NY 10021

STEPHEN T. McGARVEY PhD, MPH
Assistant Professor of Medicine, Brown University;
Program in Geographic Medicine, The Miriam Hospital,
164 Summit Ave, Providence, RI 02906

EDDIE S. MOORE MD
Professor and Chairman, Department of Pediatrics,
University of Tennessee at Knoxville, Knoxville,
TN 37920–6999

ARTHUR J. MOSS MD
Emeritus Professor, University of California, Los Angeles;
UCLA School of Medicine, Department of Pediatrics; UCLA
Medical Center, Center for the Health Sciences, PC-01, Los
Angeles, CA 90024

MARIA I. NEW MD
Professor and Chairman, Department of Pediatrics; Chief,
Pediatric Endocrinology; Program Director, Pediatric CRC,
New York Hospital–Cornell University Medical Center,
New York, NY 10021

JEFFREY M. PERLMAN MB, ChB
Associate Professor of Pediatrics and Obstetrics/
Gynecology Division of Neonatal–Perinatal Medicine, The
University of Texas, Southwestern Medical Center, Dallas,
TX 9063

MICHAEL R. PRANZATELLI MD
Director of Movement Disorders Service; Associate
Professor of Neurology, Pediatrics and Pharmacology,
George Washington University; Staff Neurologist, National
Medical Centre, 111 Michigan Avenue, Northwest,
Washington, DC 20010–2970

RONALD J. PRINEAS MB, BS, PhD
Professor and Chairman, University of Miami Department
of Epidemiology and Public Health, PO Box 016069
(R-669), 1029 Northwest 15th St, Miami, FL 33136

MAJID RASOULPOUR MD
Associate Professor, Department of Pediatrics, University
of Connecticut Health Center, School of Medicine;
Attending Physician, Hartford Hospital, Hartford,
CT 06103

NELSON REEDE COOLEY JR BA
Research Assistant, Pediatric–Perinatal Pathology,
University of South Alabama, College of Medicine,
2451 Fillingim St, Mobile, AL 36617

NORMAN D. ROSENBLUM MD
Instructor in Pediatrics, Division of Pediatric Nephrology,
The Children's Hospital, 300 Longwood Ave, Boston,
MA 02115

CURTIS A. SHELDON MD, FACS, FAAP
Associate Professor of Clinical Surgery, University of
Cincinnati College of Medicine; Director, Division of
Urology, Children's Hospital Medical Center, Elland &
Bethesda Aves, Cincinnati, OH 45229

ALAN R. SINAIKO MD
Professor of Pediatrics, Division of Clinical Pharmacology,
Departments of Pediatrics and Pharmacology, University of
Minnesota, Box 357, Mayo Building, Minneapolis,
MN 55455

PHYLLIS W. SPEISER MD
Associate Professor of Pediatrics, Division of Pediatric
Endocrinology, Department of Pediatrics, New York
Hospital–Cornell Medical Center, New York, NY 10021

ELIZABETH STONER MD
Associate Director, Clinical Research Cardiovascular/
Endocrinology, Merck, Sharp & Dohme Research
Laboratories, Rahway, NJ 07065–0914

C. FREDERIC STRIFE MD
Associate Professor of Pediatrics, University of Cincinnati
College of Medicine; Nephrologist, Children's Hospital
Medical Center, Elland & Bethesda Aves, Cincinnati,
OH 45229

WILLIAM B. STRONG MD
Charbonnier Professor of Pediatrics; Chief, Section of
Pediatric Cardiology, Medical College of Georgia, Augusta,
GA 30912

THOMAS R. WELCH MD
Associate Professor of Pediatrics, University of Cincinnati
College of Medicine; Director, Division of Nephrology,
Children's Hospital Medical Center, Elland & Bethesda
Aves, Cincinnati, OH 45229

PERRIN C. WHITE MD
Associate Professor of Pediatrics, Department of Pediatrics,
New York Hospital–Cornell Medical Center, New York,
NY 10021

STEPHEN H. ZINNER MD
Professor of Medicine, Director, Division of Infectious
Diseases, Brown University Medical Center and Rhode
Island Hospital, Providence, RI 02908

Preface

During the last 20 years it has become fairly widely accepted that essential hypertension and atherosclerosis have their origins in childhood. This information is important if effective hygienic interventions are to be devised and successfully implemented in the young, particularly those at highest risk for these conditions.

Much new information about hypertension and other coronary artery disease risk factors in children and adolescents has been collected in the past two decades from all over the world, but in the United States particularly in Bogalusa, Louisiana, and Muscatine, Iowa. The population studies conducted in these places by Dr Gerald Berenson and Dr Ronald Lauer respectively are the pediatric equivalents of the Framingham study.

However, much research is still required to further define the natural history of essential hypertension starting in childhood, as well as the efficacy of therapy in preventing its complications. One of the most important areas for study is that of the prevention and effective treatment of obesity in childhood. Obesity is a condition that is increasing in frequency in the United States in adults and in children. In our own clinical population of juveniles with essential hypertension, over 50% are 20 or more pounds (9 kg) above their ideal weight. Treatment is generally ineffective and is a source of frustration to patient and practitioner alike.

In this book, normal blood pressure control mechanisms as well as hypertension in childhood and adolescence are addressed. The first five chapters deal with the physiology of blood pressure regulation as it is known from studies in animals and humans. The next three chapters address the measurement and epidemiology of blood pressure in children.

Primary and secondary forms of hypertension, as they occur in a young population, are discussed in depth in chapters 16 through 26. There is a particularly important section of the book that deals with hypertension in special populations including blacks, pregnant females, and young athletes. In addition, there are seven chapters relating to the management of hypertension in childhood with four of these devoted to specific classes of drugs. The last two chapters of the book are related to outcome as it is presently known. Dr Blackburn's chapter (Chapter 32) on the pathology of hypertensive vascular disease is particularly provocative, and Dr Daniels provides newly accumulated data on end-organ damage from his own studies (Chapter 33).

By covering a wide range of topics, the book should be useful not only to those who have a research interest in hypertension in childhood, but also to physicians caring for children and adolescents who have high blood pressure.

Acknowledgments

For their patience and encouragement, I am indebted to all of the authors who have contributed to this book. In particular, I want to thank Dr Stephen Daniels who works with me and on whom I have leaned heavily for editorial support and advice. In addition, I am grateful to Mrs Janet Jump who has done so much of the secretarial work associated with the book in a diligent and longsuffering fashion.

Jennifer Loggie MD
Children's Hospital Medical Center
Cincinnati

1 The Integration of Blood Pressure Regulatory Mechanisms: An Overview

ARTHUR J. MOSS

Hypertension is a common disorder of the adult population in many parts of the world and it is estimated that in the United States approximately 15% of adults have hypertension of moderate or severe degree [1]. Many more have mild or borderline hypertension. Recent emphasis on the potentially serious consequences of this disorder and the likelihood that the primary (essential) form has its origins in childhood has served as a stimulus for physicians to include measurement of blood pressure as an integral part of the routine physical examination in childhood and adolescence. This is now common practice in most offices, even in children as young as 2 or 3 years of age.

The level of systemic arterial blood pressure is regulated by a number of complex and intricately interwoven factors and mechanisms (Fig. 1.1). These include cardiovascular, renal, neural, and hormonal influences. Knowledge of these forces and their integration in both health and disease is important for optimal management of the hypertensive patient, whether the disorder is primary or secondary.

The mechanisms of blood pressure control always act in concert, never in isolation. Their integration is so complex that even now, after decades of research, it is only partially understood. Basic to the comprehension of what is currently known is some degree of familiarity with the individual behavior of these forces and this is covered in great detail in subsequent chapters. However, in order to facilitate an understanding of the integration of blood pressure regulatory mechanisms to be discussed here some duplication is necessary.

THE CARDIOVASCULAR SYSTEM

The cardiovascular forces which determine and regulate the level of systemic arterial blood pressure include cardiac output (CO), blood volume, arterial elasticity, vascular resistance, and blood viscosity. As stated above, these forces do not exert their influence independently but are affected, sometimes to a profound degree, by other factors. For example, the secretion of aldosterone causes sodium and water retention and therefore increases blood volume; angiotensin is a powerful vasoconstrictor and can affect peripheral vascular resistance (PVR) in such a way that cardiac afterload is increased; the prostaglandin and kallikrein—kinin systems on the other hand are vasodilators and act to reduce afterload; other vasoactive agents are believed to include oxygen which may cause changes in blood vessel caliber and thereby affect organ flow and perfusion pressure. To complicate the picture further, blood flow and thus organ perfusion are not uniform throughout the body. For example, a rise in perfusion pressure to the kidneys by local means quickly produces a rise in vascular resistance whereas in the skin, the autoregulatory response is manifested by a fall in resistance. Add to these mechanisms the powerful influence of the central nervous system (CNS) and it is obvious that any attempt to unravel the complexities of blood pressure control is at best a difficult task.

Cardiac output

This is the driving force behind organ and tissue perfusion. It is determined by stroke volume (SV) and heart rate (HR). It has long been an accepted principle in cardiovascular laboratories that the product of SV and HR is equivalent to the volume of blood ejected by the ventricles over a given period of time (usually 1 min). Both of these parameters are major determinants of the level of blood pressure and a change in one must affect the other inversely if CO is to remain constant. For example, highly trained athletes have a very large SV but this is compensated

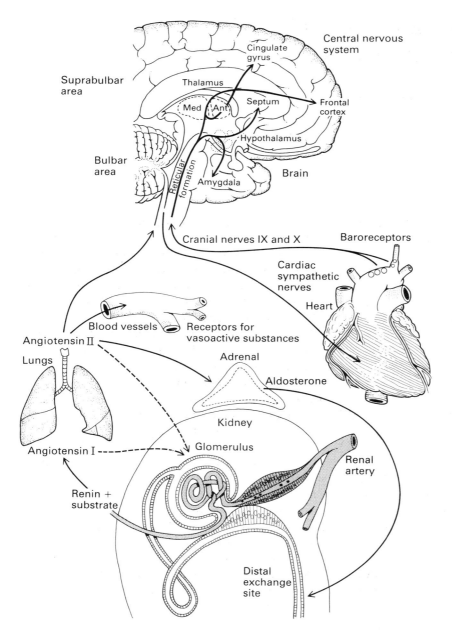

Fig. 1.1 Relationship of major systems. This rendering shows the central neural control of the circulation and the renal—adrenal axis in relation to it. (1) Cardiac output and the resultant arterial pressure monitored by the aortic and carotid baroreceptors. (2) Bulbar area (cardiorespiratory center), where the simple reflex control of the blood pressure resides (input via cranial nerves IX and X, autonomic outflow via cardiac sympathetic nerves). (3) Suprabulbar area where integrative control of the circulation occurs, based on input from all systems and appropriate changes in the arterial pressure set-point signaled to the bulbar area. (4) Renal artery vasoaction in response to neural receptors within heart and great vessels. (5) Juxtaglomerular apparatus: afferent arteriole and macula densa integration of renin release. (6) Pulmonary conversion of angiotensin I to angiotensin II. (7A) Central nervous system feedback of angiotensin. (7B) Vascular receptors for direct vasoconstriction. (7C) Angiotensin direct stimulation of adrenal for release of aldosterone. (7D) Intrarenal feedback for renin release. (8) Aldosterone release from the adrenal to effect sodium reabsorption form distal exchange site. From [2].

for by a decrease in HR. In some of these individuals, the increased SV may be reflected by an increase in *systolic* blood pressure depending on the compliance of the arterial vasculature. On the other hand, under certain circumstances, HR will affect the level of *diastolic* pressure. Diastolic blood pressure is dependent upon the rate of fall of arterial pressure during systole and the rate of fall is dependent to some extent on the interval between each systolic contraction of the heart. With a slow HR and thus a longer diastolic interval, the pressure during diastole will fall to levels lower than those seen with a rapid HR

and a shorter diastolic interval [3]. Heart rate in itself is not a very effective means of increasing CO unless other influences maintain SV. These influences may be neural, hormonal, or chemical and may exert their action directly or indirectly, in concert with one another or independently.

Changes in body position exert a profound but very transient effect on arterial pressure. But in the normal individual, the baroreceptor reflexes quickly respond and the cardiovascular adjustments consist of a rise in HR and in PVR along with a decrease in venous capacitance. Impairment of this reflex action results in orthostatic hypotension and in extreme cases syncope may ensue [4].

With the Valsalva maneuver, as in coughing or during defecation, venous return and right-sided cardiac filling are impeded by the increased intrathoracic pressure. There is also a transient increase in left-sided cardiac filling. As a result, SV and mean systemic arterial pressure rise momentarily and then fall. The latter precipitates a reflex increase in HR and in PVR. Immediately following the Valsalva maneuver, blood flow to the intrathoracic veins abruptly increases and so does cardiac filling, SV, and CO. Since PVR at that point in time is still high, there is an overshoot of arterial pressure which may be very marked. An accompanying bradycardia is reflexly produced [4].

Emotional states such as fear, anxiety, and anger are accompanied by physiologic changes in cardiovascular regulation. These are reflected by a rise in both HR and blood pressure, the latter resulting from increased resistance in the splanchnic vascular bed. Pain produces a similar reaction. In rare instances, however, bradycardia and a fall in blood pressure may occur and these may be severe enough to produce syncope (vasovagal attack) [4].

During maximal physical exercise, a significant increase in CO is needed to maintain adequate blood flow and this is accomplished by an increase in both HR and SV. As a consequence, systolic blood pressure rises, and in normotensive individuals and adolescents with borderline hypertension it has been observed to approach levels of 200 mmHg [5]. In cases of sustained primary hypertension, the peak systolic pressure rises to as high as 240 mmHg [6].

Blood volume

This is a major determinant of arterial blood pressure. Hypovolemia results in decreased venous return with diminished ventricular filling pressure and a consequent lowering of CO. Unless compensated for by other mechanisms, systemic pressure drops. With severe degrees of hypovolemia, blood pressure and perfusion fall drastically and shock may ensue. With hypervolemia, the opposite occurs; venous return is augmented, ventricular filling pressure and CO increase and systemic arterial pressure rises unless it is modulated by other mechanisms.

If the decrease in blood volume is such that a rapid fall in CO and blood pressure occurs, then an increase in PVR and a decrease in venous capacitance are reflexly produced. Blood volume is partially restored by redistribution of extracellular fluid volume (between tissue fluid and plasma) and by mobilization of blood cells from the spleen and hepatic sinusoids. Over longer periods of time, blood volume and blood pressure are restored by regulation of sodium and fluid balance by the kidneys [4]. The relationship of sodium to blood volume is, in fact, the basis for the concept that hypertension may in some cases be related to the excessive ingestion of salt [7].

Salt ingested in the diet is deposited principally in the extracellular space, resulting in an increase in plasma volume and thus in CO. It is believed that in predisposed individuals, this is reflected by an increase in blood pressure. The same sequence of events occurs when the mineralocorticoid effect of aldosterone is unopposed. Whereas an increase in blood volume may raise systemic pressure, a decrease tends to lower systemic pressure and this is partially the basis for the beneficial effects of diuretic therapy for hypertension.

Arterial elasticity

This is a principal determinant of arterial vascular response to varying degrees of left ventricular output. For example, a readily distensible aorta responds to each ventricular ejection with only a small rise in central aortic systolic pressure, whereas a rigid atherosclerotic aorta results in a much larger rise. Likewise, the peripheral vessels, whether rendered resistant by neurogenic or other stimuli or by structural changes, exert a profound effect upon arterial pressure. There is experimental evidence to suggest that decreased compliance of the aorta and carotid arteries may affect systemic pressure by inducing a readjustment of the aortic and carotid baroreceptors [8,9].

Blood viscosity

This can have a significant effect on blood flow and can therefore affect the level of blood pressure. As expressed by the Poiseuille equation, the greater the viscosity of a fluid, the less the flow and vice versa. Blood viscosity is determined by cell concentration (particularly the red cells), cell deformability, cell aggregation, and plasma viscosity. Shear stresses during circulatory flow can deform normal red blood cells and with low flow rates the cells aggregate to form rouleaux. This deformation and aggregation can alter the stream of flow and can lead to a blood viscosity which is shear-dependent. Reduction of shear rate to near stagnation has been shown to increase blood viscosity by as much as 30-fold [10]. However, the quantitative contribution of shear-dependent blood viscosity is not yet known.

It has been suggested that there is an interrelation between blood rheology and the renin—angiotensin system. Moreover, in patients with hypertension, rheological factors, because of their actions on renal reabsorption of sodium, may be responsible for changes in body fluids.

THE RENIN—ANGIOTENSIN—ADRENAL AXIS

There is a strong interplay between the kidney and the cardiovascular system in blood pressure homeostasis. Whereas the kidney may influence the action of the cardiovascular system on blood pressure by altering PVR and blood volume, so may the cardiovascular system exert its influence by altering renal blood flow. The role of renal ischemia in the activation of the renin—angiotensin—aldosterone system is now firmly established. Knowledge that this system is important in the regulation of arterial pressure and of sodium and potassium metabolism dates back to 1960 [11—13]. Research at that time not only provided evidence that a previously unknown biologic control system existed but also demonstrated that under certain conditions, the system can be responsible for the development of malignant hypertension.

Anything which lowers arterial blood pressure (i.e. heart failure, shock, hemorrhage) or which reduces distal renal tubular flow (i.e. sodium depletion) results in the secretion of renin from the kidney [14]. The major stimulus for the release of renin is reduced renal perfusion so that the performance of the cardiovascular system is intimately linked to that of the kidneys in the regulation of blood pressure. Catecholamines, by their action on β-receptors, can also stimulate renin release.

Renin is a proteolytic enzyme which has no physiologic action of its own. However it hydrolyzes angiotensinogen, a peptide substrate synthesized in the liver, to the inactive decapeptide angiotensin I. The latter, in turn, is rapidly hydrolyzed by angiotensin I converting enzyme (mainly in the lungs) to the active octapeptide, angiotensin II [14,15]. Since angiotensin II is activated in the lungs, the highest concentration is in the arterial blood. Its half-life is

very short—less than 1 min—because it is rapidly removed as it passes through the tissues.

Angiotensin II is the most powerful pressor hormone known. By means of its vasoconstrictor effect, it increases PVR and thus the afterload of the heart with a resultant rise in arterial pressure. In addition, angiotensin II is a powerful stimulant of the adrenal gland with the result that aldosterone is released into the circulation and this causes retention of sodium and excretion of potassium. The retention of sodium leads to water retention with expansion of the extracellular space. This, in turn, causes CO to increase with a tendency to increase arterial perfusion pressure and restore renal blood flow. The net result is enhancement of water and sodium excretion by the kidneys. This constellation of events thus provides a negative feedback system which effects a shutdown of the renin release system which was precipitated by reduced renal perfusion.

It has been proposed that in primary hypertension the increased peripheral vasoconstriction remains and after months or years, the arterial wall thickens and this structural change contributes further to the elevation of PVR [15].

The renin—angiotensin—aldosterone system is affected by the action of other control systems. There is evidence to suggest that renin release occurs in response to stimulation of the sympathetic adrenergic nerves which innervate the juxtaglomerular cells. It appears that these renal sympathetic nerves also receive specific connections from higher centers. It is noteworthy in this regard that renin is selectively released when certain areas in the central gray region of the brain are stimulated [4]. The complexity of the renin—angiotensin—aldosterone system is further underscored when one recognizes that angiotensin II potentiates the action of catecholamines and also has an effect on the vasomotor center with a resulting increase in sympathetic activity. In fact, as will be discussed later, it has been proposed that a separate renin—angiotensin system exists within the brain itself. The possibility has also been raised that a hormone within the heart may affect the renin—angiotensin system since a natriuretic factor which inhibits renin and aldosterone secretion has been isolated from atrial tissue [16].

THE CENTRAL NERVOUS SYSTEM

Neural forces are continuously involved in the control of the circulation. Cardiac output and consequently arterial pressure are monitored by the aortic and carotid baroreceptors. The impulses are generated by atrial pressure and are conveyed from the stretch receptors in the carotid sinus by way of cranial nerve IX and from those in the aortic arch by way of cranial nerve X. Peripheral vascular resistance is altered by excitation or inhibition of vasoconstrictor sympathetic outflow via the cardiac sympathetic nerves and this serves to regulate arterial pressure. In addition to this mechanism, the level of blood pressure may be significantly affected by a wide variety of visceral and somatic afferent impulses which converge upon the medulla oblongata.

The cardiovascular changes triggered by the baroreceptor reflexes are mediated mainly through the cardiac sympathetic and parasympathetic nerves, the sympathetic vasomotor nerves to the splanchnic area, and the splanchnic nerve to the adrenal medulla. The activity of vasomotor nerves to skin, muscle, and kidney plays only a minor role unless there is a marked fall in blood pressure. In that case, vasoconstriction in these tissues and organs becomes more important in raising the PVR [4].

Baroreceptor input is integrated by input from the limbic system, the hypothalamus, and the cerebral cortex. Thus, the level at which blood pressure is regulated may be changed by central mechanisms. An example is the so-called "defense reaction" precipitated by emotional stimuli such as pain or fright. This can be elicited by stimulation of various parts of the hypothalamus and consists of a rise in blood pressure associated with reduced renal and splanchnic blood flow and with peripheral vasodilation [16].

Of particular interest is the discovery of new neurotransmitter systems which relate to the neural regulation of the peripheral circulation [17]. The traditional view of the cholinergic and noradrenergic actions of the parasympathetic and sympathetic components of the autonomic nervous system may need to be expanded in light of recent experimental data.

Histamine and renal dopamine have both been identified as mediators of vasodilatory responses. Also, vasoactive intestinal peptides have been identified in the innervation of cerebral blood vessels but their significance is not yet known.

According to Kilcoyne [2], neural receptors in the heart and great vessels have a direct influence on the kidney. When one assumes the upright position, renal vasoconstriction occurs and the reduced blood flow to the glomeruli stimulates release of renin. This in turn activates the renin−angiotensin system which together with the cardiopulmonary, aortic, and carotid baroreceptors tends to maintain systemic pressure.

The kidney obviously has a special role in cardiovascular homeostasis and there is recent evidence to suggest that this is accomplished in part by suprabulbar reflex arcs [17]. The kidney apparently possesses a variety of mechanical and chemical receptors and it has been demonstrated that renal afferent nerves are capable of eliciting a vasoconstrictive response in the contralateral kidney. Of equal interest is the existence of a separate renin−angiotensin system within the brain. Both renin and angiotensin have been shown by immunocytochemical methods to be present in central neuronal cells of laboratory animals. Moreover, a number of areas have been identified as receptor sites for angiotensin within the CNS. Activation of these sites leads, among other things, to secretion of vasopressin and elevation of arterial pressure. Perhaps the most intriguing aspect of the central angiotensin mechanism lies in the recognition of previously unknown areas in the CNS which not only are involved in the regulation of arterial pressure but also may be involved in the development of hypertension.

Vasopressin (antidiuretic hormone), a centrally derived peptide, may also have the capability of modulating arterial pressure. This hormone is produced in the hypothalamic nuclei and is stored in the posterior lobe of the pituitary gland. It raises arterial pressure by stimulating contraction of the arteriolar musculature. Available data do not support the concept that this vasoconstrictor action is, in itself, a determinant of hypertension but there is a suggestion that vasopressin may act at the central level by reflex control of arterial pressure.

OTHER INFLUENCES

The prostaglandins

Prostaglandins were so named because they were first isolated from semen. They are a group of long-chain fatty acids which are chemically related and which are capable of lowering blood pressure. They have been found in a variety of tissues including those of the CNS. They are classified into several types, each designated by capital letters and the subscripts of each (1, 2, and 3) designate the degree of saturation of the side chain.

The relationship of prostaglandins to the kidney and to hypertension has been reviewed in detail by

Ferris [18] and is discussed at length in Chapter 2. Prostaglandins were described in renal medullary tissue in 1967, and in 1975 it was demonstrated that blood pressure could be lowered in rats suffering from a variety of hypertensive conditions when medullary interstitial tissue cells were transplanted into the peritoneum. It was also found that these cells contained lipid granules composed mainly of arachidonic acid and the cyclooxygenase enzyme necessary for the synthesis of prostaglandin.

It is believed that renal medullary prostaglandins may act as a balance to the renin−angiotensin system. Whereas angiotensin II is a powerful vasoconstrictor and a stimulator of aldosterone secretion, prostaglandin E_2 is a vasodilator and may cause natriuresis. It is tempting to postulate that prostaglandin synthesis is needed to modify or prevent vasoconstriction wherever the concentration of angiotensin II is high. Conversely, angiotensin II may be generated to modulate vasodilation in sites where prostaglandin synthesis is high. It is noteworthy in this regard that in the pregnant uterus and in the kidney, where there are high concentrations of renin, there is also a high degree of prostaglandin E_2 synthesis.

Prostaglandin I_2, which is synthesized in blood vessels, is also a vasodilating substance. It may well be involved in the control of PVR. It is now known that a variety of hormones, including angiotensin II, bradykinin, vasopressin, and norepinephrine all increase the synthesis of renal prostaglandins but the significance of this remains unclear. Perhaps in hypertensive conditions prostaglandin synthesis occurs as a secondary event whereas in pregnancy and Bartter's syndrome, where blood pressure is normal, increased prostaglandin production occurs as a primary event. Endogenous prostaglandins have a modulating effect on the vasoconstrictor action of angiotensin II and may interfere with the secretion of aldosterone [18].

The kallikrein−kinin system

Kallikrein is an enzyme of the hydrolase class and is present in plasma and in various glands. Its principal action is to liberate kinins from kininogens. Observations in humans as well as in animals suggest that the renal kallikrein−kinin system may contribute to the regulation of blood pressure but the relationship remains obscure [19−21]. It is known, however, that the kallikrein−kinin system causes vasodilation and natriuresis and this raises the possibility that chronic

depression of its activity may promote the development of hypertension. It has been shown that in human adults, kallikrein activity in the urine is lower in individuals with essential hypertension than in those who are normotensive. Also, in the black population, where the incidence of hypertension is greater than in whites, urinary kallikrein activity is considerably less than in the white population [21].

Finally, the kallikrein−kinin system probably interacts with other systems to exert its influence on blood pressure. For example, bradykinin, which has a direct effect on the vasculature, acts to release prostaglandins and may well augment its hypotensive action. Conversely, the inhibition by indomethacin of prostaglandin synthesis attenuates hypotension which has been enhanced by bradykinin [20].

Carbon dioxide

A rise in arterial carbon dioxide tension acts directly on peripheral blood vessels causing them to dilate. It also acts centrally to increase vasomotor tone and release epinephrine from the adrenal medulla [4].

Hydrogen ion

A rise in hydrogen ion concentration impairs the vascular response to a variety of vasoconstrictors. However, it does not impair the vasoconstrictor response to adrenergic nerve impulses to the same extent because neurotransmitter release is increased [4].

Catecholamines

Under conditions of mental or physical stress, catecholamines are released from the adrenal medulla. Norepinephrine causes a rise in both systolic and diastolic blood pressure due to vasoconstriction. Epinephrine causes a rise in systolic pressure and a fall in diastolic pressure [4].

Calcium

Among the local channel mediators that have recently been given increasing attention is calcium. It is now believed that changes in intracellular calcium may play an important part in the transduction of practically all hormone action. Intracellular free calcium in vascular smooth muscle can be considered the final common pathway of vascular smooth muscle contraction.

In recent years, an atrial natriuretic peptide stored in the atrial myocytes has been identified and may represent a new and important hormonal system [22]. It is apparently activated during atrial distension secondary to increased central blood volume and atrial pressures. It has a natriuretic effect and also exhibits vasorelaxant properties.

From the foregoing, it is obvious that the control of blood pressure is very complex. Although there is currently some understanding of how the various mechanisms integrate with one another, our knowledge is far from complete but is described in the chapters that follow.

REFERENCES

1 Jesse MJ. Essential hypertension in children. *Hosp Pract* November, 1982;17:81−8.

2 Kilcoyne MM. Controversies and considerations in the treatment of hypertension. *Res Staff Phys* November, 1979;114−27.

3 Rushmer RF. *Cardiovascular Dynamics*. 3rd edn. Philadelphia: WB Saunders, 1970;153.

4 Bowman WC, Rand MJ. *Textbook of Pharmacology*. Oxford: Blackwell Scientific Publications, 1980;23.1−23.

5 Riopel DA, Taylor AB, Hohn AR. Blood pressure, heart rate, pressure-rate product and electrocardiographic changes in healthy children during treadmill exercise. *Am J Cardiol* 1979;44:697−704.

6 Nudel DB, Gootman N, Brunson SC. Exercise performance of hypertensive adolescents. *Pediatrics* 1980;65:1073−8.

7 Freis ED. Salt, volume and the prevention of hypertension. *Circulation* 1976;53:589−95.

8 Hallbeck M, Lundgren Y, Weiss L. The distensibility of resistance vessels in spontaneously hypertensive rats (SHR) as compared with normotensive control rats. *Acta Physiol Scand* 1974;90:57−68.

9 Sapru HN, Wang SC. Modification of aortic baroceptor resetting in the spontaneously hypertensive rat. *Am J Physiol* 1976;230:664−74.

10 Report of the hypertension task force of the National Heart, Lung and Blood Institute. Current research and recommendations from the subgroup on local hemodynamics. *Hypertension* 1980;2:342−69.

11 Laragh JH, Ulick S, Januszewicz V, Deming QB, Kelly WG, Lieberman S. Aldosterone secretion and primary and malignant hypertension. *J Clin Invest* 1960;39:1091−106.

12 Laragh JH, Angers M, Kelly WG, Lieberman S. Hypotensive agents and pressor substances. The effect of epinephrine, norepinephrine, angiotensin II and others on the secretory rate of aldosterone in man. *JAMA* 1960;174:234−40.

13 Laragh JH. The role of aldosterone in man. Evidence for regulation of electrolyte balance and arterial pressure by a renal−adrenal system which may be involved in malignant hypertension. *JAMA* 1960;174:293−5.

14 Laragh JH. The renin system and future trends in management of high blood pressure. *Clin Exp Hypertension* 1980;2:525−52.

15 Bailie MD, Mattioli LF. Hypertension: relationships between pathophysiology and therapy. *J Pediatr* 1980;96:789−97.

16 Laragh JH. Calcium metabolism and calcium channel blockers for understanding and treating hypertension. *Am J Med* 1984;77(suppl 6B):1−23.

17 Brody MJ. New developments in our knowledge of blood pressure regulation. *Fed Proc* 1981;40:2257−61.

18 Ferris TF. The kidney and hypertension. *Arch Intern Med* 1982;142:1889−95.

19 Levinsky NG. The renal kallikrein−kinin system. *Circ Res* 1979;441−451.

20 Carretero OA, Scicli AG. The renal kallikrein−kinin system. *Am J Physiol* 1980;238:F247−55.

21 Sinaiko AR, Glasser RJ, Gillum RF, Prineas RJ. Urinary kallikrein excretion in grade school children with high and low blood pressure. *J Pediatr* 1982;100:938−40.

22 Weidmann P, Saxenhofer H, Ferrier C, Shaw SG. Atrial natriuretic peptide in man. *Am J Nephrol* 1988;8:1−14.

2 Renal and Cellular Mechanisms That Modify Blood Pressure

MICHAEL D. BAILIE AND MAJID RASOULPOUR

INTRODUCTION

Regulation of systemic blood pressure involves interactions between factors controlling cardiac output (CO) and peripheral vascular resistance [1]. Cardiac output, the product of heart rate and stroke volume, is regulated by mechanisms intrinsic to the heart muscle as well as extrinsic factors such as neurogenic influences and changes in intravascular volume and venous return (Table 2.1). Peripheral vascular resistance similarly is regulated by factors intrinsic to the precapillary vessels as well as external nonhormonal and neurogenic influences (Table 2.1). Changes in either CO or peripheral vascular resistance will modify systemic blood pressure. Therefore, hypertension will result when CO is increased, as in patients with renal failure who become fluid-overloaded, or when peripheral resistance is increased, as in patients with renovascular hypertension. In this chapter, we will discuss several elements (Table 2.2) which are thought to be important in the regulation of systemic blood pressure and which may be involved in the pathogenesis of hypertension.

It is important to note at the outset of any discussion of the etiology of essential hypertension that there are complex interactions between many metabolic and hormonal systems which may be involved in the pathogenesis of this common disease. While the elevation of blood pressure in essential hypertension may be due to a primary change in either the heart, causing increased CO or in the peripheral resistance vessels, causing increased vascular resistance, changes in the balance between vasodilatory and vasoconstrictor hormones may play an important pathogenetic role. Thus, increases in the activity of the sympathetic nervous system, the renin–angiotensin system (RAS), or levels of vasopressin, or thromboxane A_2 may all increase vascular resistance. On the other hand, the lack of vasodilators such as bradykinin, prostaglandin E_2, or prostacyclin (PGI_2) may result in increased vascular resistance.

The interaction of these various systems complicates the study of the pathogenesis of hypertension. For example, drugs which inhibit angiotensin I converting enzyme (ACE) and reduce the circulating concentration of the vasopressor, angiotensin II (AII), also inhibit the catabolism of the vasodilator, bradykinin, and therefore potentiate its action. Prostaglandins are important in modifying the vasopressor effects of AII and at the same time stimulate renin release from the kidney. A circulating inhibitor of sodium–potassium adenosine triphosphatase (Na^+-K^+-ATPase) may be natriuretic but at the same time may increase blood pressure by modifying intracellular calcium leading to increased smooth muscle tone. Many other examples may be cited and account at least in part for our inability to define clearly a single defect in the etiology of essential hypertension. The difficulties in developing a unified proposal to explain the etiology of the various forms of hypertension have been recently reviewed [2,3].

SODIUM AND HYPERTENSION

Sodium salts play a major role in the regulation of extracellular fluid (ECF) volume (see below). Since ECF volume is an important determinant of CO, the regulation of sodium homeostasis has an important impact on blood pressure control [4]. When in daily balance, the sodium intake must match its output [5]. Since only small amounts of sodium are normally lost through the skin and feces, the burden of sodium regulation falls on the kidneys where it is freely filtered and avidly reabsorbed [6].

In humans, each kidney contains about 1 million nephrons, consisting of glomerular capillaries and a renal tubule. The renal parenchyma is basically divided into cortex and medulla. Nephrons are dis-

Table 2.1 The regulation of systemic blood pressure

CARDIAC OUTPUT

Stroke volume
Intrinsic component
  Muscle fiber length
Extrinsic components
  Sympathetic stimulation, hormones, inotropic drugs, factors
    increasing venous return

Heart rate
Intrinsic component
  Sinus rhythm
Extrinsic component
  Sympathetic stimulation, hormones, chronotropic drugs

PERIPHERAL VASCULAR RESISTANCE

Intrinsic vasomotion
Local metabolites
Neural vasodilator and vasoconstrictor influences
Humoral factors
Chemical factors

Table 2.2 Hormonal and volume regulatory factors in the pathogenesis of hypertension

Renal sodium handling
Renal regulation of blood volume
Effects of blood volume and blood viscosity
The renin—angiotensin—aldosterone system
Prostaglandins and kinins
Atrial natriuretic factor
Cellular sodium—lithium countertransport
Effects of calcium

tinguished within the kidney by the locations of their glomeruli in the cortex of the kidney into superficial, midcortical and inner cortical (juxtamedullary) nephrons (Fig. 2.1).

Throughout its course, the tubule is composed of a single layer of epithelial cells that lie on a continuous layer of basement membrane. The basement membrane is considered as part of the renal interstitium. The epithelial cells are separated from each other by lateral intercellular spaces. Each cell has two distinct membranes: a luminal (apical) membrane that borders the tubular lumen and a peritubular (basolateral) membrane that separates the cell cytoplasm from the lateral intercellular and the basal interstitial spaces. Near their apical surfaces, the adjacent cells are fused by a number of strands (tight junctions) which border the luminal sides of the intercellular spaces (Fig. 2.2).

Transport of sodium between the tubular lumen and the renal interstitium occurs through two pathways: the transcellular (through the cells via apical and basolateral membranes) and the paracellular (through the tight junctions and intercellular spaces) [7]. Unlike glomerular capillaries where dissolved sodium is transported by bulk flow (filtration or convection), the transcellular transport of sodium at the apical membrane occurs as *simple diffusion* (down an electrochemical gradient); as *cotransport* (simple diffusion accelerated by transport carriers and coupled with uphill transport of other substances); and as *countertransport* (coupled with uphill transport of another substance in the opposite direction). The basolateral transport of sodium is an active process with the energy supplied from the hydrolysis of adenosine triphosphate (ATP) by Na^+-K^+-ATPase lining the basolateral borders of the epithelial cells. The active transport of sodium out of the cell into the intercellular space and renal interstitium plays the most important role in sodium reabsorption. By maintaining a low intracellular sodium concentration, the Na^+-K^+-ATPase allows sodium ions to move from its higher concentration in the tubular lumen to the lower concentration inside the cells [8]. The mechanisms involved in paracellular transport of sodium are simple diffusion and convection, the latter occurring as dissolved sodium chloride flows from the lumen into lateral intercellular spaces. If the tight junctions are highly permeable, the paracellular pathways disperse any concentration gradient generated by the transcellular transport pathway [7].

The basement membrane upon which the epithelial cells rest is basically not an effective barrier to the movement of fluid and solutes. The reabsorbed sodium in the intercellular space is, therefore, rapidly mixed with solute and water of the renal interstitium. Movement of dissolved sodium from the interstitium into the peritubular capillaries is by convection which is determined by the net balance of hydraulic and oncotic pressures across the capillary walls [9]. The hydraulic pressure of the peritubular capillaries is quite low. This capillary network is in direct continuity with the efferent arteriole. Since plasma passing through the glomerulus forms a protein-free filtrate, the oncotic pressure of the fluid in the peritubular capillary is higher than that in the afferent arteriole.

Two-thirds of the filtered sodium is reabsorbed in the proximal nephron. The proximal tubule is convoluted in its most cortical part, but as it turns toward the medulla it becomes straight (Fig. 2.1). Along its length, the proximal tubule is divided into

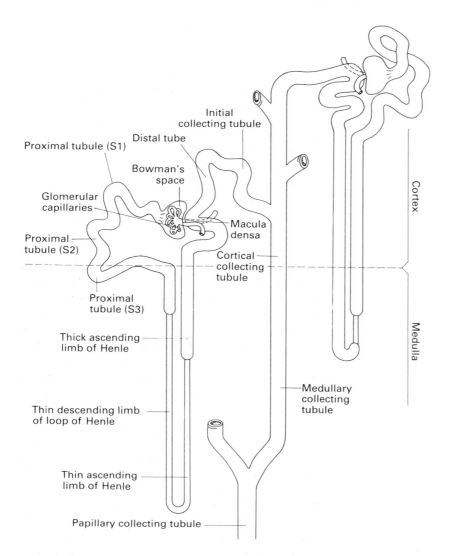

Initial
collecting tubule

Distal tube

Proximal tubule (S1)

Bowman's
space

Glomerular
capillaries

Proximal
tubule (S2)

Macula
densa

Cortical
collecting
tubule

Proximal
tubule (S3)

Thick ascending
limb of Henle

Thin descending limb
of loop of Henle

Medullary
collecting
tubule

Thin ascending
limb of Henle

Papillary collecting tubule

Cortex

Medulla

Fig. 2.1 Schematic representation of
the nephron and its various segments.

three segments: early (S1), mid (S2), and late (S3).
The proximal tubular cells possess all of the features of
salt-reabsorbing epithelia. The cells are morphologically heterogeneous. Those of the S1 segment have a
well defined brush border, extensive basal interdigitations, and numerous mitochondria. These features
gradually diminish from the S1 to the S3 segment of
the tubule [10]. Likewise, the rate of sodium transport
in the earliest segments is greater than that in later
segments [11]. Sodium is cotransported with neutral
organic solutes such as sugars and amino acids, with
organic anions such as phosphate and lactate, and it
is countertransported with hydrogen ion [9,12]. These
processes are driven by virtue of the sodium concentration gradient across the luminal membrane. The
cotransport of sodium with neutral organic solutes is

electrogenic, leading to a negative voltage in the
lumen. Farther along the proximal tubule where
chloride concentration has risen above plasma concentration, this negative voltage enhances rapid reabsorption of chloride which reverses the potential
difference to lumen-positive and, therefore, facilitates
the transport of sodium at the later sites [9]. The
basolateral transport of sodium is driven by Na^+-K^+-
ATPase. One-third of the proximal tubular sodium
reabsorption is paracellular, driven in part by:
1 convective transport produced by virtue of an osmotic gradient generated by tubular reabsorption of
glucose, amino acids, and bicarbonate;
2 the active transport of sodium into the intercellular
space; and
3 simple diffusion generated by an electric gradient

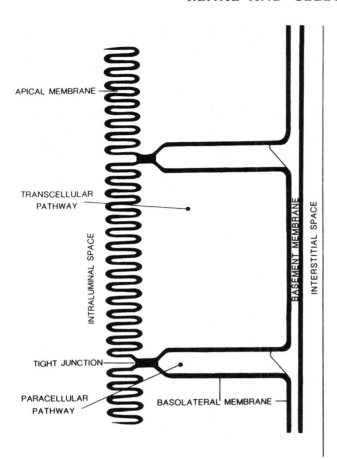

Fig. 2.2 Schematic representation of a renal tubular cell demonstrating the transcellular and paracellular pathways.

There is, however, morphologic heterogeneity among the cells along the length of the loop as well as among that of the short and long loops [13]. The basolateral membrane of the thick ascending limb has many cellular interdigitations with large mitochondria within the interdigitating processes.

The loops of Henle reabsorb about one-fourth of the filtered sodium. The descending thin limb of the loop is very permeable to water (high hydraulic conductance), far more than the proximal tubule, but it has limited sodium permeability and even less permeability to urea [14]. When intraluminal fluid is exposed to the hypertonic medullary interstitium, water flows from the intraluminal space to the interstitial space and leads to a rise in intraluminal sodium concentration. Unlike the thin descending limb, the hydraulic conductance of the thin ascending limb is negligible. This segment, however, is highly permeable to sodium, several times more than to urea [14]. Sodium is probably transported by a simple diffusion mechanism as there is no measurable Na^+-K^+-ATPase at this segment to support an active transport system. The impermeability of the thin ascending limb to water leads to a gradual dilution of luminal fluid along this segment of the nephron.

Part of the thick ascending limb of the loop is in the medulla and part in the cortex (Fig. 2.1). The cells in the cortical segments become gradually thinner along their length [15]. The hydraulic conductance of both medullary and cortical sections of the thick ascending limb of Henle is basically negligible. Both sections transport sodium from lumen to interstitium by a Na^+,K^+,$2Cl^-$ cotransport system. The energy is provided by a sodium concentration gradient across the cell membrane (driven by Na^+-K^+-ATPase at the basolateral membrane), and a lumen-positive electric gradient generated by potassium extrusion from the cell into the lumen [14,15]. The Na^+-K^+-ATPase activity of the cortical thick ascending limb of Henle is lower than that of the medullary limb, consistent with its lower capacity to reabsorb sodium [13]. Sodium transport in the thick ascending limb is, in part, through the paracellular pathway driven by lumen-positive voltage [15]. As a result of sodium reabsorption in this basically water-impermeable segment of nephron, the luminal fluid becomes further dilute. Both the sodium concentration and the osmolality of luminal fluid leaving this segment are markedly lower than those of plasma. Each of the two limbs of Henle also plays a major role in the countercurrent multiplication system [7].

(by virtue of chloride reabsorption) and a concentration gradient [9]. The proximal tubule reabsorbs the filtered water and salt to the same extent so that the concentration of sodium in the tubular fluid leaving the proximal tubule is the same as that in plasma.

The proximal tubule drains into the descending limb of the loop of Henle which bends in a hairpin turn at its distal end and becomes the ascending limb of the loop. Nephrons with superficial cortical glomeruli have short loops bending in the outer medulla, whereas juxtamedullary glomeruli have long loops bending deep in the medulla (Fig. 2.1). Nephrons in the midcortical region have both short and long loops. In the long loops, the first portion of the ascending limb is thin, whereas in short-looped nephrons, the entire ascending limb is thick. The epithelia of the thin portions of the loop of Henle have limited brush borders and few mitochondria.

As the thick ascending limb returns to its glomerulus, it passes between the afferent and efferent arterioles where they leave the glomerulus. The epithelial cells of the thick ascending limb which lie in juxtaposition to the glomerulus, the afferent and efferent arterioles, are packed densely and contain large nuclei (macula densa). The distal tubule begins at a short distance beyond the macula densa (Fig. 2.1). The earliest portion of this segment is convoluted and is shorter than the convoluted portion of the proximal tubule. Depending upon the location in the kidney, this part of the tubule gradually transforms into a connecting segment or initial collecting tubule. Until the end of the distal convoluted tubule, each nephron is separate from the others. Thereafter, they join by draining into the cortical collecting tubules through the initial collecting tubules [13]. Five to 10 nephrons drain into one cortical collecting tubule. Unlike the relatively thin cells of the terminal parts of the thick ascending limbs, the epithelia of the distal convoluted tubule and connecting segments are composed of tall and markedly interdigitating cells which are laced with many long mitochondria [13,16]. The connecting segment is composed of two types of cells: the connecting tubule cells and the intercalated cells [16]. The intercalated cells (cells that are dispersed among others) are not specific to the connecting section and their functions are beyond the scope of this discussion.

The hydraulic conductance of the distal tubule is negligible. However, since the distal convoluted tubule has the highest activity of Na$^+$-K$^+$-ATPase of any segment of the nephron, its sodium transport capacity is very high [16]. The net sodium reabsorption in the distal convoluted tubule is twice that of the connecting segment. Sodium reabsorption by the distal tubule is dose-dependent and the proportion of the filtered sodium absorbed basically remains constant [17]. Sodium reabsorption is about 99% complete when the filtrate leaves the nephron. In view of the water impermeability of this segment, the tubular fluid is further diluted [16].

The connecting segment of the distal tubule gradually transforms into the initial or cortical collecting tubule [13]. The collecting tubules run downward into the medulla to form the medullary and finally papillary collecting tubules (Fig. 2.1). Each final collecting tubule drains about 3000 nephrons. As that of the connecting segment, the epithelium of the collecting tubule is also made up of two cell types, the principal or light cells and the intercalated or dark cells [13,18]. One-third of the cortical collecting tubule epithelial cells are intercalated, while very few of this cell type are present at the lower segments of the collecting tubule [18]. The principal cells, through which sodium reabsorption most likely occurs, have no lateral interdigitations, limited numbers of mitochondria, stubby microvilli, and deep tight junctions. Sodium enters the apical membranes of the principal cells by virtue of its electrochemical gradient and it is pumped out of the cells by Na$^+$-K$^+$-ATPase [18]. Although the collecting tubules only reabsorb about 1% of the filtered sodium, they are responsible for the final adjustment of the urinary sodium concentration [18]. Hydraulic conductance of the collecting tubule is determined by antidiuretic hormone (ADH) [13]. In the absence of ADH, the cortical and medullary collecting tubules are poorly permeable to water. Continued sodium transport without water movement leads to the formation of an extremely dilute urine.

Since sodium is freely filtered at the glomerulus and reabsorbed but not secreted by the renal tubules, the final urinary sodium concentration represents the result of glomerular filtration and tubular reabsorption. Factors which modify these processes will be discussed in following sections.

EXTRACELLULAR FLUID VOLUME REGULATION

The ECF compartment contains approximately one-third of the total body water. Gain of water by this compartment leads to relative hypotonicity of the ECF and results in water moving into the intracellular space. In contrast, gain of salt by the ECF compartment leads to hypertonicity and, therefore, water moves from the intracellular into the extracellular compartment [19]. Any salt that is retained in the ECF is evenly distributed within its two divisions, the extravascular and the intravascular spaces.

As stated earlier, the arterial blood pressure is determined by the CO and the total peripheral vascular resistance. A major determinant of CO is ECF volume. To preserve circulatory integrity, the ECF volume and therefore the plasma volume should be maintained within narrow limits despite varying sodium intake. This is achieved by the integrated system of regulatory mechanisms that includes volume receptors and hormonal factors [20,21].

The ECF volume receptors are located within the vascular compartment and include: (a) the low-pressure receptors in the atria and the great intra-thoracic veins; (b) the high-pressure receptors in the aortic and carotid sinuses; and (c) the baroreceptors located in the juxtaglomerular apparatus (JGA) of the kidney. Abnormalities in the sensing mechanisms lead to an expansion of the ECF volume and may lead to hypertension. Low-pressure receptors play an important role in plasma volume regulation. A variety of maneuvers that reduce venous return, such as prolonged standing, lead to sodium and water retention by the kidney [22], whereas recumbency, which leads to increased venous return, is associated with increased renal sodium and water excretion [23]. The mechanisms for these changes in renal sodium handling are several. When stretched, by virtue of increased volume, the cardiac atria release a peptide, atrial natriuretic factor (ANF), which has a wide spectrum of hemodynamic and endocrine effects leading to natriuresis and diuresis [24] (see below). In addition to releasing ANF, distension of the atria and the great intrathoracic veins stimulates neural mechanoreceptors which reside in these regions. Signals from these receptors reach the hypothalamus [25], where an integrated reflex response, which includes inhibition of renal sympathetic nerve activity, is initiated [26]. This inhibitory effect of neural mechanoreceptors on renal sympathetic nerve activity produces natriuresis and diuresis by virtue of a direct effect of the sympathetic nervous system on tubular sodium reabsorption [27,28] and by suppressing the release of renin [29].

It has been known for several decades that closure of an arteriovenous fistula leads to natriuresis, despite a fall in the central venous pressure, whereas opening of a fistula results in the retention of sodium even though central venous filling is increased [30]. This finding has led to the concept of the effective arterial blood volume or the relative fullness of the arterial vasculature in relation to its total capacity. In response to a fall in the effective arterial volume, the kidney retains sodium, while sodium excretion increases when the effective volume rises. The high-pressure baroreceptors of the aorta and carotid sinuses sense the change in volume and relay the message to the central nervous system where sympathetic feedback modifies CO and vascular resistance [31]. In addition, since these receptors alter renal sympathetic nerve activity, they directly modify renal sodium excretion [32].

The volume-sensing device of the kidney is the JGA. The best defined receptor at this site is the baroreceptor of the afferent arteriole which plays a major role in the secretion of renin and, therefore, in the production of AII and aldosterone. Other factors involved in the regulation of the secretion of renin are discussed below [33].

As discussed earlier, about 1% of the filtered sodium is usually excreted by the kidneys. Expansion of the ECF volume by saline infusion leads to increased glomerular filtration rate (GFR) and increased renal sodium excretion [34]. The ratio of GFR to renal excretion of sodium, however, is not constant otherwise small changes in GFR would result in substantial changes in renal sodium excretion [35]. Therefore, various other mechanisms must exist to regulate renal tubular handling of sodium independently of GFR.

Since reabsorption of dissolved sodium from the renal interstitium into peritubular capillaries is determined by the net balance between hydraulic and oncotic pressure (the Starling forces), low peritubular oncotic pressure, elevated peritubular hydrostatic pressure, or both would reduce tubular sodium and water reabsorption [36]. Volume expansion, sensed by receptors which inhibit sympathetic tone, leads to a reduction of renal vascular resistance. Reduced renal vascular resistance (predominantly of the efferent arteriole) diminishes the filtration fraction (GFR/renal plasma flow) and therefore a smaller percentage of protein-free ultrafiltrate is formed at the glomerulus. This leads to a lower protein concentration in the peritubular capillaries. With the higher hydrostatic pressure induced by reduced renal vascular resistance, sodium and water reabsorption by the proximal tubule is diminished [37]. Whether the peritubular capillary hydrostatic pressure, oncotic pressure, or both are major determinants of sodium and water reabsorption of this segment of the tubule remains to be defined [21]. Recent data indicate that besides its effect on renal vascular resistance, AII also has a direct effect on proximal tubular reabsorption of sodium (see below) [38].

Extracellular fluid volume expansion may also inhibit sodium reabsorption in the loop of Henle of the medullary nephrons. As stated previously, the thin descending and ascending segments of the loop of Henle which are basically located in the renal medulla have no active transport mechanisms. Water is reabsorbed from the salt-impermeable thin descending limb by virtue of the urea and salt concentrations of the renal medulla leading to high luminal sodium chloride concentration of the thin ascending limb. This provides the driving force for sodium chloride reabsorption in this segment. Volume expansion washes out the osmotic forces of the renal medulla (urea and salt) by increasing medullary blood flow. Therefore, water reabsorption from the thin descending limb of the loop of Henle is reduced. As a result, the sodium chloride concentration of the thin ascending limb and ultimately passive reabsorption of sodium in this segment declines [36].

There are many reports supporting ECF volume regulation by virtue of a direct effect of renal nerves on tubular transport of sodium. Histochemical and ultrastructural studies have demonstrated adrenergic nerve terminals in direct contact with the tubular basement membrane of mammalian renal tubular epithelial cells [27]. Several studies have shown that stimulation of the renal nerves influences sodium transport independent of renal blood flow and GFR [39,40]. Besides the α- and β-adrenergic receptors, dopaminergic receptors are also present in the kidney. Dopamine inhibits proximal tubular reabsorption of sodium [41]. Renal sympathetic nerves appear to play a substantial role in regulating renal sodium excretion and in the maintenance of ECF volume.

Some other factors which regulate the renal excretion of sodium and thus modify plasma volume include plasma aldosterone, AII, prostaglandins, and the kallikrein−kinin system (KKS). Aldosterone plays an essential role in regulating salt reabsorption by the cortical collecting tubule. In addition, it augments ADH-mediated water permeability of the collecting duct [42]. Aldosterone is an important hormone in regulating chronic salt balance, particularly in states of sodium deprivation [21]. Its secretion from the zona glomerulosa of the adrenal gland is regulated by several factors; plasma concentration of AII plays the central role [43].

Angiotensin II modulates plasma volume via several mechanisms that include effects on the Starling forces of the peritubular capillaries [37] and its direct effect on the proximal tubular reabsorption of sodium [38]. When associated with increased renal artery pressure, high levels of AII lead to natriuresis [43].

Angiotensin II also regulates prostaglandin biosynthesis, and the renal prostaglandins have been shown to have a substantial role in mediating the release of renin (see below). Renal prostaglandins are postulated as important hormonal factors in regulating the renal excretion of sodium. Prostaglandins administered into the renal artery of dogs promote a natriuresis by inhibiting the sodium chloride reabsorption in the proximal tubule, the loop of Henle, and the collecting tubule [44]. The natriuretic effect of prostaglandins on the proximal tubule seems to be mediated by their influence on the Starling forces of the peritubular capillaries [34]. Since prostaglandins augment renal medullary blood flow, they inhibit passive sodium chloride reabsorption in the thin limbs of the loop of Henle [44]. Prostaglandin E_2 directly inhibits sodium transport across the thick ascending limb and the cortical collecting tubule [45,46]. However, despite various well understood intrarenal effects of prostaglandins, their exact role in ECF volume regulation remains to be defined. Currently, they appear to have counterregulatory roles, counterbalancing the vasoconstrictive and sodium-retaining effects of AII and norepinephrine [36].

The renal KKS has also been considered to play some role in the regulation of sodium balance. The release of renal kallikrein is stimulated by the sodium regulatory hormones (aldosterone, AII, and prostaglandins) [47]. Kallikrein is an enzyme which releases kinins from the substrate, kininogen (see below). Acute intrarenal infusion of bradykinin leads to increased renal blood flow, diuresis, and natriuresis. However, chronic infusion for 7 days had no significant effect on urinary volume and sodium excretion [48]. Beyond the interrelationship of the KKS with other hormonal modulators of sodium balance, its direct regulatory role remains unclear.

Expansion of the ECF volume of an animal whose circulatory system has been denervated would lead to increased CO and arterial blood pressure. However, when all the regulatory systems are in order, changing the salt intake over a very wide range has little effect on blood pressure [19]. Since most forms of hypertension, in their chronic phase, are characterized by normal or even slightly lowered blood volume, the relation between salt intake, volume status, and blood pressure remains to be understood [4].

LITHIUM−SODIUM COUNTERTRANSPORT

As discussed earlier, essential hypertension is characterized by increased systemic vascular resistance which may be caused, in part, by widespread alterations of cell membrane transport in vascular smooth muscle cells [49]. Since smooth muscle cells from blood vessels of living individuals are rarely obtained, human erythrocytes and leukocytes have been extensively used to investigate the cell membrane transport processes in patients with hypertension. One feature of red cell membrane transport which has been extensively studied in human hypertensive patients is the ability to exchange intracellular lithium for extracellular sodium.

Lithium (Li^+) is a monovalent cation which is abundant in many alkaline mineral-spring waters. While traces of lithium are present in tissues, it has no known physiologic role [50]. Lithium salts were introduced to psychiatry several decades ago, and they are currently considered the most effective treatment for the manic phase of affective disorders [51].

In 1974, Mendels and Frazer [52] showed that the concentration of erythrocyte lithium in patients taking lithium salts for $1\frac{1}{2}-2\frac{1}{2}$ weeks was about one-third of the plasma lithium concentration. Since a monovalent cation should be almost evenly distributed in both intracellular and extracellular fluid, this finding suggested that lithium is actively transported by cell membranes. As Maizels had shown earlier [53], Mendels and Frazer also showed that lithium is not transported by the sodium—potassium pump. The sodium—potassium pump is the most active transport mechanism across cell membranes. It requires ATPase for energy, and it is inhibited by ouabain. Lithium transport, however, is ouabain-insensitive. Hass and coworkers [54] measured the effect of external sodium on the uptake and extrusion of lithium by human red blood cells. Lithium-loaded cells suspended in a high-sodium medium promptly extruded lithium against an electrochemical potential gradient, whereas the cells in a low-sodium medium continued to gain lithium. It was concluded that transport of lithium occurs in either direction across the erythrocyte membrane. The energy required for the transport is provided by an oppositely directed electrochemical potential gradient of sodium [54]. While referring to this secondary active transport of lithium as the sodium—lithium countertransport system, Canessa and coworkers [55] showed that in a group of 36 white adult men and women with essential hypertension, the rate of lithium extrusion from lithium-loaded erythrocytes in a sodium-enriched medium was more than twofold greater than in that of a group of 26 normal control subjects. The difference between lithium extrusion into sodium-containing and sodium-free media was taken as the maximum rate (V_{max}) of sodium—lithium countertransport. Among hypertensive individuals, the V_{max} was higher in men than women. The V_{max} of the first-degree adult relatives of 8 of the patients with essential hypertension was also significantly higher than that of the first-degree adolescent relatives of 10 normal control subjects. The mean lithium extrusion value of 5 adult patients with secondary hypertension was not statistically different from the mean value of the control group. Canessa and coworkers concluded that this erythrocyte cation transport abnormality in patients with essential hypertension and their first-degree relatives may indicate that there is a hereditary abnormality in sodium transport of vascular smooth muscle cells in patients with essential hypertension and that this may somehow lead to an increased peripheral vascular resistance. This report led to considerable interest in sodium—lithium countertransport as a possible fruitful system to investigate the genetic basis, pathophysiology, and epidemiology of essential hypertension in children and adults.

In 1982, Woods and coworkers [56] showed that the rate of sodium—lithium countertransport in healthy normotensive males, ages 12—20 years, was almost twofold higher in the offspring of hypertensive parents. They found no correlation between the countertransport rate and the race, age, body size, and actual levels of blood pressure. In contrast, Ibsen and colleagues [57] found no difference in erythrocyte sodium—lithium countertransport values of 9 children (4 girls and 5 boys) with one hypertensive parent and 14 children (5 girls and 9 boys) with normotensive parents. Cooper and coworkers [58] showed that college students with mean diastolic blood pressure greater than 80 mmHg had higher sodium—lithium countertransport rates than normotensive individuals of similar age. Weight, sex, ethnicity, and age had no effect on the rates of sodium—lithium countertransport values. A positive family history of hypertension was associated with higher levels of countertransport values; however the effect could have been secondary to higher levels of blood pressure. In a separate study conducted by Cooper and colleagues [59] on high school students, it was shown that the rate of sodium—lithium countertransport in 22 students with at least one hypertensive parent was identical to 21 schoolmates with normotensive parents. Brugnara and coworkers [60] reported the sodium—lithium countertransport rate in 146 adults, of whom 58 were normotensive, 60 had essential hypertension, and 28 had secondary hypertension. Although the rates were generally higher in subjects with essential hypertension, 34 of them had normal rates of sodium—lithium countertransport.

Norling and coworkers [61] conducted a study in

45 patients, 4–18 years of age, with essential or secondary hypertension. Patients with essential hypertension had significantly higher rates of erythrocyte sodium–lithium countertransport than the normotensive control subjects. The countertransport rates of patients with secondary hypertension were intermediate, not significantly different from those of the control population or those of the patients with essential hypertension. The countertransport values did not correlate significantly with age, sex, or weight in either hypertensive or normotensive groups. In 1988, Trevisan and colleagues [62] showed that in a group of 84 randomly selected Italian schoolchildren, sodium–lithium countertransport values in boys were significantly correlated to both systolic and diastolic blood pressure. The correlation, however, lost its statistical significance when corrected for the confounding roles of weight and height. There was no correlation between the countertransport values and family history of hypertension.

It is noteworthy that blacks, who are at a higher risk for hypertension than whites, in most of the studies have shown lower levels of sodium–lithium countertransport. In a study conducted by Trevisan and coworkers [63] on the effect of race on red cell cation transport of children 11–15 years of age, the countertransport values were lower in blacks than whites. Bunker and coworkers [64] showed that the erythrocyte sodium–lithium countertransport rates of white college students were significantly higher than those of blacks of similar physical and social status. Of the blacks, 41% had sodium–lithium countertransport values lower than the lowest rate observed among white students. Norling and coworkers [61], however, did not observe statistically significant differences between the mean rates of countertransport among whites and blacks with essential hypertension. As part of a study of the genetic and environmental determinants of essential hypertension, Williams and coworkers [65] concluded that sodium–lithium countertransport is affected by both the genes and the shared family environment.

Since the inconsistencies among the studies are substantial, the erythrocyte sodium–lithium countertransport system thus far does not appear to be either a strong genetic marker or a useful diagnostic tool for essential hypertension. As pointed out by some investigators, if an abnormal sodium transport mechanism is linked to the mechanism of essential hypertension, it should be fully developed in most hypertensive individuals.

Since the endogenous lithium concentration is exceedingly low [50], the *in vivo* role of the sodium–lithium countertransport system and its relation to essential hypertension is also unclear. Canessa and colleagues [55] had suggested that the higher values of this system in erythrocytes of patients with essential hypertension and their first-degree relatives might indicate a higher rate of sodium influx through sodium–sodium exchange across the vascular smooth muscle cells, leading to an increased peripheral vascular resistance. An increased activity of sodium–sodium exchange however would not alter the net transport of sodium [66]. Because there are several *in vitro* similarities between the sodium–hydrogen antiporter of the renal brush border and the erythrocyte sodium–lithium countertransport system, Aronson [67] suggested that the erythrocyte sodium–lithium countertransport system may operate as a sodium-proton exchanger. An increased activity of this transport system may lead to increased tubular reabsorption of sodium and water which could contribute to hypertension. In a study conducted by Levine and coworkers [68], higher rates of sodium–proton exchange were noted in platelets of patients with essential hypertension than in those of normotensive control subjects. Canessa and coworkers [69] have stated that sodium–proton exchange is the main regulator of cell pH in vascular smooth muscle cells. Activation of this system may lead to an increase in sodium intake by the cells, proton extrusion from the cells, a rise in pH of the cells, and ultimately vasoconstriction.

In 1981, MacGregor and coworkers [70] suggested that normal plasma probably contains an inhibitor of Na^+-K^+-ATPase that modulates the sodium pump. They showed that the plasma activity of this inhibitor is higher in patients with essential hypertension. More recently, Haupert [71] has proposed that an augmented sodium–proton exchange in the proximal nephron leads to a transient rise in ECF volume which stimulates the release of Na^+-K^+-ATPase inhibitor. The inhibition of the sodium pump by this inhibitor promotes sodium excretion and restores the fluid volume to normal or even below normal. Similar inhibition of the ATPase-dependent sodium pump in vascular smooth muscle cells, however, leads to an increased total peripheral resistance through either a rise in intracellular free calcium concentration or an indirect effect of the inhibitor on sympathetic nerve endings. Although Canessa and coworkers [72] have suggested that the sodium–proton exchanger which is readily demonstrable in the renal brush border membrane is also present in human red cells, further investigation into its existence in erythrocytes is needed. Until more evidence is available, one concludes that the sodium—lithium countertransport and sodium—proton exchanger may not be completely identical.

NATRIURETIC HORMONES

The rate of glomerular filtration and the renal effects of aldosterone are important in the regulation of sodium excretion by the kidney. However, additional factors are involved. Therefore, investigators have focused attention on hormones that might promote natriuresis. At least two such hormones have been identified. The first is a nonpeptide, digitalis-like hormone which inhibits Na^+-K^+-ATPase ("third factor") [73,74]. The second is a peptide hormone produced in the cardiac atria which does not inhibit Na^+-K^+-ATPase [75,76]. The differences between the two hormones are outlined in Table 2.3. The reader is referred to a number of reviews for the history of the discovery and delineation of these substances [73—77].

The endogenous digitalis-like factor has been implicated in those forms of hypertension in which ECF volume is expanded, such as renal failure and low-renin essential hypertension [74,78,79]. This substance appears to have many but not all of the properties of cardiac glycosides. Strong evidence suggests that the source of this factor is the hypothalamus. The inhibition of Na^+-K^+-ATPase leads to increased cardiac and vascular smooth muscle con-

tractility, thus potentially causing increased systemic blood pressure. In addition to finding this digitalis-like factor in adults with certain forms of hypertension and other cardiovascular diseases, it has been reported to be present in human newborn infants and in amniotic fluid [80].

The ANF is produced in the cardiac atria where it is stored in secretory granules and released into the circulation when the atria are stretched [75,76]. Expansion of the ECF volume which leads to distension of the atria stimulates the release of ANF [76]. In addition, vasopressin and epinephrine also stimulate the release of ANF [76]. ANF has a number of actions [75—77] (Table 2.4) which have led investigators to speculate that it is important in the regulation of sodium excretion and may play a role in certain pathologic states such as hypertension, sodium-retaining states such as congestive heart failure, Bartter's syndrome, nephrotic syndrome, and renal failure as well as liver disease [75—77,81].

Studies on the effects of ANF in humans have been limited and few studies have been reported in children. These latter studies have been confined to determination of plasma concentrations of ANF during normal development and in pathologic states such as heart failure and respiratory distress syndrome [82—88]. Atrial natriuretic factor has been found to be present in cord blood of the human fetus between 21 and 34 weeks of gestation, and the concentration increases in response to intrauterine blood transfusion [90]. Plasma ANF appears to be highest in normal infants immediately after birth and falls rapidly to adult levels before the end of the first year of life [83,85,88]. Studies in children with various

Table 2.3 Differences between natriuretic hormones

	"Third factor"	Atrial natriuretic factor
Source	Hypothalamus	Cardiac atria
Chemistry	MW <500 Da Resists proteolysis Nonpeptide Inhibits Na^+-K^+-ATPase Binds to digoxin antibodies	MW >5000 Da Degraded by proteolytic enzymes Peptide No effect on Na^+-K^+-ATPase
Effects on: kidney	Natriuresis Diuresis	Natriuresis Diuresis
vessels	Vasoconstrictor Raises blood pressure	Vasodilator Lowers blood pressure

Table 2.4 Possible actions of atrial natriuretic factor

Heart and blood vessels
Vasodilatation
Venodilatation
Inotropic effects on the heart

Kidney
Diuresis
Natriuresis
Inhibition of tubular sodium transport
Increased glomerular filtration rate
Increased filtration fraction
Inhibition of osmotic water permeability of cortical collecting
tubule

Endocrine systems
Inhibition of aldosterone synthesis
Inhibition of renin release
Inhibition of vasopressin release

Central nervous system
Inhibition of thirst or drinking behavior

forms of heart disease indicate that levels of ANF are increased with congestive heart failure [82,83,85,88], suggesting that measurements of ANF may aid in the evaluation of this condition in children. In infants with respiratory distress syndrome [90], those receiving positive pressure ventilation had significantly higher plasma ANF values than those who required only oxygen, or normal infants matched for age. In preterm infants with respiratory distress, those on a low sodium intake had lower plasma concentrations of ANF than infants on a higher sodium intake [87]. Finally, infants with renal failure had ANF values before dialysis that were twice those found after they had been dialyzed and once fluid had been removed from the intravascular space [84,91]. On the other hand, children with idiopathic nephrotic syndrome had an increase in plasma ANF concentration following albumin infusion. Thus, in a variety of situations in children, increased intravascular volume increases the plasma concentration of ANF. The system appears to be intact even in the preterm infant.

The ontogeny and response to ANF have been studied in animals. Wei and coworkers [92] followed the developmental changes in ANF in rats. Concentrations of ANF in fetal and neonatal plasma were found to be higher than in the adult rat. However, the content of ANF in atrial tissue of the fetus was less than in ventricular tissue. During the first 2—3 weeks of postnatal life, the ventricular content of

ANF fell and the atrial content rose to that of adult levels. The authors demonstrated that control of release of ANF in the fetal rat is intact and these animals can appropriately respond to stimuli for the release of ANF. Furthermore, *in utero*, where the atria have limited physiologic importance due to shunting of blood, the ventricle appears to be more involved in the regulation of ANF. Robillard and colleagues [89] studied the response to the infusion of ANF in fetal, newborn, and adult sheep. Arterial plasma immunoreactive ANF concentrations were higher in fetal and newborn animals than in the pregnant ewe, but the same as in the nonpregnant adult animal. Atrial natriuretic factor was also found in the urine of the fetus and in the amniotic fluid. During a constant infusion of ANF, there was a rise in hematocrit in all animals as well as a stimulation of plasma renin activity. The latter finding is different than reported in other animals and humans [76,77]. The response to the infusion of ANF in the fetal sheep was different from that in the newborn and adult animals in several respects. Atrial natriuretic factor produced a significant decrease in arterial blood pressure and heart rate in the newborn and adult sheep but not in the fetal animal. Furthermore, the fetus had an increased renal response to ANF infusion with a greater increase in renal vascular resistance and decrease in renal blood flow velocity than in the older animals. Finally, ANF produced a greater increase in renal sodium excretion in the adult animals and also caused an increase in GFR which was not seen in the fetal animals. The authors suggest that both the cardiovascular and renal responses to the infusion of ANF increase as the animal matures.

Extending this work, Varille and coworkers [93] infused ANF directly into the renal artery of fetal and newborn sheep, eliminating the systemic effects. Under these circumstances they found that ANF produced consistent renal vasodilatation, suggesting that previous findings of vasoconstriction were due to the activation of compensatory mechanisms during systemic infusion of the peptide. In spite of increasing numbers of studies of the physiology of ANF in the fetus and newborn, the significance of this peptide in the homeostatic control of blood pressure remains unclear.

The link of either ANF or the endogenous Na^+-K^+-ATPase inhibitor to hypertension remains speculative [74,78,79,81]. Both are increased in hypertensive states characterized by volume expansion, including various forms of experimental low-renin hypertension and low-renin essential hypertension in man [78]. The concentration of ANF in plasma of subjects with essential hypertension appears to be higher in those with more severe elevations of blood pressure [81]. Both hormones are elevated in patients with renal failure and pregnant women — conditions that are also associated with increased intravascular volume [78]. Because of its effects on increasing cardiac and vascular reactivity, the digitalis-like hormone may well directly contribute to elevation in blood pressure under certain circumstances. On the other hand, ANF is a vasodilator and its role is less clear.

While both ANF and the digitalis-like Na^+-K^+-ATPase inhibitor appear to be important hormones, it remains to be seen what their roles are in either normal fluid and electrolyte homeostasis or in pathologic states. Atrial natriuretic factor may act as a modulator of normal day-to-day regulation of fluid balance. The evidence that the digitalis-like factor plays some role in the genesis of certain forms of hypertension seems more compelling.

VISCOSITY AND HYPERTENSION

In 1840, Jean-Louis-Marie Poiseuille formulated a mathematical expression of the flow of fluid through cylindrical tubes. Based on his formula (Poiseuille law), the steady flow of a newtonian fluid (homogeneous, such as water) through such a tube is directly proportional to the pressure gradient between the two ends of the tube and to the fourth power of the tube's diameter. It is also inversely proportional to the length of the tube and to the nature (viscosity) of the fluid:

$$Q = \pi \, \Delta P \, r^4 / 8 \, l \, \eta$$

where Q is the flow, $\pi/8$ is the proportionality constant, ΔP is the pressure gradient, r is the radius, l is the length and η is the viscosity [94].

When fluid flows at a steady rate through a tube, the velocity of flow (the rate of displacement of fluid in centimeters with respect to time in seconds, cm/s) is the lowest at the periphery of the stream, whereas it is the highest at the center, each layer of fluid moving at a faster rate than its adjacent peripheral layer (laminar flow). The faster layer tends to drag along and to be held back by the slower layer. The greater the cohesive force between adjacent layers of fluid (shear stress), the lesser the distance of one plane moving away from the other (shear rate). Viscosity (internal friction or lack of slipperiness) is

defined as the ratio of the shear stress to shear rate:

$$\eta = \text{shear stress/shear rate}$$

The shear stress is determined in units of dyne/square centimeter (dyn/cm^2) and the shear rate is determined in centimeters per second per centimeter of vertical distance between the planes (cm/s per cm) [94,95].

$$\eta = \frac{dyn \, cm^{-2}}{cm \, s^{-1} \, cm^{-1}} = dyn \, s \, cm^{-2}$$

The unit of viscosity is the poise (P). A fluid of 1 P viscosity has a cohesive force (shear stress) of 1 dyn/cm^2 between layers when flowing with a velocity gradient (shear rate) of 1 cm/s per cm. The viscosity is often expressed relative to the viscosity of water which at a temperature of approximately 20°C is 0.01 P or 1 centipoise (cP). The viscosity is measured by one of several available viscometers at various velocity gradients (shear rates) at a given temperature [96,97].

Contrary to a newtonian fluid such as water which maintains its viscosity (shear stress/shear rate) at various rates of flow, the viscosity of blood is higher at lower blood flow rates. At high rates of blood flow, the shear rate rises and the viscosity falls, whereas at lower rates of blood flow the shear rate falls and the viscosity is increased. Low rates of shear might apply to the very slow flow of blood within the microvasculature and the high rates to the flow within the large arteries. The effective viscosity of blood in capillaries, however, is very low. This occurs, at least in part, because the red cells move toward the center of the capillary where the velocity of flow is higher and the layers of blood adjacent to the capillary wall remain relatively free of cells (Fahraeus—Lindqvist effect) [94]. Besides the rate of blood flow, some other determinants of blood viscosity are the hematocrit and the concentration of plasma proteins [94—97]. Some of the conditions which may lead to blood hyperviscosity are increased number of red blood cells (polycythemia), decreased red blood cell deformability/filterability (hereditary spherocytosis), hyperproteinemia, and dysproteinemia [98,99].

As already discussed, blood pressure is basically determined by two hemodynamic factors, CO and total peripheral vascular resistance. For many decades, investigators have searched to discover whether a relationship exists between blood viscosity, which is conceivably a component of resistance to blood flow, and blood pressure. Some have concluded that a direct relationship exists, whereas others have stated that any effect of viscosity on blood pressure is counteracted by an altered CO or total peripheral resistance. In 1930, Harris and McLoughlin [100] reported higher values of blood viscosity in a group of untreated hypertensive patients (systolic blood pressure 156–170 mmHg) than in normotensive control individuals. In 1966, Tibblin and colleagues [101] showed that a group of untreated hypertensive men (blood pressure greater than 150/110 mmHg) had significantly higher values of hematocrit and blood viscosity (at a shear rate of 23/s) and slightly higher plasma protein values than control subjects. Letcher and coworkers [102] studied blood and plasma viscosity and some of its determinants in a group of untreated patients with essential hypertension. Both blood and plasma viscosity values were significantly higher in hypertensive subjects than in the control population. When blood viscosity was measured in subgroups of hypertensive subjects and control subjects with similar hematocrit values, it once again remained higher in the hypertensive subjects. Among the determinants of plasma viscosity, the concentration of plasma fibrinogen was more important than that of albumin or total globulins. Chien [103] has suggested that increased blood viscosity may be an early event in the development of essential hypertension. At a shear rate of 0.52/s, a significant correlation was observed between blood viscosity and blood pressure. Blood viscosity, plasma viscosity, hematocrit, and fibrinogen all correlated directly with blood pressure.

In the normal course of circulation of blood, solute containing water is basically lost from the arteriolar segment of the capillaries and is reabsorbed into the venular segment. Thus, viscosity will rise as water is lost from the capillaries and fall as water is reabsorbed. It has been suggested that in hypertensive individuals there is an increased leakage of plasma water from the intravascular space into the interstitium, leading to reduced plasma volume and hemoconcentration which could account for higher values of blood viscosity [102]. The high blood viscosity may impair the blood flow through arteriolar capillaries leading to an increased intracapillary pressure which may perpetuate the extravasation of plasma water and protein [104,105]. Tarazi and colleagues [106] demonstrated lower plasma volume in men with uncomplicated essential hypertension than in control subjects. The difference remained significant whether expressed in relation to body weight, height, or surface area. The values for plasma volume correlated inversely with the levels of diastolic blood pressure. Tibblin and coworkers [101] also showed that a group of untreated hypertensive men had lower values of plasma volume than control subjects. Harris and McLoughlin [100] showed that they were able to reduce both blood viscosity and blood pressure by large quantities of oral fluid intake. Chrysant and colleagues [107] reported that when they used α-methyldopa for a group of patients with essential hypertension who had relative polycythemia (hematocrit ≥51%), the reduction in blood pressure was associated with an expansion of plasma volume and a significant fall in hematocrit, blood, and plasma viscosity. Chien [103] observed similar results with prazosin, an α-adrenergic blocking agent. These results could conceivably indicate that as capillary resistance declines, transcapillary fluid influx is increased and plasma volume is restored.

Several investigators have shown that volume expanders ameliorate the blood pressure in pregnancy-associated hypertension [108]. However, in a group of men with untreated essential hypertension, Wysocki and coworkers [109] showed that hemodilution induced by saline given over 12–15 min led to a rise in mean arterial pressure as blood and serum viscosity declined. Since CO remained unchanged, they concluded that improved blood and plasma viscosity by hemodilution had no beneficial effect on total peripheral resistance. Reduced plasma volume and the resulting hemoconcentration may not entirely account for the hyperviscosity of essential hypertension. As Simpson [110] states: "The relationship between blood pressure and blood viscosity which has been known for more than 70 years requires further recognition and research."

THE RENIN–ANGIOTENSIN–ALDOSTERONE SYSTEM

Our knowledge of the RAS continues to grow rapidly and the physiology and molecular biology of the RAS have been extensively reviewed [111–113]. Renin, an aspartyl proteinase, hydrolyzes the substrate angiotensinogen to form the decapeptide, angiotensin I (AI), which is then hydrolyzed by ACE, a carboxyterminal dipeptidyl peptidase, to the octapeptide, AII (Fig. 2.3). Angiotensin II and renin are metabolized primarily in the liver and the kidney. Angiotensin I converting enzyme is found in a number of organs and tissues; however, the majority of circulating AII

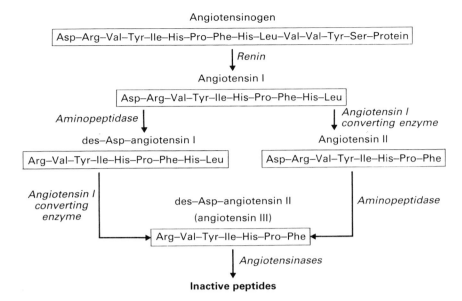

Fig. 2.3 The renin—angiotensin cascade.

is derived by the hydrolysis of AI during passage through the lung. While renin is formed in a number of organs and tissues, the major source of renin circulating in plasma is the kidney. Renin is synthesized initially as a preprorenin which is then converted into prorenin (inactive renin) [112,114]. Prorenin is converted to the active form of the enzyme and stored in granules. Inactive renin can also be released into the blood [112,114,115], although whether or not it is converted to the active renin in the circulation remains unknown [112].

The secretion of renin is regulated by multiple factors (Table 2.5) which have been reviewed extensively [111,112,116]. The baroreceptor of the kidney suppresses the secretion of renin when renal perfusion pressure increases and stimulates its secretion when the pressure falls. A second major factor in the regulation of renin release is the adrenergic nervous system: both β-adrenergic nerve stimulation and circulating catecholamines stimulate renin release. On the other hand, β-adrenergic blockade suppresses the release of renin. Additionally, dopaminergic receptor stimulation may lead to renin release [113]. While the effect of the α-adrenergic system on the regulation of renin release is less clear, it is likely that stimulation of the α-receptors suppresses it [116]. The third important factor in the regulation of renin secretion by the kidney is sodium. Sodium balance may affect renin release by leading to the expansion or contraction of the ECF volume, suppressing or stimulating renin release, respectively. However, sodium also acts through a feedback mechanism at

Table 2.5 Factors regulating the secretion of renin by the kidney

Renal baroreceptors
Changes in renal perfusion pressure
Changes in intrarenal pressure

Nervous system
β-adrenergic system
α-adrenergic system

Macula densa
Changes in sodium load or rate of delivery

Hormonal
Angiotensin II feedback
Atrial natriuretic factor
Vasopressin
Prostaglandins

Other
Calcium
Potassium

the macula densa of the distal tubule. Either the rate of delivery of sodium or the concentration of sodium or chloride reaching the macula densa cells can modify the rate of secretion of renin. Increases in sodium delivery or sodium concentration suppress renin release, while decreases have a stimulatory effect.

A number of additional factors influence the release of renin by the kidney. A decrease in serum potassium stimulates renin release as do prostaglandins, including PGI_2 and prostaglandin E_2. Vasopressin appears to inhibit renin release most likely by hemo-dynamic effects. Calcium most likely inhibits renin release, although the data are far from clear [113]. The cardiac hormone ANF has been reported to inhibit renin release [77]. Finally, there is feedback regulation of the release of renin. Angiotensin II directly inhibits renin release by its action on the juxtaglomerular cells. In addition, renin release is inhibited by the increased ECF volume associated with increased AII-stimulated aldosterone secretion and the increased renal vascular resistance stimulated in part by the pressor action of AII.

The RAS plays a role in the regulation of cardio-vascular homeostasis [117,118] as well as in the glom-erular and tubular functions of the kidney [119–121]. One of the complicating factors in attempting to determine the importance of the RAS on any given organ system is the multiple neurohormonal interac-tions in which it is involved [113,122]. For example, a fall in blood pressure secondary to blood loss not only triggers the release of renin from the kidney, but also causes a stimulation of the sympathetic nervous system, and a rise in plasma catecholamines and vasopressin. On the other hand, in normotensive sodium-depleted individuals, studies with ACE in-hibitors have demonstrated that the RAS is an import-ant factor in maintaining blood pressure with changes in posture, as when going from a supine to a standing position [117,123]. The advent of newer renin in-hibitory peptides provides new tools for study. For example, Zusman [124] has reported that one such peptide caused a dramatic decrease in blood pressure in a normotensive individual on a high sodium intake where plasma renin activity was suppressed. The mechanism of such a response needs further study.

In relation to its effects on renal function, all of the components of the RAS (angiotensinogen, renin, and converting enzyme) have been found within the kid-ney, thus allowing for the intrarenal generation of AII and its local action [121]. Angiotensin II has been demonstrated to reduce glomerular plasma flow, in-crease glomerular hydrostatic pressure, and reduce the glomerular ultrafiltration coefficient [119]. The suppression of AII formation by ACE inhibitors also affects tubular function and inhibits glomerulotubu-lar feedback [119–121]. Studies using ACE inhibitors in rats have provided evidence that AII stimulates proximal tubular reabsorption of sodium [119,120].

The role of the RAS in the genesis of certain forms of hypertension is clear. Angiotensin II is a powerful vasopressor. The elevated blood pressure in reno-vascular hypertension and malignant hypertension in humans is directly dependent on increased release of renin and the resulting elevated concentrations of plasma AII. In addition, AII is a powerful stimulator of aldosterone secretion and can lead to increased blood pressure secondary to sodium and fluid reten-tion, as in primary aldosteronism. On the other hand, in many forms of experimental renal hypertension two phases of the disease process have been ob-served. The initiation of hypertension is associated with high plasma renin activity, but then the levels fall and the chronic phase of hypertension is indepen-dent of the RAS [113].

A role for the RAS in essential hypertension has been the subject of a great deal of investigation. With the advent of ACE and renin inhibitors, it has been shown that some patients with essential hypertension do respond to blockade of AI conversion [113]. Fur-thermore, the determination of plasma renin activity has demonstrated that patients with essential hyper-tension can be categorized as being high, normal, or low renin and that the level of plasma renin activity may be related to the rate of complications associated with the hypertension [125]. Laragh and coworkers argue that the majority of forms of hypertension can be distinguished by two states of vasoconstriction, high renin with low plasma volume and low CO, and low renin with high plasma volume and high CO [125]. Even a patient with low-renin essential hyper-tension may respond to inhibition of the RAS if placed on a low-sodium diet [126]. These investi-gators propose that the vasoconstriction in both types of hypertension is related to an increase in intracellu-lar calcium (see below) [126,127].

It has been suggested that it may not be the levels of circulating renin and AII that are important in some forms of hypertension, but rather that the RAS may be active at local sites within blood vessel walls [128,129]. Renin may gain access to tissues by being synthesized locally or by entering the tissues from the circulation. For example, in a study by Loudon and coworkers, a bolus injection of renin into the circulation of rats raised arterial wall renin activity [130]. Furthermore, this increase in arterial wall renin was correlated with an elevation in blood pressure. On the other hand, direct measurements of the com-ponents of the RAS in vascular tissue suggest that it is indeed produced *in situ* [123]. Furthermore, Asaad and Antonaccio [131] have shown that arterial wall renin concentration is elevated in spontaneously hypertensive rats compared to normotensive control rats when the plasma renin activity is not different between the two groups. Captopril reduced blood pressure in both spontaneously hypertensive rats and control animals. Arterial wall renin also increased in response to captopril. Studies have also been carried out in another experimental model—two-kidney, one-clip hypertension in rats [132]. In these animals plasma renin activity is initially high and then declines although the high blood pressure is maintained, and while vascular wall renin activity follows the pattern of circulating renin, vascular wall converting enzyme concentration rises during the chronic phase of the hypertension [132]. The animals are responsive to ACE inhibitors. While direct evidence that the vascular RAS is an important factor in essential hypertension in man is lacking, this direction of study is promising and helps to explain the clinical response of many patients to ACE inhibition when plasma renin activity is not elevated.

The RAS has been extensively studied during development, and will be only briefly reviewed here. Plasma renin activity is higher in the newborn than in the adult, decreasing with age [133,134]. Hiner and colleagues [133] reported that plasma renin activity decreased by over 50% between the ages of 2—4 years to 16—17 years. Wilson and coworkers [135] reported that prorenin in cord blood and in arterial blood of infants was higher than in adults. Bailie and colleagues [115] also found that both active and inactive renin was released from the kidney of the newborn piglet in response to several stimuli and that the plasma concentrations of both active and inactive renin were greater in younger animals. Studies in lambs have also demonstrated that the fetus has higher plasma renin activity than the mother and that renin is released from the fetal kidney in response to a stimulus such as hemorrhage or suprarenal aortic constriction [136]. Wallace and coworkers [137,138] demonstrated developmental increases in pulmonary converting enzyme activity in the rat fetus and during the first 3—4 weeks of postnatal life. Gomez and colleagues [139] reported the presence of both renin and angiotensinogen messenger RNA in kidneys of 2-day-old Wistar—Kyoto and spontaneously hypertensive rats. Kidney renin messenger RNA was significantly higher in the newborn than in the adult animals. Ingelfinger and colleagues [140] determined renin activity in kidney, submandibular gland, adrenal gland, and gonads of male and female mice of three different strains. They found that during development renal renin remained unchanged but that there were developmental variations in the activity of renin in the other organs; these variations were related to strain and sex differences.

The role of the RAS and its development has been recently reviewed by Robillard and Nakamura [141]. They point out that the components of the system are intact during fetal life and that the RAS is responsive to the usual stimuli. They conclude that the magnitude of the effect of the RAS on the regulation of blood pressure, renal hemodynamics, and renal function depends on the stage of development. Our knowledge of the role of the RAS in the fetus and newborn remains fragmented and requires further study.

KALLIKREIN—KININ SYSTEM

While the KKS was described over 50 years ago [142], progress in understanding it has been slow because of difficulties in developing reliable assays and because the products of the system, the kinins, had actions which were difficult to distinguish from those of other hormones. Kallikreins are serine proteases which have been divided into two categories depending on their source: plasma kallikrein and tissue or glandular kallikrein [143,144]. Plasma and tissue kallikreins exist as zymogens, prekallikrein. Plasma kallikrein is Fletcher factor which is important in the clotting mechanism [142]. The substrate for kallikrein, kininogen, also exists in two forms; high molecular weight (HMW: 120 000 Da) and low molecular weight (LMW: 78 000 Da) kininogen. Plasma kallikrein acts on the HMW substrate to form bradykinin which is a powerful vasodilator. Tissue kallikrein can also act on the HMW substrate but in addition hydrolyzes the LMW substrate to form kallidin or lysbradykinin [144]. In addition to generating bradykinin, plasma kallikrein activates Hageman factor affecting coagulation and fibrinolysis and promoting chemotaxis for polymorphonuclear leukocytes [142]. Because of interaction with other hormonal systems, the role of the tissue kallikrein system is more complicated and will be discussed below. Finally, kinins are inactivated by two enzymes, kininase I (carboxypeptidase N) found in the plasma and kininase II (peptidyldipeptide hydrolase), which is the same as ACE [144].

As already suggested, the relationship between the KKS and regulation of blood pressure is complex. This relationship has recently been reviewed in depth [143,144]. The relationship between the rate of urinary excretion of kallikrein which is thought to reflect the activity of the renal KKS and various types of hypertension has been studied. Renal kallikrein has been localized to the distal and cortical collecting tubules [144]. It has been suggested that since bradykinin is a vasodilator which increases renal blood flow and renal sodium excretion [144,145], the KKS could play a role in the pathogenesis of hypertension [143,144]. In normotensive individuals, Margolius and colleagues [146] found that reducing dietary sodium intake resulted in increases in renal kallikrein excretion, as did treatment with mineralocorticoid agents. Patients with essential hypertension excreted kallikrein at a higher rate than did normotensive individuals on the same sodium intake [147]. Mineralocorticoid treatment in patients with essential hypertension increased urinary kallikrein excretion. In addition, patients with primary hyperaldosteronism also had increased urinary kallikrein excretion rates [147]. The authors concluded that the KKS might play a role in the response to sodium-retaining hormones as well as being important in the pathogenesis of essential hypertension.

Reduced urinary kallikrein excretion rates have been reported in other forms of hypertension including that associated with renal disease [148] and diabetes mellitus [149]. Urinary kallikrein excretion has been reported by some investigators to be increased in primary aldosteronism in humans [147] and deoxycorticosterone-salt hypertension in rats [150]. However, Holland and coworkers [151] found that some patients with primary aldosteronism did not have elevated urinary excretion rates of kallikrein, suggesting a limited use of this finding as a marker for increased mineralocorticoid activity.

Other evidence linking the KKS to hypertensive states comes from population studies. Zinner and coworkers [152] measured urinary kallikrein excretion in a study on the familial aggregation of blood pressure. They found that, like blood pressure, urinary kallikrein excretion demonstrated familial aggregation and the relationships remained over an 8-year follow-up. Urinary kallikrein excretion was found to be lower in black than in white families and correlated inversely with blood pressure [152]. In a previous study, Levy and coworkers [153] found that the rate of urinary excretion of kallikrein was greater in white normotensive individuals than it was in hypertensive patients or black normotensive patients, all on an unrestricted sodium intake. They demonstrated no difference between black normotensive and hyper-

tensive patients or between white and black hypertensive patients. They found that both racial groups of normotensive and hypertensive individuals had an increase in urinary kallikrein excretion rate when dietary sodium was restricted. This response was less in the black hypertensive population. They also found a positive correlation between kallikrein excretion and renal blood flow and suggested that the KKS as well as the RAS might be important in the regulation of renal vascular resistance and might explain the racial differences which they observed.

Holland and colleagues [151] also studied black and white normal and hypertensive individuals. They found no difference in kallikrein excretion between normotensive and hypertensive black subjects. Again, normotensive blacks had a lower rate of kallikrein excretion than did normotensive white subjects. However, they found no difference in kallikrein excretion between white normotensive and hypertensive subjects. Thus, while it appears that there is a fairly consistent racial difference between white and black normotensive individuals, differences in hypertensive patients are more variable.

A recent report does suggest a genetic component for the relationships between urinary kallikrein excretion and hypertension [154]. In a study of 57 pedigrees in the state of Utah, Berry and colleagues found a familial relationship of urinary kallikrein excretion. In relating this finding to families with a history of hypertension, they suggest that there is a dominant allele for high urinary kallikrein excretion and individuals with this allele have a decreased risk of essential hypertension.

The renal KKS might contribute to the control of blood pressure and the genesis of hypertension in two ways. First, reduced intrarenal generation of bradykinin might modify sodium excretion, or affect, renal prostaglandin, or renin production, and modify renal vascular resistance. Second, renal kallikrein might modify the circulating levels of bradykinin, a vasodilator. In a study by Mersey and coworkers [155] both kallikrein excretion and plasma bradykinin levels were determined in hypertensive patients. They found that while urinary kallikrein was reduced in subjects with normal-renin essential hypertension, plasma kinin levels were the same in both hypertensive and normal subjects. They did not subdivide their population by race and concluded that circulating kinin was unlikely to be related to the hypertensive state. However, another approach to the effects of kinins on blood pressure was that of

Carbonell and colleagues [156] who determined the effects of a kinin antagonist, DArg^0-Hyp^3-Thi^{5,8}-DPhe^7-bradykinin, on blood pressure in rats. In normal rats the intra-aortic injection of the antagonist produced an initial pressor response and then a depressor response, both of which were transient. The depressor response was inhibited by either indomethacin or nephrectomy, suggesting that it was secondary to the release of a renal prostaglandin. The authors interpret these data to suggest that kinins may be involved in the regulation of blood pressure.

While the significance is not clear, the relationship between the KKS and other hormonal systems which may modify blood pressure needs to be considered. Kinins activate phospholipase A_2, leading to the release of arachidonic acid and increased production of renal prostaglandins. Prostaglandins in turn can stimulate renin secretion by the kidney [144]. Furthermore, in addition to the fact that ACE inactivates bradykinin, renal kallikrein has been shown to activate inactive renin *in vitro* [145,157,158]. These complex interactions may be important in the regulation of blood pressure but the physiologic significance of the findings remain to be explained.

In summary, the KKS has a number of interactions which suggests that there is a potential deficiency in the system in various forms of hypertension. However, it is not clear how the changes reported in both humans and animals might lead to changes in blood pressure. In theory a genetic defect in the production of kininogen or kallikrein may be involved. On the other hand, the changes seen in the excretion of kallikrein in the urine of hypertensive individuals may be secondary to the elevated blood pressure.

PROSTAGLANDINS

Since the discovery of prostaglandins over 50 years ago, our knowledge has become more extensive about the metabolites of arachidonic acid, which now include not only the prostaglandins but also thromboxane, PGI_2, and leukotrienes. As a group, these compounds are known as eicosanoids. The biosynthesis of the prostaglandins, thromboxane, and PGI_2 has been reviewed [159]. Arachidonic acid is released from the phospholipid storage pool by phospholipase A and C, oxygenated by cyclooxygenase to form prostaglandin G_2, which is in turn converted to prostaglandins E_2 and $F_{2\alpha}$, thromboxane A_2, and PGI_2 [124,159]. Table 2.6 lists the most important renal prostaglandins and their sites of synthesis [160]. Be-

Table 2.6 The renal prostaglandins

Renal prostaglandin	Site of synthesis
Prostaglandin E_2	Glomerulus, CCT, MCT, MTHAL, MIC
Prostacyclin	Glomerulus, arterioles, MCT
Prostaglandin $F_{2\alpha}$	Glomerulus, MCT, MTHAL, MIC
Thromboxane A_2	Glomerulus, MCT

CCT = Cortical collecting tubule; MCT = medullary collecting tubule; MTHAL = medullary thick ascending limb; MIC = medullary interstitial cells.

cause of their short half-lives, ubiquity, and diversity of action, the physiology of these compounds has been difficult to study. Since prostaglandins, PGI_2 and thromboxane A_2 are synthesized and act locally, there is little evidence that they are important as circulating hormones and that they are involved in the systemic regulation of blood pressure [161]. Furthermore, since prostaglandins are not stored, the determination of increased release is taken as a measure of increased synthesis. Renal release of prostaglandins has been measured by the rate of urinary excretion of the prostaglandin itself or of its metabolites. The renal eicosanoids have been most extensively investigated for their involvement in blood pressure regulation.

With the advent of nonsteroidal anti-inflammatory agents which inhibit the synthesis of prostaglandins, the study of their physiologic as well as pathologic role in hypertension has been greatly improved. The potential role of prostaglandins in experimental and human hypertension has been reviewed [161,162]. McGiff and colleagues [163] have pointed out that within the kidney, the prostaglandins interact with both the RAS and the KKS. PGI_2 and its metabolite 6-keto-PGI_2 stimulate renin release. Studies in deoxycorticosterone-treated hypertensive rats demonstrated an association between urinary kallikrein excretion and excretion of prostaglandins E_2 and $F_{2\alpha}$. In these animals, inhibition of kallikrein with a serine protease inhibitor reduced the urinary excretion rates of the prostaglandins, kallikrein, and sodium [163]. Machida and coworkers [164] studied the chronic phase of two-kidney, one-clip hypertension in rabbits on low, normal, high, and very high sodium diets. Their data on the urinary sodium and prostaglandin E_2 excretion rates by the clipped and unclipped kidneys suggested that the hypertension in the animals on a high sodium diet was maintained by the failure of the unclipped kidney to excrete the excess salt, possibly because of an abnormal response in the renal prostaglandin system. In deoxycorticosterone- and salt-induced hypertensive rats, Roman and colleagues [165] found that renal blood flow and GFR were reduced in the hypertensive animals compared to control animals. These findings, while associated with an increase in the urinary excretion of thromboxane B_2 (a metabolite of thromboxane A_2, which is a powerful vasoconstrictor), could not be reversed by thromboxane A_2 inhibitors. On the other hand, in rats in which hypertension was induced by AII infusion and high sodium diet, the inhibition of thromboxane A_2 receptors resulted in a reduction in blood pressure, suggesting a role for vasopressor prostaglandins in this form of hypertension [166].

The role of the prostaglandins in the magnitude of the response to antihypertensive therapy has received a great deal of attention. Zusman [124] has reviewed the evidence that the antihypertensive response to captopril in states of low-renin hypertension may be related to the stimulation of vasodilator prostaglandins. Studies in a variety of forms of experimental hypertension where renin is not the mediator and in essential human hypertension support this concept. Captopril has been shown to stimulate the release of prostaglandin E_2 from the renomedullary interstitial cells *in vivo* [124]. Studies by Kudo and coworkers [167] in patients with essential hypertension demonstrated that a thromboxane A_2 synthetase inhibitor enhanced the antihypertensive effect of captopril. They suggest that thromboxane A_2 inhibits the antihypertensive effect of captopril in these patients. A study by Levens and coworkers [168] in SHR using ACE inhibitors in conjunction with thromboxane A_2 synthesis inhibitors and receptor antagonists suggests that the effect of thromboxane A_2 synthetase inhibitors is to allow the redirection of prostaglandin synthesis to vasodilatory compounds (prostaglandin E_2 and PGI_2) which enhance the effect of captopril. In a study on the effect of propranolol in essential hypertension, Beckermann and colleagues found evidence for increased PGI_2 synthesis which enhanced the response to propranolol [169].

The prostaglandins have been studied extensively in newborn and developing animals and humans. Prostaglandins are present in the plasma and urine of fetal lambs [170]. Friedman and Demers [171] studied prostaglandin synthesis in renal tissues of fetuses between 24 and 40 weeks of gestation. There was increasing synthesis of both prostaglandins E_2 and $F_{2\alpha}$ as gestational age increased. Sulyok and colleagues [172] followed the rate of urinary excretion of prostaglandin E_2 in premature infants between the first and fifth weeks of life. They found a three-fold increase in the rate of excretion over this time period. Pace-Asciak [173] has studied both the anabolic and catabolic pathways involved in maintenance of prostaglandins in the fetus and newborn. He found striking changes in the activity of several prostaglandin catabolic enzymes in the kidney of the developing rat before and after birth. His work has demonstrated the presence of prostaglandin metabolizing enzymes in a number of other organs as well as the kidney. Studies of the urinary excretion of prostaglandins E_2 and $F_{2\alpha}$ have demonstrated that there is a significant increase in the rate of excretion of both prostaglandins from birth to adult life in human subjects [174,175]. Gleason [176] has summarized the present state of knowledge about the renal prostaglandins during development. While it is far from clear what role they play in blood pressure regulation in the fetus or newborn, treatment of patent ductus arteriosus with indomethacin clearly has a suppressive effect on renal function [176].

CALCIUM AND HYPERTENSION

Calcium is an important regulator of cellular function in a wide variety of tissues including striated and smooth muscle, glandular tissue, nerve cells, and blood cells [127,177]. The contraction of vascular smooth muscle and, therefore, the regulation of peripheral vascular resistance is in part calcium-dependent. Vasoconstrictor hormones such as AII, vasopressin, and epinephrine require calcium for their activity [127].

The details of the mechanisms by which calcium acts as an intracellular mediator are too broad for this review and will be only briefly discussed here (Table 2.7). The concentration of calcium in cells can increase in two ways: movement of calcium into cells from the ECF, and the release of calcium from storage sites within cells, primarily the endoplasmic reticulum [127,177,178]. Calcium enters the cell from the ECF by at least two mechanisms: sodium−calcium exchange, and through calcium channels driven by the high extracellular calcium gradient [127]. When the calcium concentration in the cell increases, calcium is bound to calmodulin, a specific intracellular calcium-binding protein, and the events outlined in

Table 2.7 Relationship of calcium to smooth muscle contraction

1 Intracellular calcium increases either because of changes in extracellular calcium and/or release of calcium from the endoplasmic reticulum

2 Calcium is bound to calmodulin (CAL) forming Ca^2-CAL complex which changes the configuration of calmodulin

3 Ca^2-CAL activates myosin light-chain kinase which catalyzes the phosphorylation of myosin light-chain

4 The change in the myosin molecule results in increased bridging and muscle contraction

5 When intracellular calcium falls, the process is reversed and the muscle relaxes

Table 2.7 are initiated resulting in contraction of vascular smooth muscle cells [178,179].

A possible relationship between calcium and various forms of hypertension has recently received much attention [127,180−184]. The hypothesis that a deficiency of calcium is important in the genesis of hypertension is very controversial [180−182]. The association of the possible effects of calcium on blood pressure has been based on a number of observations. It has been suggested from data derived from epidemiologic studies that individuals with essential hypertension ingest less calcium than do nonhypertensive individuals [182]. However, many of these studies depend upon patient recall and have serious flaws in experimental design [181]. Other studies have demonstrated an increase in circulating parathyroid hormone in patients with essential hypertension [182,185], and it has been suggested that the hypertensive individual may have a renal calcium leak which leads to a compensatory increase in circulating parathyroid hormones. Ellison and coworkers [186] also reported that urinary cyclic adenosine monophosphate excretion was elevated in hypertensive patients, indicating increased parathyroid hormone activity. Studies on the concentration of total serum calcium and ionized calcium suggest that there is a decreased concentration of the latter in patients with hypertension. For example, Folsom and colleagues [187] reported that hypertensive individuals had lower serum concentrations of ultrafilterable calcium, as well as ionized calcium and complexed calcium, than did their normotensive, age-, sex-, and race-matched controls. Since intracellular calcium concentration appears to be important in the regulation of muscle tone, attempts have been made to determine if there are differences between normal and hypertensive individuals. Erne and coworkers [188] studied the concentration of calcium in platelets from patients with essential hypertension and in normal individuals. They found that there was a positive correlation between the intracellular concentration of calcium and both diastolic and systolic blood pressure. Furthermore, treatment with calcium channel blocking agents, β-adrenergic blocking agents, or diuretics lowered blood pressure as well as intracellular calcium. This finding, like others, however is controversial [180,181].

The question has also been asked whether increasing calcium intake will lower blood pressure. McCarron [182] has reviewed a number of studies on the effects of calcium supplementation on blood pressure and suggests that many have shown significant reductions. Hatton and colleagues [189] also reported that increased dietary calcium intake in spontaneously hypertensive rats resulted in lower levels of blood pressure. Young and coworkers [184] have recently reviewed the data relating calcium to hypertension in experimental models. They found a number of studies in which increased dietary calcium in spontaneously hypertensive rats lowers blood pressure. The data in humans were reviewed by Kaplan and Meese [181] who point out that a great deal of inconsistency remains in the findings.

Finally, an attempt has been made to relate the possible effects of calcium in essential hypertension to that of sodium and the digitalis-like natriuretic hormone [2,183,190]. This relationship is based on the fact that one of the mechanisms for calcium movement across cell membranes is a sodium−calcium exchanger [190]. It has been suggested that the effects of the natriuretic hormone which inhibits Na^+-K^+-ATPase would be to increase intracellular sodium concentration and lead to an increase in intracellular calcium which would, in turn, set off the events leading to smooth muscle contraction (Table 2.7). The system is complex and probably functions differently in different tissues [190]. Further investigation will be required to define the true nature of the relationship between calcium and the pathogenesis of essential hypertension.

REFERENCES

1 Peart WS. General review of hypertension. In: Genest J, Kuchel O, Hamet P, Cantin M, eds. *Hypertension*. 2nd edn. New York: McGraw-Hill, 1983;3−14.

2 Blaustein MP. Sodium transport and hypertension: where are we going? *Hypertension* 1984;6:445−53.

3 Córdova HR, Martínez-Maldonado M. Hormonal mechanisms in human essential hypertension. *Semin Nephrol* 1988;8:131−7.

4 Ritz E, Mann J, Schmid M. Salt and volume regulatory systems. In: Retting R, Ganten D, Luft F, eds. *Salt and Hypertension. Dietary Minerals, Volume Homeostasis and Cardiovascular Regulation*. Berlin: 1989.

5 Simpson FO. Sodium intake, body sodium and sodium excretion. *Lancet* 1988;ii:25−9.

6 Robinson BF. Sodium and calcium handling. In: Kaplan NM, Laragh JH, eds. *Perspectives in Hypertension — The Kidney in Hypertension*, vol. 1. New York: Raven Press, 1987.

7 Brenner B, Coe FL, Rector FC Jr. Transport function of the renal tubules — basic mechanisms of transport in epithelia. In: Brenner B, Coe FL, Rector FC, eds. *Renal Physiology in Health and Disease*. Philadelphia: WB Saunders, 1987.

8 Doucet A. Na-K-ATPase — general considerations, role and regulation in the kidney. *Adv Nephrol* 1985;15:876−959.

9 Schafer JA. The physiology teacher. Salt and water absorption in the proximal tubule. *Physiologist* 1982;25:95−103.

10 Koushanpour E, Kriz W. Tubular processing of glomerular ultrafiltrate: mechanisms of electrolyte and water transport. The proximal tubule. In: Koushanpour E, Kriz W, eds. *Renal Physiology — Principals, Structure and Function*. 2nd edn. New York: Springer-Verlag, 1986.

11 Jacobson HR. Transport characteristics of *in vitro* perfused proximal convoluted tubules. *Kidney Int* 1982;22:425−33.

12 Rector FC Jr. Sodium bicarbonate and chloride absorption by the proximal tubule. *Am J Physiol* 1983;244:F461−F471.

13 Jacobson HR. Functional segmentation of the mammalian nephron. *Am J Physiol* 1981;241:F203−18.

14 Kokko JP. Transport characteristics of the thin limbs of Henle. *Kidney Int* 1982;22:449−53.

15 Burg MB. Thick ascending limb of Henle's loop. *Kidney Int* 1982;22:454−64.

16 Imai M, Nakamura R. Function of distal convoluted and connecting tubules studied by isolated nephron fragments. *Kidney Int* 1982;22:465−72.

17 Khuri RN, Wiederholt M, Strieder N, Giebisch G. Effects of graded solute diuresis on renal tubular sodium transport in the rat. *Am J Physiol* 1957;228:1262−8.

18 Stokes JB. Ion transport by the cortical and outer medullary collecting tubule. *Kidney Int* 1982;22:473−84.

19 Guyton AC, Manning RD Jr, Norman RA Jr *et al*. Current concepts and perspectives of renal volume regulation in relation to hypertension. *J Hypertens* 1986;4(suppl 4): S49−56.

20 Marsden PA, Skorecki KL. Afferent limb of volume homeostasis. In: Brenner BM, Stein JH, eds. *Body Fluid Homeostasis. Contemporary Issues in Nephrology*. New York: Churchill Livingstone, 1987.

21 Raymond KH, Stein JH. Efferent limb of volume homeostasis. In: Brenner BM, Stein JH, eds. *Body Fluid Homeostasis. Contemporary Issues in Nephrology*. New York: Churchill Livingstone, 1987.

22 Epstein FH, Goodyer AVN, Lawrason FD, Relman AS. Studies of the antidiuresis of quiet standing: the importance of changes in plasma volume and glomerular filtration rate. *J Clin Invest* 1951;30:63−72.

23 Hulet WH, Smith HW. Postural natriuresis and urine osmotic concentration in hydropenic subjects. *Am J Med* 1961;39:8−25.

24 Weidman P, Saxenhofer H, Ferrier C, Shaw SG. Atrial natriuretic peptide in man. *Am J Nephrol* 1988;8:1−14.

25 Menninger RP, Frazier DT. Effects of blood volume and atrial stretch on hypothalamic single-unit activity. *Am J Physiol* 1972;223:288−93.

26 Weaver LC. Cardiopulmonary sympathetic afferent influences on renal nerve activity. *Am J Physiol* 1977;233:H592−9.

27 DiBona GF. Neurogenic regulation of renal tubular sodium reabsorption. *Am J Physiol* 1977;233:F73−81.

28 DiBona GF. Sympathetic nervous system influences on the kidney. *Am J Hypertens* 1989;2:S119−24.

29 Zehr JE, Hasbargen JA, Kurz KD. Reflex suppression of renin secretion during distension of cardiopulmonary receptors in dogs. *Circ Res* 1976;38:232−9.

30 Epspein FH, Post RS, McDowell M. The effect of an arteriovenous fistula on renal hemodynamics and electrolyte excretion. *J Clin Invest* 1953;32:233−41.

31 Mancia G, Ferrari A, Gregorini L *et al*. Control of blood pressure by carotid sinus baroreceptors in human beings. *Am J Cardiol* 1979;44:895−902.

32 DiBona GF. The kidney in the pathogenesis of hypertension:the role of renal nerves. *Am J Kidney Dis* 1985;5:A27−31.

33 Reid IA. The renin−angiotensin system and body function. *Arch Intern Med* 1985;145:1475−9.

34 Ichikawa I, Brenner BM. Mechanisms of inhibition of proximal tubule fluid reabsorption after exposure of the rat kidney to the physical effects of expansion of extracellular fluid volume. *J Clin Invest* 1979;64:1466−74.

35 Levinsky NG, Lalone RD, Moss IS. The mechanism of sodium diuresis after saline infusion in the dog. *J Clin Invest* 1963;42:1261−76.

36 Brenner B, Coe FL, Rector FC Jr. Regulation and disorders of extracellular fluid volume. In: Brenner B, Coe FL, Rector FC Jr, eds. *Renal Physiology in Health and Disease*. Philadelphia: W.B. Saunders, 1987.

37 Early LE, Friedler RM. The effects of combined renal vasodilatation and pressor agents on renal hemodynamics and the tubular reabsorption of sodium. *J Clin Invest* 1966;45:542−51.

38 Schuster VL, Kokko JP, Jacobson HR. Angiotensin II directly stimulates sodium transport in rabbit proximal convoluted tubules. *J Clin Invest* 1984;73:507−15.

39 Bello-Reuss E, Trevino DL, Gottschalk CW. Effect of renal sympathetic nerve stimulation on proximal water and sodium reabsorption. *J Clin Invest* 1976;57:1104−7.

40 Bencasth P, Szenasi G, Takacs L. Water and electrolyte transport in Henle's loop and distal tubule after renal sympathectomy in the rat. *Am J Physiol* 1985;249:F308−14.

41 Imbs JL, Schmidt M, Ehrhardt JD, Schwartz J. The sympathetic nervous system and renal sodium handling:is dopamine involved? *J Cardiovasc Pharmacol* 1984;6(suppl 1):S171−5.

42 Marver D, Kokko JP. Renal target sites and the mechanism of action of aldosterone. *Min Electrolyte Metab* 1983; 9:1−18.

43 Olsen ME, Hall JE, Montani JP et al. Mechanisms of angiotensin II natriuresis and antinatriuresis. Am J Physiol 1985;249:F299−307.

44 Levenson DJ, Simmons CE, Brenner BM. Arachidonic acid metabolism, prostaglandins and the kidney. Am J Med 1982;72:354−74.

45 Stokes JB, Kokko JP. Inhibition of sodium transport by prostaglandin E_2 across the isolated, perfused rabbit-collecting tubule. J Clin Invest 1977;59:1099−104.

46 Stokes JB. Effect of prostaglandin E_2 on chloride transport across the rabbit thick ascending limb of Henle. Selective inhibition of the medullary portion. J Clin Invest 1979;64:495−502.

47 Carretero OA, Scicli AG. The renal kallikrein−kinin system. Am J Physiol 1980;238:F247−255.

48 Granger JP, Hall JE. Acute and chronic actions of bradykinin on renal function and arterial pressure. Am J Physiol 1985;248:F87−92.

49 Blaustein MP. Sodium ions, calcium ions, blood pressure regulation, and hypertension: a reassessment and a hypothesis. Am J Physiol 1977;232:165−73.

50 Baldessarini RJ. Drugs and the treatment of psychiatric disorders. In: Goodman GA, Goodman LS, Rall TW, Murad F, eds. Goodman & Gillman's The Pharmacological Basis of Therapeutics. VII edn. New York: Macmillan, 1985:426−31.

51 Georgotas A. Affective disorder: pharmacotherapy. In: Kaplan HI, Sadock BJ, eds. Comprehensive Textbook of Psychiatry. 4th edn. Baltimore: Williams & Wilkins, 1985:821−33.

52 Mendels J, Frazer A. Alterations in cell membrane activity in depression. Am J Psychiatry 1974;131:1240−6.

53 Maizels M. Effect of sodium content on sodium efflux from human red cell suspended in sodium-free media containing potassium, rubidium, caesium or lithium chloride. J Physiol 1968;195:657−79.

54 Hass M, Schooler J, Tosteson DC. Coupling of lithium to sodium transport in human red cells. Nature 1975;258:425−7.

55 Canessa M, Adragna N, Solomon H, Connoly T, Tosteson DC. Increased sodium−lithium countertransport in red cells of patients with essential hypertension. N Engl J Med 1980;302:772−6.

56 Woods JW, Falk RJ, Pittman AW, Klemmer PJ, Watson BS, Namboodiri K. Increased red-cell sodium−lithium countertransport in normotensive sons of hypertensive parents. N Engl J Med 1982;306:539−95.

57 Ibsen KK, Jensen HA, Wieth JO, Funder J. Essential hypertension:sodium−lithium countertransport in erythrocytes from patients and from families having one hypertensive parent. Hypertension 1982;4:703−9.

58 Cooper R, LeGrady D, Nanas S et al. Increased sodium−lithium countertransport in college students with elevated blood pressure. JAMA 1983;249:1030−4.

59 Cooper R, Miller K, Trevisan M et al. Family history of hypertension and red cell cation transport in high school students. J Hypertens 1983;1:145−52.

60 Brugnara C, Corrocher R, Foroni L et al. Lithium−sodium countertransport in erythrocytes of normal and hypertensive subjects. Relationship with age and plasma renin activity. Hypertension 1983;5:529−34.

61 Norling LL, Goldring D, Hernandez A, Robson AM. Sodium−lithium countertransport in erythrocytes of children and adolescents with hypertension. Dev Pharmacol Ther 1986;9:231−40.

62 Trevisan M, Strazzullo P, Cappuccio FP et al. Red blood cell Na content, Na, Li-countertransport, family history of hypertension and blood pressure in school children. J Hypertens 1988;6:227−30.

63 Trevisan M, Cooper R, Ostrow D et al. Red cell cation transport:differences between black and white school children. J Hypertens 1983;1:245−9.

64 Bunker CH, Mallinger AG, Adams LL, Kuller LH. Red blood cell sodium−lithium countertransport and cardiovascular risk factors in black and white college students. J Hypertens 1987;5:7−15.

65 Williams RR, Hasstedt SJ, Hunt SC, Wu LL, Ash KO. Genetic studies of cation tests and hypertension. Hypertension 1978;10(suppl I):I137−41.

66 Duhm J, Becker BF. Studies on lithium transport across the red cell membrane. On the nature of the Na^+ dependent Li^+ countertransport system of mammalian erythrocyte. J Membrane Biol 1979;51:236−86.

67 Aronson PS. Red cell sodium−lithium countertransport and essential hypertension. N Engl J Med 1982;307:317.

68 Levine A, Balfe JW, Veitch R et al. Increased platelet Na^+-H^+ exchange rates in essential hypertension: application of a novel test. Lancet 1987;i:533−6.

69 Canessa M, Brugnara C, Escobales N. The Li^+Na^+ exchange and Na^+-K^+-Cl^- cotransport systems in essential hypertension. Hypertension 1987;10(suppl I):I4−10.

70 MacGregor GA, Fenton S, Alaghband-Zadeh J. Evidence for a raised concentration of a circulating sodium transport inhibitor in essential hypertension. Br Med J 1981;283:1355−7.

71 Haupert GT Jr. Circulating inhibitors of sodium transport at the prehypertensive stage of essential hypertension. J Cardiovasc Pharmacol 1988;12(suppl 3):S70−6.

72 Canessa M, Morgan K, Semplicini A. Genetic differences in lithium−sodium exchange and regulation of the sodium−hydrogen exchanger in essential hypertension. J Cardiovasc Pharmacol 1988;12(suppl 3):S92−8.

73 Buckalew VM Jr, Gruber KA. Natriuretic hormone. Annu Rev Physiol 1984;46:343−58.

74 De Wardener HE. Natriuretic and sodium-transport inhibitory factors associated with volume control and hypertension. In: Mulrow PJ, Schrier R, eds. Arterial Hormones and Other Natriuretic Factors. Bethesda, MD:American Physiological Society, 1987.

75 Adams SP. Structure and biological function of atrial natriuretic peptides. Endocrinol Metabol Clin North Am 1988;16:1−17.

76 Graham RM, Zisfein JB. Atrial natriuretic factor:biosynthetic regulation and role in circulatory homeostasis. In: Fozzard HA, Jennings RB, Haber E, Katz AM, Morgan HE, eds. The Heart and Cardiovascular System. 1st edn. New York: Raven Press, 1986.

77 Atlas SA, Maack T. Effects of atrial natriuretic factor on the kidney and the renin−angiotensin−aldosterone system. Endocrinol Metabol Clin North Am 1987;16:107−43.

78 Haddy FJ, Pamnani MB. Natriuretic factors in arterial hypertension. In: Mulrow PJ, Schrier R, eds. Atrial Hormones and Other Natriuretic Factors. Bethesda,

MD:American Physiological Society, 1987.

79 Haddy FJ, Pamnani MB. Evidence for a circulating endogenous Na$^+$K$^+$ pump inhibitor in low-renin hypertension. *Fed Proc* 1985;44:2789−94.

80 Valdes R, Graves SW, Brown BA, Landt M. Endogenous substances in newborn infants cause false positive digoxin measurements. *J Pediatr* 1983;102:947−50.

81 Genest J, Larochelle P, Cusson JR, Gutkowska J, Cantin M. The atrial natriuretic factor in hypertension:state of the art lecture. *Hypertension* 1988;11(suppl I):I-3−7.

82 Kikuchi K, Nishioka K, Ueda T *et al*. Relationship between plasma atrial natriuretic polypeptide concentration and hemodynamic measurements in children with congenital heart disease. *J Pediatr* 1987;111:335−42.

83 Matsuoka S, Kurahashi Y, Miki Y *et al*. Plasma atrial natriuretic peptide in patients with congenital heart disease. *Pediatrics* 1988;82:639−43.

84 Rascher W, Tulassay T, Lang RE. Atrial natriuretic peptide in plasma of volume-overloaded children with chronic renal failure. *Lancet* 1985;ii:303−5.

85 Rascher W, Tulassay T, Lang RE. Atrial natriuretic peptide in children. In: Murakami K, Kitagawa T, Yabuta L, Sakai T, eds. *Recent Advances in Pediatric Nephrology*. New York: Excerpta Medica, 1987.

86 Robillard JE, Weiner C. Atrial natriuretic factor in the human fetus: effect of volume expansion. *J Pediatr* 1988;113:552−5.

87 Tulassay T, Rascher W, Seyberth HW, Lang RE, Tóth M, Sulyok E. Role of atrial natriuretic peptide in sodium homeostasis in premature infants. *J Pediatr* 1986;109:1023−7.

88 Weil J, Bidlingmaier F, Döhlemann C, Kuhnle U, Strom T, Lang RE. Comparison of plasma atrial natriuretic peptide levels in healthy children from birth to adolescence and in children with cardiac diseases. *Pediatr Res* 1986;20:1328−31.

89 Robillard JE, Nakamura KT, Varille VA *et al*. Ontogeny of the renal response to natriuretic peptide in sheep. *Am J Physiol* 1988;254:F634−41.

90 Shaffer SG, Geer PG, Goetz KL. Elevated atrial natriuretic factor in neonates with respiratory distress syndrome. *J Pediatr* 1986;109:1028−33.

91 Tulassay T, Rascher W, Ganten D, Schärer K, Lang RE. Atrial natriuretic peptide and volume changes in children. *Clin Exp Hypertens − Theory Prac* 1986;A8:695−701.

92 Wei Y, Rodi CP, Day ML *et al*. Developmental changes in the rat atriopeptin hormonal system. *J Clin Invest* 1987;79:1325−9.

93 Varille VA, Nakamura KT, McWeeny OJ *et al*. Renal hemodynamic response to atrial natriuretic factor in fetal and newborn sheep. *Pediatr Res* 1989;25:291−4.

94 Berne RM, Levy MN. Hemodynamics. In: Berne RM, Levy MN, eds. *Physiology*. Washington, DC:Mosby, 1988.

95 Wells RE Jr, Merrill EW. The variability of blood viscosity. *Am J Med* 1961;31:505−9.

96 Hell KMD, Balzereit A, Diebold U, Bruhn HD. Importance of blood viscoelasticity in arteriosclerosis. *Angiology* 1987;40:539−46.

97 Jan KM, Chien S, Bigger T Jr. Observation on blood viscosity changes after acute myocardial infarction. *Circulation* 1975;51:1079−84.

98 Forconi S, Pieragalli D, Guerrini M, Galagani C, Cappelli R. Primary and secondary blood hyperviscosity syndromes, and syndromes associated with blood superviscosity. *Drugs* 1987;33(suppl 2):19−26.

99 Stoltz JF, Donner M, Larcan A. Introduction to hemorheology:theoretical aspects and hyperviscosity syndromes. *Int Angiol* 1987;6:119−32.

100 Harris I, McLoughlin G. The viscosity of the blood in high blood pressure. *Q J Med* 1930;23:451−64.

101 Tibblin G, Bergentz SE, Bjure J, Wilhelmsen L. Hematocrit, plasma protein, plasma volume and viscosity in early hypertensive disease. *Am Heart J* 1966;72:165−76.

102 Letcher TL, Chien S, Pickering TG, Sealey JE, Laragh JH. Direct relationship between blood pressure and blood viscosity in normal and hypertensive subjects. Role of fibrinogen concentration. *Am J Med* 1981;70:1195−202.

103 Chien S. Blood rheology in myocardial infarction and hypertension. *Biorheology* 1986;23:633−53.

104 Simpson LO. A hypothesis proposing increased blood viscosity as a cause of proteinuria and increased vascular permeability. *Nephron* 1982;31:89−93.

105 Simpson LO. Angina and the blood. *Lancet* 1983;i:1102.

106 Tarazi RC, Frolich ED, Dustan HP. Plasma volume in men with essential hypertension. *N Engl J Med* 1968;278:762−5.

107 Chrysant SG, Frohlich ED, Adamopoulos PN *et al*. Pathophysiologic significance of "stress" on relative polycythemia in essential hypertension. *Am J Cardiol* 1976;37:1069−72.

108 Callery EDM, Mitchell MDM, Redman CWG. Fall in blood pressure in response to volume-expansion in pregnancy-associated hypertension (pre-eclampsia): why does it occur? *J Hypertens* 1984;2:177−82.

109 Wysocki M, Persson B, Aurell M *et al*. Haemodynamics and haemorheological effects of hypervolaemic haemodilution in men with primary hypertension. *J Hypertens* 1987;5:185−9.

110 Simpson LO. Blood pressure and blood viscosity. *NZ Med J* 1988;101:581.

111 Davis JO, Freeman RH. Mechanisms regulating renin release. *Physiol Rev* 1976;56:1−56.

112 Dzau VJ, Burt DW, Pratt RE. Molecular biology of the renin−angiotensin system. *Am J Physiol* 1988;255:F563−73.

113 Dzau VJ, Pratt RE. Renin−angiotensin system: biology, physiology, and pharmacology, In: Fozzard HA, Jennings RB, Haber E, Katz AM, Morgen HE, eds. *The Heart and Cardiovascular System*. 1st edn. New York: Raven Press, 1986.

114 Sealey JE, Atlas SA, Laragh JH. Prorenin in plasma and kidney. *Fed Proc* 1983;42:2681−9.

115 Bailie MD, Derkx FHM, Schalekamp MADS. Release of active and inactive renin by the pig kidney during development. *Dev Pharmacol Ther* 1980;1:47−53.

116 Keeton TK, Campbell WB. The pharmacologic alteration of renin release. *Pharmacol Rev* 1980;32:81−228.

117 Niarchos AP, Pickering TG, Case DB, Sullivan P, Laragh JH. Role of the renin−angiotensin system in blood pressure regulation:the cardiovascular effects of converting enzyme inhibition in normotensive subjects. *Circ Res* 1979;45:829−37.

118 Sancho J, Re R, Burton J, Barger AC, Haber E. The role of the renin−angiotensin−aldosterone system in cardio-

vascular homeostasis in normal human subjects. *Circulation* 1976;53:400−5.

119 Blantz RC. The glomerular and tubular actions of angiotensin II. *Am J Kidney Dis* 1987;10(suppl 1):2−6.

120 Navar LG, Carmines PK, Huang W-C, Mitchell KD. The tubular effects of angiotensin II. *Kidney Int* 31(suppl 20):S81−8.

121 Navar LG, Rosivall L. Contribution of the renin−angiotensin system to the control of intrarenal hemodynamics. *Kidney Int* 1984;25:857−68.

122 Brunner HR, Waeber B, Nussberger J. Renin secretion responsiveness: understanding the efficacy of renin−angiotensin inhibition. *Kidney Int* 1988;34 (suppl 26):S80−5.

123 Rosenthal JH, Pfeifle B, Michailov ML *et al.* Investigations of components of the renin−angiotensin system in rat vascular tissue. *Hypertension* 1984;6:383−90.

124 Zusman RM. Renin- and non-renin-mediated antihypertensive actions of converting enzyme inhibitors. *Kidney Int* 1984;25:969−83.

125 Laragh JH, Resnick LM. Recognizing and treating two types of long-term vasoconstriction in hypertension. *Kidney Int* 1988;34(suppl 25):S162−74.

126 Haber E, Zusman R, Burton J, Dzau VJ, Barger AC. Is renin a factor in the etiology of essential hypertension? *Hypertension* 1983;5(suppl V):V8−15.

127 Exton JH. Calcium signaling in cells − molecular mechanisms. *Kidney Int* 1987;32(suppl 23):S68−76.

128 Dzau VJ. Significance of the vascular renin−angiotensin pathway. *Hypertension* 1986;8:553−9.

129 Dzau VJ. Vascular renin−angiotensin system in hypertension. *Am J Med* 1988;84(suppl 4A):4−8.

130 Loudon M, Bing RF, Thurston H, Swales JD. Arterial wall uptake of renal renin and blood pressure control. *Hypertension* 1983;5:629−34.

131 Asaad MM, Antonaccio MJ. Vascular wall renin in spontaneously hypertensive rats: potential relevance to hypertension maintenance and antihypertensive effect of captopril. *Hypertension* 1982;4:487−93.

132 Okamura T, Miyazaki M, Inagami T, Toda N. Vascular renin−angiotensin system in two-kidney, one-clip hypertensive rats. *Hypertension* 1986;8:560−5.

133 Hiner LB, Gruskin AB, Baluarte HJ, Cote ML. Plasma renin activity in normal children. *J Pediatr* 1976;89:258−61.

134 Kotchen TA, Strickland AL, Rice TW, Walters DR. A study of the renin−angiotensin system in newborn infants. *J Pediatr* 1972;80:938−46.

135 Wilson DM, Stevenson DK, Luetscher JA. Plasma prorenin and renin in childhood and adolescence. *Am J Dis Child* 1988;142:1070−2.

136 Smith FG, Lupu AN, Barajas L, Bauer R, Bashore RA. The renin−angiotensin system in the fetal lamb. *Pediatr Res* 1974;8:611−20.

137 Wallace KB, Bailie MB, Hook JB. Angiotensin-converting enzyme in developing lung and kidney. *Am J Physiol* 1978;3:R141−5.

138 Wallace KB, Bailie MD, Hook JB. Development of angiotensin-converting enzyme in fetal rat lungs. *Am J Physiol* 1979;236:R57−60.

139 Gomez RA, Lynch KR, Chevalier RL *et al.* Renin and angiotensinogen gene expression in maturing rat kidney.

Am J Physiol 1988;254:F582−7.

140 Ingelfinger JR, Pratt RE, Dzau VJ. Regulation of extra-renal renin during ontogeny. *Endocrinology* 1988;122:782−6.

141 Robillard JE, Nakamura KT. Neurohormonal regulation of renal function during development. *Am J Physiol* 1988;254:F771−9.

142 Movat HZ. The kinin system: its relation to blood coagulation, fibrinolysis and the formed elements of blood. *Rev Physiol Biochem Pharmacol* 1978;84:143−88.

143 Mills IH. Kallikrein, kininogen and kinins in control of blood pressure. *Nephron* 1979;23:61−71.

144 Sharma JN. Interrelationships between the kallikrein−kinin system and hypertension: a review. *Gen Pharmacol* 1988;19:177−87.

145 Sealey JE, Atlas SA, Laragh JH. Linking the kallikrein and renin systems via activation of inactive renin:new data and a hypothesis. *Am J Med* 1978;65:994−9.

146 Margolius HS, Horwitz D, Keller RG *et al.* Urinary kallikrein excretion in normal man: relationship to sodium intake and sodium-retaining steroids. *Circ Res* 1974;35:812−19.

147 Margolius HS, Geller R, Pisano JJ, Keiser HR. Urinary kallikrein excretion in hypertensive man: relationships to sodium intake and sodium-retaining steroids. *Circ Res* 1974;35:820−5.

148 Mitas JA, Levy SB, Holle R, Frigon RP, Stone RA. Urinary kallikrein activity in the hypertension of renal parenchymal disease. *N Engl J Med* 1978;299:162−5.

149 Marre M, Alhenc-Gelas F, Menard J, Passa P. Reduced urinary kallikrein in hypertensive diabetic patients. *J Diabetic Compl* 1988;2:88−91.

150 Margolius HS, Geller R, deJong W, Pisano JJ, Sjoerdsma A. Altered urinary kallikrein excretion in rat with hypertension. *Circ Res* 1972;30:358−62.

151 Holland OB, Chud JM, Braunstein H. Urinary kallikrein excretion in essential and mineralocorticoid hypertension. *J Clin Invest* 1980;65:347−56.

152 Zinner SH, Margolius HS, Rosner B, Kass EH. Stability of blood pressure rank and urinary kallikrein concentration in childhood: an eight-year follow up. *Circulation* 1978;58:908−15.

153 Levy SB, Lilley JJ, Frigon RP, Stone RA. Urinary kallikrein and plasma renin activity as determinants of renal blood flow; the influence of race and dietary sodium intake. *J Clin Invest* 1977;60:129−38.

154 Berry TD, Hasstedt SJ, Hunt SC *et al.* A gene for high urinary kallikrein may protect against hypertension in Utah kindreds. *Hypertension* 1989;13:3−8.

155 Mersey JH, Williams GH, Emanuel R, Dluhy RG, Wong PY, Moore TJ. Plasma bradykinin levels and urinary kallikrein excretion in normal renin essential hypertension. *J Clin Endocrinol Metab* 1979;48:642−7.

156 Carbonell LF, Carretero OA, Madeddu P, Scicli AG. Effects of a kinin antagonist on mean blood pressure. *Hypertension* 1988;11(suppl I):I84−8.

157 Derkx FMH, Bouma BN, Schalekamp MPA, Schalekamp MADH. An intrinsic factor XII-prekallikrein-dependent pathway activates the human plasma renin−angiotensin system. *Nature* 1979;280:315−16.

158 Sealey JE, Atlas SA, Laragh JH, Oza NB, Ryan JW. Human urinary kallikrein converts inactive to active renin and is a possible physiological activator of renin. *Nature*

1978;275:144—5.

159 Zusman RM. Eicosanoids: prostaglandins, thromboxane and prostacyclin. In: Fozzard HA, Jennings RB, Haber E, Katz AM, Morgan HE, eds. *The Heart and Cardiovascular System*. 1st edn. New York: Raven Press, 1986.

160 Dunn MJ. Renal prostaglandins. In: Dunn MJ, ed. *Renal Endocrinology*. 1st edn. Baltimore: Williams & Wilkins, 1983.

161 Cinotti GA, Pugliese F. Prostaglandins in blood pressure regulation. *Kidney Int* 1988;34(suppl 25):S57—60.

162 Dunn MJ, Gröne H-J. The relevance of prostaglandins in human hypertension. *Adv Prostagl Thrombox Leukotr Res* 1985;13:179—87.

163 McGiff JC, Schwartzmam M, Ferreri NR. Renal prostaglandins and hypertension. *Adv Prostagl Thrombox Leukotr Res* 1985;13:161—9.

164 Machida J, Ueda S, Yoshida M, Soejima H, Ikegami K. Role of sodium and renal prostaglandin E₂ in the maintenance of hypertension in the chronic phase of two-kidney one-clip renovascular hypertension in rabbits. *Nephron* 1988;49:74—80.

165 Roman RJ, Kaldunski ML, Mattson DL, Mistry M, Nasjletti A. Influence of eicosanoids on renal function of DOCA-salt hypertensive rats. *Hypertension* 1988;12:287—94.

166 Mistry M, Nasjletti A. Role of pressor prostanoids in rats with angiotensin II-salt-induced hypertension. *Hypertension* 1988;11:758—62.

167 Kudo K, Abe K, Chiba S *et al*. Role of thromboxane A₂ in the hypotensive effect of captopril in essential hypertension. *Hypertension* 1988;11:147—52.

168 Levens NR, Ksander GM, Zimmerman MB, Mullane KM. Thromboxane synthase inhibition enhances action of converting enzyme inhibitors. *Hypertension* 1989;13:51—62.

169 Beckermann ML, Gerber JG, Byyny RL, LoVerde M, Nies AS. Propranolol increases prostacyclin synthesis in patients with essential hypertension. *Hypertension* 1988;12:582—8.

170 Walker DW, Mitchell MD. Presence of thromboxane B₂ and 6-keto-prostaglandin F₁ alpha in the urine of fetal sheep. *Prostagl Med* 1979;3:249—50.

171 Friedman Z, Demers LM. Prostaglandin synthetase in the human neonatal kidney. *Pediatr Res* 1979;14:190—3.

172 Sulyok E, Ertl T, Csaba IF, Varga F. Postnatal changes in urinary prostaglandin E excretion in premature infants. *Biol Neonate* 1980;37:192—6.

173 Pace-Asciak CR. Developmental aspects of the prostaglandin biosynthetic and catabolic systems. *Semin Perinatol* 1980;4:15—21.

174 Goddard C, Vallotton MB, Favre L. Urinary prostaglandins, vasopressin, and kallikrein excretion in healthy children from birth to adolescence. *J Pediatr* 1982;100:898—902.

175 Ignatowska-Switalska M, Januezewicz P. Urinary prostaglandin E₂ and F₂α in healthy newborns, infants, children and adults. *Prostagl Med* 1980;5:289—96.

176 Gleason CA. Prostaglandins and the developing kidney. *Semin Perinatol* 1987;11:12—21.

177 Exton JH. Mechanisms of action of calcium-mobilizing agonists: some variations on a young theme. *FASEB J* 1988;2:2670—6.

178 Walsh MP. Calcium regulation of smooth muscle contraction. In: Marmé D, ed. *Calcium and Cell Physiology*. New York: Springer-Verlag, 1985.

179 Kerreck WGL, Hoar PE. Smooth muscle: regulation by calcium and phosphorylation. In: *Ciba Foundation Symposium 122*. New York: John Wiley, 1986.

180 Bianchi G, Cusi D, Vezzoli G. Role of cellular sodium and calcium metabolism in the pathogenesis of essential hypertension. *Semin Nephrol* 1988;8:110—19.

181 Kaplan NM, Meese RB. The calcium deficiency hypothesis of hypertension: a critique. *Ann Intern Med* 1986;105:947—55.

182 McCarron DA. Calcium metabolism and hypertension. *Kidney Int* 1989;35:717—36.

183 van Zweiten PA. Pathophysiology of hypertension with regard to calcium and the sympathetic nervous system. In: Rosenthal J, ed. *Calcium Antagonists and Hypertension: Current Status*. Princeton, NJ: Excerpta Medica, 1986.

184 Young EW, Bukoski RD, McCarren DA. Calcium metabolism in experimental hypertension. *Proc Soc Exp Biol Med* 1988;187:123—41.

185 Grobbee DE, Hackeng WHL, Birkenhager JC, Hofman A. Intact parathyroid hormone (1—84) in primary hypertension. *Clin Exp Hyperten* 1986;A8:299—308.

186 Ellison HD, Shneidman R, Morris C, McCarron DA. Effects of calcium infusion on blood pressure in hypertensive and normotensive humans. *Hypertension* 1986;8:497—505.

187 Folsom AR, Smith CL, Prineas RJ, Grimm RH Jr. Serum calcium fractions in essential hypertensive and matched normotensive subjects. *Hypertension* 1986;8:11—15.

188 Erne P, Bolli P, Bürgisser E, Bühler FR. Correlation of platelet calcium with blood pressure: effect of antihypertensive therapy. *N Engl J Med* 1984;310:1084—8.

189 Hatton DC, Muntzel M, McCarron DA, Pressley M, Bukoski RD. Early effects of dietary calcium on blood pressure, plasma volume, and vascular reactivity. *Kidney Int* 1988;34(suppl 25):S16—18.

190 Baker PF. The sodium—calcium exchange system. In: *Ciba Foundation Symposium 122*. New York: John Wiley, 1986.

3 Cardiovascular and Autonomic Influences on Blood Pressure

PEDRO A. JOSE, GERARD R. MARTIN, AND ROBIN A. FELDER

The cardiovascular system provides appropriate organ and tissue perfusion at rest and at times of stress by regulation of blood pressure. The arterial pressure level reflects the composite activities of the heart and the peripheral circulation.

CONTROL OF BLOOD PRESSURE

Although the relationship between pressure and flow through the vascular tree is not linear, blood pressure can be expressed as the product of cardiac output (CO) and peripheral resistance [1,2] (Table 3.1). These variables are closely intertwined and the control mechanisms for pressure regulation involve more than simply a direct change in either CO or peripheral resistance [3]. The major determinant of blood

Table 3.1 Factors influencing arterial pressure as the product of cardiac output and peripheral resistance [2]

Cardiac output
Heart rate
Stroke volume
  Venous return
  Myocardial contractility
Blood volume

Peripheral resistance
Adrenergic nervous system activity
Circulating catecholamines
Other vasoactive substances
  Angiotensin II
  Prostaglandins, leukotrienes, thromboxanes
  Vasopressin (antidiuretic hormone)
  Kallikreins
  Neuropeptides (e.g. substance P, neurotensin)
  Acetylcholine
  Endothelium derived hemodynamic factors
  Mineralocorticoids
Ions and cellular regulations (e.g. calcium, sodium, chloride, potassium, magnesium, manganese, and trace metals, pH, etc.)
Hematocrit (viscosity)

pressure at rest is arteriolar resistance; during exercise, CO assumes a more important role. [4]

Cardiac output

Cardiac output is defined as the quantity of blood moved per minute from the great veins to the aorta into the arterial system. Control of CO is governed by two kinds of mechanisms: primary mechanisms, which operate quickly for acute regulation, and secondary mechanisms, which have a slower onset and regulate long-term aspects of cardiac function. The primary components which contribute to CO are preload, afterload, heart rate and rhythm, and myocardial contractility. Each of these factors in turn is modified by secondary mechanisms in response to the physiologic state of the individual. While each primary factor governing CO will be discussed in turn, it must be noted that these factors are operating concurrently and are interrelated.

PRELOAD

The output of the heart is determined primarily by the volume of venous blood which fills the ventricle during diastole, the preload. The adult heart has the capability to pump up to 15 l/min, but the usual resting CO is only 5 l/min. It is the preload that sets the level of CO. The Frank—Starling law of intrinsic autoregulation describes the inherent ability of the heart to regulate its output despite a rapidly varying venous return. Contractile force is directly proportional to muscle fiber length, which is determined by both the end-diastolic volume and the compliance of the myocardial tissue. The energy output of a heart muscle fiber increases with increasing fiber length up to a point, beyond which further extension of the fiber results in a decrease in the fiber contractile force. One of the most important aspects of the

Frank—Starling relationship is that a change in the afterload (or outflow resistance) has almost no influence on CO. Essentially, stroke work of the myocardium increases with increasing venous inflow and, conversely, decreases with decreasing venous return in order to maintain the CO equal to the input.

AFTERLOAD

One of the factors counteracting CO is the afterload or force that opposes ventricular emptying. After the ventricle has ejected its contents, the rise in aortic pressure forces the aortic valve closed and maintains a back-pressure that the next cycle of systole has to overcome. Components of the aortic back-pressure include the tension developed in the aortic walls, peripheral vascular resistance, and even the reflected pressure waves within the ventricle. Because the afterload does not allow the ventricle to empty completely, a percentage of the original venous return remains in the heart. The term *ejection fraction* (EF) describes the amount of blood ejected from the ventricle during one systolic wave (stroke volume, SV) divided by the amount of blood in the ventricle at the end of diastole (left ventricular end-diastolic volume, LVEDV).

$$EF = SV/LVEDV$$

Typically the ejection fraction for a normal adult is 0.50—0.75.

HEART RATE AND RHYTHM

One of the mechanisms available to increase CO is to increase heart rate. During periods of tachycardia, peak ejection velocity is increased. The net effect of the tachycardia is an increased CO because the stroke volume is occurring at a faster rate. Outside the normal adult physiologic range, large increases or decreases in heart rate result in a decrease in the net CO. In the adult, tachycardia of 170 beats/min or greater allows too little time for ventricular filling. The small ejection volume cannot be overcome by the increased heart rate. Lower than normal heart rate, or bradycardia, causes a decreased CO because of a reduced stroke volume relative to the requirements of the individual. In the case of reduced heart rate below 40 beats/min (in the adult) the increase in preload due to increased filling time is limited because major ventricular filling, which occurs early

in diastole, is not maintained throughout the extent of the diastolic period. Cardiac output decreases because stroke volume does not increase sufficiently.

MYOCARDIAL CONTRACTILITY

Myocardial contractility accounts for the increases in contractile force of a muscle fiber with no accompanying change in fiber length. Biochemical events allow for greater influx of calcium which results in an increase in inotropy due to an increase in the formation of force-generating sites and enhanced energy conversion in the myocardial muscle. *Homeotropic regulation* is the term used to describe the ability of the heart to change contraction force independent of muscle fiber length, and is dependent on balancing forces within the autonomic nervous system. Sympathetic stimulation causes a positive inotropic effect, presumably through the stimulation of β-adrenergic receptors residing on the surface of the myocardial membrane. Normal sympathetic input to the heart maintains myocardial contractility at about a 20% greater force than the denervated heart. Increased sympathetic input to the heart can significantly enhance both heart rate and contractile force, up to 100%. Parasympathetic innervation, on the other hand, reduces both heart rate and contractile force through nerve fibers supplying mainly the atria; however, myocardial contractility can only be decreased by 20%, which is a relatively small amount when compared to the influence of the sympathetic nerves.

SECONDARY REGULATION OF CARDIAC OUTPUT

A variety of factors operate in the normal individual to regulate CO over the long term. These secondary control mechanisms do not have as great an influence on the heart as the components previously described. Secondary controls include cardiovascular reflexes and hormonal influences. Mechanoreceptors are present in the atria and ventricles. An increase in distension of the atria results in a decrease in circulating levels of vasopressin, aldosterone, and renin, among other hormones, but causes an increase in the natriuretic factor synthesized by the atrium (atriopeptin or atrial natriuretic factor). Depressor reflexes in the heart originating mainly from the inferoposterior wall of the left ventricle promote bradycardia, vasodilatation, and hypotension (Bezold—Jarisch reflex).

These are mediated by increased parasympathetic and decreased sympathetic activity. Left ventricular mechanoreceptor stimulation can also attenuate arterial baroreflex control of heart rate. Decreased activity of cardiac vagal afferents results in enhanced sympathetic activity and increased vascular resistance, renin release, and vasopressin secretion [5]. Alterations in extracellular fluid volume influence CO via changes in venous return and blood pressure (Fig. 3.1).

Peripheral resistance

Blood flow through a vessel is determined by two primary factors: the amount of pressure forcing the blood through the vessel, and the resistance to flow. The resistance to flow in a blood vessel is best described as impedance because this takes into account elastic properties of blood vessels, viscosity of blood, the inertial properties of blood, and the variable geometrics of blood vessels during phasic flow. One of the most important factors influencing the flow through the arteries is the vessel diameter, since the conductance is proportional to the fourth power of the diameter. Therefore flow is influenced more by changes in vascular resistance than by pressure changes. The different variables influencing peripheral resistance are listed in Table 3.1.

CONTROL MECHANISMS FOR BLOOD PRESSURE REGULATION

The short-term adjustment and long-term control of blood pressure are supplied by a hierarchy of pressure controls [3]. The cardiovascular reflexes are the most rapidly acting pressure control mechanisms. They are activated within seconds and the effect may last a few minutes to a few days. The pressure controls acting with intermediate rapidity include capillary fluid shifts, stress relaxation, and hormonal control that includes the angiotensin and vasopressin systems. These systems, like the cardiovascular reflexes, function to buffer acute changes in pressure. Long-term control is afforded by long-term regulation of body fluids [3].

ARTERIAL BARORECEPTORS

The degree of arteriolar constriction is determined by a balance between tonic output from the pressor areas of the cardiovascular center and the degree of

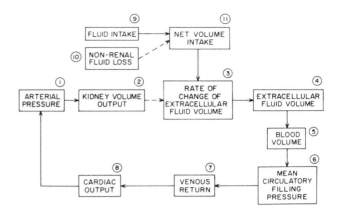

Fig. 3.1 The basic kidney—blood volume—pressure regulatory mechanism. A solid arrow means that a change in the first factor causes a change in the next factor in the same direction. A dashed line indicates an opposite change [3].

inhibition from the baroreceptors. The arterial baroreceptors are the major fast-reacting, slowly adapting feedback elements to the central—neural cardiovascular regulatory system and operate to limit sudden changes in blood pressure. Their endings are located at the medial—adventitial border of blood vessels with elastic structure, mainly at the aortic arch and carotid sinuses. The receptors respond to deformation of the vessel in any direction, i.e. circumferential and longitudinal stretch. The pressure—diameter relationship is concave with the greatest distensibility at about 120—140 mmHg. There are two types of receptors in the carotid sinus: type I receptors are thin myelinated fibers and type II receptors are thick myelinated fibers with fine end-branches terminating in neurofibrillar end-plates. The latter receptors are also seen in the aortic arch.

Sensory innervation of the aortic arch is derived from the vagus while the carotid sinus nerve originates from the glossopharyngeal nerve. The majority of the afferent nerves are medullated type A fibers. These fibers have large and intermediate spikes of 40—120 μV corresponding to the high distensibility region. At normal pressure levels, these fibers transmit mainly the dynamic components of blood pressure, pulse pressure (dp/dt), and pulse frequency. The receptor sensitivity is highest at the lower end (60—100 mmHg) of the high distensibility region of the blood vessel. There are a few non-medullated type C fibers, located mainly in the sinus nerve. The spikes are small (5—10 μV), have a higher static threshold (120—150 mmHg), correspond to the low distensibility region, and mainly transmit mean pressure. The type C fibers can be activated independently by sympathetic stimuli.

The arterial baroreceptors are more effective in compensating for a fall than a rise in mean arterial pressure. The interaction between mean and pulsatile components can be of considerable importance in the hemodynamic response to hemorrhage [6]. For example, the initial response to moderate hemorrhage results in a decrease in pulse pressure with maintenance of mean arterial pressure. Decreasing pulse pressure results in a redistribution of CO to the mesenteric and cardiac circulations with no effect on the renal circulation.

Information carried by the afferent limb of the reflex arc from the baroreceptors is relayed to the lower brainstem via the vagus and glossopharyngeal nerves. Most secondary neurons are located at the nucleus of the tractus solitarius and projections are directed to various regions of the brainstem (see Chapter 4 for central mechanisms for blood pressure control). The effectors of the baroreceptors include systems that have an immediate but short-term effect on circulatory function and those that have delayed but long-term effects. Examples of the former are resistance vessels—arterioles throughout the systemic circulation—the capacitance vessels—veins and arteries—and the heart. An example of a system with a long-term effect is kidney. In addition, neural reflexes may influence circulating levels of several hormones (e.g. renin, vasopressin) with short- and long-term effects on cardiovascular regulation [7]. The effect of neural reflexes on the kidneys may be direct through renal sympathetic nerve activity or indirect through circulating catecholamines.

Norepinephrine-containing nerve endings are found in the carotid sinus and aortic arch and may influence the sensitivity of the sinus reflex. Norepinephrine given intravenously decreases distensibility of the sinus at low pressures but increases distensibility at high pressure. In the conscious dog, sinus hypotension induces a reflex tachycardia and sympathetic vasoconstriction of the skeletal resistance vessels. The changes in the renal and mesenteric beds (45% of total peripheral resistance) seem to be solely due to autoregulation. In the anesthetized dog, sinus hypotension induces a greater magnitude and more generalized pattern of sympathetic vasoconstriction and may include both resistance and capacitance vessels. Logan and coworkers [8] reported that unilateral carotid sinus hypotension resulted in a redistribution of renal blood flow from outer to inner cortex. After bilateral carotid artery occlusion, there is a redistribution of blood flow to the outer cortex as a result of the increase in perfusion pressure.

ADAPTATION OF THE BARORECEPTORS

The baroreceptors exert a tonic inhibitory influence on peripheral sympathetic activity. Baroreceptor nerves interact by mutual inhibitory addition; with a decrease in pressure, there is less reflex inhibition and a resultant increase in sympathetic outflow. While transient baroreceptor-induced changes in heart rate are primarily mediated by the parasympathetic nervous system, steady-state responses are due to a greater involvement of the sympathetic nervous system. A sudden increase in pressure (with resultant stretching of the receptors) causes an immediate increase in baroreceptor firing rate. With continued elevation of the pressure, however, there is a decrease in the rate of baroreceptor firing. Initially the decrease is rapid, and during the succeeding hours and days it slows down. This adaptation, or resetting, in response to a lower or higher pressure seems to be complete in 2 days. This adaptation can occur at the receptor and nervous signal pathway [3].

ARTERIAL BARORECEPTORS DURING DEVELOPMENT

Studies in humans and experimental animals suggest that arterial baroreceptors are present in the fetus and undergo postnatal maturation [9,10]. In adults with intact arterial baroreceptors, a rapid head-up tilt is accompanied by an immediate increase in heart rate and peripheral vascular resistance with maintenance of mean arterial pressure in the upper body. In preterm and term human infants, a 45° head-up tilt results in an increase in peripheral resistance without any significant changes in heart rate. In the conscious newborn dog the magnitude of the increase in mean arterial pressure and peripheral resistance following bilateral carotid occlusion is less than in the adult. In addition these changes occur without alterations in heart rate, similar to the effects noted in infants. Newborn lambs exhibit the classic inverse relationship between heart rate and blood pressure but the sensitivity is only about 50% that of the adult. A similar response to small changes in blood pressure is noted in fetal lambs. However when the change in blood pressure is greater than 15% the responses are different. In newborn lambs a progressive tachycardia accompanies the increasing hypotension, due to a combination of increased sympathetic outflow and parasympathetic withdrawal. There is no progressive tachycardia in the fetus; in fact when the blood pressure change is greater than 50% bradycardia occurs, apparently due to augmentation of vagal parasympathetic tone [11]. Similar patterns are apparently seen in hypoxia.

There are age-dependent differences in the ability of the piglet to compensate for arterial but not venous hemorrhage; neonatal swine are able to compensate with greater facility for venous than arterial hemorrhage [12]. Increasing arterial pressure by intravenous administration of vasoconstrictor agents results in smaller changes in heart rate in the newborn animal as well. Completion of sympathetic efferent pathways occurs before baroreceptor reflex activity is capable of modulating cardiac sympathetic activity. Thus, maturation of baroreceptor reflex activity may be dependent on development of baroreceptor function or of connections between baroreceptor and sympathetic efferents [13].

Autonomic regulation of blood pressure

Regulation of the distribution of CO and maintenance of blood pressure are major functions of the autonomic nervous system. The arterioles are normally in a continuous state of partial constriction, largely determined by an equilibrium between vasoconstrictor influences from the cardiovascular centers and the inhibitory input from the peripheral baroreceptors. The veins also receive autonomic innervation. Adrenergic nerves induce venous constriction with a resultant decrease in capacitance which increases venous return and CO. The effects of the adrenergic nervous system are conveyed by the neurotransmitters norepinephrine, epinephrine, and dopamine. Epinephrine is released mainly from the adrenal medulla, while norepinephrine is released mainly in terminal nerve endings. In organs with dopaminergic nerves, a greater proportion of catecholamine released is dopamine.

Norepinephrine synthesized at peripheral nerve endings is stored in subcellular granules. After a specific stimulus, it is released into the synaptic cleft where it interacts with specific receptors at the effector cell. The neurotransmitter is inactivated to a large extent by re-uptake into the storage granules. This re-uptake process (re-uptake-1) is stereoselective, sodium-dependent, and of high affinity. A presynap-

tic re-uptake that is of low affinity and nonsodium-dependent has been termed re-uptake-2. Although the enzymatic degradation of the neurotransmitter by monoamine oxidase and catechol-O-methyl transferase is much less important in termination of neurotransmitter action in nervous tissue, in vascular smooth muscles this metabolism plays an important role [14]. The remainder of the neurotransmitter which escapes re-uptake-1 and -2 is released into the circulation. Since only about 20% of the total appears in the circulating pool the plasma levels of catecholamines are merely a rough index of adrenergic activity [15].

For the neurotransmitter to exert its specific effect, it must occupy a specific receptor on the cell surface. Catecholamines can occupy specific pre- and post-synaptic receptors (Fig. 3.2). Each receptor has different subtypes. Sub subtypes of α_1-and α_2-adrenoceptors have also been described [17,18]. Table 3.2 lists some drugs that have relative selectivity

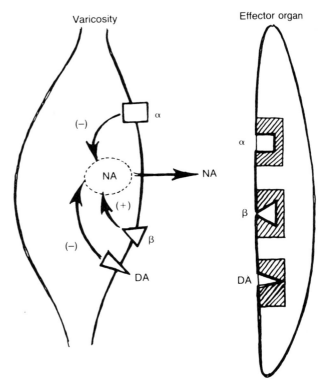

Fig. 3.2 Schematic representation of a nonadrenergic—neuroeffector junction in the peripheral nervous system. Pre- and postsynaptic adrenergic and dopamine receptors are depicted [16].
NA = Noradrenaline; DA = dopamine receptor; α = α-adrenoceptor; β = β-adrenoceptor.

Table 3.2 Some drugs showing selectivity for adrenergic and dopamine receptor subtypes

Drug name	Agonists	Antagonists
α-*Adrenoceptor*		
Nonselective	Norepinephrine	Phentolamine
α_1	Methoxamine	Prazosin
α_2	UK 14304	Idazoxan
		Rauwolscine
		Yohimbine
β-*Adrenoceptor*		
Nonselective	Isoproterenol	Propranolol
		Pindolol
β_1	Prenalterol	Metoprolol
		Atenolol
		ICI 89,406
β_2	Salbutamol	Butoxamine
	Terbutaline	ICI 118,551
Dopamine receptor (DA)		
Nonselective	Dopamine	Haloperidol
DA-1	Fenoldopam	SCH 23390
DA-2	LY 171555	YM 09151
	SKF103376	Domperidone

to each particular receptor subtype in the peripheral vascular bed. Occupation of presynaptic α_2-adrenergic and dopamine$_2$ receptors inhibits norepinephrine release. Occupation of presynaptic β-receptors enhances norepinephrine release. At low levels of nerve stimulation norepinephrine release is increased; at high levels of stimulation, the inhibitory effects of presynaptic α_2-adrenoceptors predominate, acting as a short-loop feedback. The antihypertensive effects of dopamine agonists and β-adrenergic antagonists may be due in part to their ability to decrease release of norepinephrine at the terminal nerve endings.

Occupation of postsynaptic α_1- and α_2-adrenoceptors leads to arterial and venous constriction [19]. α_1-but not α_2-adrenoceptors have been described in the heart [20,21]. Postsynaptic α_1- and extrasynaptic α_2-receptors are associated with renal tubular sodium reabsorption [22–26] as well as with stimulation or inhibition of renin release respectively. The effects of extrasynaptic α_2-receptors on sodium reabsorption may be complex; some report a decrease rather than an increase in transport while others have reported no effect [23–25]. Postsynaptic β-adrenoceptors are associated with cardiac stimulation. β_1-Adreno-

ceptors predominate in ventricular and atrial muscles; β_2-adrenoceptors are also present in the atria and atrioventricular node [27]. β_1-Adrenoceptors mediate the inotropic response of the ventricles while both β-adrenoceptor subtypes affect the chronotropic response of the atria. β_2-Adrenoceptors are linked to vasodilatation. Vasodilatory β_1-adrenoceptors are also present [28]. The β-adrenoceptor has also been linked to renal tubular sodium transport. Postsynaptic dopamine$_1$ receptors are associated with arterial vasodilatation in mesenteric, renal, and cerebral beds, while dopamine$_2$ receptors may mediate femoral arterial vasodilatation. Dopamine receptors have also been described in the heart. While dopamine$_1$ receptors decrease renal sodium transport [29], dopamine$_2$ receptors are linked to increased sodium reabsorption in small intestines of the rabbit. Adrenal dopamine$_2$ receptors also inhibit aldosterone secretion.

Postsynaptic adrenoceptors may influence each other. In the kidney, occupancy of α_1-adrenoceptors decreases β-adrenoceptor affinity. Clearance of catecholamines is modulated by β-but not by α-adrenoceptors. Hormones such as estrogen and thyroxin, ions such as sodium and magnesium, and other factors regulate adrenergic receptor density and affinity. Several neurotransmitter receptors have been cloned and sequenced; expression of gene coding and transmembrane domains has been reported [30,31].

The signal resulting from occupation of cell membrane receptors is amplified by intervention of other agents called second messengers. Occupation of either β-adrenoceptor subtype or the dopamine$_1$ receptor by agonists stimulates adenylate cyclase activity; agonist occupancy of α$_2$-adrenoceptors or dopamine$_2$ receptors leads to inhibition of adenylate cyclase activity [29,32,33]. The changes in intracellular cyclic adenosine monophosphate levels alter activity of certain enzymes, e.g. protein kinase A, and mediate the eventual response of the effector cell. Certain drugs (e.g. nitrites) exert their vasodilatory effect by stimulation of guanylate cyclase activity. Another second messenger is associated with the polyphosphoinositide system. The α$_1$-adrenoceptor and the dopamine$_1$ receptor are linked to phospholipase C; stimulation leads to an increase in formation of inositol phosphates and diacylglycerol [34]. Inositol phosphates increase intracellular calcium while diacylglycerol stimulates protein kinase C [35,36]. Occupation of α$_1$-adrenoceptors may also result in the activation of phospholipase A$_2$ increasing the formation of biologically active arachidonate metabolites [37].

Catecholamines can influence blood pressure not only by direct effects on resistance vessels but also indirectly, by modulating the secretion of other vasoactive agents such as angiotensin II (via renin), vasopressin, prostaglandins, substance P, and other neuropeptides. In addition to direct chronotropic and inotropic effects on the heart, catecholamines can modulate CO indirectly by affecting blood volume and venous return. Blood volume can be regulated by direct effects on sodium and water transport through renal nerves, by antagonizing effects of other hormones (e.g. vasopressin), and indirectly by modulating vasopressin and aldosterone secretion.

ADRENERGIC SYSTEM DURING DEVELOPMENT

The low blood pressure at birth, due to low CO and peripheral resistance, increases rapidly in the first 6 weeks of life, remains at a constant level until age 6, and increases gradually until age 18 years. The increase in blood pressure with age is due to a rise in both CO and total peripheral resistance. The age-related changes in vascular resistance are selective since in the perinatal period there is a rapid fall in resistance in the lungs and the kidney. The newborn infant increases its CO mainly by increasing heart rate. The high heart rate may be due to differential sympathetic and parasympathetic effects, hypersensitivity of the cardiac receptors, and peripheral vasodilatation. The low precapillary resistance, and low venous capacitance are conducive to high systemic blood flow per unit body weight, and provide increased tissue perfusion for growth.

Study of the role of the adrenergic nervous system in the control of cardiovascular dynamics is complicated by species differences. Some studies have suggested that pigs and dogs provide the closest model to the newborn human in terms of cardiovascular development [38]. Ruggles and coworkers suggest that the renal adrenergic system of the dog is similar to the human [39]. On the other hand, the sheep fetus is a very useful model for chronic conscious studies [40].

DEVELOPMENT OF THE SYMPATHETIC NERVOUS SYSTEM

The development of the sympathetic nervous system can be divided into two stages. In the first stage, the neural crest cells migrate to their positions within the body tissues. The second stage is concerned with the differentiation and selection of the neurotransmitter. Cholinergic development generally takes place prior to adrenergic differentiation; however, transition from adrenergic to cholinergic function can also occur. A critical event in the development of the adrenergic nervous system is the establishment of functional innervation of the different organs. Function requires that central nervous pathways to the preganglionic neurons be established, that information be relayed to postganglionic neurons, and that neurotransmitter synthesis, release, and re-uptake, and postreceptor mechanisms be operative. Effector organ innervation involves the outgrowth of new axons, appearance of intense fluorescence, and differentiation of adrenergic nerve varicosities. Maturation of the nerve−terminal−effector complex occurs before ganglionic transmission is fully developed and is largely independent of neural connections. In the heart, the development of β-adrenoceptors and responsiveness to catecholamines is not closely linked to innervation. Nonsympathetic hormonal factors appear to control early maturation of receptors and the growth and development of the nervous system [41].

Birth is associated with an increase in circulating catecholamines. There is no difference in plasma concentrations between infants delivered vaginally and those by cesarean section, suggesting that stress *per se* is not responsible for the levels. Studies in the fetal sheep indicate a surge in plasma catecholamines with the onset of parturition, and accentuated by cord-cutting [42]. The half-life of circulating catecholamines in the preterm infant may be longer than in older children, due in part to lower levels of catecholamine-degrading enzymes. However, children may metabolize catecholamines more rapidly than adults. Preterm infants have greater levels of epinephrine in umbilical arterial plasma than full-term human infants. Preterm fetal sheep also have higher circulating catecholamine levels than their full-term counterparts. The circulating levels of catecholamines decrease with maturation, but beyond 20 years of age plasma norepinephrine increases. Adrenal medullary activity, when compared to adrenergic nervous activity, is also lower at birth and increases with maturation.

Urinary catecholamines are low at birth and increase with age. Urinary catecholamines and metabolites are higher in preterm human infants (31 weeks' gestational age) than in full-term infants; these values are still lower than the levels in adults, however. Small-for-gestational-age babies have greater sympathoadrenal activity than babies of the same gestational age [43]. However, different results are reported by Nicolopoulos and colleagues [44]; newborn preterm infants excrete less norepinephrine and more dopamine than term infants; epinephrine excretion is comparable. At 2 weeks of age, urinary dopamine and metabolites are greatly increased in preterm infants. Beyond 1 year of life, the developmental patterns of adrenergic nervous and adrenal medullary activity are similar and reach mature values at 5 years of age. When expressed as a function of surface area or weight no changes in urinary catecholamines and metabolites occur after 1 year of age. In the first 5 years of life, however, sympathoadrenal activity is less in girls than in boys. It should be kept in mind, though, that circulating and urinary levels of catecholamines are only rough indices of adrenergic activity.

Catecholamine secretion at birth may be important in the adaptation of the fetus to extrauterine life [42,45]. Complete ganglionic blockade before delivery of the lamb does not attenuate the normal postnatal rise in blood pressure, indicating that the autonomic nervous system may not play a significant role in the increase in systemic pressure after birth. However, although clamping of adrenal vessels did not alter mean blood pressure of very young puppies [46], in the newborn dog adrenalectomy leads to hypotension and bradycardia. In addition, adrenergic blockade in the newborn lamb reduces systemic pressure whereas no effect is seen in adult sheep. Other evidences for the importance of the adrenergic nervous system during the neonatal period include both impaired myocardial contractile responses to adrenergic agents and hypoxia after adrenalectomy.

The time of development of adrenergic innervation and responses to adrenergic stimulation varies not only with species but also among vessels in the same animal. Some of the reported differences in results may also be due to experimental conditions (anesthetized versus unanesthetized state, *in vitro* versus *in vivo* studies). In the heart, responses to β-adrenergic and dopamine stimulation increase with age while the response to α-adrenergic stimulation decreases with age. While the decreasing responsiveness to α-adrenergic stimulation with maturation has been linked to similar directional changes in myocardial α_1-adrenoceptors, the changes in myocardial β-adrenoceptors are not linked. For example, in the dog heart there is an increased β-adrenoceptor density in the newborn period. The decline in cardiac β-adrenoceptor density with age is accompanied by decreased β-adrenergic responsive adenylate cyclase activity. Other studies however have shown that cardiac β-adrenoceptors increase with age but the proportions of β-adrenergic subtypes do not.

In the mature heart, responsiveness to β-adrenergic agonists can be regulated trans-synaptically by neurotransmitter concentrations in the synaptic cleft. High levels of β-adrenergic stimulation result in depressed cardiac responsiveness and reduction in receptor density (down-regulation) while the converse occurs with low levels of stimulation with up-regulation of receptor density. However, this does not occur during the period in which receptor numbers and cardiac sensitivity to agonists are undergoing marked developmental increases [41]. The developmental changes in cardiac responsiveness to dopamine have not been correlated with dopamine receptor density or adenylate cyclase activation.

β-Adrenergic-induced relaxation of the aorta of

rabbits increases with age, reaching a maximal level at 1 month; thereafter a decline in responsiveness occurs. In dogs stimulation of lumbar sympathetics induces femoral vasodilatation early in life; after 2 months a greater vasoconstriction is noted. This corresponds to a marked increase in adrenergic innervation. In the piglet, the renal vascular response to β-adrenergic stimulation is also less in the immediate newborn period compared to adults but may be markedly increased some time before maturation [47]. These changes in renal β-adrenergic responsiveness have been correlated with β-adrenoceptor density in the dog [48]. However, β_2-adrenergic vasodilatory effects are enhanced in the renal vascular bed of the fetal lamb [49].

There is much disagreement on the maturation of blood vessel reactivity to α-adrenergic stimulation. In general, during the neonatal period there is a lesser responsiveness of the canine aorta and sheep carotid to norepinephrine compared to the adult. After the immediate newborn period, the neonatal renal circulation is more sensitive to α-adrenergic stimulation in dogs, pigs, and guinea pigs. The isolated renal vessels of fetal lamb studied in vitro are more reactive to α-adrenergic stimulation than their newborn or adult counterparts [50]. Studies in vivo (intrarenal arterial administration) however showed no age-related differences in renal vascular responsiveness to α-adrenergic agonists [51]. Thus in the fetal lamb studied in vivo, inherent renal vascular adrenergic hypersensitivity may be masked by counterregulatory vasodilator mechanisms. The rabbit seems to be an exception, in that the renal vasculature in the adult is more sensitive to catecholamines compared to that of the newborn animal.

The neonatal renal circulation is also more responsive to the effects of renal nerve stimulation in some species [47,52]. In addition, renal nerve transection in piglets leads to an increase in renal blood flow [52]. In the fetal sheep, however, renal nerve transection does not affect renal blood flow. Moreover, renal nerve stimulation during α-adrenergic blockade actually increases renal blood flow [49]. In the neonatal dog kidney increased α-adrenergic effects are related to increased α-adrenoceptor density [48]. Dopamine mainly induces a vasoconstrictor response (an α-adrenoceptor effect) in the early neonatal period [48]. Even low dosages, which produce renal vasodilatation in the adult kidney, are associated with renal vasoconstriction in the newborn period. The

vasodilator effects of dopamine become evident in the femoral circulation before being noted in the kidney. When α and β-adrenoceptors are blocked during dopamine infusion, the renal vasodilator effect of dopamine is still less in the fetus and the newborn animal compared to the adult. In contrast to the correlation between renal vascular responses and α- and β-adrenoceptor density, no correlation is observed with dopamine receptors and the age-related changes in renal dopamine responsiveness. In general, the pressor changes induced by α-adrenergic or dopaminergic stimulation seem to be greater in the newborn animal than in the adult. The converse is true for the vasodilatory effects of β-adrenergic and dopaminergic agonists.

SYSTEMIC HEMODYNAMICS AND HYPERTENSION

For arterial pressure to rise there must be an increase in CO or peripheral resistance or both. Established hypertension in adults is characterized by increased vascular resistance and normal CO [53]. Adults with more severe or long-standing hypertension have been reported to have a reduction in CO [54]. However, in early or borderline hypertension, heart rate and stroke volume and hence CO may actually be elevated [55,56]. The mechanism for the increased CO is a matter of debate. Guyton [3] has suggested that a defect in renal regulation of salt and water leads to increased plasma volume (Fig. 2.1). The increased cardiac filling pressures result in an increase in CO. In an attempt to normalize the high CO, possible responses are increases in vascular resistance due to structural changes of the blood vessels; an increase in vascular reactivity, or autoregulatory vasoconstriction. Alternatively, the increased CO may be due to central redistribution of blood volume, increased adrenergic activity [57,58], or decreased parasympathetic activity. Korner [54] has presented evidence against the autoregulation theory, based on studies showing that long-term changes in blood pressure can be due solely to independent changes in CO or peripheral resistance. Low, normal, or elevated CO can occur in hypertensive individuals as young as 6 years old [56,59,60]. In children cardiac index is negatively correlated with blood pressure [56]. Hofman and colleagues found no association between blood pressure and CO in teenagers [61]. However Blake and coworkers [62] reported evidence for a role of tissue autoregulation of blood flow as a mechanism for the increased peripheral resistance in hypertensive humans.

Ventricular function

The cardiac manifestations of hypertension may include diastolic or systolic abnormalities. Concentric hypertrophy and occasional ventricular dysfunction or a hyperkinetic hypertrophied heart with or without outflow obstruction may occur. In children, high blood pressure is associated with increased ventricular septum, left atrium, and left ventricular wall mass that is detected by echocardiography but not with electrocardiography [63–66]. Left ventricular hypertrophy (involving ventricular septum and posterior wall) is a common and early finding in hypertension and has been described in adolescents and offspring of hypertensive parents [67]. Left ventricular mass may be an important predictor of subsequent hypertension in children [68]. In adults ventricular mass and wall thickness correlate with elevation of blood pressure during working hours and at home on workdays [69]. Ventricular systolic and diastolic volumes are usually normal. Cardiac contractility estimated from echocardiographic studies has not been consistently abnormal. Systolic time intervals show a normal relationship between ventricular ejection rate and stroke volume but with a prolongation of electromechanical systole. With hypertension, left ventricular mass may increase by 30% without affecting stroke volume or ejection fraction. Right ventricular hypertrophy is associated with left ventricular hypertrophy (LVH) in patients with hypertension [70].

Diastolic abnormalities can precede systolic abnormalities in hypertension [71]. The rapid filling of the ventricle in early diastole is decreased but is increased in late diastole. These events are present even when CO, ejection fraction, and maximal velocity of ejection are normal [72]. Indeed there is an inverse relationship between diastolic blood pressure and peak flow velocity in early diastole [73]. The first clinical evidence of cardiac involvement in hypertension may be a left atrial abnormality, apparently due to decreased compliance of the hypertrophying left ventricle. This may be preceded by an impaired emptying index of the left atrium [70]. It must be noted, however, that left atrial dimensions can also be normal even in the presence of ventricular hypertrophy.

Left ventricular hypertrophy in hypertension is due to multifactorial causes but may be primarily related to the hemodynamic factor of increased left ventricular afterload [74–76]. However, there may be a lack of association between the rate of development of hypertension and LVH. Thus, there are additional nonhemodynamic factors associated not only with the development of LVH but also with its regression with antihypertensive therapy. There is a genetic predisposition in some with a strong family history of hypertension that facilitates the development of LVH. Left ventricular hypertrophy may be in part a phenotypic expression rather than a result of blood pressure elevation [68]. Both hypertrophy and hyperplasia occur. Pressure overload induces the myocardium to increase protein sythesis; decreased proteolysis may also occur [77]. However, the increase in protein synthesis may not be due to increased pressure alone but to the effect of pressor substances (e.g. angiotensin II and catecholamines) on protein synthesis. Adrenergic stimulation can lead to cardiac hypertrophy, accentuate its development, and prevent its regression despite optimal blood pressure control [78]. Subpressor doses of norepinephrine and the β-adrenergic agonist isoproterenol have produced ventricular hypertrophy. The hypertrophied left ventricle is more likely to regress in mass when blood pressure is controlled with drugs that blunt or at least do not stimulate adrenergic activity [79,80]. Altered purine metabolism and elevated serum uric acid have been associated epidemiologically with increased risk of cardiac enlargement and increased cardiovascular morbidity and mortality [74]. Gruskin and coworkers have reported increased serum uric acid levels in young hypertensive patients [81]. This was positively correlated with high plasma renin activity. Interestingly, angiotensin II can also increase myocardial protein synthesis. Other nonhemodynamic factors influencing left ventricular function are listed in Table 3.3 [74]. The greater prevalence of LVH in males than in females disappears at the time of menopause. Aging, high salt intake, racial factors, and obesity may be additional risk factors.

The cardiac hypertrophy that develops in response to or associated with hypertension increases the force of contraction at the cost of diminished compliance. This initial increase in cardiac performance may become harmful in the long run. As hypertension becomes more severe cardiac dilatation ensues, systolic wall tension rises, ejection fraction falls, and end-diastolic ventricular pressure rises, first during exercise and later at rest. A syndrome of severe

Table 3.3 Factors associated with development of left ventricular hypertrophy in clinical and experimental forms of hypertension

Hemodynamic factors
Volume overload
Pressure overload
Other considerations
  Faster heart rate
  Augmented ventricular contractility
  Increased total peripheral resistance
  Blood viscosity

Nonhemodynamic factors
Aging
Collagen deposition
Coexisting diseases
  Atherosclerosis
  Myocarditis
  Diabetes mellitus
  Other
Race
Sex
Obesity
Hormones
  Catecholamines
  Angiotensin II
  Growth hormone
Therapy

concentric LVH with reduced cavity size, excessive systolic emptying, impaired diastolic function, and clinical signs of heart failure has been described in elderly hypertensive patients [76]. Cardiac hypertrophy may also alter coronary flow, compounding the problem.

The effects of acute preload and afterload stress on the myocardium may differ in the young and in the adult [82]. The neonatal heart increases CO mainly by increasing heart rate. A high level of myocardial performance exists after birth in both animals and humans [83]. However, the response of the heart of a newborn infant to stress is less. In the adult, acute preload stress causes a small but consistent improvement in left ventricular contraction; the effect in the perinatal period is limited. The decreased preload reserve in the newborn infant has been thought to be due to decreased ventricular compliance and high resting heart rate. There are studies that suggest that the newborn heart is at upper limits of the Starling curve; this situation may limit the cardiac response to volume loading [84]. Acute afterload stress has a greater effect in neonatal than in

adult hearts. Afterload stress due to a postnatal increase in systemic vascular resistance secondary to congenital heart disease or vasoconstrictor drugs may compromise myocardial function sooner in the newborn infant than in the adult.

Role of the heart in hypertension

The heart can initiate hypertension by several mechanisms [57,76,85]. The hypertension can be initiated by reflexes from the heart and large vessels. These pressor reflexes can be triggered by distension of the coronary vessels, myocardial ischemia, specific chemoreceptors, or stretch of the aortic walls. Activation of the aortic pressor reflex may decrease baroreceptor sensitivity (a mechanism implicated in essential hypertension and increased blood pressure during exercise). Clinical expression of these reflexes includes coronary insufficiency, hypertension after coronary bypass surgery, dissecting aortic aneurysm, and aortic insufficiency. However, whether a cardiac reflex-related increase in blood pressure can be chronic is not proved. The heart can also increase blood pressure by influencing volume regulation via renal hemodynamics and renin release and by its modulation of the release of hormones such as atrial natriuretic factor, aldosterone, and vasopressin.

Receptors in the ventricle, atrium, and pulmonary bed may exert tonic restricting influences on cardiovascular centers. In borderline hypertension, reduction of cardiopulmonary volume was associated with a greater increase in forearm vascular resistance than in normotensive subjects. Increased CO has been shown in several forms of hypertension (Table 3.4) [57]. The high CO in borderline hypertension due to enhanced myocardial function may be related to increased adrenergic drive. Whether this eventually leads to increased peripheral resistance in hypertension is, as discussed earlier, controversial.

In hypertension, the hypertrophied heart and vessels have different amplifying capacities, which determines why blood pressure eventually comes to be maintained by peripheral resistance. In the early stages of hypertension the amplifying capacity of the heart and blood vessels is evenly matched so that hypertension can be maintained by either CO or peripheral resistance. When vascular hypertrophy becomes greater than cardiac hypertrophy total peripheral resistance becomes predominant in maintaining the hypertension. Subsequently CO declines.

Table 3.4 Types of hypertension associated with high cardiac output [57]

Essential hypertension
Borderline hypertension
Subset of established severe hypertension with marked
   hyperkinetic circulation

Secondary hypertension
Renal arterial disease
Primary aldosteronism
Pheochromocytoma

Hypertension associated with
Anemia (uremic hypertensive patients)
Hyper-β-adrenergic state
?Hyperthyroidism

Hypertension treated with vasodilators

Baroreceptors and hypertension

Numerous studies have demonstrated an abnormal baroreflex control of the circulation in hypertension. A resetting and a decrease in baroreflex sensitivity have been described in essential hypertension [86]. These abnormalities have been shown for both heart rate and control of the peripheral vasculature. A correlation has been described among the age-related (in adults) increase in plasma norepinephrine levels, rise in systolic blood pressure, and decrease in baroreflex sensitivity. There is a negative relationship between plasma norepinephrine levels and baroreflex sensitivity in both hypertensive and normotensive subjects. The abnormalities in baroreflex control of blood pressure in hypertension may be due to changes in smooth muscle electrolyte and water content or in vessel mechanics, especially when there are hypertensive vascular lesions. Additionally, there may be changes in the baroreceptor receptors themselves, central neural integration, or efferent autonomic pathways. Whether abnormalities in baroreceptor control of blood pressure can initiate or maintain hypertension is a controversial issue. High blood pressure *per se* can reduce the sensitivity of the baroreflex.

CARDIOVASCULAR RESPONSE TO STRESS

Physical stress

The effects of exercise on the cardiovascular system depend upon the type, intensity, and duration of the exercise [87] and on the physical condition, training, and hemodynamic status of the individual. Dynamic exercise involves repetitive activities of large muscle groups performing against a constant load, and results in changes in muscle length with little change in muscle tension. This type of exercise has also been termed "aerobic" because a major source of energy is from oxidative phosphorylation, and "isotonic" because of the relative constant muscle tension involved. Examples of dynamic exercise include jogging, rowing, swimming, and cycling. Static exercise involves a sustained activity that changes muscle tension without altering muscle length (isometric). This type of exercise is fueled largely by the anaerobic breakdown of glucose to lactate. Examples of static exercise include holding a heavy object, pushing against an immovable surface, and extended handgrip. Resistive training is used to describe a wide variety of muscular strength and power-building methods which may incorporate elements of both static and dynamic exercise. The most familiar example of resistive training is weight-lifting.

ACUTE PHYSICAL STRESS (see also Chapter 27)

The acute hemodynamic effects of dynamic and static exercise differ (Fig. 3.3) [88]. Among normotensive adults, dynamic exercise increases systolic blood pressure mainly due to an increase in CO. Diastolic blood pressure may not change, or decreases slightly [88–91]. Mean arterial pressure may not change or slightly increases while total peripheral resistance decreases [88,89,91]. Cardiac output increases to a similar extent whether the dynamic exercise is performed in the upright or supine position. However during maximal exercise heart rate is lower and stroke volume greater in supine than in upright exercise [91]. In static exercise the increase in blood pressure is due to both an increase in CO and peripheral resistance. Stroke volume is unchanged or even decreased in static exercise while it is increased in dynamic exercise [88,89]. Although weight-lifting is a form of dynamic exercise the cardiovascular effects are similar to those of static exercise.

The task of the cardiorespiratory system during sustained dynamic exercise is to supply oxygen to the site of oxygen extraction and energy production, to transport the metabolic products resulting from exercise, and to dissipate heat. To accomplish this task the cardiovascular system operates in an integrated fashion to increase CO, perfusion pressure,

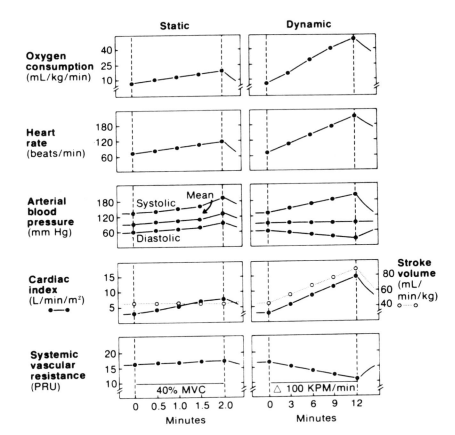

Fig. 3.3 Comparison of cardiovascular responses to static and dynamic exercise. The comparison is made of the acute effects that static and dynamic exercise have on oxygen consumption, heart rate, arterial blood pressure, stroke volume, and systemic vascular resistance. Static (isometric) exercise was performed at 40% of maximum voluntary contraction (MVC); dynamic exercise was performed on a bicycle by increasing the workload by 100 kilopond meters/minute (kPm/min) for the duration of exercise. PRU = Peripheral resistance unit.

and muscle blood flow (Fig. 3.4) [92]. Oxygen in cells is sufficient to support exercise for only a few seconds. Therefore blood flow has to increase immediately for aerobic metabolism to continue.

Under conditions of aerobic metabolism there is a linear increase in blood pressure with graded exercise; a nonlinear relationship occurs during anaerobic metabolism [93]. Despite the differences in cardiovascular adaptations that occur with the type of exercise, the CO response is tightly coupled to the absolute oxygen consumption [89]. During dynamic exercise, the increase in CO is nearly linear to the rise in metabolic demand and is due mainly to the increase in stroke volume secondary to increased venous return, decreased systemic vascular resistance, and myocardial contractility. Beyond 50% maximal work capacity the increase in CO is mainly due to an increase in heart rate. The increase in heart rate early in exercise is due to parasympathetic withdrawal and later to adrenergic stimulation of CO affecting rate, contractility, and venous return (by vasoconstriction). The venous return is further augmented by the pumping action of the contracting muscles. The increased sympathetic activity (neural

and humoral) induces arteriolar constriction but is overridden by local vasodilatation in the exercising muscle. The perfusion pressure is maintained by redistribution of blood flow from nonexercising muscle, splanchnic areas, and the skin. Absolute blood flow is maintained, however, because of the marked increase in CO. Cerebral blood flow is also maintained. The increase in CO is also associated with an increase in coronary flow. Myocardial flow is increased to all layers of the heart but with abolition of the gradient of flow between the endocardium and epicardium. Catecholamine response to static and dynamic exercise differs. During maximal dynamic exercise in normal young subjects, plasma norepinephrine may increase from 1.4 to 20 nmol/l while epinephrine increases from 0.25 to 2 nmol/l. During static exercise there are only small increments in plasma norepinephrine. However, the rise in plasma norepinephrine is larger relative to that of epinephrine during static exercise than during dynamic exercise. This apparently is due to a greater increase in sympathetic activity in visceral organs than muscle in static exercise.

During exercise the blood pressure rises towards a

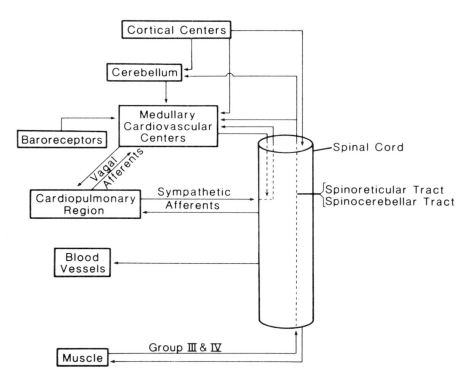

Fig. 3.4 Schematic representation of current knowledge concerning the regulation of the cardiovascular system during exercise. Both central command and feedback loops are included. Heart, baroreceptors, and muscle compose the feedback loops in the peripheral system and the cerebellum forms a central feedback loop [92].

new level which is determined by the vigor and the mass of the contracting muscle. After this new level is attained further rises are blunted because of a negative feedback control system. This system has been related to receptors in the exercising muscle sensing the level of blood flow necessary to fulfill metabolic demands, and to homeostatic reflexes from arterial and left ventricular mechanoreceptors. The muscular activity initiated by centers in the cerebral cortex with direct input into the brainstem where the cardiovascular centers are located (central command) is modified by afferent fiber information from the cardiovascular system and active tissues. These afferent nerves are thought to be the group III (A δ) fibers which have diameters of 1−6 μm and conduct impulses at 31−70 m/s and group IV fibers (C) which have diameters of 1 μm or less and conduct at 2.5 m/s or less. These afferent fibers from muscles of group III or IV can be further classified into ergoreceptors and nociceptors. Ergoreceptors cause the pressor reflex and are stimulated by static contraction of the muscle. Nociceptors perceive pain and are stimulated by algesic chemicals (bradykinin, serotonin, potassium, capsaicin etc.) and direct pain. The increase in muscle blood flow with exercise, however, can occur even in the denervated state.

The steep rise in blood pressure at the start of exercise does not produce bradycardia but rather is accompanied by tachycardia. This has led to the hypothesis that the set point or sensitivity of the baroreceptor reflex is decreased in exercise. Most of the evidence, however, points to a preservation of the ability of the baroreflex to regulate blood pressure during exercise [94]. Thus nonbaroreflex mechanisms are thought to be responsible for the increase in blood pressure during exercise. Additional central modulation of the baroreflex is possible.

CHRONIC PHYSICAL STRESS

With training there is reduced activation of the sympathetic tone at the same absolute submaximal workload [95]. The decreased vasoconstrictor activity results in a greater increase in blood flow to nonexercising muscle, splanchnic and renal beds. Circulating catecholamines at rest are similar in trained and untrained individuals; with training, the increase in circulating catecholamines at similar workloads is less [96]. The negative inotropic effect of propranolol is also less after chronic exercise, suggesting changes in adrenoceptor characteristics. However the changes in the characteristics of β-adrenoceptor binding in lymphocytes after chronic exercise are not consistent. The lesser increase in heart rate after exercise in the trained subject may be due not only to a decrease in sympathetic drive but also to an increase in parasympathetic activity. For example, the myocardial concentrations of acetylcholine are increased with training and the effects of atropine are lessened.

The hypertrophy of the myocardium after chronic dynamic exercise is global, of the volume overload type, with maintenance of the usual wall thickness to internal diameter ratio. This contrasts with the concentric afterload type noted in strength-trained athletes. Weight training increases left ventricular mass, wall thickness, septum thickness, and septum to free wall ratio.

Physical stress and hypertension

The hemodynamic consequences of exercise among hypertensive patients are influenced by age, myocardial function, and state of the peripheral vasculature. Dynamic exercise increases systolic blood pressure to a similar extent in young subjects with borderline hypertension and normotensive age-matched controls [87,90,97—99]. Diastolic blood pressure decreases or is unchanged compared to controls [97,98]. Elderly patients and those with long-standing hypertension have a greater increase in systolic blood pressure during exercise than age-matched control subjects. Diastolic pressure fails to decrease appropriately or may actually increase.

Static exercise increases systolic and diastolic blood pressure to a similar extent in normotensive and hypertensive adolescents [98]. In subjects with normal hearts static exercise increases systemic vascular resistance and causes a small increase in heart rate with little or no change in cardiac index. Blood pressure response to stress testing has been claimed to be a good indication of subjects who eventually develop hypertension [68]. However, Fixler and co-workers report that dynamic or static exercise is not a valid method for predicting eventual persistent hypertension [100].

Cardiac output increases normally in relation to oxygen consumption with exercise in hypertensive individuals. In subjects with borderline hypertension the high CO seen at rest disappears with exercise. The mean systolic ejection rate during supine exercise is lower than in normotensive people, and the normal shortening of the systolic ejection time is absent in those with hypertension. Like CO, stroke index in borderline hypertension moves to the normal range with exercise. This is due to the fact that the increase in stroke index with dynamic exercise in people with mild hypertension is less than in age-

matched normotensive controls. Although CO for a given workload may be normal in individuals with hypertension, it is achieved with a higher filling pressure. While systemic vascular resistance decreases during exercise in hypertensive people, the decrease does not normalize systemic resistance which cannot be overcome by the intense metabolic demand.

Although dynamic exercise acutely raises blood pressure, repeated dynamic physical exercise reduces blood pressure in both normotensive and hypertensive adults and adolescents. Resistive exercise (weight training) causes a marked increase in both systolic and diastolic pressure acutely. However, chronic resistive exercise, like chronic dynamic exercise, can also decrease both systolic and diastolic blood pressure [101].

Dynamic exercise increases plasma catecholamines in individuals with borderline and established hypertension as well as in normotensive people. Plasma norepinephrine increases to the greatest extent when borderline hypertension is present, while epinephrine increases to the greatest extent in the presence of established hypertension [102]. Static exercise increases plasma epinephrine and norepinephrine to a greater extent in people with established hypertension than in those who are normotensive or who have borderline hypertension. Intravenous infusion of norepinephrine may also increase blood pressure to a greater extent in hypertensive than in normotensive subjects. This increased vascular reactivity may be due to adrenergic receptor abnormalities (e.g. increased α-adrenoceptors), to enhanced intracellular messenger activity, or to the vascular smooth muscle *per se*.

Mental stress

The cardiovascular response to behavioral demands varies depending upon the resultant adaptive reaction. When the environmental stimulus results in inhibition of behavioral activity, the blood pressure increase is mainly due to a rise in total peripheral resistance. Heart rate and CO decrease. There is vasoconstriction of the skeletal and renal vascular beds. In dogs the preavoidance cardiovascular reactions are not prevented by α- or β-adrenergic blockade. The fight or flight reaction is mediated by the sympathetic nervous system in response to adversive stimulation [102]. Similar reactions have been described during mental stress [103]. While heart rate is invariably increased, the changes in CO and resistance are variable. Three hemodynamic patterns occur in response to mental stress [104]:

1 increased CO with little change or a decrease in total peripheral resistance;

2 increased peripheral resistance with no change or a decrease in CO, or

3 an increase in both CO and peripheral resistance.

Although there is marked overlap, the first pattern is more common in normotensive subjects, while the second and third patterns are more common in hypertensive patients. Humoral responses include an increase in plasma catecholamines, adrenocorticotrophic hormone, gluco- and mineralocorticoids, and vasopressin. The increase in renal nerve activity is associated with an elevation in plasma renin activity and a decrease in renal blood flow and sodium excretion. Electrolyte absorption in the gastrointestinal tract may also be increased. The increase in renal sodium reabsorption is mediated by renal α-adrenergic activity and controlled by central β-adrenoceptors in the posterior hypothalamus.

Irrespective of the hemodynamic patterns, the regional changes in blood flow are the same following mental stress. There is vasoconstriction of the renal, skin, and splanchnic beds, whereas there is vasodilatation of coronary vessels, and vessels in muscle and brain. Compared to normotensive subjects, those with hypertension demonstrate a greater degree of vasoconstriction and a greater increase in heart rate. In addition, the pressor responses last longer in hypertensive subjects. After mental stress, the increase in plasma norepinephrine is noted only in individuals with established hypertension while plasma epinephrine increases in both borderline and established hypertension. There is also a greater increase in the heart rate–pressure product (index of CO) and the diastolic blood pressure in borderline hypertension. Plasma cyclic adenosine monophosphate and glycerol however were similar in normotensive subjects and those with borderline or established hypertension. In contrast to mental stress, the cold pressor test increases blood pressure and peripheral resistance while CO shows no change or decreases in normotensive and hypertensive subjects. There are also differences among patients in changes in plasma norepinephrine or epinephrine after an orthostatic cold pressor test [105]. Norepinephrine increases in normotensive people as well as in those with borderline or established hypertension while epinephrine increases in hypertensive but not in normotensive subjects.

The buffering of cardiac reflexes from baro- and cardiac receptors is largely overridden by the limbic–hypothalamic discharge. The baroreflex control is inhibited during mental stress. The cardiac component of the baroreflex during emotional stress may also be inhibited. In contrast to dynamic exercise, shock avoidance behavior leads to lesser changes in heart rate and an increase in CO in excess of metabolic demands.

A role for stress-related behavioral changes in cardiovascular and renal hemodynamics has been implicated in the neurogenic mediation of hypertension in both humans and experimental animals. A greater cardiovascular response to behavioral stress has been reported not only in patients with borderline and established hypertension but also in the offspring of hypertensive parents [106,107]. Moreover salt-loading further increased these differences [107]. Falkner [107,108] and others have suggested that those normotensive patients with a family history of hypertension and a greater cardiovascular response to stress are at risk for developing sustained hypertension later in life.

REFERENCES

1 Conway J. Hemodynamic aspects of essential hypertension in humans. *Physiol Rev* 1984;64:617–60.

2 Jose PA. Hypertension and hypotension. In: Colon AR, Ziai M, eds. *Pediatric Pathophysiology*. Boston: Little, Brown, 1982.

3 Guyton AC. *Arterial Pressure and Hypertension*. Philadelphia: Saunders, 1980.

4 Little RC. *Physiology of the Heart and Circulation*. 3rd edn. Chicago: Year Book, 1985.

5 Mark AL. The Bezold–Jarisch reflex revisited: clinical implications of inhibitory reflexes originating in the heart. *J Am Coll Cardiol* 1983;1:90–102.

6 Bagshaw RJ. Evolution of cardiovascular baroreceptor control. *Biol Rev* 1985;60:121–62.

7 Bishop VS, Hasser EM. Arterial and cardiopulmonary reflexes in the regulation of the neurohormonal drive to the circulation. *Fed Proc* 1985;44:2377–81.

8 Logan A, Jose P, Eisner G, Lilienfield L, Slotkoff L. Intracortical distribution of blood flow in hemorrhagic shock in dogs. *Circ Res* 1971;29:257–66.

9 Holden K, Morgan JS, Krauss AN, Auld PAM. Incomplete baroreceptor responses in newborn infants. *Am J Perinatol* 1985;2:31–4.

10 Gootman PM, Gootman N, Buckley BJ. Maturation of central autonomic control of the circulation. *Fed Proc* 1983;42:1648–55.

11 Walker AM, Cannata JP, Ritchie BC, Maloney JE. Hypotension in fetal and newborn lambs; different patterns of reflex heart rate control revealed by autonomic blockade. *Biol Neonate* 1983;44:358−65.

12 Buckley BJ, Gootman N, Nagelberg JS, Griswold PR, Gootman PM. Cardiovascular response to arterial and venous hemorrhage in neonatal swine. *Am J Physiol* 1984;247:R626−33.

13 Bartolome J, Mills E, Lau C, Slotkin TA. Maturation of sympathetic neurotransmission in the rat heart. V. Development of baroreceptor control of sympathetic tone. *J Pharmacol Exp Ther* 1980;215: 596−600.

14 Bevan JAA, Su C. Sympathetic mechanisms in blood vessels: nerve and muscle relationships. *Annu Rev Pharmacol* 1973;13:269−85.

15 Hoeldke RB, Cilmi KM, Reichard GA, Boden G, Owen OE. Assessment of norepinephrine secretion and production. *J Lab Clin Med* 1983;101:772−82.

16 Jose PA. Adrenergic regulation of blood pressure. In: Loggie JMH, Horan MH, Gruskin AB, Hohn AR, Dunbar JB, Havlik RJ, eds. *NHLBI Workshop on Juvenile Hypertension*. New York: Biomedical Information, 1984.

17 Bylund DB. Heterogeneity of α_2-adrenergic receptors. *Pharmacol Biochem Behav* 1985;22:835−43.

18 Flavahan NA, Vanhoutte PM. α_1-adrenoceptor subclassification in vascular smooth muscle. *Trends Pharmacol Sci* 1986;7:347−9.

19 Langer AZ, Hicks PE. α-Adrenoceptor subtypes in blood vessels: physiology and pharmacology. *J Cardiovasc Res* 1984;6:S547−58.

20 Muntz KH, Garcia C, Hagler HK. α_1-Receptor localization in rat heart and kidney using autoradiography. *Am J Physiol* 1985;249:H512−19.

21 Muntz KH, Meyer L, Gadol S, Callianos TA. α_2-Adrenergic receptor localization in the rat heart and kidney using autoradiography and tritiated rauwolscine. *J Pharmacol Exp Ther* 1986;236:542−7.

22 Koepke JP, DiBona GF. Functions of renal nerves. *Physiologist* 1985;28:47−52.

23 Smyth DD, Umemura S, Pettinger WA. Renal nerve stimulation causes α_1-adrenoceptor-mediated sodium retention but not α_2-adrenoceptor antagonism of vasopressin. *Circ Res* 1985;57:304−11.

24 Pettinger WA, Umemura S, Smyth DD, Jeffries WB. Renal α_2-adrenoceptors and the adenylate cyclase-cAMP system: biochemical and physiological interactions. *Am J Physiol* 1987;252: F199−208.

25 DiBona GF, Sawin LL. Role of renal α_2-adrenergic receptors in spontaneously hypertensive rats. *Hypertension* 1987;9:41−8.

26 Fildes RD, Eisner GM, Calcagno PL, Jose PA. Renal α-adrenoceptors and sodium excretion in the dog. *Am J Physiol* 1985;17:F128−33.

27 Saito K, Kurihara M, Cruciani R, Potter WZ, Saavedra JM. Characterization of β_1- and β_2- adrenoceptor subtypes in the rat atrioventricular node by quantitative autoradiography. *Circ Res* 1988;62:173−77.

28 Taira N, Yabuuchi Y, Yamashita B. Profile of β- adrenoceptors in femoral, superior mesenteric and renal vascular beds of dogs. *Br J Pharmacol* 1977;59:577−83.

29 Felder RA, Felder CC, Eisner GM, Jose PA. Renal dopamine receptors. In: McGrath B, Bell C, eds. *Peripheral Actions of Dopamine*. London: Macmillan, 1988;124−140.

30 Kobilka BK, Matsui H, Kobilka TS et al. Cloning, sequencing, and expression of the gene coding for the human platelet α_2-adrenergic receptor. *Science* 1987;238:650−9.

31 Kobilka BK, Kobilka TS, Daniel K, Regan JW, Caron MG, Lefkowitz RJ. Chimeric α_2-, β_2- adrenergic receptors: delineation of domains involved in effector coupling and ligand binding specificity. *Science* 1988;240:1310−16.

32 Gillman AG. G proteins and dual control of adenylate cyclase. *Cell* 1984;36:577−9.

33 Lefkowitz RJ, Caron LM. Adrenergic receptors: molecular mechanisms of clinically relevant regulation. *Clin Res* 1985;33:395−405.

34 Berridge MJ, Irvine RF. Inositol trisphosphate, a novel second messenger in cellular signal transduction. *Nature* 1984;312:315−21.

35 Exton JH. Mechanisms of action of calcium-mobilizing agonists: some variations on a young theme. *FASEB J* 1988;2:2670−6.

36 Kikkawa U, Nishizuka Y. The role of protein kinase C in transmembrane signaling. *Annu Rev Cell Biol* 1986;2: 149−78.

37 Slivka SR, Insel PA. α_1-Adrenergic receptor-mediated phosphoinositide hydrolysis and prostaglandin E$_2$ formation in Madin−Darby canine kidney cells. Possible parallel activation of phospholipase C and phospholipase A$_2$. *J Biol Chem* 1987;262:4200−7.

38 Duckles SP, Banner W Jr. Changes in vascular smooth muscle reactivity during development. *Annu Rev Pharmacol Toxicol* 1984;24:65−83.

39 Ruggles BT, Murayama N, Werness JL, Gapstur SM, Bentley MD, Dousa TP. The vasopressin-sensitive adenylate cyclase in collecting tubules and thick ascending limb of Henle's loop of human and canine kidney. *J Clin Endocrinol Metab* 1985;60:914−21.

40 Robillard JE, Nakamura KT, Ayres NA. Control of fluid and electrolyte balance during fetal life. In: Jones CT, Nathanielsz PW eds. *Physiological Development of the Fetus and Newborn*. London: Academic Press 1985.

41 Lau C, Burke SP, Slotkin TA. Maturation of sympathetic neurotransmission in the rat heart: IX. Development of transsynaptic regulation of cardiac adrenergic sensitivity. *J Pharmacol Exp Ther* 1982;233:675−80.

42 Padbury JF, Polk DH, Newham JP, Lam RW. Neonatal adaptation: greater sympathoadrenal response in preterm than full-term fetal sheep at birth. *Am J Physiol* 1985;248: E443−9.

43 Dalmaz YL, Peyrin L, Dutruge J, Sann L. Neonatal pattern of adrenergic metabolites in urine of small for gestational age and preterm infants. *J Neural Trans* 1980;49:151−65.

44 Nicolopoulos D, Agathopoulos A, Galanakos-Tharouniati M, Stergiopoulos C. Urinary excretion of catecholamines by full term and premature infants. *Pediatrics* 1969;44: 262−5.

45 Heymann MA, Iwamoto HS, Rudolph AM. Factors affecting changes in the neonatal systemic circulation. *Annu Rev Physiol* 1981;43:371−83.

46 Gauthier P, Nadeau RA, de Champlain J. The development

of sympathetic innervation and functional state of the cardiovascular system in newborn dogs. *Can J Physiol Pharmacol* 1975;53:763−76.

47 Gootman N, Gootman PM. *Perinatal Cardiovascular Function.* New York: Marcel Dekker, 1983.

48 Felder RA, Jose PA. Development of adrenergic and dopamine receptors in the kidney. In: Strauss J, ed. *Electrolytes, Nephrotoxins, and the Neonatal kidney.* The Hague: Martinus-Nihjoff, 1985.

49 Robillard JE, Nakamura KT. Neurohormonal regulation of renal function during development. *Am J Physiol* 1988;254: F771−9.

50 Matherne GP, Nakamura KT, Alden BM, Robillard JE. Regional variation of postjunctional α-adrenoceptor responses in the developing renal vascular bed. *Pediatr Res* 1988;23:261A.

51 Matherne GP, Nakamura KT, Robillard JE. Ontogeny of α-adrenoceptor responses in renal vascular bed of sheep. *Am J Physiol* 1988;254:R277−83.

52 Gootman PM, Buckley NM, Gootman N. Postnatal maturation of neural control of the circulation. In: Scarpelli EM, Cosmi EV, eds. *Reviews in Perinatal Medicine* vol. 3. New York: Raven Press, 1979:1−72.

53 Freis ED. Hemodynamics of hypertension. *Physiol Rev* 1960;40:27−54.

54 Korner PI. Causal and homeostatic factors in hypertension. *Clin Sci* 1982;63:5s−26s.

55 Messerli HF, Ventura HO, Reisin E *et al.* Borderline hypertension and obesity: two prehypertensive states with elevated cardiac output. *Circulation* 1982;66:55−66.

56 Schieken RM, Lauer RM, Clarke WR. Hemodynamics in childhood hypertension. *Hypertens Clin Exp* 1986;A8: 703−20.

57 Tarazi RC, Fouad FM, Ferrario CM. Can the heart initiate some forms of hypertension? *Fed Proc* 1983;42:2691−7.

58 Esler M, Julius S, Zweifler A *et al.* Mild high-renin essential hypertension. *N Engl J Med* 1977;296:405−11.

59 Dustan HP, Tarazi RC. Hemodynamic abnormalities of adolescent hypertension. In: New MI, Levine LS, eds. *Juvenile Hypertension.* New York: Raven Press, 1977.

60 Davignon A, Rey C, Payot M, Biron P, Mongeau JG. Hemodynamic studies of labile essential hypertension in adolescents. In: New MI, Levine LS, eds. *Juvenile Hypertension.* New York: Raven Press, 1977.

61 Hofman A, Ellison RC, Newberger J, Miettinen OS. Blood pressure and haemodynamics in teenagers. *Br Heart J* 1982; 48:377−80.

62 Blake S, Carey M, McShane A, Walley T. Autoregulation of tissue blood flow in essential hypertension. *Hypertension* 1985;7:1003−7.

63 Schieken RM, Clark WR, Prineas R, Klein W, Lauer R. Electrocardiographic measures of left ventricular hypertrophy in children across the distribution of blood pressure; the Muscatine study. *Circulation* 1982;66:428−32.

64 Schieken RM. Measurement of left ventricular wall mass in pediatric populations. *Hypertension* 1987;9(suppl II):II-47−52.

65 Culpeper WS, Sodt PC, Messerli FH, Ruschhaupt DG, Arcilla RA. Cardiac status in juvenile borderline hypertension. *Ann Intern Med* 1983;98:1−7.

66 Berenson GS, Cresanta JL, Webber LS. High blood pressure in the young. *Annu Rev Med* 1984;35:535−60.

67 Culpeper WS. Cardiac anatomy and function in juvenile hypertension: current understanding and future concerns. *Am J Med* 1983;75:57−61.

68 Mahoney LT, Schieken RM, Clarke WR, Lauer RM. Left ventricular mass and exercise responses predict future blood pressure. The Muscatine study. *Hypertension* 1988;12:206−13.

69 Devereux RB, Pickering TG, Harsfield GA *et al.* Left ventricular hypertrophy in patients with hypertension: importance of blood pressure to regularly recurring stress. *Circulation* 1983;68:470−6.

70 Nunez BD, Masserli FH, Amodeo C, Garavaglia GE, Schmeider RE, Frohlich ED. Biventricular hypertrophy in essential hypertension. *Am Heart J* 1987;114:813−18.

71 Snider AR, Giddening SS, Rocchini AP *et al.* Doppler evaluation of left ventricular diastolic filling in children with systemic hypertension. *Am J Cardiol* 1985;56:921−6.

72 Fouad FM, Tarazi RC, Gallagher JH, MacIntyre WJ, Cook SA. Abnormal left ventricular relaxation in hypertensive patients. *Clin Sci* 1980;59 (suppl):411s−14s.

73 Graettinger WF, Weber MA, Gardin JM, Knoll ML. Diastolic blood pressure as a determinant of Doppler left ventricular filling indexes in normotensive adolescents. *J Am Coll Cardiol* 1987;16:1280−385.

74 Frohlich ED. Hemodynamics and other determinants in development of left ventricular hypertrophy. *Fed Proc* 1983;42:2709−15.

75 Trimarco B, De Luca N, Cuocolo A *et al.* β Blockers and left ventricular hypertrophy in hypertension. *Am Heart J* 1987;144:975−83.

76 Devereux RB, Pickering TG, Alderman MH, Chien S, Borer JS, Laragh JH. Left ventricular hypertrophy in hypertension. Prevalence and relationship to pathophysiologic variables. *Hypertension* 1987;9(suppl II):II 53−60.

77 Morgan HE, Gordon EE, Kira Y *et al.* Biochemical mechanisms of cardiac hypertrophy. *Annu Rev Physiol* 1987;49:533−43.

78 Tarazi RC, Sen S, Saragoca M, Khairallah PA. The multifactorial role of catecholamines in hypertensive cardiac hypertrophy. *Eur Heart J* 1982;3(suppl A):103−10.

79 Sen S, Tarazi RC, Khairallah PA, Bumpus FM. Cardiac hypertrophy in spontaneously hypertensive rats. *Circ Res* 1974;35:751−81.

80 Fouad FM, Nakashima Y, Tarazi RC, Salcedo EE. Reversal of left ventricular hypertrophy in hypertensive patients treated with methyldopa. *Am J Cardiol* 1982;49:795−801.

81 Gruskin AB, Perlman SA, Baluarte JH, Morgenstern BZ, Polinsky MS, Kaiser BA. Primary hypertension in the adolescent: facts and unresolved issues. In: Loggie JMH, Horan MH, Gruskin AB, Hohn AR, Dunbar JB, Havlik RJ, eds. *NHLBI Workshop on Juvenile Hypertension.* New York: Biomedical Information, 1984.

82 Berman W, Christensen D. Effects of acute preload and afterload stress on myocardial function in newborn and adult sheep. *Biol Neonate* 1983;43:61−6.

83 Teitel D, Rudolph AM. Perinatal delivery and cardiac function. *Adv Pediatr* 1985;32:321−47.

84 Klopfenstein HS, Rudolph AM. Postnatal changes in the circulation and responses to volume loading in sheep. *Circ Res* 1978;42:839−45.

85 Frohlich ED. The heart in hypertension: unresolved conceptual challenges. *Hypertension* 1988;11(suppl I):I-19−24.

86 Floras JS, Hassa O, Vann Jones J, Osikowska BA, Sever PS, Sleight P. Factors influencing blood pressure and heart rate variability in hypertensive humans. *Hypertension* 1988;11:273−81.

87 McMahon M, Palmer RM. Exercise and hypertension. *Med Clin North Am* 1985;69:57−70.

88 Longhurst JC, Mitchell JH. Does endurance training benefit the cardiovascular system? *J Cardiovasc Med* 1983;8: 227−36.

89 Hanson P, Nagle F. Isometric exercise: cardiovascular responses in normal and cardiac populations. *Cardiol Clin* 1987;5:157−70.

90 Pickering TG. Exercise and hypertension. *Cardiol Clin* 1987;5:311−18.

91 Hossack KF. Cardiovascular responses to dynamic exercise. *Cardiol Clin* 1987;5:147−56.

92 Stone HL, Dormer KJ, Foreman RD, Theis R, Blair RW. Neural regulation of the cardiovascular system during exercise. *Fed Proc* 1985;44:2271−8.

93 Spence DW, Peterson LH, Friedewald VE Jr. Relation of blood pressure during exercise to anaerobic metabolism. *Am J Cardiol* 1987;59:1342−4.

94 Lubdrook J. Reflex control of blood pressure during exercise. *Annu Rev Physiol* 1983;45:155−68.

95 Hammond HK, Froelicher VF. The physiologic sequelae of chronic dynamic exercise. *Med Clin North Am* 1985;69: 21−39.

96 Cristensen NJ, Galbo H. Sympathetic nervous activity during exercise. *Annu Rev Physiol* 1983;45:139−53.

97 Fixler DE, Pennoch L, Browne R, Fitzgerald V, Wilson S, Vance R. Response of hypertensive adolescents to dynamic and isometric exercise stress. *Pediatrics* 1979;64:579−83.

98 Nudel DB, Gootman N, Brunson SC, Stenzler A, Shenker R, Gauthier BG. Exercise performance of hypertensive adolescents. *Pediatrics* 1980;65:1073−8.

99 McCrory WW, Klein AA, Fallo F. Predictors of blood pressure: humoral factors. In: Loggie JMH, Horan MJ, Gruskin AB, Hohn AR, Dunbar JB, Havlik RJ, eds. *NHLBI Workshop on Juvenile Hypertension*. New York: Biomedical Information, 1984:181−202.

100 Fixler DE, Laird WP, Dana K. Usefulness of exercise stress testing for production of blood pressure trends. *Pediatrics* 1985;75:1071−5.

101 Hagberg JM, Ehsani AA, Goldring D, Hernandez A, Sinacore DR, Holloszy JO. Effect of weight training on blood pressure and hemodynamics in hypertensive adolescents. *J Pediatr* 1984;104:147−51.

102 Anderson DE. Interactions of stress, salt, and blood pressure. *Annu Rev Physiol* 1984;46:143−53.

103 Herd JA. Cardiovascular response to stress in man. *Annu Rev Physiol* 1984;46:177−85.

104 Brod J. Haemodynamic basis of acute pressor reactions and hypertension. *Br Heart J* 1963;25:227−245.

105 Eliasson K. Borderline hypertension. Circulatory sympatho-adrenal and psychological reactions to stress. *Acta Med Scand* 1985; 692(suppl):1−90.

106 Light KC, Obrist PA. Cardiovascular reactivity to behavioral stress in young males with and without marginally elevated systolic pressures: comparison of clinic, home and laboratory measures. *Hypertension* 1980;2:802−8.

107 Falkner B. Cardiovascular reactivity and psychogenic stress in juveniles. In: Loggie JMH, Horan MH, Gruskin AB, Hohn AR, Dunbar JB, Havlik RJ, eds. *NHLBI Workshop on Juvenile Hypertension*. New York: Biomedical Information, 1984:161−71.

108 Falkner B. Is there a black hypertension? *Hypertension* 1987;10:551−4.

4 The Role of the Central Nervous System in Blood Pressure Regulation

MICHAEL R. PRANZATELLI AND DARRYL C. DE VIVO

INTRODUCTION

Blood pressure and the central nervous system (CNS) are usually discussed clinically in the context of the neurologic complications of hypertension, which will not be covered here. Our understanding of the CNS role in cardiovascular physiology and pathophysiology has emerged only recently. The brain, besides exerting a unique role in regulating its own perfusion, is in many ways the guardian of systemic perfusion. Central regulatory mechanisms, like blood pressure itself, are a composite of reflexes and integrated responses at many levels. Anatomic, electrophysiologic, and pharmacologic probes have helped to reveal how the CNS acts to regulate blood pressure. The reader is referred to several reviews for details beyond the scope of this chapter [1–4].

Anatomic, neurophysiologic, and pharmacologic studies have provided strong evidence for a role in the regulation of blood pressure by the CNS. Studies of animal models such as the spontaneously hypertensive rat (SHR) have identified several neurochemical abnormalities in brain, for which a causal relation with hypertension must be established. The pharmacologic substrate of the neuroanatomic pathways and nuclei which subserve physiologic reflexes such as the baroreceptor reflex arc includes multiple neurotransmitter systems. Of these, brainstem adrenergic neurotransmission is most clearly involved, and is targeted by many centrally active antihypertensive drugs. Neuropeptides have been identified more recently in structures which influence blood pressure, where they may act as neurotransmitters or neuromodulators. The mechanisms by which brain pathology alters blood pressure are still elusive. Animal models suggest that central mechanisms are involved in the etiology of essential hypertension, but evidence in humans is lacking. Discrete lesions in animals involving structures important to blood pressure regulation within the brainstem or hypothalamus induce hypertension. In humans, hypertension is an uncommon association of several neurologic disorders which cause increased intracranial pressure or affect central or peripheral components of the autonomic nervous system. The exact human counterpart of experimental neurogenic hypertension is unclear, but new imaging techniques may allow clinicopathologic correlation *in vivo*. Some forms of experimental hypertension can be pharmacologically reversed. The possibilities of clinical therapeutic intervention in neural regulation have only begun to be explored.

PHYSIOLOGY AND ANATOMY

Medullary centers

As early as 1870, it was recognized by Dittmar and Owsjannikow that intact medullary function was necessary for normal cardiovascular homeostasis. Peripheral afferent nerves were found to contain pressor and depressor fibers [5]. The hypothesized vasoreflex and vasotonic bulbar centers [6] were present in the floor of the fourth ventricle [7]. Later these centers were thought to be in deeper structures within the medullary reticular formation [8,9]. Using a stereotactic device, Alexander [10] mapped a pressor center to the lateral reticular formation in the rostral two-thirds of the medulla and a separate depressor center (tonically inhibiting spinal centers) in the medial reticular formation of the caudal medulla. Neuronal activity in the rostral ventrolateral medulla appears to be necessary for processing of afferent signals [11]. The existence of tonic vasomotor activity is disputed [12,13].

Forebrain centers

The concept of a medullary cardiovascular center which maintains blood pressure has been expanded in recent years to encompass the suggested role of the forebrain in integrating the appropriate cardiovascular response with a behavior (Table 4.1). Hypothalamus and limbic structures modify blood pressure in the defensive reaction [13,14]. Nonbrainstem influences on blood pressure were recognized at least as early as 1941 with the finding that electrical stimulation of various hypothalamic nuclei, amygdala, and related cortical structures evokes increases or decreases in blood pressure and heart rate [15]. Tracing of the involved pathways reveals a longitudinal brainstem organization for central blood pressure regulation [16,17]. Midpontine transection allows normal basal control of arterial pressure but prevents its modulation by higher centers. Transection below the medulla dramatically reduces arterial blood pressure [18].

Mechanisms for regulating blood pressure

The nervous system regulates blood pressure by reflex mechanisms originating outside the brain. They include baroreceptor feedback, the CNS ischemic response, and chemoreceptors [19]. These neural responses are rapid. Centrally mediated pressor responses are transmitted through the autonomic nervous system to end-organs via postganglionic nerve fibers. The release of norepinephrine stimulates cardiovascular adrenergic receptors.

The baroreceptor reflex arc (Fig. 4.1) in the brain has been identified by lesions in the CNS as well as by electrophysiologic studies. The reflex arc consists of baroreceptor centers and their afferent and efferent connections [1]. A short loop and a long loop

Table 4.1 Central nervous system regulation of blood pressure

Seat of autonomic nervous system
  Parasympathetic (anterior hypothalamus)
  Sympathetic (posterior hypothalamus)
Steady-state response to cardiovascular mechanoreceptors
Coupling of circulatory changes with behavior
Effects on hypothalamopituitary axis (fluid, electrolyte, endocrine balance)

have been identified anatomically. In the short-loop reflex, baroreceptor afferents directly access vasomotor cells located in the medulla. In the long-loop reflex arc, hypothalamic and limbic centers are interposed. These forebrain structures modulate cardiovascular centers in the lower brainstem as well as integrating neurohumoral aspects of cardiovascular regulation with fluid and electrolyte homeostasis. The glossopharyngeal (IX) and vagus (X) nerves carry baroreceptor afferent stimuli from the aortic depressor and carotid sinus nerves to the medulla (20). In the medulla, the brainstem or nucleus of the solitary tract (NTS) is the primary baroreceptor center, containing the principal synapses of the baroreceptor reflex arc [21]. NTS sends axons to the vasomotor cells (short-loop) or to modulatory forebrain centers (long-loop). The vasomotor cells (Fig. 4.2) are located in the medulla (nucleus ambiguus and dorsal vagal nucleus) and spinal cord (intermediolateral cell column) [22]. Efferent preganglionic fibers from the vasomotor cells project to postganglionic autonomic neurons and to the heart and vessels. The structural organization of the brainstem allows multiple access for cardiovascular information at numerous levels [23].

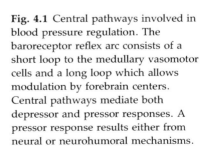

Fig. 4.1 Central pathways involved in blood pressure regulation. The baroreceptor reflex arc consists of a short loop to the medullary vasomotor cells and a long loop which allows modulation by forebrain centers. Central pathways mediate both depressor and pressor responses. A pressor response results either from neural or neurohumoral mechanisms.

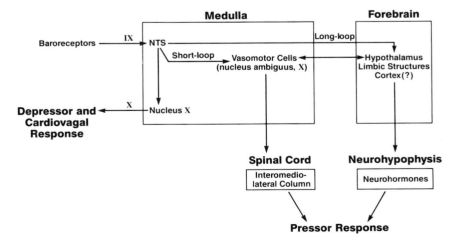

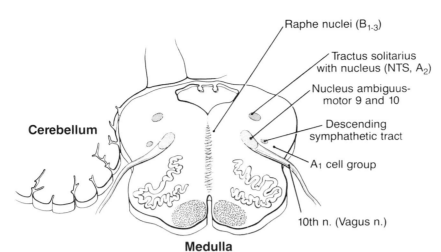

Raphe nuclei (B$_{1-3}$)

Tractus solitarius
with nucleus (NTS, A$_2$)

Nucleus ambiguus-
motor 9 and 10

Descending
symphathetic tract

A$_1$ cell group

Cerebellum

10th n. (Vagus n.)

Medulla

Fig. 4.2 Schematic cross-section of medulla showing localization of principal blood pressure regulatory centers and adjacent monoamine cell bodies.

The baroreceptor reflex evokes hypotension, bradycardia, and apnea. Baroreceptor impulses inhibit the medullary vasoconstrictor center and excite the vagal center, with the net result of lowering blood pressure. Low pressure stimulates the opposite baroreceptor response. Interruption of the reflex by removing baroreceptor input (deafferentation) also increases blood pressure. The baroreceptor system opposes acute changes in blood pressure. However, it has less importance in chronic blood pressure regulation because it adapts to a sustained change in blood pressure.

Chemoreceptors, responding presumably to acidosis or hypercarbia, increase blood pressure in hypoxia [24]. The CNS ischemic response is one of the most powerful activators of sympathetic vasoconstriction. An ischemic mechanism also may be activated by increased intracranial pressure by compromising the cerebral perfusion pressure. Neural and hormonal (norepinephrine–epinephrine, renin–angiotensin, vasopressin) responses produce vasoconstriction. Sympathetic nerves on cerebral blood vessels, once regarded as functionless, have a role in cerebral blood flow [25].

PHARMACOLOGY

Recent investigation has attempted to identify the pharmacologic correlates of various brainstem centers of physiologic importance to blood pressure regulation. The abundance of neurotransmitter- and neuropeptide-containing cell bodies and pathways in the brainstem has complicated this task. Identification of central sites of action of some antihypertensive drugs has helped to assess the functional significance of neurochemical data.

Monoamines

Cell bodies for monoamine (catecholamine and indoleamine) systems are located predominantly in the brainstem (Fig. 4.2) and project diffusely to forebrain, spinal cord, and within the hindbrain. The trend begun by early workers of labeling these monoaminergic nuclei with a letter and number has persisted; some also have a name. However, these nuclei seldom contain a pure population of monoamine neurons. Noradrenergic nuclei (A1–8) extend longitudinally throughout the brainstem [26,27]. Descending noradrenergic nerves arise from A5 and A7 [28]. A6 is the locus ceruleus. Anatomic connections between the locus ceruleus (tonic excitatory input) and dorsal raphe nucleus (B7) have been demonstrated [29,30]. Descending serotonergic projections arise mainly from the medullary raphe nuclei B1–3 [31], which terminate especially in sympathetic intermediolateral cell columns between segments T1 and L2 [32]. Epinephrine-containing cells in the brainstem, denoted C1–3, extensively innervate the hypothalamus [33]. The C1 (lateral tegmentum) and C2 (dorsal medulla) subgroups in the NTS overlap partially with A1 and A2, respectively [34]. Epinephrine fibers also innervate A6, the intermediolateral spinal column, and the periventricular region of the fourth ventricle. A role for brain dopamine (A8–14) in blood pressure regulation has not been established. More recent extensions of classical monoamine fluorescence studies, such as the horseradish peroxidase

Table 4.2 Putative transmitter innervation of central blood pressure centers

NTS, DVN	A2, A6, C2
Pressor area	A6 (?)
Depressor area	A1, A3–A5 (?)

NTS = Nucleus of the solitary tract; DVN = dorsal vagal nucleus; A6 = locus ceruleus.

technique, have revealed the greater complexity of monoaminergic projections [28].

The correlation of specific monoamine nuclei with blood pressure centers in brain is still uncertain (Table 4.2). However, there is a dense catecholaminergic innervation of the area of the first synapse in the baroreceptor reflex arc (A2) [35]. Data support the importance of an inhibitory α-adrenergic pathway within the NTS in the control of blood pressure [36]. A1 may correspond to the ventrolateral vasomotor cells, and A2 to both the NTS and vagal complex [37,38]. The pontomedullary pressor area may be the locus ceruleus. A2 neurons have been presumed to have vasodepressor function, possibly facilitating baroreceptor reflexes. Stimulation of α-adrenergic receptors in the vasomotor centers inhibits peripheral sympathetic centers.

The complex effects of central serotonin (5-HT) on blood pressure have been reviewed recently [39]. Powerful central and peripheral serotonergic effects on blood pressure have been observed experimentally. Heterogeneity of central and peripheral 5-HT receptors may explain some of the conflicting results. Generally, intracerebrally administered 5-HT is mainly pressor, while systemic precursors or agonists cause depressor effects. 5-HT neurotoxins and 5-HT synthesis inhibitors have different effects on blood pressure. They suggest the presence of descending pressor pathways in cervical cord. Increased spinal and brainstem 5-HT and 5-HIAA in rabbits with neurogenic hypertension and young SHR have been described [40,41]. 5-HT-1A agonist receptors may mediate 5-HT-induced hypotension, and may act in part centrally. However, 5-HT-2 antagonists (with α-adrenergic effects) have useful peripheral antihypertensive effects.

Transmitter amino acids

Glutamate has been proposed as a neurotransmitter of baroreceptor afferent fibers in the NTS [42]. Microinjected L-glutamate in the NTS (intermediate third)

stimulates the baroreceptor reflex, an effect reversed by the glutamate antagonist glutamate diethylester. Blockade of the baroreceptor reflex and hypertension are produced by bilateral microinjection of kainic acid, a rigid glutamate analog. Baroreceptor deafferentation to the NTS reduces high-affinity L-glutamate uptake.

γ-Aminobutyric acid (GABA) agonists have opposing effects on blood pressure and heart rate in the rostral and caudal ventrolateral medullary neurons [11]. GABAergic mechanisms in ventrolateral medulla may be tonically involved in maintenance and reflex regulation of vasomotor activity, possibly providing reciprocal inhibition between vasopressor and vasodepressor neuron pools [11].

Neuropeptides

An increasing number of vasoactive peptides have been identified in brain centers which are influential in the regulation of blood pressure (Table 4.3). The exact regional and subcellular localization of peptides in the baroreceptor reflex arcs has been the focus of research. By immunocytochemistry, five neuropeptides have been localized in the vagus nerve and 14 in the NTS [43]. Pharmacologic manipulations have not established a physiologic role for these neuropeptides. Many peptides exert their effects through brainstem

Table 4.3 Neurochemistry of blood pressure control*

Neurotransmitters	Neuropeptides
Norepinephrine	Angiotensin II
Epinephrine	Vasopressin
Serotonin	Oxytocin
Glutamate	Enkephalin
γ-Aminobutyric acid	Thyrotropin-releasing hormone
	Somatostatin
	Neurotensin
	Vasoactive intestinal peptide
	Adrenocorticotrophic hormone
	Substance P
	β-Endorphin
	α-Melanocyte-stimulating hormone
	Cholecystokinin
	Bombesin

* Vasoactive substances identified in brainstem centers or pathways involved in blood pressure regulation which alter blood pressure when administered centrally. The direction of effect on blood pressure is not indicated here because the route of administration, dose, and animal species are critical variables which do not allow generalizations.

catecholamine neurons by altering synthesis, turn-over, and rates of firing. Circulating peptides cross the blood−brain barrier poorly, but may access the brain through barrier-free areas such as the area postrema.

Peptide abnormalities are not present in all animal models of hypertension, suggesting lack of a crucial role in the pathogenesis of hypertension. The cardio-vascular effects of peripheral and centrally adminis-tered neuropeptides are often opposite. The argument that any single peptide plays a key role in blood pressure homeostasis in the medulla is weakened by the plethora of peptides localized to this region.

The NTS contains both enkephalinergic cell bodies and nerve terminals, unlike several other brain nuclei [43]. Leucine-enkephalin and α-endorphin have the highest opioid pressor activity; β-endorphin and enkephalin analogs decrease blood pressure [44]. Intracisternal morphine has a biphasic effect on blood pressure, only one part of which is naloxone-antagonized. It has been suggested that release of a β-endorphin-like peptide in the brainstem con-tributes to the antihypertensive action of central α-adrenergic stimulation.

Cisternal substance P increases blood pressure and might have a role in the first baroreceptor reflex [28]. Neuropeptides of the neurohypophyseal system do not affect basal blood pressure and heart rate on intracerebroventricular administration but do inhibit the pressor response evoked by mesencephalic electric stimulation.

Vasopressin and angiotensin are best supported as physiologic neurohormones in blood pressure regu-lation [45, 46]. Angiotensin II acts on the CNS to increase blood pressure and cardiac output. It may be synthesized in the CNS. Angiotensin receptors have been localized to lateral septum, midbrain, hypo-thalamus, and medulla in the rat [47]. Within the medulla, the greatest density of sites is in the area postrema and ventral medulla. Cerebrospinal fluid angiotensin is increased 50% in the SHR. Little is known about physiologic control of renin secretion by brain. Renin secretion is increased by electric stimulation of brainstem and posterior hypothalamus and decreased by anterior hypothalamic stimulation. Hypertensive effects of angiotensin II can be me-diated by both the area postrema and by the subfor-nical organ (anteroventral third ventricle) [48]. Renin release is inhibited by central catecholaminergic pathways and stimulated by serotonergic pathways [49,50]. The CNS control of renin secretion is me-diated by renal sympathetic nerves, circulating catecholamines, and vasopressin. During renin-mediated hypertension, neurogenic tone is maintained at a high level in spite of prevailing hypertension; peripherally derived angiotensin may induce sympathetic excitation by a central mech-anism [48]. Experimental one-kidney hypertension (renin-independent) is prevented by lesions of the anteroventral third ventricle.

Acetylcholine

The role of cholinergic systems in blood pressure regulation has not been well characterized. Cholino-mimetic drugs injected into the cerebral ventricles evoke excitatory cardiovascular responses. Injections within the lateral medullary pressor area or posterior hypothalamus reveal inhibitory muscarinic cholino-receptors in the lateral medullary pressor area and excitatory nicotinic receptors in both areas [51]. Intravertebral artery injections of muscarinic or nic-otinic agonists induce hypotension. In contrast, nic-otine given systemically causes a pressor response [51].

Central effects of clinical antihypertensive drugs

Many antihypertensive drugs access the brain at clinical dosages and produce central side-effects, but only some have a central mechanism of action, and essentially all also have peripheral effects. Most anti-hypertensive drugs with central activity are sympath-olytic and are sedative [52]. They act by interfering with the CNS regulation of blood pressure (Table 4.4). Clonidine, reserpine, and α-methyldopa are well studied examples.

Systemic administration of clonidine at low doses suppresses norepinephrine neuron firing in the locus ceruleus and 5-HT neuron firing in the dorsal raphe nucleus [53]. Clonidine decreases sympathetic ac-tivity, increases vagal tone, and inhibits the secretion of pressor hormones (renin, vasopressin, adrenocorti-cotrophic hormone) [54−56]. Clonidine also alters brain serotonergic and dopaminergic neurotrans-mission through effects on central noradrenergic neurons [57]. It is primarily an α$_2$-adrenergic agonist within the CNS [53]. α-Adrenergic receptor effects may not be of sole importance, however, since in the medullary lateral reticular nucleus, imidazolines (such as clonidine) but not α$_2$-selective catecho-lamines induce hypotension [58]. The projections of

Table 4.4 Central nervous system action of antihypertensive drugs

Drug	Action
Clonidine	Decreased neuron firing in LC, NTS (?) α_2-Adrenergic agonist
α-Methyldopa	Metabolism to α-methylnorepinephrine, an α-adrenergic agonist
Reserpine	Decreased monoamines available for synaptic release
Propranolol (?)	Blockade of prejunctional β-adrenergic receptors (?)

LC = locus ceruleus; NTS = nucleus of solitary tract.

the locus ceruleus are especially diffuse, throughout the reticular activating system and forebrain. Another site in the brain mediating the antihypertensive action of drugs such as clonidine and α-methyldopa may be the NTS [59].

Reserpine irreversibly depletes monoamines in storage granules centrally and peripherally. Most of the catecholamines are deaminated intraneuronally.

α-Methyldopa enters brain, where it is decarboxylated and β-hydroxylated to α-methyl-norepinephrine in central adrenergic neurons [60]. α-Methylnorepinephrine, a powerful agonist at α_2-adrenergic receptors, inhibits sympathetic outflow [61,62]. These observations revise the older false transmitter hypothesis which stated that these agents were ineffective.

The importance of the CNS effects of β-blockers in their antihypertensive properties is uncertain. Lipophilicity and the antihypertensive properties of β-blockers do not correlate despite the occurrence of centrally mediated side-effects, such as vivid dreams and nightmares [63].

Other drugs, such as analeptics and analgesics, suppress pressor responses to stimulation of different pontomedullary structures unequally, further supporting pharmacologic and anatomic differences between these structures [64,65].

PATHOPHYSIOLOGY

Absence of structural lesions in the brain to explain the pathophysiology of essential hypertension has directed a search for neurochemical and neurotransmitter abnormalities.

Animal models

Abnormalities have been found in central neurotransmitter mechanisms in different animal models of hypertension, particularly in the early stages of the condition. Animal models range from renin- and nonrenin-dependent renal hypertension, salt-mediated hypertension, and neurogenic hypertension to genetically mediated models. The SHR model has been particularly well studied. A diversity of neurochemical changes has been found, but cause and effect have not been established (Table 4.5). Many studies have focused on brainstem regions. A unifying characteristic of many of these models is the existence of exaggerated sympathetic nervous system participation in the maintenance of high arterial pressure. Abnormal catecholamine levels or turnover and enzyme activities have been found. The patterns of abnormalities differ among animal models. A 20% increase in the number of epinephrine nerve cells with a similar increase in phenylethanolamine-N-methyltransferase has been reported in the SHR [66]. An increase in hypothalamic and medullary epinephrine and vasopressin precedes the development of hypertension [4]. In renal hypertension, norepinephrine increases instead. In some models, neurotransmitters, precursors, agonists, and antagonists have been administered systemically, intrathecally, and stereotactically into discrete nuclei. Neurotoxins

Table 4.5 Diversity of central neurochemical changes found in the spontaneously hypertensive rat

Increased
Tryptophan hydroxylase (spinal cord, pons, medulla)
NE (A1); NE, DA, EPI (A2); NE (cord, cerebellum)
NE turnover rate
PNMT (A1, A2, spinal cord)*
EPI nerve cell numbers (medulla)
β-Endorphin (neurointermediate lobe)
Angiotensin II (CSF)
Vasopressin (hypothalamus, medulla)
Sympathetic nerve discharge

Decreased
Dynorphin (hypothalamus, pituitary)
EPI (A1, A2)*

* Young animals only.
NE = norepinephrine; DA = dopamine; EPI = epinephrine; PNMT = phenylethanolamine-N-methyltransferase; CSF = cerebrospinal fluid.
Regions or compartments where changes were found appear in parentheses.

such as 6-hydroxydopamine (6-HDA) and 5,7-dihydroxytryptamine (DHT) have been used to lesion monoamine terminals selectively. Intracisternal 6-HDA in neonatal SHR prevents hypertension but does not block it once it has developed [67].

Evidence that the brain renin−angiotensin system helps regulate blood pressure is controversial. In genetically hypertensive rats, differences in the concentration of angiotensin and distribution of angiotensin receptors have been found [46,47].

INCREASED INTRACRANIAL PRESSURE

The rise in blood pressure caused by increased intracranial pressure has been known for 100 years. Cushing [68] described the graded elevation of blood pressure and fall in heart rate when intracranial pressure exceeds blood pressure, and the response bears his name. Widespread activation of sympathetic neurons occurs, inducing vasoconstriction in most vascular beds. This response is due to central adrenergic discharge since it persists in adrenalectomized animals [2,69]. The receptive area has been mapped in the lower brainstem [70]. Direct pressure or axial displacement may cause local ischemia [71]. Initially, cardiac output is increased. As vasoconstriction is enhanced, cardiac output may fall, leading to cardiac failure and pulmonary edema [72]. The Cushing response persists after prepontine decerebration and transection of all cranial nerves. It disappears with cervical (C1) spinal transection. The stimulus or receptors for the Cushing phenomenon have not been adequately defined. However, pressure delivered with a fine metal probe along the floor of the fourth ventricle or by rapid delivery of 1−3 μl of artificial cerebrospinal fluid in the rostral medulla and caudal pons below the fourth ventricle evokes the response. The stimulus is rapid brainstem distortion [73].

NEUROGENIC HYPERTENSION

Removal of inhibitory baroreceptor input to the CNS elevates blood pressure (Table 4.6). The hypertension, if sustained, is termed "neurogenic," and may be fulminant. Bilateral NTS lesions, sectioning of baroreceptor afferents, and sinoaortic deafferentation result in neurogenic hypertension, which is caused by loss of inhibitory baroreceptor input on sympathetic excitatory centers in brain [74]. Hypertension induced by NTS lesions is not associated with generalized

Table 4.6 Central neurogenic hypertension

Clinical features
Typically labile
Stimulus-sensitive

Possible mechanisms
Cushing response
Sympathetic discharge
Central deafferentation

sympathetic activation and is independent of the adrenal glands and kidneys [75]. Higher centers are requisite, since mid collicular decerebration will block NTS lesion-induced hypertension.

Acute experimental brainstem ischemia, hypoxia, or hypercarbia evokes elevated blood pressure, bradycardia, and apnea. These responses occur independently of baroreceptor reflex mechanisms, via neurogenic sympathetic and vagal activity and the adrenal glands [24].

A role for the forebrain in central hypertension has been supported by electrical stimulation and by lesion studies [76−78]. Bilateral anterior hypothalamic lesions induce acute fulminating hypertension in the rat via the adrenal glands [78−80]. However, certain forebrain lesions may result in hypotension [77,81].

Bilateral lesions of the NTS, induced by procaine, kainic acid, or electrolytic lesions, induce acute fulminating hypertension in the rat, which is blocked by α-adrenergic blocking agents (phentolamine), clonidine, or ganglionic blocking agents, systemic 6-HDA, anteroventral third ventricle lesions, but not by adrenalectomy or nephrectomy (Table 4.7). In the rat, NTS hypertension is acute, labile, displays exaggerated reactivity, loss of baroreceptor reflexes, and enhanced conditioned arterial pressure responses. In the dog, NTS hypertension is chronic and sustained.

A selective neurochemical abnormality in the brain can simulate human hypertension. Electrolytic lesions of A2 abolish the cardiovagal (but not depressor) component of the baroreceptor reflex; labile blood pressure but not sustained hypertension results. This is of interest since labile blood pressure may be an early sign of essential hypertension [82]. After A2 lesions, the activity of dopamine β-hydroxylase falls to 50% of control in the NTS [83] or in 6-HDA lesions of the NTS. Unlike A2 lesions, 6-HDA lesions of NTS decrease the gain but do not abolish baroreceptor reflexes. These data suggest that norepinephrine release from A2 terminals into the

Table 4.7 Central nervous system lesions that reduce or block experimental hypertension

Lesion	Hypertensive model
Mid collicular decerebration Anteroventral third ventricle	NTS
Posterior hypothalamus	SHR
Central nucleus of amygdala* Anteroventral third ventricle	Other models†

* Bilateral lesions.
†Renin and non-renin renal hypertension, mineralocorticosteroid salt-hypertension.
NTS = lesions or deafferentation of the nucleus of the solitary tract; SHR = spontaneously hypertensive rat.

NTS stabilizes blood pressure. A1 lesions, which induce hypertension and pulmonary edema via release of vasopressin in the rabbit, do not abolish the baroreceptor reflex. This is a model of neuro-endocrine-mediated hypertension [38].

Humans

Compared to the extensive studies in animals, there are few data in humans on the role of the CNS in the development of essential hypertension, and of the consequences of CNS pathology on blood pressure.

There has been renewed interest in a neural etiologic role in the pathophysiology of essential hypertension. One of the earliest hypotheses of a neural mechanism for essential hypertension was a dysfunction of the baroreceptor reflex, since 1927 when Hering discovered that sinoaortic denervation resulted in hypertension [84]. Subsequent work demonstrated that baroreceptor changes were secondary to the hypertension [85]. In 1936, Foerster described lowering of blood pressure in hypertensive patients by bilateral section of the ventrolateral and presumably sympathetic pathways of the spinal cord [86]. Since then, many measurements of circulating catecholamines have been marshaled in the argument for increased sympathetic activity, particularly in younger individuals with hypertension or patients with labile blood pressure [87]. Recent evidence also renews support for an important influence of psychologic factors on blood pressure [28,82]. Supporters of the neural hypothesis argue from animal studies that these changes would occur early, and that the hypothalamus may be an important site.

Several types of CNS lesions are associated with hypertension (Table 4.8). Clinicopathologic correlation has been generally lacking, and most studies in survivors antedate the era of computerized tomography. Increased intracranial pressure in humans may be associated with massive sympathetic discharge. Posterior fossa tumors, especially of the fourth ventricle, may induce hypertension with symptoms suggestive of a pheochromocytoma [88−90]. The distinction between medullary infiltration and increased intracranial pressure in these cases has not been made. The localizing value of hypertension in brain lesions is disputed [75,91].

Central autonomic discharges are a recognized manifestation of limbic epilepsy [92]. Direct pressure on the hypothalamus by third ventricular cysts may also induce hypertension. Intrinsic hypothalamic lesions which produce hypertension usually also give other evidence of hypothalamic dysfunction.

Centrally induced autonomic hypotension occurs in Shy−Drager syndrome (diffuse degenerative changes in central preganglionic autonomic neurons). These patients do not manifest signs of sympathetic discharge in the face of syncope-producing hypotension. Loss of cardiovascular regulation may occur in brain death. Mixed central and peripheral autonomic lesions are found in familial dysautonomia (Riley−Day syndrome). This syndrome may represent denervation supersensitivity in its hyper-responsiveness to sympathomimetic agents. The CNS may also be the selective target of various endotoxins, such as *Shigella*, which induce endotoxic shock by a central mechanism.

Hypertension may be a paroxysmal feature of several dysautonomias primarily affecting the peripheral autonomic nervous system, such as diabetes mellitus, chronic alcoholism, amyloidosis, acute intermittent

Table 4.8 Neurologic disorders associated with hypertension

Central mechanism likely	Peripheral mechanism likely
Convulsions	Polyneuropathy
Diencephalic epilepsy	Familial dysautonomia
Basilar artery ectasia	Reye syndrome
Syringobulbia	Tetanus
Bulbar poliomyelitis	
Ischemic brainstem lesions	
Decerebrating lesions	
Hypothalamic lesion	
Posterior fossa tumors	
Spinal cord lesions	
Intracranial hypertension	

porphyria, botulism, paraneoplastic syndrome, and Fabry's disease. In Fabry's disease, renal involvement is contributory. In acute idiopathic polyneuropathy (Guillain−Barré syndrome), hypertension may develop during the acute illness, with reports in a 6-year-old boy of levels as high as 230/190 mmHg [93]. Sympathetic overactivity and involvement of the afferent baroreceptor nerves by the neuropathy have been implicated. Neurologic conditions with autonomic involvement commonly are associated with postural hypotension.

Hypertension may be the result of systemic disorders which secondarily involve the CNS, such as hypercalcemia, sympathomimetic intoxication, mercury or thallium poisoning, and neuroblastoma, in which case the distinction between central and peripheral mechanisms may be blurred. Adrenocorticotrophic hormone, used to treat several neurologic disorders, induces adrenal-dependent hypertension, probably by a peripheral mechanism [54].

The NTS, IX, and X cranial nerve nuclei, and nucleus ambiguus fall within a watershed area supplied by the ipsilateral posterior inferior cerebellar artery (less often from the vertebral artery), the superior cerebellar artery, and the basilar artery. Lateral medullary infarctions do not give rise to hypertension, but the NTS is not always included in the lesion. Unilateral involvement may be part of the reason. Hypertension in basilar artery ectasia has been attributed to medullary compression [94].

The authors have observed hypertension with evidence of sympathetic overactivity in children with decerebrating lesions of various etiologies [95].

In severe acute poliomyelitis, hypertension is common (see Chapter 26). Differential involvement of brain versus spinal cord has been suggested, but not all series agree. Bulbar lesions have been found in some of these patients [96]. Hypertension may become chronic in many patients [97].

Spinal cord injuries can increase or decrease blood pressure. When control by the brain of sympathetic outflow is lost below a complete spinal transection, the autonomous cord exhibits reflex activity. Complete and partial loss of outflow are seen with lesions above T1 and T6, respectively [92]. The phase of autonomic hyperreflexia can result in severe hypertension in response to minimal stimuli (such as bladder distension), sometimes also associated with increased vagal activity [98,99].

In humans, bilateral vagal block by local anesthetic, neuropathy, or sectioning elevates blood pressure [100]. Bilateral sectioning of glossopharyngeal nerves in the posterior fossa induces permanent hypertension.

REFERENCES

1 Palkovits M, Mezey E, Zaborszky. Neuroanatomical evidences for direct neural connections between the brain stem baroreceptor centers and the forebrain areas involved in the neural regulation of the blood pressure. In: Meyer P, Schmitt H, eds. *Nervous System and Hypertension*. New York: John Wiley, 1979:18−30.

2 Reis DJ, Talman WT. Brain lesions and hypertension. In: de Jong W, ed. *Handbook of Hypertension*, vol 4: *Experimental and Genetic Models of Hypertension*. Amsterdam: Elsevier Science, 1984:451−76.

3 Reis DJ, Doba N. The central nervous system and neurogenic hypertension. *Prog Cardiovasc Dis* 1974;17:51−71.

4 Versteeg DHG, Petty MA, Bohus B, de Jong W. The central nervous system and hypertension: the role of catecholamines and neuropeptides. In: de Jong W, ed. *Handbook of Hypertension*, vol 4: *Experimental and Genetic Models of Hypertension*. Amsterdam: Elsevier Science, 1984:398−430.

5 Hunt R. The fall of blood pressure resulting from the stimulation of afferent nerves. *J Physiol* 1985;18:381−410.

6 Porter WT. The vasotonic and the vasoreflex center. *Am J Physiol* 1915;36:418−22.

7 Ranson SW, Billingsley PR. Vasomotor reactions from stimulation of the floor of the fourth ventricle. III. Studies in vasomotor reflex arcs. *Am J Physiol* 1916;41:85−90.

8 Wang S-C, Ranson SW. Autonomic responses to electrical stimulation of the lower brainstem. *J Comp Neurol* 1939; 71:437−55.

9 Scott JMD. The part played by the ala cinera in vasomotor reflexes. *J Physiol* 1925;590:443−54.

10 Alexander RS. Tonic and reflex functions of medullary sympathetic cardiovascular centers. *J Neurophysiol* 1946; 9:205−17.

11 Willette RN, Barcas PB, Krieger AJ, Sapru HN. Endogenous GABAergic mechanisms in the medulla and regulation of blood pressure. *J Pharmacol Exp Ther* 1984;230:34−8.

12 Dampney RAL, Moon EA. Role of the ventrolateral medulla in vasomotor response to cerebral ischemia. *Am J Physiol* 1980;239:H349−358.

13 Hilton SM. Ways of viewing the central nervous control of circulation—old and new. *Brain Res* 1975;87:213−19.

14 Mancia G, Zanchetti A. Hypothalamic control of autonomic functions. In: Morgane PJ, Panksepp J, eds. *Behavioral Studies of the Hypothalamus. Handbook of the Hypothalamus*, vol 3-B. New York: Marcel Dekker, 1981. 147−202.

15 Pitts RF, Larrabee MG, Bronk DW. An analysis of hypothalamic cardiovascular control. *Am J Physiol* 1941; 134:359−83.

16 Hilton SM, Spyer KM. Participation of the anterior hypothalamus in the baroreceptor reflex. *J Physiol* 1971; 218:271−93.

17 Miura M, Reis DJ. Cerebellum: a pressor response elicited from the fastigial nucleus and its efferent pathway in brainstem. *Brain Res* 1969;13:595−9.

18 Manning JW. Cardiovascular reflexes following lesions in medullary reticular formation. *Am J Physiol* 1965;208:283−8.

19 Dickinson CJ ed. *Neurogenic Hypertension*. Oxford: Blackwell Scientific Publications, 1965.

20 Coote JH, Macleod VH. Evidence for the involvement in the baroreceptor reflex of a descending inhibitory pathway. *J Physiol* 1974;241:477−96.

21 Palkovits M, Zaborsky L. Neuroanatomy of central cardiovascular control. Nucleus tractus solitarii: afferent and efferent neuronal connection in relation to the baroreceptor reflex arc. *Prog Brain Res* 1977;47:9−34.

22 McAllen RM, Spyer KM. Baroreceptor neurones in the medulla of the cat. *J Physiol* 1965;222:68P−9P.

23 Korner PI. Integrative role of the central nervous system in cardiovascular control. In: Kovach AGB, Sandor P, Kollai M, eds. *Advances in Physiological Science*, vol 9. *Cardiovascular Physiology: Neural Control Mechanisms*. Oxford: Pergamon Press, 1981.

24 Downings SE, Mitchell JH, Wallace AG. Cardiovascular responses to ischemia, hypoxia, and hypercapnia of the central nervous system. *Am J Physiol* 1963;204:881−7.

25 Reis DJ. Central neural control of cerebral circulation and metabolism. In: Mackenzie ET, Seylaz J, Bes A, eds. *Neurotransmitters and the Cerebral Circulation*. New York: Raven Press, 1984:91−119.

26 Bjorklund A, Skagerberg G. Descending monoaminergic projections to the spinal cord. In: Sjolund B, Bjorklund A, eds. *Brain Stem Control of Spinal Mechanisms*. New York: Elsevier Biomedical Press, 1982:55−88.

27 Lightman SL, Todd K, Everitt BJ. Ascending noradrenergic projections from the brainstem: evidence for a major role in the regulation of blood pressure and vasopressin secretion. *Exp Brain Res* 1984;55:145−51.

28 Chalmers JP, West MJ. The nervous system in the pathogenesis of essential hypertension. In: Robertson JIS, ed. *Handbook of Hypertension*, vol 1. New York: Elsevier Science, 1983:64−96.

29 Sakai K, Salvert D, Touret M, Jouvet M. Afferent connections of the nucleus raphe dorsalis in the cat as visualized by the horseradish peroxidase technique. *Brain Res* 1977; 137:11−35.

30 Descarrier L, Leger L. Serotonin nerve terminals in the locus ceruleus of the adult rat. In: Garattini S, Pujol JF, Samamin R, eds. *Interactions between Putative Neurotransmitters in the Brain*. New York: Raven Press, 1978: 355−67.

31 Fuxe K, Hokfelt T, Ungerstedt U. Localization of indolealkylamines in CNS. *Adv Pharmacol* 1968;6A:235−51.

32 Dahlstrom A, Fuxe K. Evidence for the existence of monoamine neurones in the central nervous system. II. Experimentally induced changes in the intraneuronal amine levels of bulbospinal neurone systems. *Acta Physiol Scand* 1965; 64(suppl 247):1−37.

33 Hokfelt T, Johansson O, Fuxe K, Goldstein M, Park D. Immunohistochemical studies on the localization and distribution of monoamine neuron systems in the rat brain. I. Tyrosine hydroxylase in the mes- and diencephalon. *Med Biol* 1976;54:427−53.

34 Ross CA, Delbo A, Reis DJ. Effect of electrical stimulation of the C1 adrenergic cell group and the Kolliker−Fuse nucleus on sympathetic vasomotor activity and adrenal

35 Fuxe K, Bolme P, Jonsson G *et al*. On the cardiovascular role of noradrenaline, adrenaline, and peptide-containing neuron systems in the brain. In: Meyer P, Schmitt H, eds. *Nervous System and Hypertension*. Davis, Wiley-Flammarion, 1979.

36 DeJong W, Zandberg P, Bohus B. Central inhibition of noradrenergic cardiovascular control. *Prog Brain Res* 1975; 42:285−98.

37 Chalmers JP. Brain amines and models of experimental hypertension. *Circ Res* 1975;36:469−80.

38 West MJ, Blessing WW, Chalmers J. Arterial baroreceptor reflex function in the conscious rabbit after brainstem lesions coinciding with the A1 group of catecholamine neurons. *Circ Res* 1981;49:959−70.

39 Kuhn DM, Wolf WA, Lovenberg W. Review of the role of the central serotonergic neuronal system in blood pressure regulation. *Hypertension* 1980;2:243−55.

40 Smith ML, Browning RA, Myers JH. *In vivo* rate of serotonin synthesis in brain and spinal cord of young spontaneously hypertensive rats. *Eur J Pharmacol* 1979;53:301−5.

41 Wing LMH, Chalmers JP. Effects of p-chlorophenylalanine on blood pressure and heart rate in normal rabbits and rabbits with neurogenic hypertension. *Clin Exp Pharmacol Physiol* 1974;1:219−26.

42 Talman WT, Granata AR, Reis DJ. Glutaminergic mechanisms in the nucleus tractus solitarius in blood pressure control. *Fed Proc* 1984;43:39−44.

43 Palkovits M. Neuropeptides in the central regulation of blood pressure. In: Villarreal H, Sambhi MP, eds. *Topics in Pathophysiology of Hypertension*. Boston: Martinus Nijhoff Publishers, 1984:282−90.

44 Olson GA, Olson RD, Kastin AJ. Review. Endogenous opiates: 1984. *Peptides* 1985;6:769−91.

45 Reis DJ. Central neural control of cerebral circulation of blood pressure and vasopressin secretion. *Exp Brain Res* 1984;55:145−51.

46 Ganten D, Hutchinson JS, Schelling P. The intrinsic brain iso-renin angiotensin system in the rat: its possible role in central mechanisms of blood pressure regulation. *Clin Sci Mol Med* 1975;48:265s−8s.

47 Sirett NE, McLean AS, Bray JJ, Hubbard JI. Distribution of angiotensin II receptors in rat brain. *Brain Res* 1977; 122:299−312.

48 Brody MJ, Hartle DK, Lind W, Johnson AK. Evidence for the participation of specific hypothalamic pathways in the pathogenesis of hypertension. In: Villarreal H, Sambhi MP, eds. *Topics in Pathophysiology of Hypertension*. Boston: Martinus Nijhoff 1984:275−81.

49 Zimmermann H, Ganong WF. Pharmacological evidence that stimulation of central serotonergic pathways increases renin secretion. *Neuroendocrinology* 1980;30:101−7.

50 Blair ML, Reid IA, Ganong WF. Effect of L-dopa on plasma renin activity with and without inhibition of extracerebral dopa decarboxylase in dogs. *J Pharmacol Exp Ther* 1977;202:209−15.

51 Tangri KK, Jain IP, Bhargava KP. Role of central cholinoceptors in cardiovascular regulation. In: De Jong W, Provoost AP, Shapiro AP. *Hypertension and Brain Mechanisms*. Amsterdam: Elsevier Scientific, 1977:123−30.

medullary catecholamine secretion in rat. *Soc Neurosci Abst* 1981;7:210.

52 Hansson L. Drug treatment of hypertension. In: Robertson JIS, ed. *Handbook of Hypertension*, vol 1. *Clinical Aspects of Essential Hypertension*. Amsterdam: Elsevier Science, 1983:397–436.

53 Svensson TH, Bunney BS, Aghajanian GK. Inhibition of both noradrenergic and serotonergic neurons in brain by the α-adrenergic agonist clonidine. *Brain Res* 1975; 92:291–306.

54 Reid IA. The brain, centrally acting drugs, the renin system and blood pressure regulation. In: Laragh JH, Buhler FR, Seldim DW, eds. *Frontiers in Hypertension Research*. New York: Springer-Verlag, 1981:329–37.

55 Kobinger W, Walland AW. Evidence for central activation of a vagal cardiodepressor reflex by clonidine. *Eur J Pharmacol* 1972;19:203–9.

56 Sweet GS, Columbo JM, Gaul SL. Central antihypertensive effects of inhibition of the renin-angiotensin system in rats. *Am J Physiol* 1976;231:1794–9.

57 Geyer MA, Lee EHY. Effects of clonidine, piperoxane and locus ceruleus lesion on the serotonergic and dopaminergic systems in raphe and caudate nucleus. *Biochem Pharmacol* 1984;33:3399–404.

58 Bousquet P, Felman J, Schwartz J. Central cardiovascular effects of α-adrenergic drugs: differences between catecholamines and imidazolines. *J Pharmacol Exp Ther* 1984;230:232–7.

59 Haeusler G. Brain centers for pharmacologic control of the cardiovascular system. In: Laragh JH, Buhler FR, Seldin DW, eds. *Frontiers in Hypertension Research*. New York: Springer-Verlag, 1981:344–7.

60 Henning M, Rubenson A. Evidence that the hypotensive action of methyldopa is mediated by central action of methylnorepinephrine. *J Pharm Pharmacol* 1971;23:407–11.

61 Freed CR, Quintero E, Murphy C. Hypotension and hypothalamic amine metabolism after longterm α-methyldopa infusions. *Life Sci* 1978;23:313–22.

62 Langer SZ. The role of α- and β-presynaptic receptors in the regulation of noradrenaline release elicited by nerve stimulation. *Clin Sci Mol Med* 1976;51:423s–6s.

63 Amer MS. Mechanism of action of β-blockers in hypertension. *Biochem Pharmacol* 1977;26:171–5.

64 Kovalyov GV. Localization and characteristics of the influence of some neurotrophic drugs on the bulbar vasomotor centre. In: Valdman AV, ed. *Pharmacology and Physiology of the Reticular Formation*. Amsterdam: Elsevier, 1967:187–209.

65 Bondaryvov MG. The influence of analeptic drugs on the pontine vasomotor center. In: Valdman AV, ed. *Pharmacology and Physiology of the Reticular Formation. Progress in Brain Research*, vol 20. Amsterdam: Elsevier, 1967;171–186.

66 Howe PRC, Lovenberg W, Chalmers JP. Increased number of PNMT-immunofluorescent nerve cell bodies in the medulla oblongata of stroke-prone hypertensive rats. *Brain Res* 1981;205:123–30.

67 Yamori Y, Yamahe H, DeJong W, Loveberg W, Sjoerdsma A. Effect of tissue norepinephrine depletion by 6-hydroxydopamine on blood pressure in spontaneously hypertensive rats. *Eur J Pharmacol* 1973;17:135–40.

68 Cushing H. Some experimental and clinical observations concerning states of increased intracranial tension. *Am J Med Sci* 1902;124:374–400.

69 Jeffers WA, Lindauer MA, Lukens FDW. Adrenalectomy in experimental hypertension from kaolin. *Proc Soc Exp Biol Med* 1937;37:260–2.

70 Doba N, Reis DJ. Localization within the lower brainstem of a receptive arc mediating the pressor response to increased intracranial pressure (the Cushing response). *Brain Res* 1972;47:487–91.

71 Doba N, Reis DJ. Role of central and peripheral adrenergic mechanisms in neurogenic hypertension produced by brainstem lesions in the rat. *Circ Res* 1974;34:293–300.

72 Ducker TB, Simmons RL, Anderson RW. Increased intracranial pressure and pulmonary edema. III. The effect of increased intracranial pressure on the cardiovascular hemodynamics of chimpanzee. *J Neurosurg* 1968;29:475–83.

73 Thompson RK, Malina S. Dynamic axial brainstem distortion as a mechanism explaining the cardiovascular changes in increased intracranial pressure. *J Neurosurg* 1959;16:664–76.

74 Brody MJ, Faber JE, Mangiapane ML, Porter JP. The central nervous system and prevention of hypertension. In: DeJong W, ed. *Handbook of Hypertension*, vol 4. *Experimental and Genetic Models of Hypertension*. Amsterdam: Elsevier, 1984:474–94.

75 Reis DJ, Doba N. Hypertension as a localizing sign of mass lesions of brain stem. *N Engl J Med* 1972;287:1355–6.

76 Hartle DK, Brody MJ. Hypothalamic vasomotor pathways mediating development of hypertension in the rat. *Hypertension* 1982;4:68–71.

77 Yamori Y. Hypothalamic hyper- and hypotension induced by the destruction of the tuberomammillary region of the rat. *Jpn Circ J* 1967;31:743–80.

78 Nathan MA, Reis DJ. Fulminating arterial hypertension with pulmonary edema from release of adrenomedullary catecholamines after lesions of the anterior hypothalamus in the rat. *Circ Res* 1975;37:226–35.

79 Gauthier P, Reis DJ, Nathan MA. Arterial hypertension elicited either by lesions or by electrical stimulations of the rostral hypothalamus in the rat. *Brain Res* 1981;211:91–105.

80 Nosaka S. Hypertension induced by extensive medial anteromedian hypothalamic destruction in the rat. *Jpn Circ J* 1966;30:509–23.

81 Okamoto K, Nosaka S, Yamori Y. Experimental hypertension and hypotension induced by hypothalamic damage in the rat. *Jpn Circ J* 1967;31:743–80.

82 Caris TN ed. *A Clinical Guide to Hypertension*. Littleton, Massachusetts: PSG, 1985.

83 Talman WT, Synder DW, Reis DJ. Chronic lability of arterial pressure produced by destruction of A_2 catecholamine neurons in rat brainstem. *Circ Res* 1980;46:842–53.

84 Wang S-C. Central autonomic nervous system—cardiovascular functions at the bulbar level. In: *Physiology and Pharmacology of the Brainstem*. New York: Futura Publishing, 1980:5–80.

85 Magnus O, Koster M, Van Der Drift JHA. Cerebral mechanisms and neurogenic hypertension in man, with special reference to baroreceptor control. *Prog Brain Res* 1977;47:199–228.

86 Wang S-C. Central autonomic system cardiovascular functions at diencephalic (suprabulbar) level. In: *Physiology and Pharmacology of the Brainstem*. New York: Futura, 1980:81–113.

87 De Chaplain J. Evaluation of the neurogenic component in

human hypertension. In: Julius S, Esler MD, eds. *The Nervous System in Arterial Hypertension*. Springfield, Illinois: Charles C Thomas, 1976;267−300.

88 Cameron SJ, Doig A. Cerebellar tumors presenting with clinical features of astrocytoma. *Lancet* 1970;i:492−4.

89 Evans CH, Westfall V, Atuk NO. Astrocytoma mimicking the features of pheochromocytoma. *N Engl J Med* 1972; 286:1397−9.

90 Meyer BC. Neoplasms of the posterior fossa simulating cerebral vascular disease: report of five cases with reference to the role of the medulla in the production of arterial hypertension. *Arch Neurol Psychiatry* 1941;45:468−80.

91 Plum F, Posner JB. *The Diagnosis of Stupor and Coma*. Philadelphia: FA Davis, 1980:30−2.

92 Johnson RH, Spalding JMK. *Disorders of the Autonomic Nervous System*. Philadelphia: FA Davis, 1974:33−58,67−78.

93 Spalding JMK, Smith AC. *Clinical Practice and Physiology of Artificial Respiration*. Oxford: Blackwell Scientific Publications, 1963.

94 Montgomery BM. The basilar artery syndrome. *Arch Intern Med* 1961;108:115−25.

95 Pranzatelli MR, Pavlakis SG, Gould RJ, De Vivo DC. Hypothalamic-midbrain dysregulation syndrome: hypertension, hyperthermia, hyperventilation, and decerebration. *J child Neurol.* 1991;6:115−22.

96 Baker AB, Matze HA, Brown JR. Poliomyelitis. III. Bulbar poliomyelitis: a study of medullary function. *Arch Neurol Psychiatry* 1950;63:257−81.

97 Perlstein MA, Andelman MB, Rosner DC, Wehrle P. Incidence of hypertension in poliomyelitis. *Pediatrics* 1953;11:628−33.

98 Appenzeller O. Autonomic function, its pathophysiology and clinical assessment in paraplegia and tetraplegia. In: *The Autonomic Nervous System*. New York: Elsevier Biomedical Press, 1982:397−409.

99 Appenzeller O. The neurogenic control of the circulation. In: *The Autonomic Nervous System*. New York: Elsevier Biomedical Press, 1982:109−99.

100 Holt GW. *The Vagi in Medicine and Surgery*. Springfield, Illinois: Charles C Thomas, 1968:55−9.

5 Steroid Modulation of Blood Pressure and Mineralocorticoid Hypertension

PHYLLIS W. SPEISER, ELIZABETH STONER, PERRIN C. WHITE, CHRISTOPHER CRAWFORD, AND MARIA I. NEW

INTRODUCTION

Blood pressure is regulated through the interaction of intravascular volume, cardiac output, and peripheral resistance. Hormones involved in blood pressure regulation may effect a change in any or all of these parameters. Secretion of renin by the juxtaglomerular apparatus of the kidney results in the production of angiotensin II (AII), a powerful vasoconstrictor; AII also induces aldosterone secretion by the adrenal zona glomerulosa. Adrenocorticotropic hormone (ACTH) plays a minor stimulatory role in aldosterone production. Mineralocorticoids, including aldosterone, cause expansion of intravascular volume and an acute increase in blood pressure by increasing renal distal tubular sodium reabsorption. (A detailed discussion of the renin–angiotensin–aldosterone axis can be found in Chapter 2.) These hemodynamic changes then affect peripheral resistance and cardiac output, which in turn influence blood pressure.

Steroid hormones, particularly the glucocorticoids, directly accentuate the response of vascular smooth muscle to pressor agents. Mineralocorticoids, and exceptionally glucocorticoids, act via the type I (mineralocorticoid) receptor to promote sodium reabsorption. Water retention and expansion of intravascular volume follow from the vasopressin-mediated mechanism preserving serum osmolality, while a counter-controlling mechanism, chiefly effected by atrial natriuretic factor, aims to reduce intravascular volume and permits cardiac output and blood pressure to be kept within normal range. Aberrant intravascular volume, electrolyte concentration, or blood pressure should result in appropriate hormonal responses to restore homeostasis. This chapter reviews the major primary disturbances in steroid hormonal synthesis and action that alter the modulation of blood pressure and lead to hypertension.

SYNTHETIC DEFECTS OF STEROIDOGENESIS ASSOCIATED WITH HYPERTENSION

Decreased synthesis of the essential glucocorticoid, cortisol, results in increased hypothalamic corticotropin-releasing hormone (CRH) and pituitary ACTH secretion and overstimulation of the adrenal cortex (Fig. 5.1). A defect in any of the five enzymes in the biosynthesis of cortisol from cholesterol (all are inherited as autosomal recessive traits) results in the disorder called congenital adrenal hyperplasia (CAH) in which excess production of other steroid products occurs via unimpeded synthetic pathways (Fig. 5.2). Two specific forms of CAH result in accumulation of mineralocorticoid hormones characteristically producing hypertension: steroid 11β-hydroxylase deficiency and 17α-hydroxylase/17,20-lyase deficiency [3]. Patients with these forms of CAH are usually identified by clinical features resulting from

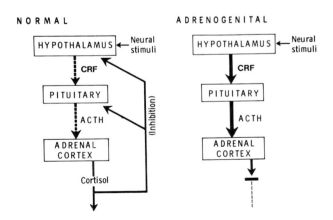

Fig. 5.1 Regulation of cortisol secretion in normal subjects and in patients with congenital adrenal hyperplasia (or adrenogenital syndrome). From New and Levine [1], with permission.

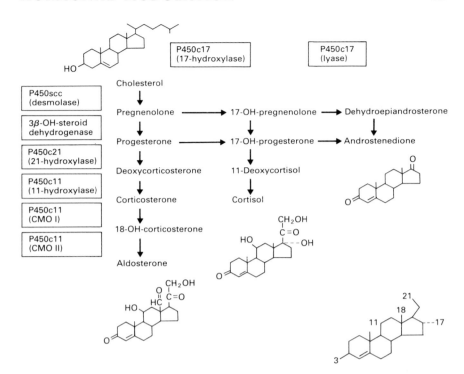

Fig. 5.2 Adrenal steroidogenesis. Biosynthetic pathways from cholesterol to mineralocorticoids (aldosterone), glucocorticoids (cortisol), and androgens (androstenedione) are shown, as are the structures of cholesterol, aldosterone, cortisol, and androstenedione (small amounts of testosterone and estrogen are also synthesized in the adrenal gland). The 3, 11, 17, 18, and 21 positions are marked on the diagram of a steroid molecule (bottom right). Arrows indicate individual biosynthetic conversions. The enzyme specifically mediating each step is indicated at the top or left, with the name of the enzymatic activity in parentheses; note that one protein can mediate more than one step. OH denotes hydroxy- and CMO corticosterone methyl oxidase. From White and coworkers [2], with permission.

altered sex steroid production. In the 11β-hydroxylase defect steroid precursors are channeled into androgenic pathways, resulting in excess adrenal androgen secretion and virilization of genetic females (female pseudohermaphrodites with normal female internal genitalia). Isosexual precocity is seen in males with 11β-hydroxylase deficiency. If untreated, these children have rapid somatic growth and appearance of secondary sexual characteristics associated with adrenarche; early epiphyseal fusion results in short stature. The 17α-hydroxylase/17,20-lyase defect (this enzyme is expressed in the gonads also) blocks androgen production and results in genital underdevelopment in genetic males (male pseudohermaphroditism) at birth. Since androgens are required as substrates for aromatase in the formation of estrogens, there is impairment of pubertal changes in genetic females affected with 17α-hydroxylase/17,20-lyase deficiency, who have primary amenorrhea, hypoplastic breasts, and little sexual hair.

The adrenal 11β-hydroxylase deficiency produces high plasma concentrations of deoxycorticosterone (DOC) and 11-deoxycortisol (compound S), and high levels in urine of the respective tetrahydro (TH) metabolites, tetrahydro-DOC (THDOC) and tetrahydro-S (THS). Plasma DOC is also high in 17α-hydroxylase/17,20-lyase deficiency, in which the abnormal pattern of adrenal steroid synthesis generates elevated

plasma levels as well of 18-hydroxy-DOC (18-OH-DOC) and corticosterone (compound B). Aldosterone is extremely low, but can over time rise to normal on treatment as suppression of the fasciculata lowers DOC levels, allowing the glomerulosa to gain secretory function.

The mechanism for the development of hypertension is similar in the two enzyme defects. DOC is a precursor in the aldosterone biosynthetic pathway and is itself a potent mineralocorticoid. Only small quantities of DOC are normally secreted by the adrenals, and the hypertension that results in 11β-hydroxylase- and 17α-hydroxylase-deficiency CAH is attributed to the elevated plasma DOC levels. Circulating levels of DOC do not correlate entirely with blood pressure values [4], however, suggesting that other factors [5,6] contribute to development of hypertension in these conditions.

In the untreated deficiencies of 11β-hydroxylase and 17α-hydroxylase/17,20-lyase, elevated DOC causes sodium retention, kaliuresis, and plasma volume expansion, suppressing renin and aldosterone. Since circulating DOC is largely a product of the cortisol-producing zone, the zona fasciculata, of the adrenal cortex [7], the lowering of ACTH levels that occurs with glucocorticoid replacement therapy, which suppresses adrenal androgen overproduction, also reduces DOC secretion. Ensuing natriuresis

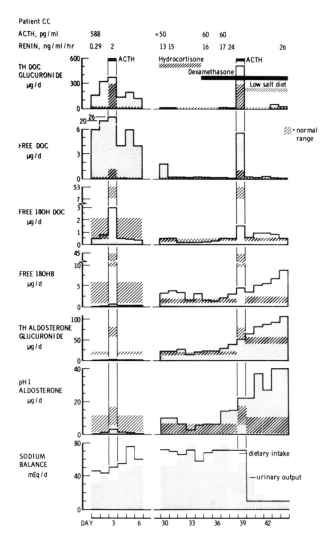

Fig. 5.3 Metabolic balance and urinary hormone excretion in a prepubertal boy with 11β-hydroxylase deficiency during baseline, adrenocorticotrophic hormone (ACTH), dexamethasone, and dexamethasone and low salt (marked with*) periods. ▨ Patient's response; ▨ normal control response. From Levine and coworkers [8], with permission.

brings about a rise in renin and stimulation of the aldosterone-producing adrenal zona glomerulosa (Figs 5.3 and 5.4).

Molecular biology of adrenal steroid 11β-hydroxylase and 17α-hydroxylase/17,20-lyase enzymes

Steroid 11β-hydroxylase and steroid 17α-hydroxylase/17,20-lyase are both cytochrome P450 hemeproteins, termed P450c11 and P450c17. The single

P450c17 protein has two functions, 17α-hydroxylating corticosteroids as well as cleaving the short fragment at the $C_{17}-C_{20}$ bond to yield androgens. There are two closely related P450c11 isozymes. The three activities of 11β-hydroxylation, 18-hydroxylation [corticosterone methyl oxidase (CMO) I] and 18-oxidation (CMO II) represent the steps converting DOC to aldosterone [10]. Only one isozyme carries out the 18-oxidation step which yields aldosterone — this isozyme is called aldosterone synthase or $P450_{aldo}$ [11].

The two genes encoding the two P450c11 isozymes — genes CYP11B1 and CYP11B2 — have been cloned and sequenced and have been mapped to the long arm of chromosome 8 [12,13]. A point mutation in CYP11B1 (not arising by conversion from the 95% concordant CYP11B2 sequence) has been identified in a cohort of 11β-hydroxylase deficiency patients [14]. Isolated defects in the 18-oxidation step (CMO II) of P450c11 have been observed [15]. A linkage analysis has been performed on six families with this variant defect of P450c11. Consistent segregation of one restriction fragment length polymorphism (RFLP) in the CYP11B gene with the disease trait demonstrated that the mutation was in or very near the CYP11B gene loci [16].

Human cDNA corresponding to P450c17 has been characterized [17] and the CYP17 gene locus is situated on chromosome 10 [18]. Several mutations in CYP17 have been identified in DNA from patients, with 17α-hydroxylase/17,20-lyase deficiency [reviewed in 1].

OTHER GENETIC FORMS OF STEROID HORMONE-INDUCED HYPERTENSION

Dexamethasone-suppressible hyperaldosteronism (DSH)

Hypertension secondary to DSH was recognized two decades ago [20,21] and has since been reported by investigators from several continents [22–27]. The salient feature of this autosomal dominant disorder (Fig. 5.5) distinguishing it from primary aldosteronism (usually a non-genetic disorder found rarely in children) is complete and rapid suppression of moderate aldosterone hypersecretion within 48 h of dexamethasone administration (Fig. 5.6). Accompanying changes include elevation of suppressed plasma renin activity to the normal range, and restoration of the normal aldosterone responsiveness to

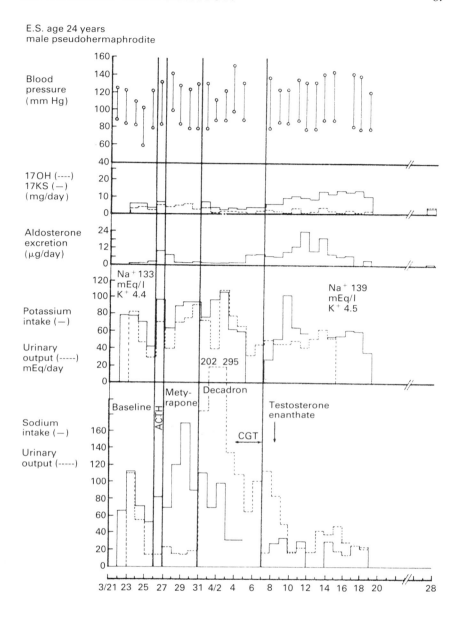

Fig. 5.4 Metabolic balance of sodium and potassium in a patient with 17α-hydroxylase deficiency, correlated with various periods of therapy and hormonal measurements. From New [9], with permission.

changes in posture [22] and dietary sodium manipulation [23]. In addition to glucocorticoid suppressibility, the usual aldosterone escape from chronic ACTH stimulation is lacking [29]. It is apparent that aldosterone *per se* is not the hypertensinogenic steroid in this disorder. Infusion of ACTH in a glucocorticoid-treated patient caused recrudescence of the hypertension, whereas separate infusions of the known mineralocorticoids [aldosterone, DOC and 18-hydroxy-deoxycorticosterone (18-OHDOC)] did not effect significant changes in blood pressure [30]. Studies using an *in vitro* receptor assay have shown total mineralocorticoid activity in plasma of untreated

DSH patients in excess of that accounted for by the combined immunoreactive values of aldosterone, DOC, and cortisol (unlike the case for both normal subjects and patients with other forms of hypertension) [31,32]. It was further shown with stimulation and suppression tests that this excess mineralocorticoid activity is under ACTH control [32]. Indeed, plasma ACTH levels are sometimes elevated in patients with DSH, and where radiographic imaging or direct pathologic examination has been performed, adrenal hyperplasia or nodularity has been noted.

Although a pituitary-derived aldosterone-stimu-

Pedigree A

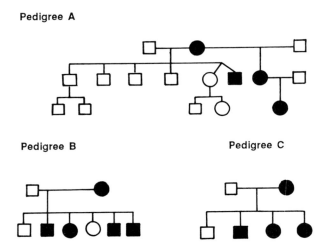

Pedigree B   **Pedigree C**

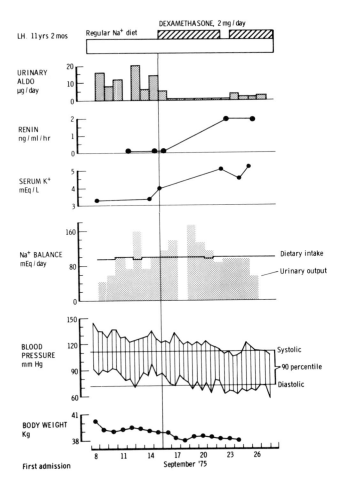

Fig. 5.5 Three families, in which individuals affected with dexamethasone-suppressible hyperaldosteronisn (DSH) are indicated by darkened symbols. The finding of affected individuals of either sex in two successive generations is consistent with autosomal dominant transmission. Adapted from New and coworkers [28], with permission.

lating factor has been implicated in the pathogenesis of hyperaldosteronism [33,34], a consistent relationship between a novel peptide hormone and disorders of aldosterone excess has not been demonstrated. Alternatively, the finding of abnormally high concentrations of the 17α-hydroxylated analogs of 18-hydroxycorticosterone (18-OHB) and aldosterone, that is, 18-hydroxycortisol and 18-oxocortisol [35], in urine from patients with DSH, along with the clinical hormonal findings, suggest that many of the features of DSH can be explained on the basis of defective functional zonation of the adrenal cortex. One hypothesis posits the abnormal persistence of aldosterone-synthesizing capacity in cells of a transitional zone intermediate between the glomerulosa (cells possessing CMO II activity and synthesizing aldosterone mainly in response to renin and angiotensin II) and fasciculata (cells lacking CMO II and responsive to ACTH), which then causes exaggerated mineral-ocorticoid synthesis in response to ACTH [36]. A recent analysis of the patterns of steroid C-18 oxidation in DSH theorizes that a defect involving gene regulation could affect enzyme expression in the zone fasciculata itself [37]. The high index of activity of the cortisol C-18 oxidation pathway in DSH is important in differential diagnosis and contrasts with other forms of aldosteronism.

In children with DSH the hypertension resolves within 10 days to 2 weeks after initiation of glucocor-

Fig. 5.6 Response to dexamethasone in a patient with dexamethasone-suppressible hyperaldosteronism (DSH) (patient 3 in reference [23]). Note the suppression of aldosterone excretion within 24 h of dexamethasone administration, the natriuresis which ensues, followed by weight loss, rise in renin, and the consequent aldosterone rise.

ticoid treatment. In adults, however, the response to glucocorticoids is variable and management of hypertension may require the additional use of one of the standard antihypertensive drugs. This should be a potassium-sparing agent—either spironolactone, which blocks the action of aldosterone by occupying the type I (mineralocorticoid) receptor, or one of either triamterene or amiloride. These act at the distal tubule by a distinct mechanism affecting electrogenic sodium transfer across the membrane. It should be stated that although the etiology of the hypertension in DSH is mineralocorticoid excess, hypokalemia, metabolic alkalosis, and hypervolemia may be absent.

Diagnostically DSH can be distinguished from the above-discussed synthetic defects of steroidogenesis associated with low-renin hypertension by normal growth and sexual development, normal levels of urinary adrenal hydroxycorticoid and ketosteroid metabolites. Apparent mineralocorticoid excess (AME), to be discussed below, differs from DSH in that the hypertension in children with AME is usually exacerbated by administration of glucocorticoids, and patients with AME have minimal to undetectable aldosterone levels.

In summary, DSH is an autosomal dominant form of low-renin hypertension characterized by excess adrenal mineralocorticoid synthesis which is responsive chiefly to factors which traditionally stimulate and suppress glucocorticoid synthesis. The gene causing DSH has not been identified, but molecular genetic techniques of linkage analysis with selected cDNA probes may provide a clue in the future.

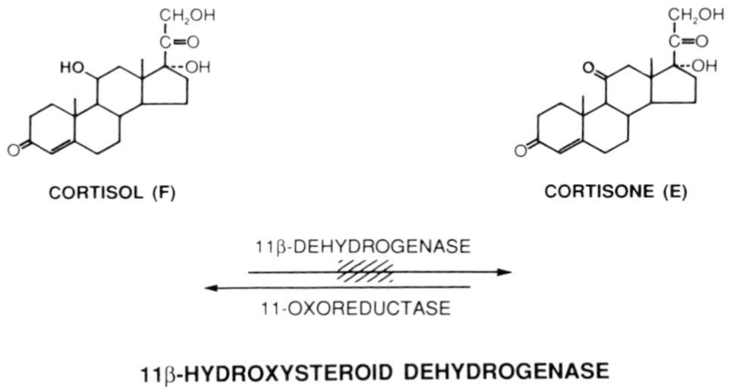

Apparent mineralocorticoid excess

The syndrome of AME (hyporeninemic hypoaldosteronism) results from a deficiency of 11β-hydroxysteroid dehydrogenase, a microsomal enzyme composed of independent 11β-dehydrogenase and 11-oxoreductase components [38] necessary for the interconversion of cortisol (compound F) and cortisone (compound E) (Fig. 5.7). This enzyme deficiency was originally described in a Zuñi Indian girl in whom failure to thrive associated with severe hypertension and hypokalemia was recognized within the first year of life [39]; this patient subsequently died in early adolescence as a result of complications related to intractable hypertension and metabolic abnormalities. Additional salient physiologic derangements found among approximately 24 patients identified to date include delayed plasma clearance of cortisol with normal absolute cortisol levels due to low cortisol secretion rate [40], reduced secretion of all known mineralocorticoids, and suppressed renin unresponsive to low-sodium diet. The urinary steroid profile diagnostic of this condition is a depressed ratio of 11-oxo (cortisone) metabolites relative to 11β-hydroxy metabolites (e.g. the tetrahydrocortisone: tetrahydrocortisol [THE:THE] ratio, normally >1, is ≪1). Of note is the fact that patients with AME are capable of normal conversion of cortisone to cortisol [40,41]. Nephrocalcinosis appears to be more common in AME than in any other form of hypertension and may relate to the severe hypokalemia. A high fatality rate in this disorder has been observed.

It has further been shown that the hypertension,

11β-HYDROXYSTEROID DEHYDROGENASE

Fig. 5.7 Interconversion of cortisol (F) and cortisone (E) by 11β-hydroxysteroid dehydrogenase. In apparent mineralocorticoid excess (AME) there is a defect in the conversion of cortisol to cortisone (11β-dehydrogenase activity) but no defect in conversion of cortisone to cortisol (11-oxoreductase activity).

which is due only in part to sodium retention and volume expansion, is exacerbated by low-dose hydrocortisone or ACTH administration, but not by aldosterone infusion [42]. Type I (i.e. mineralocorticoid) receptor blockade and inhibition of steroid synthesis one step proximal to cortisol are effective in lowering blood pressure. An extensive search for mineralocorticoid activity in blood and urine using bioassay and radioreceptor assay techniques has revealed no excess activity, suggesting that there are no unmeasured mineralocorticoids. It is hypothesized that in this disorder cortisol itself, which cannot be normally metabolized to cortisone, acts as the mineralocorticoid [43,44]. Cortisone is not a ligand for either the mineralocorticoid or glucocorticoid receptor due to the conformational change that occurs when cortisol is converted to cortisone.

Recent advances in the understanding of steroid hormone receptors have shed light on the pathophysiology of AME. Classic aldosterone-binding or type I receptors have been shown to possess equal affinity for glucocorticoids in cytosol preparations devoid of cortisol-binding globulin. *In vivo* studies have repeatedly shown preservation of the classic hierarchy of ligand specificity [45]. Extensive sequence homology has been found for cDNA encoding the mineralocorticoid and glucocorticoid receptors, and expression of the mineralocorticoid cDNA has demonstrated lack of binding specificity, as is seen in cytosol preparations [46]. Clearly some extrinsic factor determines affinity of the type I receptor for various steroid ligands. The observation that licorice ingestion produces an acquired defect in the ability to convert cortisol to cortisone, resulting in a syndrome of hypertension and mineralocorticoid excess which closely mimics AME, has provided strong evidence that this extrinsic factor common to both disorders is the failure to convert intrarenal cortisol to cortisone [47]. Thus, apparent mineralocorticoid excess results from abolition of the physiologic mechanism which protects the renal type I receptors from a 1000-fold excess concentration of cortisol relative to aldosterone. This mechanism also explains why hypertension in AME is extraordinarily severe compared to the hypertension of glucocorticoid excess in Cushing's syndrome where presumably 11β-hydroxysteroid dehydrogenase activity is intact [48] (Table 5.1).

The hypertension and metabolic abnormalities of AME are usually responsive to treatment with mineralocorticoid receptor antagonists, but may re-

Table 5.1 Apparent mineralocorticoid excess (AME)

___

Primary defect
Abnormal 11β-hydroxysteroid dehydrogenase: reduced 11β-dehydrogenase but not 11-oxoreductase activity

Cortisol cannot be metabolized to cortisone

Secondary defects
All cortisol secreted is bioactive since it cannot be converted to cortisone which has no affinity for type I (mineralocorticoid) receptors

Cortisol half-life is prolonged, resulting in normal serum levels

There is suppression of adrenocorticotrophic hormone by the active serum cortisol and decreased secretion of all other corticosteroids

Pathogenesis of hypertension in AME
Because of the 11β-dehydrogenase defect within the cell, type I receptors are not protected from cortisol occupancy

All cortisol entering the cell acts as a mineralocorticoid agonist

Evidence in favor of this model
Hypertension of apparent mineralocorticoid excess (AME) is largely Na$^+$- and volume-dependent

Reversal of symptoms by sodium restriction or type I receptor blockade with spironolactone; exacerbation of symptoms with glucocorticoid administration.

Failure to detect excess mineralocorticoid activity in serum or urine from AME patients in several bioassay systems.

Licorice intoxication produces a syndrome similar to AME; the compound carbenoxolone in licorice has been shown *in vitro* to inhibit 11β-dehydrogenase activity of the 11β-hydroxysteroid dehydrogenase enzyme.

___

quire additional antihypertensive medication. Supplemental potassium is usually also required.

MOLECULAR GENETICS OF 11β-HYDROXYSTEROID DEHYDROGENASE

Enzyme purification [48] and antibody production led to cloning and sequencing of a cDNA for the messenger sequence of rat corticosteroid 11β-dehydrogenase (interconverting corticosterone, or compound B, and 11-dehydrocorticosterone, or compound A [compare Fig. 5.7]). Cell expression of this clone yielded enzyme with both dehydrogenase and reductase activity. Glycyrrhetinic acid, an active principle in licorice, inhibited dehydrogenase activity by 50% and did not affect reductase activity [49]. Cloning and structural analysis have now been achieved for the gene encoding human 11β-hydroxysteroid dehydrogenase [50]. It remains to be determined whether mutations in this gene can be identified in patients with AME. No consistent defect has been identified in obligate heterozygote patients [40,44,51].

Primary hyperaldosteronism

Primary hyperaldosteronism (autonomous overproduction of aldosterone) results in high serum aldosterone levels producing hypertension with low plasma renin activity and hypokalemia. In children, primary hyperaldosteronism is very rare. To date, fewer than 25 cases have been reported [52—58].

In the majority of cases, bilateral adrenal hyperplasia is found in presentations of primary hyperaldosteronism; underlying adrenal adenoma or carcinoma can also be found. Administration of dexamethasone, which causes the complete and rapid suppression of aldosterone secretion that distinguishes DSH, fails to cause any reduction in serum aldosterone levels in primary hyperaldosteronism. In addition, administration of a high-sodium diet does not result in decreased aldosterone excretion as it does in normal children [59]. Twenty-four-hour urinary aldosterone levels can only be interpreted as elevated when sodium excretion is similarly elevated (Fig. 5.8). A study of mineralocorticoid receptors on mononuclear leukocytes has shown that the number of binding sites per cell is significantly lower in patients with primary hyperaldosteronism than in normal subjects [60]. Thus there is down-regulation of the mineralocorticoid receptor in hyperaldosteron-

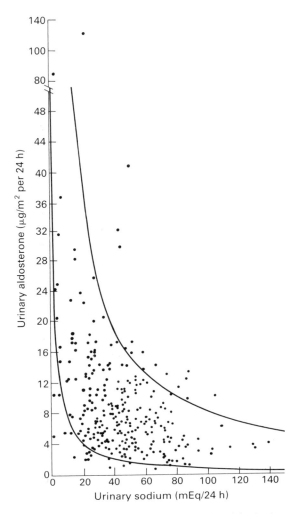

Fig. 5.8 Daily aldosterone excretion (normalized for body surface area) plotted against sodium excretion in 60 normal children aged 1 month to $17\frac{1}{2}$ years. The hyperbolas indicate the 5th and 95th percentiles. From New and coworkers [53], with permission.

ism similar to that documented for some other chronic hormone excess states [61,62]. (Leukocytes from DSH patients in contrast were found to have a normal number of binding sites per cell. This difference may be a function of cyclic as opposed to sustained aldosterone elevation.)

Nuclear magnetic resonance imaging, computerized tomography scan, radioiodocholesterol scans, and bilateral adrenal vein sampling are the diagnostic tools used in the identification and characterization of primary hyperaldosteronism [63,64].

In patients in whom an adrenal adenoma is found, surgery is the treatment of choice. This mode of treatment is less satisfactory in patients with bilateral adrenal hyperplasia, in whom spironolactone at times achieves a better therapeutic result.

SUMMARY

Among the many factors regulating blood pressure are the adrenal steroid hormones. While aldosterone is the classic mineralocorticoid in humans, other precursors to aldosterone may act as mineralocorticoid agonists; examples of such clinical conditions are found in hypertensive congenital adrenal hyperplasia due to 11β-hydroxylase deficiency and 17α-hydroxylase deficiency and in DSH. The regulation of mineralocorticoid receptor specificity by the 11β-hydroxysteroid dehydrogenase enzyme in target tissues appears to provide the most coherent explanation for the syndrome of AME in which cortisol cannot be converted to cortisone due to congenital deficiency of this enzyme. Primary hyperaldosteronism is rare in children, but should be suspected in cases where elevated mineralocorticoid secretion fails to respond to dexamethasone administration and radiographic studies show adrenal enlargement.

ACKNOWLEDGMENTS

Sections of work reported in this chapter have been supported by USPHS grants HD00072, AM06354, and HL17749 from the National Institutes of Health (NIH), and by grant RR47 from the General Clinical Research Centers Program of the Division of Research Resources (NIH). Support from the Horace Goldsmith Foundation is also gratefully acknowledged.

REFERENCES

1 New MI, Levine LS. Congenital adrenal hyperplasia. In: Harris H, Hirschhorn K, eds. *Advances in Human Genetics*, vol 4. New York: Plenum Press, 1973;251–326.

2 White PC, New MI, Dupont B. Congenital adrenal hyperplasia. *N Engl J Med* 1987;316:1519–24.

3 New MI, White PC, Pang S, Dupont B, Speiser PW. The adrenal hyperplasias. In: Scriver CR, Beaudet AL, Sly WS, Valle D, eds. *The Metabolic Basis of Inherited Disease*. 6th edn. New York: McGraw-Hill, 1989;1881–917.

4 Zachmann M, Tassinari D, Prader A. Clinical and biochemical variability of congenital adrenal hyperplasia due to 11β-hydroxylase deficiency. A study of 25 patients. *J Clin Endocrinol Metab* 1983;56:222–9.

5 Ulick S. Diagnosis and nomenclature of the disorders of the terminal portion of the aldosterone biosynthetic pathway. *J Clin Endocrinol Metab* 1976;43:92–6.

6 Griffing GT, Wilson TE, Holbrook MM *et al.* Plasma and

urinary 19-nor-DOC in 17α-hydroxylase deficiency syndrome. *J Clin Endocrinol Metab* 1984;59:1011−15.

7 New MI, Seaman MP. Secretion rates of cortisol and aldosterone precursors in various forms of congenital adrenal hyperplasia. *J Clin Endocrinol Metab* 1970;30:361−71.

8 Levine LS, Rauh W, Gottesdiener K *et al.* New studies of the 11β-hydroxylase and 18-hydroxylase enzymes in the hypertensive form of congenital adrenal hyperplasia. *J Clin Endocrinol Metab* 1980;50:258−63.

9 New MI. Male pseudohermaphroditism due to 17α-hydroxylase deficiency. *J Clin Invest* 1970;49:1030−941.

10 Yanagibashi K, Haniu M, Shively JE, Shen WH, Hall P. The synthesis of aldosterone by the adrenal cortex. *J Biol Chem* 1986;261:3556−61.

11 Kawamoto T, Mitsuuchi Y, Ohnishi T. *et al.* Cloning and expression of a cDNA for human cytochrome P450$_{aldo}$ as related to primary aldosteronism. *Biochem Biophys Res Comm* 1990;173:309−16.

12 Chua SC, Szabo P, Vitek JK, Grzeschik K-H, John M, White PC. Cloning of cDNA encoding steroid 11β-hydroxylase (P450c11). *Proc Natl Acad Sci USA* 1987;84:7193−7.

13 Mornet E, Dupont J, Vitek A, White PC. Characterization of two genes encoding human steroid 11β-hydroxylase (P-45011β). *J Biol Chem* 1989;264:20961−67.

14 White PL, Dupont J, New MI, Leiberman E, Hochberg Z, Rösler A, A mutation in CYP11β1 (Arg$_{448}$→His) associated with steroid 11β-hydroxylase deficiency in Jews of Moroccan origin. *J Clin Invest* 1991 [in press].

15 Rosler A, Leiberman E. Enzymatic defects of steroidogenesis: 11β-hydroxylase deficiency congenital adrenal hyperplasia. In: New MI, Levine LS, eds. *Adrenal Diseases in Childhood.* Basel: S Karger, 1984;47−71.

16 Globerman H, Rösler A, Theodor R, New MI, White PC. An inherited defect in aldosterone biosynthesis caused by a mutation in or near the gene for steroid 11-hydroxylase. *N Engl J Med* 1988;319:1193−7.

17 Chung BC, Picardo-Leonard J, Haniu M *et al.* Cytochrome P450c17 (steroid 17β-hydroxylase/17,20-lyase): cloning of human adrenal testis cDNAs indicates the same gene is expressed in both tissues. *Proc Natl Acad Sci USA* 1987;84:407−11.

18 Matteson KJ, Picardo-Leonard J, Chung B-C, Mohandas TK, Miller WL. Assignment of the gene for adrenal P-450$_{17α}$- (steroid 17α-hydroxylase/17,20 lyase) to human chromosome. *J Clin Endocrinol Metab* 1986;63:789−91.

19 Yanase T, Simpson ER, Waterman MR. 17α-Hydroxylase/17,20-lyase deficiency: from clinical investigation to molecular definition. *Endocrine Rev* [in press].

20 New MI, Peterson RE. A new form of congenital adrenal hyperplasia. *J Clin Endocrinol Metab* 1967;27:300−5.

21 Sutherland DJA, Ruse JL, Laidlaw JC. Hypertension, increased aldosterone secretion, and low plasma renin activity relieved by dexamethasone. *Can Med Assoc J* 1966;95:1109−19.

22 Ganguly A, Grim CE, Weinberger MH. Anomalous postural aldosterone response in glucocorticoid-suppressible hyperaldosteronism. *N. Engl J Med* 1981;305:991−3.

23 Oberfield SE, Levine LS, Stoner E *et al.* Adrenal glomerulosa function in patients with dexamethasone-suppressible hyperaldosteronism. *J Clin Endocrinol Metab* 1981;53:158−64.

24 New MI, Siegal E, Peterson RE. Dexamethasone-suppressible hyperaldosteronism. *J Clin Endocrinol Metab* 1973;37:93−100.

25 Miura K, Yoshinaga K, Goto K *et al.* A case of glucocorticoid-responsive hyperaldosteronism. *J Clin Endocrinol Metab* 1968;28:1807−15.

26 Giebink GS, Gotlin RW, Biglieri EG, Katz FH. A kindred with familial glucocorticoid-suppressible aldosteronism. *J Clin Endocrinol Metab* 1973;36:715−23.

27 Fallo F, Sonino N, Armanini D *et al.* A new family with dexamethasone-suppressible hyperaldosteronism: aldosterone unresponsiveness to angiotensin II. *Clin Endocrinol* 1985;22:777−85.

28 New MI, Oberfield SE, Levine LS. Hypertension in children. In: Genest J, Kuchel O, Hamet P, Cantin M, eds. *Hypertension: Pathophysiology and Treatment.* 2nd edn. New York: McGraw-Hill, 1983;853−89.

29 Fallo F, Boscaro M, Sonino N, Mantero F. Abnormal adrenal responsiveness in dexamethasone-suppressible hyperaldosteronism: further evidence. In: New MI, Borelli P, eds. *Dexamethasone-suppressible Hyperaldosteronism. Serono Symposia Review no. 10.* Rome: Ares Symposia, 1986;105−17.

30 New MI, Peterson RE, Saenger P, Levine LS. Evidence for an unidentified ACTH-induced steroid hormone causing hypertension. *J Clin Endocrinol Metab* 1976;43:1283−93.

31 Lan NC, Matulich DT, Stockigt JR, Biglieri EG, New MI, Baxter JD. Role of steroids in various states of mineralocorticoid excess hypertension: analysis by mineralocorticoid receptor assay. In: Giovannelli G, New MI, Gorini S, eds. *Hypertension in Children and Adolescents.* New York: Raven Press, 1981;165−75.

32 Speiser PW, Martin KO, Kao-Lo G, New MI. Excess mineralocorticoid receptor activity in patients with dexamethasone-suppressible hyperaldosteronism is under adrenocorticotropin control. *J Clin Endocrinol Metab* 1985;61:297−302.

33 Mulrow PJ. Glucocorticoid-suppressible hyperaldosteronism: a clue to the missing hormone? *N Engl J Med* 1981;305:1012−14.

34 Carey RM, Sen S, Dolan LM, Malchoff CD, Bumpus FM. Idiopathic hyperaldosteronism: a possible role for aldosterone-stimulating factor. *N Engl J Med* 1984;311:94−100.

35 Ulick S, Chan CK. Physiological insights derived from the search for unknown steroids in low renin essential hypertension. In: Montero F, Scoggins BA, Takeda R, Biglieri EG, Funder JW, eds. *The Adrenal and Hypertension: From Cloning to Clinic* (Serono Symposia, vol. 57). New York: Raven Press, 1989;313−22.

36 Gomez-Sanchez CE, Gill JR Jr, Ganguly A, Gordon RD. Glucocorticoid-suppressible aldosteronism: a disorder of the adrenal transitional zone. *J Clin Endocrinol Metab* 1988;67:444−8.

37 Ulick S, Chan CK, Gill JR Jr, Gutkin M, Letcher L, Mantero F, New MI. Defective fasciculata zone function as the mechanism of glucocorticoid-remediable aldosteronism. *J Clin Endocrinol Metab* 1990;71:1151−7.

38 Lakshmi V, Monder C. Evidence for independent 11-oxidase and 11-reductase activities of 11β-hydroxysteroid dehydrogenase: enzyme latency, phase transitions, and lipid requirements. *Endocrinology* 1985;116:552−60.

39 New MI, Levine LS, Biglieri EG, Pareira J, Ulick S. Evidence for an unidentified steroid in a child with apparent mineralocorticoid excess hypertension. *J Clin Endocrinol Metab* 1977;44:924—33.

40 Ulick S, Levine LS, Gunczler P *et al*. A syndrome of apparent mineralocorticoid excess associated with defects in the peripheral metabolism of cortisol. *J Clin Endocrinol Metab* 1979;49:757—64.

41 Monder C, Shackleton CHL, Bradlow HL *et al*. The syndrome of apparent mineralocorticoid excess: its association with 11β-dehydrogenase and 5β-reductase deficiency and some consequences for corticosteroid metabolism. *J Clin Endocrinol Metab* 1986;63:550—7.

42 Oberfield SE, Levine LS, Carey RM, Greig F, Ulick S, New MI. Metabolic and blood pressure responses to hydrocortisone in the syndrome of apparent mineralocorticoid excess. *J Clin Endocrinol Metab* 1983;56:332—9.

43 New MI, Oberfield SE, Carey R, Greig F, Ulick S, Levine LS. A genetic defect in cortisol metabolism as the basis for the syndrome of apparent mineralocorticoid excess. In: Mantero F, Biglieri EG, Edwards CRW, eds. *Endocrinology of Hypertension* (Proceedings of the Serono Symposia, vol. 50). New York: Academic Press, 1982:85—101.

44 Stewart PM, Corrie JET, Shackleton CHL, Edwards CRW. Syndrome of apparent mineralocorticoid excess, a defect in the cortisol—cortisone shuttle. *J Clin Invest* 1988;82:340—9.

45 Funder JW, Pearce PT, Smith R, Smith AI. Mineralocorticoid action: target tissue specificity is enzyme, not receptor, mediated. *Science* 1988;242:583—5.

46 Arriza JL, Weinberger C, Cerelli G *et al*. Cloning of human mineralocorticoid receptor complementary DNA: structural and functional kinship with the glucocorticoid receptor. *Science* 1987;237:268—75.

47 Stewart PM, Wallace AM, Valentino R, Burt D, Shackleton CHL, Edwards CRW. Mineralocorticoid activity of liquorice: 11-β-hydroxysteroid dehydrogenase deficiency comes of age. *Lancet* 1987;ii:821—4.

48 Lakshmi V, Monder C. Purification and characterization of the corticosteroid 11β-dehydrogenase component of the rat liver 11β-hydroxysteroid dehydrogenase complex. *Endocrinology* 1988;123:2390—8.

49 Agarwal AK, Monder C, Eckstein B, White PC. Cloning and expression of rat cDNA encoding corticosteroid 11β-dehydrogenase. *J Biol Chem* 1989;264:18939—43.

50 Tannin GM, Agarwal AK, Monder C, New MI, White PC. The human gene for 11β-hydroxysteroid dehydrogenase: structure, tissue distribution and chromosomal localization.

[*J Biol Chem*, submitted, (1991)]

51 DiMartino-Nardi J, Stoner E, Martin K, Balfe JW, Jose PA, New MI. New findings in apparent mineralocorticoid excess. *Clin Endocrinol* 1987;27:49—62.

52 Baer L, Sommers SC, Krakoff LR, Newton MA, Laragh JH. Pseudoprimary aldosteronism. *Circ Res* 1970;26/27 (suppl 1):203—16.

53 Bryer-Ash M, Wilson D, Tune BM, Rosenfeld RG, Shochat SJ, Leutscher J. Hypertension caused by an aldosterone secreting adrenal. *Am J Dis Child* 1986;128:673—6.

54 Decsi J, Soltesz G, Harangi F, Nemes J, Szabo M, Pinter A. Severe hypertension in 10-year-old boy secondary to an aldosterone producing tumor identified by adrenal sonography. *Acta Pediatr Hung* 1986;27:233—8.

55 George JM, Wright L, Bell NH, Bartter FC. The syndrome of primary aldosteronism. *Am J Med* 1970;48:343—56.

56 Grim CE, McBryde AC, Glenn JF, Gunnells JC. Childhood primary aldosteronism with bilateral adrenocortical hypertension: plasma renin activity as an aid to diagnosis. *J Pediatr* 1967;71:377—83.

57 New MI, Peterson RE. Aldosterone in childhood. In: Levine SZ, ed. *Advances in Pediatrics*. Chicago: Year Book, 1968;111—36.

58 Oberfield SE, Levine LS, Firpo A *et al*. Primary hyperaldosteronism in childhood due to unilateral macronodular hyperplasia. *Hypertension* 1984;6:75—84.

59 New MI, Baum CJ, Levine LS. Nomograms relating aldosterone excretion to urinary sodium and potassium in the pediatric population: their application to the study of childhood hypertension. *Am J Cardiol* 1976;37:658—66.

60 Armanini D, Witzgall H, Wehling M, Kuhnle U, Weber PC. Aldosterone receptors in different types of primary hyperaldosteronism. *J Clin Endocrinol Metab* 1987;65:101—4.

61 Clayton RN (ed). Receptors in health and disease. *Clin Endocrinol Metab* 1985;12:1.

62 Schlechte JA, Ginsberg BH, Sherman BM. Regulation of the glucocorticoid receptor in human lymphocytes. *J Steroid Biochem* 1982;16:69.

63 Melby JC. Diagnosis and treatment of primary aldosteronism and isolated hypoaldosteronism. In: DeGroot LJ, ed. *Endocrinology*, vol 2. Philadelphia: WB Saunders, 1989:1705—13.

64 Herd GW, Semple PF, Parker D, Davidson JK, Hilditch TE, Fraser R. False localization of an aldosteronoma by dexamethasone-suppressed adrenal scintigraphy. *Clin Endocrinol* 1987;26:699—705.

6 Measurement of Blood Pressure

DAVID E. FIXLER

During the 1970s considerable research was directed toward elucidating those factors that determine blood pressure levels in children. Knowledge of the factors that affect the measurement of blood pressure is important not only to the epidemiologist who is primarily interested in identifying precursors of high blood pressure but also to the clinician who relies upon epidemiologic data to define the normal range of blood pressure in children. Unfortunately, in the past, methodologic differences have resulted in inconsistent findings among various studies and it has become apparent that in order to make group comparisons or to track blood pressures in individuals over time, proper measurement requires meticulous attention to methodologic details. The purpose of this chapter is to provide the reader with a better understanding of the technical and physiologic factors that influence results of blood pressure measurements.

STANDARD METHODS OF MEASUREMENT

Auscultation sphygmomanometry

Accurate determinations of blood pressure can be carried out in infants and children provided attention is paid to specific details. Most important is the selection of a properly sized inflatable bladder within the blood pressure cuff. The bladder should be long enough to encircle the extremity completely or nearly completely. There is no evidence that a bladder which slightly overlaps leads to erroneous measurements. For infants and young children, it has been demonstrated that it is necessary to use a bladder cuff whose width equals or exceeds two-thirds the length of the extremity [1]. The recommended ideal bladder dimensions according to arm size are listed in Table 8.4 (p. 94). It is emphasized

that the selection of the proper cuff-bladder is based on the size of the arm, not the age group of the child. When narrower or shorted cuff-bladders are used, spuriously high blood pressure measurements are obtained.

The blood pressure cuff should be wrapped snugly around the extremity since falsely elevated readings will also result when the cuff is applied loosely. While palpating the brachial arterial pulse, the cuff should be inflated above the point where the pulse disappears. During deflation, at a rate of 2–3 mmHg/beat, the point when the pulse is first palpated approximates systolic pressure. After complete deflation, the stethoscope is placed lightly over the brachial artery. The cuff is then rapidly inflated to about 30 mmHg above the estimated systolic pressure level. The pressure is slowly released and the onset of a clear tapping sound defines the systolic blood pressure. With further release of cuff pressure, the tap becomes low-pitched, muffled, and less intense; this indicates the phase IV level. All three values should be recorded: systolic, diastolic (muffling), and diastolic (disappearance). Phase IV has been recommended as the measure of diastolic blood pressure in infants and preadolescent children [2]. With further cuff deflation, the phase V is characterized by the disappearance of these sounds altogether. The phase V blood pressure level has been recommended as a measure of diastolic blood pressure in adolescent children and adults [3]. Although the choice of diastolic Korotkoff phases in children may be controversial, the 1987 normal standards for children's blood pressure are based on using phase IV for children under 13 years of age and phase V for older adolescents.

Since the level of arterial pressure is profoundly influenced by anxiety, the child should be approached in a nonthreatening manner and sufficient time should be allowed for recovery from recent

74

stimuli. The child should be reassured by having the procedure fully explained and should be sitting in a comfortable position with the right arm fully exposed at the level of the heart. The examiner should be comfortable and have an unobstructed view of the sphygmomanometer at eye level to avoid errors of parallax. Sufficient time should elapse between cuff inflations, since rapid successive inflations lead to venous congestion and increased pressure measurements.

The aneroid and the mercury manometers are the most common instruments in general use. Both give accurate results; however, the mercury manometer does not require recalibration. Mercury needs to be added to the reservoir when the edge of the meniscus is below the zero mark. Although less bulky, the aneroid manometer requires regular calibration against a mercury manometer depending on the frequency of use. For example, in a hypertension clinic it may have to be done monthly. The calibrations should be made at several points over the entire pressure range. If after complete deflation the needle does not rest on zero, the instrument needs to be adjusted and recalibrated. Aneroid manometers constructed with stop-pins should not be used as they may be out of calibration when they are on zero and this will not be apparent to the user.

Flush method

This method has been used to estimate arterial pressure when difficulty is encountered in hearing the Korotkoff sounds in small infants [4]. It is still a useful method when more modern instrumentation is not available. The blood pressure cuff is applied just proximal to the wrist or ankle and the hand or foot is wrapped snugly with an elastic bandage to drain it of blood. Wrapping should start at the distal portion of the extremity and proceed toward the blood pressure cuff. Following firm wrapping, the cuff is inflated to above systolic levels and the elastic bandage is quickly removed. The pressure is slowly released at a rate of 2−3 mmHg/s and the pressure level is noted at the point where there is definite flushing of the previously blanched extremity. The procedure requires two examiners, one to observe the distal extremity and the other to observe the level of cuff pressure. Moss and Adams [5] have reported that during the first 9 months of life, flush blood pressure may be slightly greater in the hand than in the foot.

Doppler ultrasound

The Doppler method is preferable to the flush method for measurement of bood pressure in infants since it is simpler to perform and provides a more accurate measure of systolic blood pressure. This method is based on the Doppler phenomenon, i.e. when sound waves are reflected off a moving object, a shift in frequency occurs. For this technique, a small transducer is placed over a systemic artery and ultrasonic waves are transmitted through the subcutaneous tissue, muscle, arterial wall, and blood cells. During blood pressure determination, the cuff is applied in the conventional manner and inflated above systolic pressure. During deflation, systolic and diastolic pressures are determined by the change in frequency of the sound beam reflected off the pulsatile vessel wall or off the moving blood cells.

The simplest Doppler device uses a small skin transducer that is applied over an artery distal to the blood pressure cuff (Parks Electronics Laboratory, Beaverton, OR). In this method, the Doppler ultrasound beam is reflected off blood cells flowing in the artery. When the cuff is inflated above systolic pressure, blood flow ceases; therefore no change in sound frequency occurs and no audible signal is generated. At the systolic pressure level flow commences and the ultrasonic beam undergoes a shift in frequency producing an audible signal which is proportional to blood flow velocity. Systolic pressure is taken at the first audible signal. However, diastolic pressure cannot be determined since blood flow velocity does not change at this pressure level.

Despite this limitation, the method is particularly suitable for measuring systolic blood pressure in infants under office conditions. Elseed and coworkers [6] performed validation studies in small infants and children using direct intra-arterial measurements for standard reference. They demonstrated that the Doppler technique was more accurate than standard auscultation, palpation, or flush methods (Table 6.1). In this study, flush pressure was significantly correlated with systolic blood pressure but not with mean pressure. The Doppler technique was also found to be useful in measuring lower-extremity systolic pressure in the presence of aortic coarctation.

A second Doppler technique has been developed for measuring both systolic and diastolic blood pressure based on ultrasonic detection of arterial wall motion. The small movement of an uncompressed artery does not generate an audible ultrasonic signal;

Table 6.1 Comparisons of indirect sphygmomanometry: differences from intra-arterial measurements of systolic pressure [6]

Indirect methods	Mean ± SD (mmHg)	P
Flush	41.8 ± 10.5	<0.001
Palpation	10.3 ± 7.6	<0.001
Auscultation	2.9 ± 6.5	NS
Doppler*	2.2 ± 7.1	NS

* Doppler signal generated by intra-arterial blood flow.

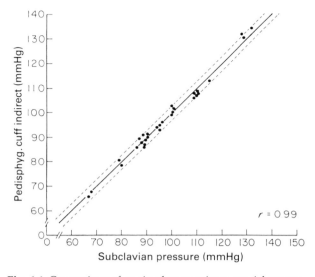

Fig. 6.1 Comparison of 30 simultaneous intra-arterial versus Parks Ultrasonic Doppler flow detector systolic pressure determinations. The solid line is the line of identity; broken lines represent ±3 mmHg from the line of identity. From Reder and coworkers [7].

however, when the cuff is inflated to a pressure level between systolic and diastolic blood pressure, the artery opens and closes with each pulse. When the cuff is inflated above systolic pressure the artery remains closed and no Doppler signal is generated. As the cuff pressure falls to the level of systolic pressure, the first movement of the arterial wall occurs and produces opening and closing signals. As the cuff pressure continues to drop, the opening and closing signals come closer together, becoming one at the diastolic pressure point. When the Doppler signals are graphically recorded, cuff pressure at the first signal equals systolic pressure; at the first merging of the opening and closing signals it equals diastolic pressure.

Validation studies of this technique have been carried out in children comparing the Arteriosonde instrument (Roche Medical Electronics, Cranberry, NJ) and the Parks Ultrasonic Doppler flow detector with simultaneously recorded intra-arterial pressures [7]. Figure 6.1 demonstrates that the Parks Doppler flow detector accurately estimated intra-arterial systolic pressure (*r* = 0.99). Figures 6.2 and 6.3 show a similar comparison for the Arteriosonde instrument. Although significant correlations were found, note that for systolic blood pressure, the Arteriosonde tended to underestimate intra-arterial systolic pressure. Diastolic pressure could be measured with the Arteriosonde instrument but it was less accurately determined than systolic pressure. These data indicate that in children, Doppler devices based on detection of blood flow velocity give more reliable estimates of systolic blood pressure. Doppler devices which detect arterial wall motion tend to yield less accurate systolic pressure but do provide estimates of diastolic pressure.

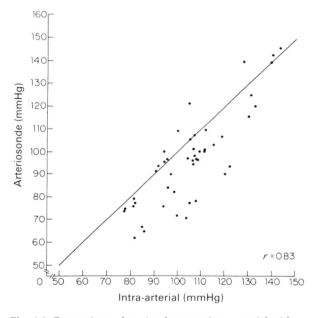

Fig. 6.2 Comparison of 47 simultaneous intra-arterial with Arteriosonde systolic pressure measurements. The solid line is the line of identity. Note that the Arteriosonde tends to underestimate intra-arterial systolic pressure. From Reder and coworkers [7].

Oscillometry

This method is based on the fact that arterial pulsations may be transmitted through a partially in-

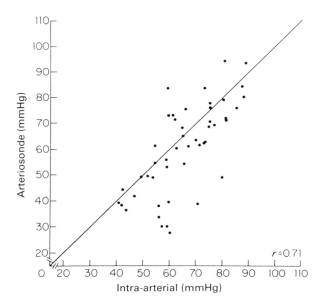

Fig. 6.3 Comparison of 48 simultaneous intra-arterial with Arteriosonde diastolic pressure measurements. The solid line is the line of identity. Note the wide scatter on both sides of the line of identity. From Reder and coworkers [7].

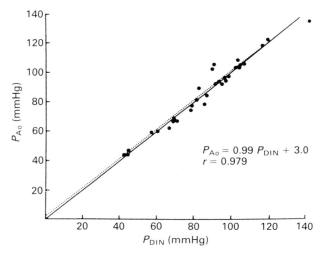

Fig. 6.4 Comparison of simultaneous central aortic with Dinamap systolic pressure measurements. The linear regression equation and correlation coefficient (r) are given. The solid line is the line of identity, the dotted line is the regression line. From Colan and coworkers [8].

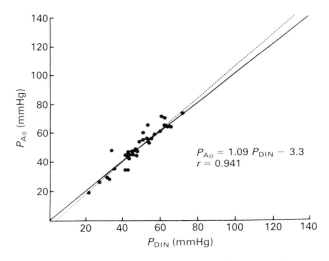

Fig. 6.5 Comparison of simultaneous central aortic with Dinamap diastolic pressure measurements. The linear regression equation and correlation coefficient are given. The solid line is the line of identity; the dotted line is the regression line. From Colan and coworkers [8].

flated blood pressure cuff and produce oscillations in the mercury column or the needle of an aneroid manometer. In standard oscillometry, as cuff pressure is lowered, the artery expands slightly as the systolic pressure wave arrives at the constricting cuff and causes the first oscillations to appear, indicating the systolic pressure level. As cuff pressure reaches the diastolic level, the oscillations become maximal since the artery is fully open at systole and closed at diastole. Unfortunately, with the simple standard technique, the arterial pulse pressure often impinges on the edge of the cuff, giving rise to oscillations at pressures above systolic levels. More sophisticated instruments have been developed that use the oscillometric principle (Dinamap, Critikon, FL) to record systolic, diastolic, and mean blood pressures automatically. Colan and colleagues [8] have compared measurements using this instrument with those recorded simultaneously in the central aorta (Figs 6.4 and 6.5). The correlation coefficient for systolic pressure was 0.98 and for diastolic pressure 0.94. In all, 75% of the systolic pressures by Dinamap were within 5 mmHg of the central aortic values, and 84% of the diastolic pressure measurements were within 5 mmHg of the aortic diastolic values. These data indicate that the Dinamap measures diastolic pressure more accurately in infants and small children than any currently available Doppler instrument.

This device also has the advantage of not using a transducer, which may be displaced by patient movement.

Infrasonic method

The Physiometrics recorder (Sphygmetrics) uses the following method to detect Korotkoff sounds. A small microphone transducer is positioned under the bladder of the blood pressure cuff directly over the artery. The low-frequency vibrations of the Korotkoff sounds activate the transducer and are converted to electronic signals which move a mechanical pen. The signals are recorded on a circular paper disc, along with the decreasing cuff pressure. Systolic and diastolic pressures are determined by comparing the Korotkoff signals with the cuff pressure signals. The Physiometrics automatic blood pressure recorder uses a rigid cuff with an inner inflatable bladder. The subject's arm is inserted into the cuff. When the rigid cuff is used in small children, systolic and diastolic blood pressures are underestimated because the bladder is too large.

Validation studies comparing the Physiometrics instrument with a standard mercury sphygmomanometer are shown in Figure 6.6 [9]. Note that both systolic and diastolic pressure readings were lower in younger children and higher in older children when determined by the Physiometrics recorder as compared to conventional mercury sphygmomanometer. Other studies in children 2–5 years of age have indicated an even greater underestimation

of systolic and diastolic blood pressure by the Physiometrics instrument [10].

Random-zero sphygmomanometer

This instrument is similar in principle to the standard mercury sphygmomanometer except that a mechanical device is interposed between the mercury reservoir and the mercury column [11]. When measuring the blood pressure, the observer spins a wheel which alters the height of the mercury column between 0 and 60 mm. As a result, the true zero cannot be determined by the observer until the end of the reading. After spinning the wheel, the blood pressure is taken in the standard manner, recording the height of the mercury column at the systolic and diastolic pressure points. The observer then determines the zero offset and subtracts this value from the observed readings. A major disadvantage of this instrument in children is that, in the unmodified device, the cuff pressure must be inflated 60 mmHg above systolic pressure; this often causes discomfort that may alter the child's blood pressure. The device may be purchased with a smaller variable chamber so that the

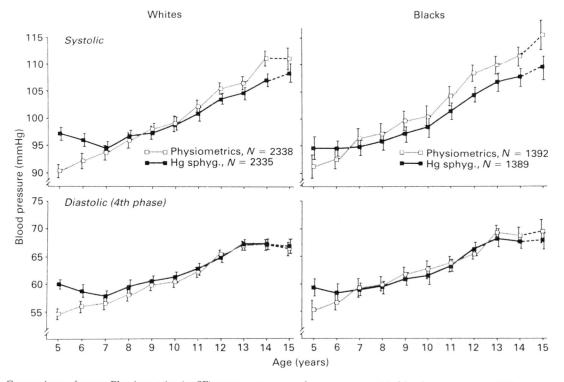

Fig. 6.6 Comparison of mean Physiometrics (± SE) versus mercury sphygmomanometric blood pressures in children 5–15 years of age. From Voors and coworkers [9].

zero offset is reduced to 0 and 30 mmHg, which lessens the chance of inflation artifact. This instrument was designed to be used in research studies to reduce observer bias.

Barker and coworkers [12] have compared blood pressures measured by a standard mercury sphygmomanometer (Baumanometer) with those obtained by using Doppler ultrasound (Arteriosonde 1216), infrasound (Physiometrics SR-2), and random-zero (Gelman-Hawksley) devices in adolescents. Concurrent validity was estimated by computing the average of three serial readings with each instrument in all subjects. The data in Table 6.2 from this study allow comparisons of the measurements recorded by the four instruments. The random-zero device yielded results closest to those obtained with the standard mercury manometer. The Physiometrics measurements of systolic and diastolic pressure were significantly lower than the Baumanometer, probably due to the use of oversized, rigid cuffs.

SOURCES OF VARIABILITY IN BLOOD PRESSURE

Since 1970, several large blood pressure surveys have been performed in pediatric populations to determine the range of normal values for children. In 1977, the Task Force on blood pressure control in children published normal standards for school-age children [2]. Since this publication, several other pediatric surveys have reported results which are significantly different from those of the Task Force [13]. After reviewing the various reports, it is evident that the discrepancies between the studies were due in large part to methodologic differences. When comparing an individual child's blood pressure to normal standards, it is important to consider whether the conditions of measurement were similar. If conditions were significantly different from those under which the standards were obtained, then a child's blood pressure status may be misclassified. Therefore, one needs to be familiar with the standard conditions and to reproduce those conditions as closely as possible.

Variability due to techniques of measurement

The potential for error in measuring blood pressure may be greater in children because the wide range of arm sizes makes selection of proper blood pressure cuffs critical. The effect of arm size on blood pressure may be eliminated when the width of the bladder is appropriate and the length encircles at least 90% of the arm circumference. High readings may also result if the cuff is re-inflated before venous congestion is relieved. During cuff deflation, re-inflation should never be done to ascertain a pressure point. The cuff should be completely deflated first and the arm held vertically for several seconds to relieve venous congestion before re-inflation. The arm itself should be supported at the level of the heart to prevent venous pooling. The pressure exerted on the head of the stethoscope affects the accuracy of auscultatory blood pressure measurement. Londe and colleagues [14] have demonstrated that as little as 10 mmHg pressure exerted on the head of the stethoscope produces a significant lowering of diastolic blood pressure. With firm pressure, it is common to obtain diastolic readings down to zero. If review of records reveals frequent zero diastolic readings, then the examiners need to be cautioned about this measurement artifact.

Observer bias is another important source of measurement error. Many examiners have an unconscious preference for certain digits. This will result in higher frequencies of certain terminal digit readings on their blood pressure records. Examination of the records for this tendency may be useful in identifying those examiners who need further training. When a specific blood pressure level is used as a cutpoint for classifying subjects, some examiners may unconsciously put marginal readings consistently above or below the cutpoint. This type of bias led to the development of the random-zero device which blinds the examiner to the true level of blood pressure.

Table 6.2 Instrument comparisons of measured pressures (mmHg) in 24 adolescent girls [12]

Instrument	Systolic	Diastolic phase IV	Diastolic phase V
Baumanometer	108.2 ± 7.5 (SD)	70.3 ± 8.0	57.3 ± 11.6
Random-zero	104.1 ± 6.7	68.4 ± 10.0	53.8 ± 12.0
Arteriosonde 1216	104.0 ± 9.4	67.6 ± 9.8	
Physiometrics SR-2	100.3 ± 8.9	61.2 ± 8.6	

The number of measurements taken at a single examination is also a factor which affects the average and variability of blood pressure readings. In the Bogalusa study [15] the first systolic reading averaged 2 mmHg higher than the third systolic reading, while diastolic pressures did not differ. Cases with high readings on the first measurement tend to show a larger decrease on the next reading. Such cases may be misclassified if the average value is compared to normal tables of single blood pressure determinations. The 1987 normal values published by the Task Force on blood pressure control in children [3] are based on single blood pressure measurements recorded in seated children. If these tables are chosen as a reference standard, then single measurements should be recorded.

Environmental factors at the location of examination have been shown to affect blood pressure levels. In the Minneapolis study [16] room temperature, time of day, and season were found to be significant variables. Systolic blood pressure decreased, whereas diastolic pressure increased with higher room temperatures. However, in the moderate range of 68–76°F, room temperature did not have an important effect on the blood pressure level of children. With regard to seasonal variations, systolic pressures were significantly higher in the spring than those recorded in winter, whereas diastolic pressures in the spring were lower than those in winter. Although diastolic pressures exhibited minimal daytime differences, systolic pressures measured in the morning were approximately 2 mmHg lower than those measured in the afternoon, reflecting normal diurnal variation in pressure.

Variability due to variation in the state of the subject

Controversy remains as to whether casual or basal blood pressures should be recorded. The answer to this controversy depends upon how the measurements are going to be used. If it is essential for the investigator to minimize the intra-individual variability in blood pressure, then basal blood pressures should be recorded. If the measured values, collected in a clinical setting, are to be compared with the 1987 standards, then casual pressures are most appropriate. With casual determinations, it is important to measure pressure after the child has been reassured and has been positioned comfortably for at least 3 or 4 min. When these precautions are taken, little differences are found between average casual and basal values [13].

Situations which evoke apprehension in children result in higher blood pressure levels. Blood pressures may be affected by performing venipunctures or exercise stress tests on the day of examination. Data from the National Health Survey [17] indicate that mean systolic pressure prior to venipuncture was approximately 5 mmHg higher than pressures measured after venipuncture. Physical activity is known to influence blood pressure, therefore it is imperative that sufficient time elapses before the pressure is measured. During the National Health Survey examinations submaximal exercise tests were performed, consisting of a 5-min walk on a treadmill surface. Among the adolescents, systolic pressure measured within 20 min of exercise averaged 7 mmHg higher than pressures measured either before the exercise or after a recovery period of longer than 20 min. Therefore, the carryover effect of physical activity should be taken into consideration before a measurement is made.

Measurement of blood pressure in infants warrants special consideration. Vigorous crying in the infant is comparable to physical exertion in the older child and its effects will carry over for several minutes. Blood pressures recorded in newborn infants while they were sucking have shown that systolic pressures averaged 6 mmHg and diastolic 3 mmHg higher than pressures taken when they were awake but not sucking [18]. The 1987 standards for blood pressures in infants were derived primarily from data obtained on infants from Pittsburgh [19], London [20], and Providence [21]. Measurements were made with the infants resting quietly or sleeping. In the London study, awake infants had systolic blood pressures that were higher than sleeping infants. During the first week of life, the difference was approximately 5 mmHg and at 6 weeks it averaged 7 mmHg. Beyond 1 year of age, the infants were awake but neither crying nor feeding at the time of the measurement. This indicates that an infant needs to be resting quietly at the time of the pressure measurement for meaningful comparisons with normal standards.

AMBULATORY BLOOD PRESSURE MEASUREMENT

Over the past several years medical technology has developed methods for measuring ambulatory blood pressures during routine activities throughout a 24-h period. Some children may be apprehensive enough to give falsely high readings under the usual clinical conditions and this could result in their being misclassified as hypertensive. One rationale for using ambulatory blood pressure monitoring in children is to identify those children who may be misclassified by office measurements. Also the technique can be used to verify that a child is receiving effective antihypertensive therapy.

The equipment for ambulatory monitoring of pressure consists of a standard blood pressure cuff taped around the upper arm. Some instruments use a small microphone transducer positioned under the cuff and over the brachial artery. Cuff inflation is either automatic over preselected intervals, usually 7.5 or 15 min or semiautomatic, whereby the patient activates the cuff inflation by pushing a button. The microphone over the artery senses the appearance and disappearance of the Korotkoff sounds. Signals from the transducer are stored on tape or a solid-state memory. The 24-h recordings are processed and edited by computer programs designed to eliminate spurious readings, e.g. diastolic pressure greater than systolic pressure, diastolic pressure less than 30 mmHg, pulse pressure less than 10 mmHg, change in pressure from previous or subsequent readings greater than 40 mmHg. Since editing programs vary, it is essential for the user to know the specific editing criteria. The output formats available provide printouts of 24-h average systolic/diastolic pressure, average systolic/diastolic pressure during sleep, average systolic/diastolic pressure during work, frequency of elevated pressures during these periods, and graphic display of hourly average systolic/diastolic pressures. Prior to starting the 24-h recordings, pressures need to be recorded simultaneously with a standard manometer for calibration. Recalibration should be performed at the end of the 24-h period to ensure that the cuff and transducer have not been displaced. During the day the compact pressure monitor is carried with a shoulder strap and at night the device is placed on the night table during sleep. Since some individuals complain of having their sleep disturbed during cuff inflation, less frequent measurements can be taken during sleep.

Berglund and coworkers [22] tested the validity of a Del Mar Avionics Pressurometer by comparing the automatic and the conventional auscultatory measurement of blood pressure before and during exercise. Their results showed very good agreement between systolic and diastolic blood pressures measured by these two methods. The reproducibility of ambulatory blood pressure measurements was evaluated by Weber and colleagues [23] who compared blood pressure recordings from two 24-h study periods, 2–8 weeks apart. The average of all systolic pressures measured during the second study day was within 10 mmHg of the average measured on the first day in 79% of the subjects; diastolic pressure averages were within 5 mmHg in 65% of the subjects. Pickering [24] has discussed the role of ambulatory blood pressure monitoring in adults with hypertension.

Scanty information has been published on ambulatory blood pressures in children. Kennedy and co-authors [25], in their studies of ambulatory blood pressure in 72 healthy males, included 7 subjects who were 10–19 years old. The 24-h mean systolic pressure was 115 ± 11 (SD) mmHg; diastolic pressure was 60 ± 12 mmHg. In this study the frequency of elevated readings in normal children was based on adult criteria, i.e. systolic pressure above 140 mmHg or diastolic pressure above 90 mmHg. Use of adult criteria in children should be avoided since it will underestimate the frequency of elevated pressures in an individual child. Figure 6.7 displays the hourly average systolic and diastolic pressures in 10 hypertensive and 9 normotensive 17-year-old boys [26]. Note that the diurnal trends parallel each other, with systolic pressure being higher in the afternoon and evening, and lowest during sleep. The systolic pressure difference between the normotensive and hypertensive boys was greatest in the afternoon. However, among individual boys there was considerable overlap between the two groups. During afternoon classes 11% of the normotensive and 80% of the hypertensive boys had average systolic or diastolic pressures above the 95th percentile. Also, during this time period, individual normotensive boys frequently had elevated blood pressure, ranging from 4 to 75% of the recordings.

Unfortunately no single criterion from ambulatory blood pressure data clearly classifies individuals as being normotensive or hypertensive. For adults, most authors have defined abnormal as being a level 2 SD above the average pressure for 24-h, daytime, or nighttime periods. To estimate the average and the standard deviations, it was necessary to record 24-h ambulatory pressures in a large number of adults. This approach with children is impractical since it would require doing 24-h ambulatory blood pressure monitoring in a large sample of children at each age. It was difficult enough to obtain a concensus for normal standards of resting blood pressure in children. Since the 1987 Task Force standards [3] for resting pressure in school-age children were derived from measurements recorded at school, it seems

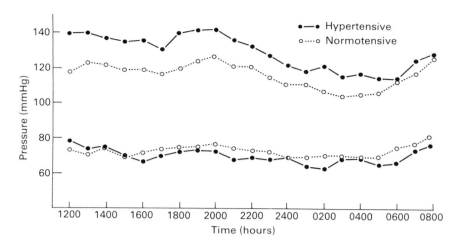

Fig. 6.7 Diurnal hourly average systolic and diastolic blood pressures in hypertensive (solid line) and normotensive (dotted line) 17-year-old boys. Note that the systolic pressures are highest in the afternoon and evening, and systolic pressure differences between the two groups are greatest during these times. From Fixler and coworkers [26].

reasonable to compare the average ambulatory blood pressures at school with these normal standards. However, validation studies of ambulatory blood pressures in children are needed to provide more specific guidelines for their interpretation.

REFERENCES

1 Steinfeld L, Dimich I, Reder R, Cohen M, Alexander H. Sphygmomanometry in the pediatric patient. *J Pediatr* 1978;92:934–8.

2 Report of the Task Force on Blood Pressure Control in Children. National Heart, Lung, and Blood Institute. *Pediatrics* 1977;59:797–820.

3 Report of the Second Task Force on Blood Pressure Control in Children. National Heart, Lung, and Blood Institute. *Pediatrics* 1987;79:1–25.

4 Goldring D, Wohltmann H. Flush method for blood pressure determinations in newborn infants. *J Pediatr* 1952;40:285–9.

5 Moss AJ, Adams FH. *Problems of Blood Pressure in Childhood.* Springfield, Illinois: Charles C. Thomas, 1962.

6 Elseed AM, Shinebourne EA, Joseph MC. Assessment of techniques for measurement of blood pressure in infants and children. *Arch Dis Child* 1973;48:932–6.

7 Reder RF, Dimich I, Cohen ML, Steinfeld L. Evaluating indirect blood pressure measurement techniques: a comparison of three systems in infants and children. *Pediatrics* 1978;62:326–30.

8 Colan SD, Fuji A, Borow KM, MacPherson D, Sanders SP. Noninvasive determination of systolic, diastolic, and end-systolic blood pressure in neonates, infants, and young children: comparison with central aortic pressure measurements. *Am J Cardiol* 1983;52:867–70.

9 Voors AW, Foster TA, Frerichs RR, Webber LS, Berenson GS. Studies of blood pressures in children, ages 5–15 years, in a total biracial community: the Bogalusa heart study. *Circulation* 1976;54:319–27.

10 Voors AW, Webber LS, Berenson GS. Blood pressure of children, ages $2\frac{1}{2}$–$5\frac{1}{2}$ years, in a total community—the Bogalusa heart study. *Am J Epidemiol* 1978;107:403–11.

11 Labarthe DR, Hawkins CM, Remington RD. Evaluation of performance of selected devices for measuring blood pressure. *Am J Cardiol* 1973;32:546–53.

12 Barker WF, Hediger ML, Katz SH, Bowers EJ. Current validity studies of blood pressure instrumentation. *Hypertension* 1984;6:85–91.

13 Fixler DE, Kautz JA, Dana K. Systolic blood pressure differences among pediatric epidemiological studies. *Hypertension* 1980;2(suppl I):I-3–7.

14 Londe S, Klitzner TS, Moss AJ. Effects of pressure exerted on the stethoscope head on auscultatory blood pressure. In: Loggie JMH, Horan MJ, Gruskin AB, Hohn AR, Dunbar JB, Hanlik RJ, eds. *NHLBI Workshop on Juvenile Hypertension.* New York: Biomedical, 1984.

15 Berenson GS, McMahan CA, Voors AW et al. *Cardiovascular Risk Factors in Children.* New York: Oxford University Press, 1980.

16 Prineas RJ, Gillum RF, Horibe H, Hannan PJ. The Minneapolis blood pressure study: standards of measurement for children's blood pressure. *Hypertension* 1980;2(suppl I):I-18–24.

17 *Blood Pressure of Youths 12–17 Years: United States Vital and Health Statistics: series 11. Data from the National Health Survey,* no. 163. DHEW publication no. (HRA) 77–1645. Washington, DC: US Government Printing Office, 1977.

18 Lee YH, Rosner B, Gould JB, Lowe EW, Kass EH. Familial aggregation of blood pressure of newborn infants and their mothers. *Pediatrics* 1976;58:722–9.

19 Schachter J, Kuller LH, Perkins JM, Radin ME. Infant blood pressure and heart rate: relation to ethnic group (black or white), nutrition, and electrolyte intake. *Am J Epidemiol* 1979;110:205–17.

20 de Swiet M, Fayers P, Shinebourne EA. Systolic blood pressure in a population of infants in the first year of life: the Brompton study. *Pediatrics* 1980;65:1028–35.

21 Zinner SH, Kass EH. Epidemiology of blood pressure in infants and children. In: Loggie JMH, Horan MJ, Gruskin AB, Hohn AR, Dunbar JB, Hanlik RJ, eds. *NHLBI Workshop on Juvenile Hypertension.* New York: Biomedical, 1984.

22 Berglund G, deFaire U, Castenfors J et al. Monitoring 24-hour blood pressure in a drug trial: evaluation of a non-invasive device. *Hypertension* 1985;7:688–94.

23 Weber M, Drayer J, Nakamur D, Wyle F. The circadian blood pressure pattern in ambulatory normal subjects. *Am J Cardiol* 1984;54:115–19.

24 Pickering TG, Harshfield GA, Devereux RB, Laragh JH. What is the role of ambulatory blood pressure monitoring in the management of hypertensive patients? *Hypertension* 1985;7:171–7.

25 Kennedy HL, Horan MJ, Sprague MK, Padgett NE, Shriver KK. Ambulatory blood pressure in healthy normal males. *Am Heart J* 1983;106:717–22.

26 Fixler DE, Wallace JM, Thornton WE, Dimmitt P. Ambulatory blood pressure monitoring in hypertensive adolescents. *Am J Hypertension* 1990;3(4):288–92.

7 Epidemiology of Blood Pressure in the First 2 Years of Life

STEPHEN T. McGARVEY AND STEPHEN H. ZINNER

INTRODUCTION

Research on blood pressure in infants and young children has increased in the past two decades since familial aggregation of blood pressure was demonstrated in young children [1] and reliable methods were developed to measure blood pressure early in life [2,3]. One of the goals of such research is the detection of the origins of essential hypertension. Epidemiologic efforts that involve infant blood pressure include:

1 studies of familial aggregation of blood pressure with an eye toward the integration of genetic and environmental factors;

2 tracking of blood pressures throughout infancy and early childhood to examine the predictive value of infant blood pressures for those in later childhood and adolescence; and

3 examination of the roles of biologic factors such as body size, and environmental factors such as diet and socioeconomic status in the determination of blood pressure.

This chapter focuses on epidemiologic investigations of blood pressure during the first 2 years of life and concentrates on studies of healthy full-term, appropriate-for-gestational-age newborn infants. This chapter does not address special issues concerning blood pressure in preterm or small-for-gestational-age babies or in those with pre-eclamptic mothers [4,5].

BLOOD PRESSURE MEASUREMENT

As reviewed in Chapters 6 and 8, blood pressure must be measured with meticulous attention to detail. Correct bladder and cuff sizes are essential to avoid artifact. The sleep/awake status must be similar for all infants or should be accurately recorded and used to adjust the measured blood pressure. Awake babies have blood pressure values 7–10 mmHg higher than sleeping babies [6].

Doppler ultrasound instruments are generally used in epidemiologic studies of blood pressures of infants and young children. Ultrasonic measurements of systolic blood pressure closely resemble intra-arterial determinations and yield reasonable diastolic readings. Thus, ultrasonic devices are recommended as the standard instrument for blood pressure studies in children from birth to 2 years of age. Systolic (Korotkoff phase I) and muffling (Korotkoff phase IV) diastolic blood pressures are the usual measurements reported in infancy [6,7].

INFANT AGE AND BLOOD PRESSURE

In infancy, blood pressure is strongly associated with age. Most studies report a rapid and steady increase in blood pressure from birth to approximately 1–2 months of age with a subsequent small increase to about 6 months and then little or no consistent increase through the first 2 years. Several studies have reported varying mean systolic and diastolic blood pressures in newborn infants that range from 69.7 ± 7.3/52.7 ± 7.5 mmHg [7], to 63 ± 10/40 ± 9 mmHg [8] to 59 ± 8/43 ± 8 mmHg [9]. These values were adjusted to or taken during an "awake and quiet" status.

Blood pressure increases from birth to 1 week of age to values ranging from 70 to 80 mmHg systolic and from 45 to 55 mmHg diastolic [6,7,9]. Much of the variation between different studies may stem from the use of dissimilar methods for recording and adjusting for the activity state of the infants during the blood pressure measurements [6,10].

Systolic and diastolic blood pressures continue to increase gradually until about 6 months of age when there is a leveling off, with reported mean values that include 92.2 ± 8.9/54.8 ± 8.6 mmHg [7], 101 ± 9/59 ± 8 mmHg [8], 86.9 ± 7.7/48.3 ± 7.4 mmHg (for whites only) [11] and 93 ± 13 mmHg (for systolic only) [12]. Blood pressures at 1 year of age are about 1−2 mmHg higher than those at 6 months [7,8,13], with a typical mean value of 94.9 ± 7.9/55.6 ± 7.5 mmHg as reported from our laboratory [7].

At 2 years of age both systolic and diastolic blood pressures are approximately 4 and 2 mmHg higher respectively than at 1 year of age. For example, in our previously published population study the mean systolic and diastolic blood pressures among 2-year-olds were 98.7 ± 7.5 and 57.9 ± 7.4 mmHg, respectively [7]. From five separate studies, Schachter and co-authors [11] presented mean blood pressures for 2-year-olds ranging from 92 to 102 mmHg for systolic and 55 to 66 mmHg for diastolic pressures.

A more comprehensive summary of infant blood pressure distribution by age is available from the 1987 Report of the Second Task Force on blood pressure control in children [14]. Blood pressure values were combined from several studies and smoothed age-specific percentiles were generated from birth to 2 years of age. These show similar trends to those described above for individual studies. The percentile graphs enable clinicians to observe blood pressure over time and to evaluate the need for intervention in very young children with persistently elevated age-specific blood pressure.

SEX, RACE, AND SOCIOECONOMIC STATUS

In general, blood pressure values in male and female children are comparable in the first 2 years of life [6,7,9−11,15,16], although in two studies males had slightly higher blood pressure than females from 6 months to 1 year [8] and from 1 to 3 years [16].

Almost all studies have found no differences in blood pressure between black and white children from birth to 2 years of age [7,8,10,15,16]. However, Schachter and colleagues [6] reported that systolic blood pressure was lower in black children aged 15 and 24 months and diastolic blood pressure was higher in black newborn infants but the mean differences were only about 2.5 mmHg. In a later report these authors concluded that there were no clear differences in blood pressures between black and white children in the first 2 years of life [11].

A more recent study of 3-month-old South African infants found a statistically significant (2 mmHg) higher mean systolic blood pressure in blacks relative to mixed-race (triracial) infants, and a trend for higher systolic blood pressure in mixed-race compared to white infants [17]. More research is needed to clarify whether there are genetically based ethnic group differences in blood pressure in infancy. Such studies should include observations on parental blood pressures and prenatal and infant dietary factors.

Family socioeconomic status has not been associated with blood pressure from birth to 2 years of age [6,7,11]. Thus environmental factors related to socioeconomic status such as physical activity, diet, education, stress, and access to medical care presumably exert their effects only later in life.

FAMILIAL AGGREGATION

Familial aggregation of blood pressure can be demonstrated in the first 2 years of life. This may be due to shared genes, shared environments, and/or the interaction of these factors. A variety of family designs are used to separate these effects. In a study of monozygotic and dizygotic twin infants there was no significant genetic variance of blood pressure before 6 months of age [8,18]. Over the age span from birth to 1 year approximately 25% of systolic blood pressure variation was due to additive genetic variance with a slight reduction after body weight adjustment. From 6 months to 1 year genetic variance explained 33% of systolic and 24% of diastolic blood pressure variation. These heritability estimates are quite similar to those found among older children in different ethnic populations and environments [19−21], and support a role for genetic effects on blood pressure in infancy. The likelihood of simultaneous environmental effects and gene−environment interactions stemming from strong maternal prenatal or familial postnatal influences must be considered as well. For example, the reduction in heritability with weight adjustment indicates that a small but significant amount of familial blood pressure resemblance is due to weight [8].

Familial aggregation studies of blood pressure in infants have employed nuclear families with parent−offspring, sibling−sibling, and adopted−natural children pairs. The majority of the findings support the fact that moderate blood pressure aggregation occurs in infants, in some cases beginning at birth.

Lee and colleagues [10] found significant mother—newborn regression coefficients for diastolic but not systolic blood pressure. Schachter and co-authors [22] reported a significant correlation, $r = 0.23$, between the blood pressure of mothers during pregnancy and the systolic pressures of their newborn babies. De Swiet and colleagues [23] found no parent—newborn blood pressure correlations.

In a recent report from our Providence cohort, significant correlations were found in the blood pressures of parents and their infants starting days after birth and extending to 2 years of age [7]. Correlation coefficients ranged from 0.19 to 0.25 for parent—infant pairs, including newborn infants and mothers. We found significant correlations ranging from 0.15 to 0.33 between infants and older siblings starting at 6 months of age [7]. There were no correlations between siblings and newborn infants, or at 1 week and 1 month of age. Significant infant—sibling blood pressure correlations were reported by Hennekens and co-authors [16] at 1 month for systolic and diastolic blood pressure. There were no significant correlations of siblings' blood pressures with those of newborn infants. These investigators also reported that in a subset of families with full and half-siblings, full sibling—infant correlations were significantly higher than half-sibling—infant correlations [24]. The absence of sibling—infant correlations very early in life may be due to a rapid increase in blood pressure in the first month or might reflect a lack of sufficient time for significant environmental interactions. Statistically significant infant—sibling correlations by 6 months suggest the expression of the effects of shared genes but certainly do not exclude the effects of shared environmental factors or gene—environment interactions.

Studies of adopted children provide additional evidence for the role of shared genes in blood pressure variance. One study included a small number of children aged 1–3 years and found that adopted children had smaller, nonsignificant blood pressure correlations with parents and siblings than did natural children [25]. However, it is possible that these correlations might increase with longer periods of shared environments.

Another argument supporting the family aggregation of blood pressure is the association of blood pressure in infancy with parental hypertension. Schachter and coworkers [11] reported that in children 0–2 years of age, those with blood pressures consistently above the 80th percentile had a higher percentage of hypertensive parents (2/8 or 25%) than did children whose pressures were consistently below the 20th percentile (0/6).

In summary, several studies have reported a consistent and significant familial aggregation of blood pressures in infancy. Moreover, studies in twin infants indicate a significant contribution of shared genes to blood pressure variance, and suggest body size as an important variable. Newborn—maternal correlations suggest an influence of both genetic and prenatal environmental factors. The appearance at 6 months of stable paternal—infant and sibling—infant blood pressure correlations also argues strongly for an environmental effect. The magnitude of the familial correlations among 0–2-year-olds is of the same order as those reported in studies of older children and adults [26].

Blood pressure in infancy appears to be determined by both genetic and environmental factors. Furthermore, it may be argued that familial blood pressure aggregation stems from complex patterns of gene—environment interactions such as genetically susceptible subgroups exposed to specific dietary nutrients.

BIOLOGIC CORRELATES

Body size

The first 2 years of life are characterized by rapid growth in height and weight. Height and weight have been associated with infant blood pressure in many studies [11,13,27–29]. However, these associations are not entirely consistent at each age point. For example, birth weight or neonatal weight has been related to blood pressure in several [9,10,13,28], but not all studies [11]. The range of significant correlations is from 0.15 to 0.30. At later ages, weight was moderately correlated with blood pressure in most studies [9,11,13]. Weight change from 6 to 15 months was significantly related to systolic and diastolic blood pressure and relative weight change was related only to systolic pressure in studies by Schachter and colleagues [11]. We have found a significant effect of weight change from birth to 6 months on systolic blood pressure at 6 months, but not at other ages in the first 2 years of life [30].

The body length of healthy newborn infants was significantly related to their blood pressure in some studies [9,28], but not others [10,11]. Later in infancy Schachter and coworkers [11] found a significant relationship between body length and blood pressure at 15 and 24 months. Webber and co-authors [29] found that change in length from 6 months to 1 year was significantly related to systolic blood pressure at 1 year and we [30] found that length at 12 months and change in length from 12 to 18 months were significantly related to systolic blood pressure at 18 months.

Since weight and length both increase markedly from birth to 2 years and since both are highly correlated, weight/height indices are often used to assess adiposity and overall body size. Schachter and colleagues [11] reported that weight/height correlated with systolic blood pressure at 24 months and with diastolic blood pressure at 6, 15, and 24 months. Quetelet's index—(weight/height^2) $\times$ 100—was also related in the same pattern, although with smaller correlation coefficients. In preliminary analysis of the Providence infant cohort, no relationship was found between blood pressure at any infant age and change in Quetelet's index [30].

Height and weight relations with blood pressure in different studies are not universally consistent but do suggest that body size is positively related to blood pressure from birth to 2 years of age. This is similar to results in older children and adults. The inconsistent age-specific results may be the consequence of measurement error of infant height and weight, inadequate statistical techniques to model the dynamic change in height and weight, and/or the inability to separate the independent effects of height and weight.

Heart rate

Heart rate is related to blood pressure in many adult studies. A similar relationship may exist in infants. Several studies have not been able to demonstrate such a relationship in newborn babies or during the first year of life [10,13,28,31,32]. Schachter and co-workers [27] found positive heart rate and blood pressure correlations in white children at 15 and 24 months, but negative correlations in black children at 24 months.

In several studies, black newborn babies and infants have had higher heart rates than whites [32, 33]. The reverse is the case later in childhood and adolescence. The relation of this finding to blood pressure is not clear, although Schachter and colleagues [33] speculate about possible ethnic/racial differences in heart rate, blood volume, and blood pressure.

NUTRITION AND RELATED FACTORS

Dietary electrolyte intake

Research on sodium intake in infants has attempted to detect an association between sodium intake and blood pressure by taking advantage of the relative lack of exposure to excess dietary sodium and salted foods in early life. Schachter and co-authors [6] found no association between blood pressure and sodium intake calculated from a 2-day dietary record in 6-month-old infants. However, in white infants whose mothers' blood pressures were above the median, sodium intake did correlate with their blood pressure. In a follow-up study at 15 and 24 months of age there was no relationship between estimated sodium intake and blood pressure regardless of parental blood pressure [34]. However, among those with a high sodium intake at 24 months, there was a trend among infants with low potassium intake for higher systolic blood pressure [34].

There were no significant differences in blood pressure in 27 black male infants divided into two groups and fed a low (15 mmol Na/day) or a high (81 mmol Na/day) sodium diet from age 3 to 8 months [35]. The high-sodium diet was similar to commercially available salted baby food available in 1969. The blood pressure differences at the end of the 5 months were 2 mmHg systolic and 1 mmHg diastolic higher in the high-sodium group, but these were not statistically significant. The very small sample size must be considered in evaluating these results.

Hofman and others [36] studied the blood pressure effects over 6 months of a normal- versus low-sodium infant formula in 476 newborn babies who were randomly assigned to the formulas. At the end of the study, systolic blood pressure was statistically significantly greater in the normal-sodium group than in the low-sodium group by 2.1 mmHg and the group difference increased significantly during the 6 months. However, in a follow-up at 1 year of age, Hofman [37] found the mean systolic blood pressure difference was a nonsignificant 1 mmHg. Although few studies are available it appears that sodium intake in the usual range may relate to infant blood pressure. These data might become even more impressive if analyses were stratified by parental blood pressure and/or family history of hypertension.

Because of the controversy about dietary calcium and adult blood pressure [38] we studied the association between maternal prenatal calcium, potassium and magnesium intakes, and blood pressures in infancy [39]. Dietary intake in pregnancy was assessed by a validated food-frequency questionnaire in 212 women, and their infants were followed up to 1 year of age. Preliminary results revealed consistent negative relations between maternal prenatal calcium intake and infant blood pressure at 1, 6, and 12 months of age. For example, pregnancy calcium intake was related to 6-month diastolic blood pressure ($r = -0.23$, $p<0.01$, $n = 114$). Maternal prenatal potassium intake was inversely related to 6- and 12-month blood pressure and magnesium intake to 1- and 6-month blood pressure. It appears that prenatal dietary exposures, especially to calcium, may exert detectable and important influences on blood pressure in infancy. We are continuing studies of the association of diet and blood pressure in infancy and childhood.

Salt-taste responsiveness

One of the current theories about nutritional factors and blood pressure is that some individuals have a greater pressor response to sodium intake than others. We are conducting a study in infants to test the hypothesis that neonatal salt-taste responsiveness is related to sodium/salt sensitivity and is associated with blood pressure in infancy [40]. Sucking responses of healthy newborn babies, 2−4 days of age, to water and saline solutions indicate that they can clearly discriminate salt from water. Neonatal salt-taste responses were significantly related to systolic blood pressure at 2−4 days of age [41]. Infants who exhibited salt-taste preferences had significantly higher systolic blood pressures. Among infants with a positive family history of hypertension, salt-taste responses were more strongly and significantly related to both systolic and diastolic blood pressure. Neonatal salt-taste responses may be a detectable risk factor for later blood pressure elevations. In addition, this relationship may be stronger in families with a positive history of hypertension. We are continuing studies of the interrelation of salt-taste responsiveness and diet with blood pressure in infancy and childhood.

BLOOD PRESSURE TRACKING

Although there is evidence for familial aggregation of blood pressure in infancy and a variety of biologic and environmental blood pressure correlates and predictors, it is crucial to know whether blood press-

ures are reproducible during the first 2 years of life and whether they predict blood pressure later in life.

Several studies have found significant tracking correlations of blood pressure starting at 6 months of age, but not before [7,11,16]. Schachter and colleagues [11] reported consistent tracking correlations between systolic blood pressure at 6, 15, and 24 months. The tracking correlations for systolic blood pressure ranged from 0.23 to 0.32. Blood pressures in newborn infants did not relate to later blood pressures. De Swiet and coworkers [12,23] demonstrated significant systolic blood pressure tracking correlations ranging from 0.09 to 0.26 in a large cohort of infants followed throughout the first 2 years of life. Two studies not measuring blood pressure in the neonatal period reported significant correlations for systolic and diastolic blood pressure between 6 and 12 months [16,29]. In a study of Norwegian infants Uhari [9] found significant correlations between 1 and 4−5 days for both systolic and diastolic blood pressure and for diastolic between 4−5 days and 4 months. No significant correlations were detected between 4 and 12 months.

We found a consistent predictive relation between activity-adjusted blood pressure at 6 months and those obtained later in the first 2 years of life [7]. There were only a few significant correlations between blood pressures obtained in the newborn period and those later in life. Tracking correlations ranged from 0.14 to 0.22 for both systolic and diastolic blood pressures [7].

The Bogalusa study demonstrated that systolic blood pressure at 6 months correlated with that at 1 year ($r = 0.24$), and at 2 years ($r = 0.16$), of age [42]. Furthermore, infant blood pressures at 6 months, 1, and 2 years were significantly related to later blood pressures at 3, 4, and 7 years of age. For example, 2-year systolic blood pressure correlated with that at 7 years ($r = 0.35$, $p<0.01$), as did diastolic blood pressure ($r = 0.23$, $p<0.01$).

The tracking data show that blood pressure from birth to 2 years of age is reproducible and that prior blood pressure levels predict later levels, although at low levels of correlation, ranging from 0.15 to 0.30. The correlations between serial blood pressures in infants and young children increase with age. The stability of rank demonstrated by the significant correlations seems to begin at 6 months of age and to continue until 7 years. Sufficient long-term observations have not been made to allow us to conclude that blood pressure in newborn babies and infants is a reliable predictor of blood pressure level later in life. However, the tracking correlations do increase with age, suggesting that a gradual reduction of blood pressure variability might begin early in life.

SUMMARY

Evidence from several different studies indicates that blood pressures in infancy aggregate in families, begin to track, are associated with genetic variance, and are subject to environmental influences such as those related to body size and dietary sodium.

Although the evidence suggests that there are ample genetic and environmental correlates and predictors of blood pressure from birth to 2 years, the predictive value of blood pressure this early in life for the ultimate detection of essential hypertension is still unknown. At the present time there are not enough data to allow clinicians fully to interpret or predict the impact of blood pressure measurements in infants on the future health of the child. The obvious exception is the presence of persistently high blood pressure for a specific age. This should lead to appropriate diagnostic studies designed to detect a secondary form of hypertension [43]. Available evidence suggests that epidemiologic studies of blood pressure in very young children 0–2-years-old should remain a fruitful area for further research. Such studies may provide insights into the origins of essential hypertension.

ACKNOWLEDGMENT

This work was supported in part by grants 5-R01-HL-22298 and 5-R01-HL-33221 from the National Heart, Lung, and Blood Institute.

REFERENCES

1 Zinner SH, Levy PS, Kass EH. Familial aggregation of blood pressure in childhood. *N Engl J Med* 1971;284:401–4.

2 Hochberg HM, Saltzman MB. Accuracy of ultrasound blood pressure instrument in neonates, infants, and children. *Curr Ther Res* 1971;13:482–83.

3 Dweck HS, Reynolds DW, Cassady G. Indirect blood pressure measurement in newborns. *Am J Dis Child* 1974;127:492–4.

4 Moscoso P, Goldberg RN, Jamieson J, Bancalari E. Spontaneous elevation in arterial blood pressure during the first hours of life in the very-low-birth-weight infant. *J Pediatr* 1983;103:114–17.

5 Cabral LA, Read J, Miller F. Elevated blood pressure in infants of pre-eclamptic mothers. *Pediatr Res*

1981;15:549–53.

6 Schachter J, Kuller LH, Perkins JM, Radin ME. Infant blood pressure and heart rate: relation to ethnic group (black or white), nutrition, and electrolyte intake. *Am J Epidemiol* 1979;110:205–18.

7 Zinner SH, Rosner B, Oh W, Kass EH. Significance of blood pressure in infancy. Familial aggregation and predictive effect on later blood pressure. *Hypertension* 1985;7:411–16.

8 Levine RS, Hennekens CH, Perry A, Cassady J, Gelband H, Jesse MJ. Genetic variance of blood pressure levels in infant twins. *Am J Epidemiol* 1982;116:759–64.

9 Uhari M. Changes in blood pressure during the first year of life. *Acta Paediatr Scand* 1980;69:613–7.

10 Lee YH, Rosner B, Gould JB, Lowe EW, Kass EH. Familial aggregation of blood pressure of newborn infants and their mothers. *Pediatrics* 1976;58:722–9.

11 Schachter J, Kuller LH, Perfetti C. Blood pressure during the first two years of life. *Am J Epidemiol* 1982;116:29–41.

12 De Swiet M, Fayers P, Shinebourne EA. Value of repeated blood pressure measurements in children—the Brompton study. *Br Med J* 1980;280:1567–9.

13 De Swiet M, Fayers P, Shinebourne EA. Systolic blood pressure in a population of infants in the first year of life: the Brompton study. *Pediatrics* 1980;65:1028–35.

14 Report of the Second Task Force on Blood Pressure Control in Children—1987. *Pediatrics* 1987;79:1–25.

15 Levine RS, Hennekens CH, Klein B et al. Tracking correlations of blood pressure levels in infancy. *Pediatrics* 1978;61:121–5.

16 Hennekens CH, Jesse MJ, Klein BE, Gourley JE, Blumenthal S. Aggregation of blood pressure in infants and their siblings. *Am J Epidemiol* 1976;103:457–63.

17 Herman AAB, Irwig LM. Systolic blood pressure differences in black, colored, and white infants. *Am J Epidemiol* 1987;125:221–30.

18 Levine RS, Hennekens CH, Duncan RC et al. Blood pressure in infant twins: birth to 6 months of age. *Hypertension* 1980;2(suppl I):29–33.

19 Annest JL, Sing CF, Biron P, Mongeau JG. Familial aggregation of blood pressure and weight in adoptive families II. Estimation of the relative contributions of genetic and common environmental factors to blood pressure correlations between family members. *Am J Epidemiol* 1979;110:492–503.

20 Ward R, Chin PG, Prior IAM. Genetic epidemiology of blood pressure in a migrating isolate: prospectus. In: Sing CF, Skolnick M, eds. *Genetic Analysis of Common Diseases: Applications to Predictive Factors in Coronary Disease.* New York: A R Liss, 1979.

21 MCGarvey ST, Schendel DE, Baker PT. Modernization effects on familial aggregation of Samoan blood pressure: a preliminary report. *Med Anthropol* 1980;4:321–38.

22 Schachter J, Lachin JM, Kerr JL, Wimberly FC, Ratey JJ. Heart rate and blood pressure in black newborns and in white newborns. *Pediatrics* 1976;58:283–7.

23 De Swiet M, Shinebourne EA. Blood pressure in infancy. *Am Heart J* 1977;9:399–401.

24 Klein BE, Hennekens CH, Jesse MJ, Gourley JE, Blumenthal S. Longitudinal studies of blood pressure in offspring of hypertensive mothers. In: Paul O, ed. *Epidemiology and*

Control of Hypertension. New York: Symposia Specialists, 1975.

25 Biron P, Mongeau JJ. Familial aggregation of blood pressure and its components. *Pediatr Clin North Am* 1978;25:29−37.

26 Tyroler HA. The Detroit project studies of blood pressure. A prologue and review of related studies and epidemiological issues. *J Chron Dis* 1977;30:613−24.

27 Schachter J, Kuller LH, Perfetti C. Blood pressure during the first five years of life: relation to ethnic group (black or white) and to parental hypertension. *Am J Epidemiol* 1984;119:541−53.

28 Zinner SH, Lee YH, Rosner B, Oh W, Kass EH. Factors affecting blood pressures in newborn infants. *Hypertension* 1980;2(suppl I):I-99−101.

29 Webber LS, Srinivasan SR, Voors AW, Berenson GS. Persistence of levels for risk factor variables during the first years of life: the Bogalusa heart study. *J Chron Dis* 1980;33:157−67.

30 McGarvey ST, Rosner B, Kass EH, Oh W, Zinner SH. Blood pressure change from birth to 24 months in relation to growth in height and weight. *Cardiovasc Dis Epidemiol Newsletter* 1986;39:53(abstract).

31 Long M, Dunlop JR, Holland WW. Blood pressure recording in children. *Arch Dis Child* 1971;46:636−42.

32 Schachter J, Lachin JM, Wimberly FC. Newborn heart rate and blood pressure: relation to race and to socioeconomic class. *Psychosom Med* 1976;38:390−8.

33 Schachter J, Kuller LH, Perfetti C. Heart rate during the first five years of life: relation to ethnic group (black or white) and to parental hypertension. *Am J Epidemiol* 1984;119:554−63.

34 Schachter J, Kuller LH, Perfetti C. Blood pressure and sodium intake in the first two years of life. In: Fregly MJ, Kare MR, eds. *The Role of Salt in Cardiovascular Hypertension*. New York: Academic Press, 1982.

35 Whitten CF, Stewart RA. The effect of dietary sodium in infancy on blood pressure and related factors. Studies of infants fed salted and unsalted diets for five months at eight months and eight years of age. *Acta Paediatr Scand* 1980;279(suppl):1−17.

36 Hofman A, Hazebroek A, Valkenburg HA. A randomized trial of sodium intake and blood pressure in newborn infants. *JAMA* 1983;250:370−3.

37 Hofman A. Sodium intake and blood pressure in newborns: Evidence for a causal connection. In: Filer RJ, Lauer RM, eds. *Children's Blood Pressure. Report of the 88th Ross Conference on Pediatric Research*. Columbus, Ohio: Ross Labs, 1985: 91−4.

38 Kaplan NM, Meese RB. The calcium deficiency hypothesis of hypertension: a critique: *Ann Intern Med* 1986;105:947−55.

39 McGarvey ST, Zinner SH, Rosner B, Willett WC, Oh W. Maternal prenatal dietary potassium calcium, magnesium, and infant blood pressure. *Hypertension* 1991;17:218−224.

40 McGarvey ST, Zinner SH, Lipsitt LP, Rosner B, Oh W. Neonatal salt taste and infant blood pressure: report of work in progress. In: Hofman A, ed. *International Symposium on the Early Pathogenesis of Primary Hypertension*. Amsterdam: Elsevier, 1987.

41 McGarvey ST, Lipsitt LP, Rosner B, Oh W, Zinner SH. Neonatal salt taste and infant blood pressure. *Cardiovasc Dis Epidemiol Newsletter* 1987;41:21(abstract).

42 Burke GL, Voors AW, Shear CL *et al*. Blood pressure. *Pediatrics* 1987;80(suppl):784−8.

43 Adelman RD. Neonatal hypertension. In: Loggie JHH, Heran MJ, Gruskin AB, Hohn AR, Dunbar JB, Havlik J, eds. *NHLBI Workshop on Juvenile Hypertension*. New York: Biomedical Informatics, 1984.

8 Epidemiology and Measurement of High Blood Pressure in Children and Adolescents

RONALD J. PRINEAS AND ZEINAB M. ELKWIRY

High blood pressure in children is important for two reasons. First, it may be a sign of primary (or essential) hypertension. Although specific, identifiable cellular and/or organ dysfunction may not be identified, it carries the potential of future end-organ damage (principally cardiovascular–renal), the likelihood of a shortened lifespan if left untreated, and is a major risk factor for atherosclerotic disease in later life. Second, it may be an indication of secondary hypertension or hypertension resulting from organ dysfunction or damage that may be correctable. Before considering high blood pressure it is necessary to understand normal blood pressure and its determinants in children.

LEVELS OF BLOOD PRESSURE IN CHILDHOOD AND ADOLESCENCE

The distribution of blood pressure levels in children, as in adults, is unimodal at any given age. That is, there is no clear separation of a hypertensive subset of individuals. Blood pressure rises rapidly in the first month of life and then very little until age 5 years, after which it rises at the rate of 1–2 mmHg per year of life throughout childhood and adolescence for systolic, and 0.5–1 mmHg for diastolic blood pressure.

In Tables 8.1–8.3 (adapted from [1]), distributions of mean blood pressure by age are shown for males and females for mean systolic and phase IV diastolic blood pressure through 18 years of age, and for diastolic Vth phase for ages 13–18 years. Most screening studies of children have shown only minimal differences between blood pressure levels in boys and girls until around the age of puberty, when the levels for boys rise more steeply than for girls between ages 13 to 18 years—probably reflecting their later maturation to adult size and greater body size.

The data in Tables 8.1–8.3 are derived from nine studies [2–17] used by the Report of the Second Task Force. The studies included more than 70 000 children (with approximately even numbers of males and females) in the USA and UK including African-American, Mexican-American, and Caucasian children. The first seated blood pressure measurement from each of the childhood studies was used to develop the Task Force data. All measurements were obtained with a standard mercury sphygmomanometer except for one study [10] that used a modified random-zero device. Infant blood pressures were measured using a Doppler device.

USE OF STANDARD TABLES AND NOMOGRAMS

When comparing clinic measurements of blood pressure in children with standard tables of nomograms such as those published by the Second Task Force [1] (adapted in Tables 8.1–8.3 and Figures 8.1–8.8), impediments to precise equivalence and ranking need to be kept in mind. Most standard tables are derived from multiple studies. Soon, a European standard compiled from measurements on 18 000 European children will also be published (A. Hofman, personal communication). Examination of the age-specific values for mean blood pressures from each of the nine contributing studies to the Second Task Force Report shows considerable variation of these values from study to study. This variation is unlikely to be due substantially to significant biologic differences of the respective populations. The variability more likely derives from differences in measurement technique and conditions of measurement. The Second Task Force [1] studies are more similar in measurement methodology than those used for the first Task Force Report [18]. However, notable differences exist among the nine studies used for the Second Task Force Report.

Table 8.1 Systolic blood pressure (mmHg). Means and standard deviations based on available data from nine studies of males and females, ages from newborn to 18 years. Adapted from [1]

Age Group	Males Mean	SD	n	Females Mean	SD	n
Less than 7 days	72.7	9.6	1435	71.8	9.3	1365
8 days—<1 month	82.0	11.1	334	81.7	12.0	352
1—<6 months	93.0	12.9	1212	92.0	12.2	1162
6—<12 months	95.4	14.8	906	94.5	14.6	877
1 year	93.6	12.2	1104	93.0	12.8	1046
2 years	95.0	10.8	1044	94.6	10.9	1001
3 years	93.5	12.7	996	92.6	12.7	943
4 years	90.8	12.1	459	90.7	13.1	449
5 years	94.3	10.9	1143	94.1	10.6	1204
6 years	96.2	10.1	1362	95.5	10.6	1272
7 years	97.8	10.4	1308	96.4	10.3	1310
8 years	98.7	10.0	1362	98.3	10.3	1289
9 years	100.7	10.1	1309	100.2	10.8	1284
10 years	101.9	10.5	1453	101.8	10.9	1351
11 years	103.2	10.8	1301	104.6	11.1	1234
12 years	105.8	10.8	1352	107.5	11.5	1303
13 years	107.8	12.6	4056	107.2	12.1	4248
14 years	110.1	12.9	3469	107.8	11.8	3042
15 years	113.0	12.5	3734	107.5	11.4	3963
16 years	114.7	12.3	2650	109.1	11.2	2364
17 years	117.6	12.2	3010	109.9	11.1	3089
18 years	118.7	12.4	1336	110.0	10.9	1157

Table 8.2 Diastolic (Korotkoff phase IV) blood pressure (mmHg). Means and standard deviations based on available data from nine studies of males and females, ages from newborn to 18 years. Adapted from [1]

Age group	Males Mean	SD	n	Females Mean	SD	n
Less than 7 days	51.1	8.9	480	50.5	8.4	489
8 days—<1 month	50.3	11.2	329	50.7	11.5	341
1—<6 months	47.8	11.2	342	49.5	10.6	352
6—<12 months	53.3	9.9	339	52.5	9.6	376
1 year	53.0	9.0	395	52.4	9.2	392
2 years	56.5	8.6	419	57.0	8.8	431
3 years	54.3	9.4	588	55.1	9.8	575
4 years	53.9	9.4	459	54.5	9.2	449
5 years	57.4	9.7	1136	57.3	9.9	1202
6 years	58.5	10.0	1245	59.3	10.2	1152
7 years	60.7	10.2	1159	59.7	10.5	1155
8 years	61.6	10.0	1220	61.0	10.1	1162
9 years	62.6	10.0	1165	62.7	10.2	1130
10 years	63.6	9.5	1290	63.1	9.9	1222
11 years	63.4	9.8	1151	64.5	10.1	1092
12 years	65.6	9.8	1205	67.1	9.7	1158
13 years	65.5	10.8	3891	67.4	10.7	4094
14 years	66.2	10.9	3280	67.6	10.6	2861
15 years	66.2	11.0	3555	66.2	10.2	3816
16 years	67.4	11.1	2471	67.0	10.7	2193
17 years	70.2	10.4	2827	67.6	10.1	2953
18 years	71.9	10.1	1179	67.4	10.4	993

Sphygmomanometer

A standard mercury sphygmomanometer was used in eight of the nine studies in the latest report, but one study [10], which contributed the most values for children 13—18 years of age, used a random-zero sphygmomanometer. This latter device is used in experimental and epidemiologic studies to reduce the effect of digit preference and remove some of the effect of bias due to observer expectation of blood pressure level. Blood pressure measurement with the random-zero device gives values systematically lower (approximately 1 mmHg for systolic and 2 mmHg for IVth and Vth phase diastolic) than the standard manometer [19].

Posture and arm position

All blood pressures in the nine studies were measured on the right arm with the children in the seated position (infants were lying). This is important because many clinic measurements in children and adolescents are made in the supine posture. This last

Table 8.3 Diastolic (Korotkoff phase V) blood pressure (mmHg). Means and standard deviations based on available data from nine studies of males and females, age from 13 to 18 years.

Age group	Males Mean	SD	n	Females Mean	SD	n
13 years	57.5	12.2	3142	59.7	12.0	3424
14 years	57.9	12.7	2627	60.3	12.3	2267
15 years	60.8	11.6	3116	60.9	10.5	3332
16 years	62.7	12.1	2107	62.0	11.0	1842
17 years	63.7	11.4	2548	61.4	10.6	2640
18 years	66.0	11.7	1146	62.3	10.8	967

Adapted from [1].

position produces systematically higher levels of blood pressure. In addition to posture, the arm position, with the cubital fossa at the level of the fourth intercostal space, is important for standardization. Higher positions of the arm will elevate, and lower positions will depress the blood pressure level measurement. This point is often neglected when the same table and chair are used for children of differing heights.

Repeated measurements

The first measurement of blood pressure was used to standardize the Task Force Study comparisons. Yet most authorities advocate repeated measures of blood pressure before characterizing an individual as having high or normal blood pressure level. This is because blood pressure at the high levels tends to fall on repeat measurement from one occasion to the next due to an accommodation effect, i.e. due to a reduction of anxiety as the measurement situation is experienced, and because of regression to the mean, a nonbiologic phenomenon that derives from mathematical considerations. Blood pressure level is not static but varies even under standard resting conditions. Therefore, a more precise characterization of an individual's blood pressure level is an average of multiple blood pressure measurements. If, by chance, a level from the high end of an individual's blood pressure distribution is measured first, then by chance alone there is a higher probability that a level from the lower end of that individual's blood pressure distribution will be recorded on a subsequent occasion. Therefore, an average of repeated measurements gives a lower estimate than the first high measurement. Both accommodation and regression to the mean operate between repeat measurements made at the same clinic visits. As a consequence, repeated clinic measures can be expected to yield lower blood pressure values in any given child with elevated blood pressure than those provided by the Second Task Force Report. Thus, the Task Force distribution tables provide a conservative approach for the further clinical investigation of children with high blood pressure.

OTHER FACTORS AFFECTING BLOOD PRESSURE MEASUREMENT

Other factors that affect blood pressure variability could not be standardized between studies that contributed data to the Second Task Force Report. Nevertheless, such factors should be accounted for if properly comparable blood pressure measurements are to be obtained for individuals on separate occasions. Blood pressure varies in a circadian fashion; values obtained in the morning will be lower than those obtained in the afternoon, and still lower values will be obtained during sleep. The room temperature as well as season of the year also affect blood pressure levels. Levels are lower in summer than winter, and change significantly at a room temperature outside the range of 65–78°F [20]. Multiple observers and their age, race, sex, and professional status may all interact to give systematic differences in measured blood pressure levels. A light pressure of the stethoscope head [21] and use of the bell rather than the diaphragm, either in the cubital fossa or over the brachial artery just medial to the cubital fossa and posterior to the biceps tendon, are also useful standardizations to reduce measurement variation [22].

Cuff-bladder size

A major problem for standardization of blood pressure is choice of the correct cuff size. Cuff-bladders wider than appropriate for arm circumference cause an underestimate and those narrower than the appropriate size an overestimate of the blood pressure level. Cuff-bladder length is also important. Long cuffs that encircle the full circumference of the arm reduce some of the variability due to variations of cuff-bladder width.

Recommended lengths and widths of cuff-bladders for blood pressure measurement in children have expanded and contracted and overlapped over the years due, no doubt, to the changing views of experimental evidence, the vagaries of commercial cuff size availability, and possibly to committee members' fatigue [1,18,23–27]. No consistent recommendations exist. Cuff size is important in children because as the upper arm grows, cuff artifact (falsely high or low blood pressure due to the use of an inappropriate cuff size) will cause systematic errors in measurement that could lead to wrongly labeling a child as hypertensive or falsely reassuring a child whose blood pressure is truly elevated. Systematic errors may also be introduced to longitudinal studies of children's blood pressure because of increasing arm size during maturation. For this reason it is useful to consider the guidelines for appropriate cuff size in some detail.

Width

Cuff-bladder width should be equal to 120% of the diameter of the upper arm [24–28], which translates to 38% of the circumference [$120\%D = (C \times 120\%)/\pi = 38\%C$, where C = circumference and D =

diameter of arm]. Cuff-bladder widths also need to accommodate a reasonable range of arm circumferences to obviate the need for a specific arm cuff for every small increment in arm circumference. Therefore, a standardization should be adopted for each specified cuff-bladder width to encompass a range of arm circumferences such that the cuff-bladder width ranges equally above and below 38% of the arm circumference. A reasonable range might be 33–43%, i.e. 38 ± 5%. A larger range than this could lead to unacceptable systematic blood pressure differences between the smallest and largest arm circumference measured by the same cuff-bladder [29]. It should be further noted that cuff-bladder width should not be determined *both* by arm circumference and arm length. This would only be possible if the ratio of arm circumference to length was constant. This is not the case. Among more than 10 000 children aged 6–10 years, measured in the Minneapolis Children's Blood Pressure Study [unpublished data], the arm circumference: length ratio varied from 0.4 to 1.9 and was not linearly related to age or height.

A possible range of appropriate cuff-bladder widths for given arm circumferences is proposed in Table 8.4. The range of arm circumferences includes more than 90% of school-age children and adolescents measured in the Minneapolis Children's Blood Pressure Study [20]. The widths are chosen with some rounding off to give whole numbers, and to avoid overlapping ranges of arm circumference. It would also be practical to suggest cuff-bladder sizes that are readily commercially available. Unfortunately, this is not possible because of the inappropriate width–length combinations of most commercially available cuffs. We have reviewed 10 of the largest purveyors of blood pressure cuffs in the USA and have been unable to make a set that meets the above specifications.

Very precise specifications of cuff dimensions (to the nearest 0.25 cm) are probably futile because of the current manufacturing quality of available cuff-bladders which is limited, no doubt, by inexact control of vulcanized rubber used in most cuff-bladders. We have found manufacturers' cuff-bladder stated widths and lengths to vary by as much as 5% from measurements on hundreds of cuffs obtained by us on the current market-place.

Length

There is less experimental evidence to support a standard specification for length of cuff-bladder than for width. Voors [30] concluded that cuffs which encircled at least 90% of the arm should be used for measuring children's blood pressure. Table 8.4 suggests cuff-bladder lengths that would encircle all arms by at least 90%. Using these recommendations, some arms would be encircled completely with overlap of the cuff-bladder ends. There is no evidence to suggest that such overlap causes systematic differences of blood pressure measurement.

Recommendations

Rational standardization of cuff sizes needs to be established by responsible institutions, regulatory agencies, and manufacturers working in concert to replace the current imperfect recommendations from other groups [1,23,24].

In the face of the difficulty of obtaining commercial cuffs that meet the precise dimensions of an ideal cuff-bladder, a range of cuff-bladders should be obtained and marked so that the cuff-bladder width meets the requirement of being close to 38% (± 5%) of the arm circumference on which the cuff is to be used and is long enough to encircle at least 90% of the arm. The cuffs can be used for an acceptable range of arm circumferences by marking two permanent vertical lines on the inside of the cuff at the appropriate distance from the end of the cuff and separated by a distance encompassed by that range. Then the cuff itself can be used to judge the correct size without the need for measuring the mid upper arm circumference on each occasion. Commercial cuffs are available with such markings but the ranges marked on them are sometimes inappropriate and,

Table 8.4 Possible ideal cuff-bladder sizes*

Midpoint upper arm circumference[†] (cm)	Bladder width (cm) 33–43% of arm circumference	Bladder length (cm) ≥90% of arm circumference
14–18	6	16
19–24	8	22
25–30	10	27
31–39	13	35
40–52	17	47

* See text for discussion.

[†] Measured at the midpoint of the circumference between the olecranon and the acromion.

therefore, should be checked before clinical or screening use.

Blood pressure level should be established by at least two measurements made on at least two occasions. The average of these values greatly reduces the within-subject variability of blood pressure. This more precise characterization allows true differences to be more readily established to guide change in drug treatment or dietary interventions and for studying etiologic links with possible environmental and genetic factors.

PREVALENCE OF HYPERTENSION

The definition of hypertension for children continues to evolve although it is defined by measured blood pressure level. Primary hypertension is rarely found in children when using adult blood pressure level criteria of repeated measurements equal to or greater than 140 mmHg systolic and/or equal to or greater than 90 mmHg diastolic IVth phase. Among more than 10 000 school-children aged 6–10 years in Minneapolis [20] measured in the supine position with a random-zero sphygmomanometer in 1977–1978, less than 0.25% could be classified as hypertensive using blood pressure measurements made on two occasions within 2 weeks. The first Task Force Report [18] introduced the idea of blood pressure rank and suggested that high blood pressure levels in children were those above the 95th percentile for age and sex according to the values presented in nomograms. This concept presumes a tracking effect of children's blood pressure, as discussed below.

Defining high blood pressure as greater than the 95th percentile means that the prevalence of hypertension in children would be expected to be 5% if there were no significant biologic variations from the Task Force's study populations and if the techniques and methods of measurement were identical. Not surprisingly, the latter caveats have not prevailed and following the first Task Force Report, estimated prevalence rates for hypertension in population-based childhood groups have ranged from 1 to 9%, using Task Force nomograms. Using other definitions, estimates of hypertension in children have been published that range up to more than 60% in some subgroups. For published individual studies, blood pressure measurements have generally been internally consistent so that repeated observations of elevated blood pressure levels have enabled certain subgroups of "at-risk" children to be identified with some confidence. However, geographic differences in childhood hypertension cannot be estimated until the same standardized methods and conditions of measurement are repeated in different geographic areas. Blood pressure was measured at the first screening in 10 446 black and white Minneapolis/St Paul school-children, aged 10–16 years in grades 5–8 with two blood pressure measurements and on two occasions, approximately 3 weeks apart, for those in the upper 30 percentiles of first-screening blood pressure (2808). "Significant" hypertension was found in 6.3% after the first screening measurement; this was reduced to 4.5% after averaging the first two screening measurements; this was further reduced to 1% after one rescreening measurement, and finally was reduced to 0.8% after averaging two rescreening measurements [31].

Clinic studies have generally shown that among children under the age of 13 years referred for evaluation of high blood pressure, secondary hypertension (usually related to kidney pathology) is more common than primary hypertension, but that this quickly reverses in adolescents past the age of 13 years [32]. Estimates of secondary hypertension from children's population studies or general pediatric clinics are much lower than those from hypertension clinics.

Figures 8.1–8.8 display the mean blood pressure level at each age from infancy to 18 years and levels for the 50th, 75th, 90th, and 95th percentile distributions for systolic and diastolic blood pressure. Diastolic blood pressure graphs are based on the IVth phase diastolic to age 12 years and on the Vth phase diastolic level from ages 13–18 years. Tables 8.2 and 8.3 give IVth and Vth phase mean diastolic values for this latter age group. The Vth phase (rather than IVth phase) diastolic was recommended to match general practice for adults as the children move to adult size. Fourth phase diastolic blood pressure has generally been used by pediatricians because the Vth phase diastolic in younger children more often reached 0 mmHg and therefore misrepresents intra-arterial blood pressure. The nomograms may be used to indicate that a child with a blood pressure at or above the 90th or 95th percentile should receive particular attention for future regular screening.

These nomograms do not take account of body size. Others have already noted that in children, age is not an important factor in explaining blood pressure variability if measurements are adjusted for

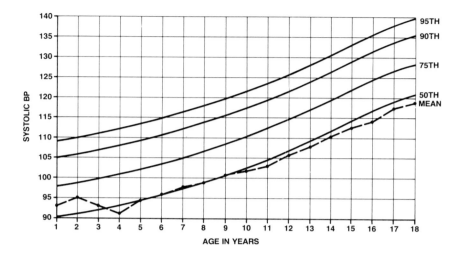

Fig. 8.1 Boys: age-specific means and percentiles of systolic blood pressure measurements. Ages 1–18 years. Adapted from the Second Task Force Report [1].

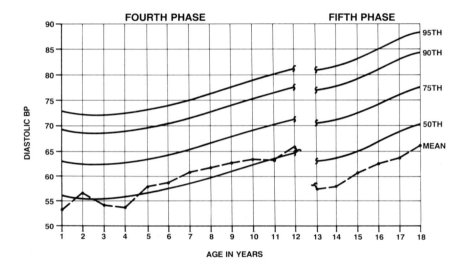

Fig. 8.2 Boys: age-specific means and percentiles of diastolic blood pressure measurements: phase IV, ages 1–12 years; phase V, ages 13–18 years. Adapted from the Second Task Force Report [1].

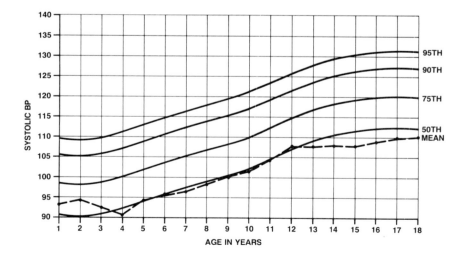

Fig. 8.3 Girls: age-specific means and percentiles of systolic blood pressure measurements. Ages 1–18 years. Adapted from the Second Task Force Report [1].

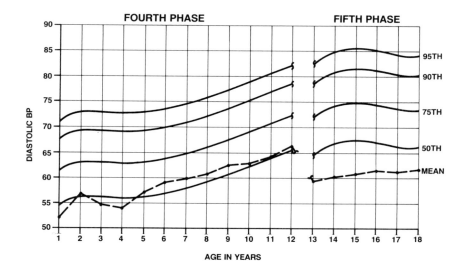

Fig. 8.4 Girls: age-specific means and percentiles of diastolic blood pressure measurements: phase IV, ages 1–12 years; phase V, ages 13–18 years. Adapted from the Second Task Force Report [1].

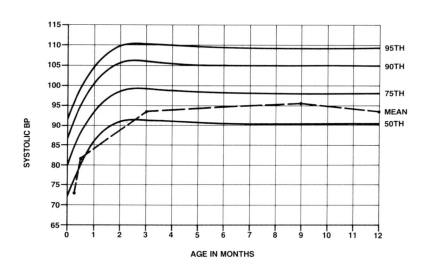

Fig. 8.5 Boys: age-specific means and percentiles of systolic blood pressure measurements. Ages from birth to 12 months. Adapted from the Second Task Force Report [1].

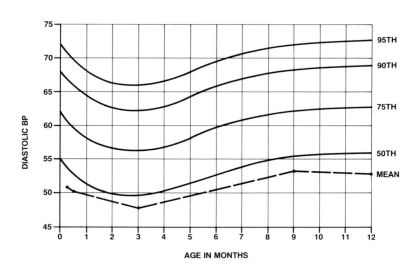

Fig. 8.6 Boys: age-specific means and percentiles of Korotkoff phase IV diastolic blood pressure measurements. Ages from birth to 12 months. Adapted from the Second Task Force Report [1].

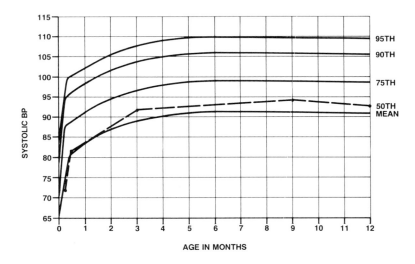

Fig. 8.7 Girls: age-specific means and percentiles of systolic blood pressure measurements. Ages from birth to 12 months. Adapted from the Second Task Force Report [1].

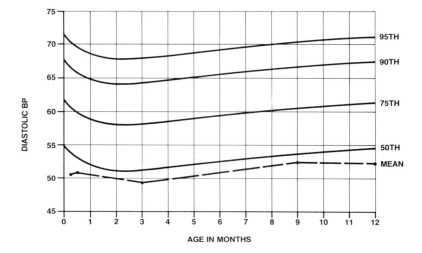

Fig. 8.8 Girls: age-specific means and percentiles of Korotkoff phase IV diastolic blood pressure measurements. Ages from birth to 12 months. Adapted from the Second Task Force Report [1].

height [33,34]. Therefore, nomograms based on height may be more useful for ranking children's blood pressure because they are not confounded by different levels of maturity for children of the same age. The Second Task Force Report [1] does publish sex-specific 90th percentile values for height and weight at each age to indicate that some children will be in the highest blood pressure percentiles because of body size. Those who are obese with relatively high blood pressure need to be followed closely because the elevated blood pressure may be modified by reducing obesity.

DETERMINANTS OF HIGH BLOOD PRESSURE

Many other surveys in the USA and around the world have shown a similar increase in blood pressure throughout childhood, even among populations unlike that of the USA that show no increase in blood pressure among aging adults. In other words, the observed increase in blood pressure throughout childhood is a natural phenomenon of growth and maturation. In cross-sectional studies the major contribution to the variability of blood pressure in children is body size—whether indexed as height or weight or some combined index [33,34]. This is not to say that the increased blood pressure that accompanies obesity, in childhood as well as adults, is a "natural" or desirable phenomenon; the increase, with increase in height and lean body mass, is normal in children. The increase in blood pressure at puberty has not been shown to be independently due to the accompanying body size change, hormonal change, or the maturation process itself. Children have not been shown to be at any special increased risk for developing hypertension during this period of development.

Generally, in cross-sectional studies, no more than 40% of the variability (between children in a population) of systolic blood pressure, in multiple regression analysis, can be "explained" by physical and biochemical variables. Most of these variables relate to body size but include heart rate and blood pressure levels of parents, especially mothers. Much less of the variability of diastolic blood pressure can be so explained [35]. Large heritability indexes have indicated powerful effects of genetics on blood pressure variability. A reasonable estimate of the proportion of phenotypic variability of blood pressure attributed to genes has been placed at approximately 0.3 [36]. This estimate is much lower than that derived from twin studies. The latter, however, overestimate gene effects [36], because of the strongly shared environment of twins — greater for monozygotic than dizygotic. Much of systolic blood pressure variability and most of diastolic blood pressure variability in childhood remains unexplained. This indicates that other environmental factors and specific environmental/genetic interactions may remain to be identified, or identified factors need to be more precisely quantified. In other words, if blood pressure was more precisely characterized by the mean of multiple measurements, the identified factors might "explain" more of the variability between individuals than is the case from present longitudinal studies.

Race

There is a well documented excess of hypertension among adult African-Americans compared to whites. Yet, among children under the age of 12 years, differences in mean blood pressures and prevalence of hypertension, however defined, are not substantially different between African-Americans and whites in the USA. This has been found to be so in studies from many different regions of the country. Studies of adolescents in the USA have provided conflicting results. The blood pressures of African-American teenagers have been reported to be higher than those of white teenagers in the east and south, but many of these studies are confounded by differences in weight and obesity between ethnic groups. In the south, rural African-American adolescents generally have higher blood pressures than urban African-American

adolescents. Much of the geographic difference is likely to be due to socioeconomic-related factors and dietary differences, as recently reviewed [37].

Studies of blood pressure difference between African and US blacks by the same investigative team are rare. Such studies are important because they use standard methods of measurement to enable comparison between groups. In a study by Akinkugbe [38] using standardized methods in both study locations, it was found that the blood pressures of Nigerian children were higher than those of black or white children in Boston. This is in contrast to reported lower blood pressures for Nigerian adults than for adult African-American. All of this underscores the theory that environmental differences, which may include diet (see below), are strongly related to socioeconomic factors, and are likely causes for US black/white differences in blood pressure level. Low socioeconomic class, estimated by income and educational level, is strongly and significantly related to the prevalence and incidence of hypertension in both African-American and white adults.

Diet

The major dietary influences promoting high blood pressure have been identified as excess sodium and decreased potassium intake [39]. The genetic influences mentioned earlier imply that sodium sensitivity will vary between individuals and that the metabolism of other electrolytes linked to blood pressure control and sodium metabolism in adults (including potassium, calcium, magnesium, and chloride) may be equally affected.

There is no satisfactory way at present to quantify sodium sensitivity. Nevertheless, it is likely to be a common phenomenon given that hypertension is highly prevalent in societies with the greatest dietary salt intake. There is a vast literature linking sodium intake with elevated blood pressure within and between populations, worldwide [39].

The importance of sodium in promoting high blood pressure as early as infancy was demonstrated by Hofman and coworkers [40]. They provided 476 infants with free formula and solid foods; 245 of these infants were given formula and solid food containing 50% less sodium than the other group. A significantly lower systolic blood pressure was observed by 21 weeks in the sodium-restricted group, without any differences in growth patterns observed between the two groups. If these differences could be maintained during biologic development, the impact on the incidence of primary hypertension is obvious. In another study, a short-term clinical trial of dietary sodium restriction among normotensive adolescents, it was found that a significant reduction of blood pressure during a 1-month period was achieved by the leanest adolescents, but not by the others [41]. This observation may be important in light of obesity-related tracking of blood pressures, as noted below.

Increasingly, alcohol ingestion has been implicated in the genesis and maintenance of hypertension in adults in population studies and clinical trials. Similar studies have not been conducted among adolescents. Other dietary factors related to high blood pressure in adults have not been studied in children. These include the electrolytes noted earlier (calcium, magnesium, and chloride) and relatively high dietary saturated fat or low polyunsaturated fat.

Obesity

Obesity has been shown to be a predictor and concomitant of hypertension among adults in many clinical and population studies. As with sodium, obesity is governed both by environmental and genetic factors. Obese children also have higher mean blood pressures than non obese children of the same age. In population studies, black girls have generally been shown to be more obese than white girls, and than boys of either race. As a consequence, blood pressures in black girls have been shown to be higher than those of white girls in some studies, with most of the blood pressure difference explained by the difference in body mass between the two groups. Obesity-related high blood pressure in black girls, then, may have strong environmental and sociological causes and may be preventable.

Reduction of obesity in adults has been shown to reduce blood pressure but there have been no randomized, controlled trials among children to test such an effect. It is not at all certain which children should be included in such a study. There is evidence from longitudinal blood pressure studies in normal children to suggest that weight reduction among children consistently in the upper tertile of body mass index and triceps skinfold thickness could bring about only a modest reduction in systolic blood pressure but little, if any, change in diastolic blood pressure [42]. It should also be aknowledged that a potential complication of dietary control of obesity may be the onset of eating disorders that occur more frequently among girls [43].

TRACKING AND PREDICTION

The concept of tracking of blood pressure, or the maintenance of blood pressure rank in relation to peers, has been applied to children for about 10 years and double that time for adults (Figure 8.9). Repeated studies in children have shown statistically significant and sizeable Pearson linear correlation coefcients between blood pressures measured on multiple occasions years apart, between infancy and adolescence. The correlations are higher for older children and for shorter durations between measurements. For studies using carefully standardized measurement methods, the correlation coefficient for systolic blood pressure is of the order of 0.6 between measurements separated by as long as 5 years. The coefficients are much smaller for diastolic blood pressures which are far more variable and less subject to prediction over time [35]. Indeed the greater variability of diastolic blood pressure than systolic blood pressure on repeat measurement has prompted the authors of one detailed study [44] to recommend that in the "screening of children [for high blood pressure] under the age of 13 years...systolic blood pressure [rather than diastolic blood pressure] may be more useful as the primary tool" for classification.

Another way of estimating tracking in groups is to divide the blood pressure distributions at each occasion into equal intervals and to observe how individuals remain within these intervals over time. Such an estimate, using the κ statistic, calculated for age−sex-specific quintiles of nine successive biannual school screening among Minneapolis schoolchildren, gave higher "tracking" values for systolic blood pressure than a similar statistic calculated for adults in the Framingham Heart Study [45]. Lauer and colleagues [3] have also suggested another tracking index based on "level," "trend," and "variability" of age−sex-specific ranks of a given population, and have found that a significant, but small proportion of children "track" in relation to blood pressure. Such studies show that genetic/environmental influences on later levels of blood pressure are operational in childhood, and thus tracking may provide clues to identify groups at risk for the development of primary hypertension. These studies also demonstrate that the adult rank of an individual's blood pressure cannot be accurately predicted from childhood rank alone, whether one uses study-specific or national nomograms to establish rank. This is true despite repeated evidence that the best predictor of blood pressure level in a child in the future is the blood

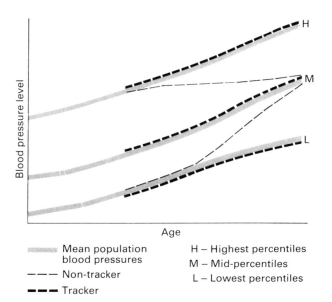

Blood pressure level

Age

- ▨▨▨ Mean population blood pressures
- – – – Non-tracker
- ▰▰▰ Tracker

- H – Highest percentiles
- M – Mid-percentiles
- L – Lowest percentiles

Fig. 8.9 Classification of tracking of blood-pressure level in childhood.

pressure level in a child measured on a previous occasion. Nevertheless, children of parents with high blood pressure track at higher levels of blood pressure through adolescence than those whose parents have normal blood pressures [46]. Families with high blood pressure could be targeted for preventive environmental activities such as increasing exercise, and decreasing calories and dietary sodium as possible counteractants to the family genetic/environmental susceptibility.

It has been shown that lean children in the upper quintile of blood pressure at an initial exam were more likely than obese children in the same quintile to maintain this blood pressure rank 4 years later [28]. As with the sodium reduction trial in children, noted above, lean children with elevated blood pressure may represent a group with primary hypertension with specific genetic/environmental determinants different from those among obese hypertensive children. These findings need to be tested in other population studies and clinical trials.

Other

Myriad other factors have been linked to elevated blood pressure in children in clinical and metabolic ward studies and cross-sectional field studies. The studies have generally been aimed at establishing differences in stress exposure and response, sensitivity of the sympathetic nervous system, and hormonal and enzymatic differences controlling

vasodilation and sodium metabolism. A number of studies have also sought a genetic explanation for these differences. None of these factors has been satisfactorily established in longitudinal population studies as a predictor of the development of hypertension in children.

One of the more extensively studied physiologic phenomena is the rate of cellular influx of sodium, tested in red and white blood cells in humans and smooth muscle cells in some rat models of hypertension. A low flux rate with accumulation of intracellular sodium has been linked to one possible cause of inherited primary hypertension that may be mediated by an increase in concentration of a circulating sodium transport inhibitor [47–49]. A link between the latter, obesity and hyperinsulthemia may also exist [50].

SUMMARY

The epidemiologic study of elevated blood pressure in childhood will continue to provide data to aid the development of strategies for child-specific and community-wide primary prevention. Because we are, as yet, unable to predict a definite hypertensive outcome for individual normotensive children, and because adult hypertension is so ubiquitous, safe measures for behavior change for the whole population should be promulgated. These measures include dietary and physical activity changes to prevent obesity, to reduce sodium intake, and to prevent regular alcohol ingestion.

Any obesity reduction programs in children must be accompanied by long-term follow-up. The safest and probably most effective approach to obesity reduction, a mass phenomenon in our society, is through community interventions that modify societal behaviors.

Given the widespread use of alcohol by teenagers, alcohol ingestion should be considered when caring for adolescents with hypertension.

Black children and adolescents, because of the high prevalence and incidence of hypertension among black adults, should be considered at risk and special efforts should be made to obtain routine blood pressure measurements at their places of medical care.

Much has been learned about blood pressure distribution and determinants of normal blood pressure level in children in the past decade. We are now moving into an era when controlled clinical trials and intervention studies need to be carried out to determine preventable causes of elevated blood pressure in children. These studies should be based on data derived from epidemiologic, experimental, and clinical studies that have identified subgroups at risk of hypertension due to modifiable nutritional and behavioral factors.

ACKNOWLEDGMENT

This chapter was funded in part by support from National Heart, Lung, and Blood Institute grants HL-19877 and HL-34659.

REFERENCES

1 Task Force on Blood Pressure Control in Children. Report of the Second Task Force on blood pressure control in children. *Pediatrics* 1987;79:1–25.

2 Clarke WR, Schrott HG, Leaverton PE, Connor WE, Lauer RM. Tracking of blood lipids and blood pressures in school age children: the Muscatine study. *Circulation* 1978;58:626–34.

3 Lauer RM, Clarke WR, Beaglehole R. Level, trend, and variability of blood pressure during childhood: the Muscatine study. *Circulation* 1984;69:242–9.

4 Lackland DT, Riopel DA, Shepard DM, Wheller FC. Blood pressure and anthropometric measurement results of the South Carolina dental health and pediatric blood pressure study. South Carolina Dental Health and Pediatric Blood Pressure Study, 1985. Described in [1].

5 Gutgesell M, Terrell G, Labarthe D. Pediatric blood pressure: ethnic comparison in a primary care center. *Hypertension* 1981;3:39–46.

6 Berenson GS, McMahan CA, Voors AW et al. *Cardiovascular Risk Factors in Children—The Early Natural History of Atherosclerosis and Essential Hypertension*. New York: Oxford University Press, 1980.

7 Berenson GS. *Causation of Cardiovascular Risk Factors in Children—Perspectives on Cardiovascular Risk in Early Life*. New York: Raven Press, 1986.

8 Voors AW, Foster TA, Frerichs RR, Webber LS, Berenson GS. Studies of blood pressure in children, ages 5–14 years in a total biracial community—the Bogalusa heart study. *Circulation* 1976;54:319–27.

9 McDowell A, Engel A, Massey JT, Maurer K. *Plan and Operation of the Second National Health and Nutrition Examination Survey, 1976–1980*. DHSS Publication no. (PHS) 81–1317 series 1 no. 15. London: DHSS, 1981.

10 Fixler DE, Laird WP. Validity of mass blood pressure screening in children. *Pediatrics* 1983;72:459–63.

11 Baron AE, Freyer B, Fixler DE. Longitudinal blood pressure in blacks, whites and Mexican Americans during adolescence and early adulthood. *Am J Epidemiol* 1986;123:809–17.

12 Schachter J, Kuller LH, Perfetti C. Blood pressure during the first five years of life: relation to ethnic group (black or white) and to parental hypertension. *Am J Epidemiol* 1984;119:541–53.

13 Zinner SH, Rosner B, Oh WO, Kass EH. Significance of blood pressure in infancy. *Hypertension* 1985;7:411–16.

14 De Swiet M, Fayers P, Shinebourne EA. Blood pressure survey in a population of newborn infants. *Br Med J* 1976;2:9–11.

15 De Swiet M, Fayers P, Shinebourne EA. Systolic blood pressure in a population of infants in the first year of life: the Brompton study. *Pediatrics* 1980;65:1028–35.

16 De Swiet M, Fayers P, Shinebourne EA. Value of repeated blood pressure measurement in children: the Brompton study. *Br Med J* 1980;280:1567–9.

17 De Swiet M, Fayers P, Shinebourne EA. Blood pressure in four and five year old children: the effects of environment and other factors in its measurement: the Brompton study. *J Hypertension* 1984;2:501–5.

18 Report of the Task Force on Blood Pressure Control in Children. *Pediatrics* 1977;59:797–820.

19 DeGuademaris R, Folsom AR, Prineas RJ, Luepker RV. The random-zero versus the standard mercury sphygmomanometer: a systematic blood pressure difference. *Am J Epidemiol* 1985;121:282–90.

20 Prineas RJ, Gillum RF, Horibe H, Hannan PJ. The Minneapolis children's blood pressure study. Part 1: standards of measurement for children's blood pressure. *Hypertension* 1980;2(suppl I):I-18–24.

21 Londe S, Klitzner TS, Moss AJ. Effects of pressure exerted on the stethoscope head on auscultatory blood pressure. In: Loggie JMH, Horan MJ, Gruskin AB, Hohn AR, Dunbar JB, Havlik RJ, eds. *Workshop on Juvenile Hypertension*. New York: Biomedical Information, 1984.

22 Prineas RJ, Jacobs D. Quality of Korotkoff sounds: bell vs diaphragm, cubital fossa vs brachial artery. *Prev Med* 1983;12:715–19.

23 Kirkendall WM, Burton AC, Epstein FH, Freis ED. Recommendations for human blood pressure determination by sphygmomanometer: report of a subcommittee of the post graduate education committee. American Heart Association, 1980;28.

24 Frohlich ED, Grim C, Labarthe DR, Maxwell MH, Perloff D, Weidman WH. Recommendations for human blood pressure determination by sphygmomanometers. Report of a special Task Force appointed by The Steering Committee, American Heart Association. *Circulation* 1988;77:502A–14A.

25 Guntheroth WG, Nadas AS. Blood pressure measurements in infants and children. *Pediatric Clin North Am* 1955;2:257–63.

26 Park MK, Guntheroth WG. Direct blood pressure measurements in brachial and femoral arteries in children. *Circulation* 1970;41:231–7.

27 Park MK, Kawabori I, Guntheroth WG. Need for an improved standard for blood pressure cuff size. *Clin Pediatr* 1976;15:784–7.

28 Burke GL, Freedman DS, Webber LS, Berenson GS. Persistence of high diastolic blood pressure in thin children: the Bogalusa heart study. *Hypertension* 1986;8:24–9.

29 Rastam L, Prineas RJ, Gomez-Marin O. Ratio of cuff width/arm circumference as a determinant of arterial blood pressure measurements in adults. *J Intern Med* 1990;227:225–32.

30 Voors AW. Cuff bladder size in a blood pressure survey of children. *Am J Epidemiol* 1975;101:489–94.

31 Sinaiko AR, Gomez-Marin O, Prineas RJ. "Significant" diastolic hypertension in pre-high school black and white children: the children and adolescent blood pressure program. *Am J Hypertens* 1988;1−178−80.

32 Loggie JMH. Epidemiology of childhood hypertension. In: Giovanneli G, New MI, Gorini S, eds. *Hypertension in Children and Adolescents*. New York: Raven Press, 1981.

33 Voors AW, Webber LS, Frerichs RR, Berenson GS. Body weight and body mass as determinants of basal blood pressure in children: the Bogalusa heart study. *Am J Epidemiol* 1977;106:101−8.

34 Prineas RJ, Gillum RF, Horibe H, Hannan PJ. The Minneapolis children's blood pressure study part 2: multiple determinants of children's blood pressure. *Hypertension* 1980;2(suppl 1):I-24−28.

35 Prineas RJ, Gillum RF, Gomez-Marin O. The determinants of blood pressure levels in children: the Minneapolis children's blood pressure study. In: Loggie JMH, Horan MJ, Gruskin AB, Hohn AR, Dunbar JB, Havlik RJ, eds. *NHLBI Workshop on Juvenile Hypertension*. New York: Biomedical Information, 1984.

36 Mongeau JG, Biron P, Sing CF. The influence of genetics and household environment on the variability of normal blood pressure: the Montreal adoption survey. In: Filer LJ, Lauer RM, eds. *Children's Blood Pressure—Report of the Eighty-Eighth Ross Conference on Pediatric Research*. Columbus, Ohio: Ross Laboratories, 1985.

37 Prineas RJ, Gillum RF. US epidemiology of hypertension in blacks. In: Hall WD, Saunders E, Shulman NB, eds. *Hypertension in Blacks: Epidemiology, Pathophysiology, and Treatment*. Chicago: Year Book, 1985.

38 Akinkugbe OO. World epidemiology of hypertension in blacks. In: Hall WD, Saunders E, Shulman NB, eds. *Hypertension in Blacks: Epidemiology, Pathophysiology, and treatment*. Chicago: Year Book, 1985.

39 Prineas RJ, Blackburn H. Clinical and epidemiologic relationships between electrolytes and hypertension: dietary electrolytes in hypertension. In: Horan MJ, Blaustein M, Dunbar JB, Kachadorian W, Kaplan NM, Simopoulos AP, eds. *NIH Workshop on Nutrition and Hypertension*. New York: Biomedical Information, 1985.

40 Hofman A, Hazebroek A, Valkenburg HA. A randomized trial of sodium intake and blood pressure in newborn infants. *JAMA* 1983;250:370−3.

41 Cooper R, Van Horn L, Liu K *et al*. A randomized trial on the effect of decreased dietary sodium intake on blood pressure in adolescents. *J Hypertens* 1984;2:361−6.

42 Prineas RJ, Gomez-Marin O, Gillum RF. Children's blood pressure: dietary control of blood pressure by weight loss. In: Filer LJ, Lauer RM, eds. *Children's Blood Pressure: Report of the Eighty-eighth Ross Conference on Pediatric Research*. Columbus, Ohio: Ross Laboratories, 1985.

43 Wooley SC, Wooley OW. Should obesity be treated at all? In: Stunkard AJ, Stellar E, eds. *Eating and its Disorders*. New York: Raven Press, 1984.

44 Rosner B, Cook NR, Evans DA *et al*. Reproducibility and predictive values of routine blood pressure measurements in children. Comparison with adult values and implications for screening children for elevated blood pressure. *Am J Epidemiol* 1987;126:1115−25.

45 Prineas RJ, Gomez-Marin O, Gillum RF. Tracking of blood pressure in children and nonpharmacologic approaches to the prevention of hypertension. *Ann Behav Med* 1985;7:25−9.

46 Munger RG, Prineas RJ, Gomez-Marin O. Persistent elevation of blood pressure among children with a family history of hypertension: the Minneapolis children's blood pressure study. *J Hypertens* 1988;6:647−53.

47 DeWardener HE, MacGregor GA. The natriuretic hormone and essential hypertension. *Lancet* 1982;i:1450:4.

48 Canessa M, Adrana N, Solomon HS, Connolly TM, Tosteson DC. Increased sodium−lithium countertransport in red cells of patients with essential hypertension. *N Engl J Med* 1980;302:772−6.

49 Blaustein MP, Hamlyn JM. The basic science of electrolytes and hypertension: the natriuretic hormone—Na/Ca exchange hypertension hypothesis. In: Horan MJ, Blaustein M, Dunbar JB, Kachadorian W, Kaplan NM, Simopoulos AP, eds. *Workshop on Nutrition and Hypertension*. New York: Biomedical Information, 1985.

50 Donahue RP, Skyler JS, Schneiderman N, Prineas RJ. Hyperinsulinemia and elevated blood pressure: cause, confounder, or coincidence. *Am J Epidemiol* 1990;132:827−36.

9 Definition, Prevalence, and Distribution of Causes of Hypertension

WALLACE W. McCRORY

DEFINITION OF HYPERTENSION

The identification of a significantly elevated blood pressure (BP) level in childhood poses special problems since the level of BP varies with age into adulthood. Virtually every adult patient with a diastolic BP which persistently exceeds 90 mmHg is a candidate for diagnostic studies and for subsequent treatment. The finding on physical examination of elevated BP in an infant or a child constitutes an abnormal finding but not one considered as representing hypertension unless found to be sustained on subsequent examinations. We cannot use a single BP level to define elevated BP in childhood because modest but continuous increases in BP are a universal accompaniment of growth until pubertal maturation. This pattern is found in all societies including such populations as the Tokelau Islands [1] and the Yanamamo Indians [2], no-salt cultures where adult pressure levels were low and did not increase appreciably with aging after pubertal maturation.

Until recently, we did not have data describing the normal distribution of BP levels from birth to maturity. Normative data derived from sampling more than 70 000 children have now been provided by the report of the Second Task Force on BP control in children [3]. This document also provided advice on methodology and instrumentation for BP measurements and guidelines for detecting children with high BP.

The Task Force defines normal BP as systolic and diastolic levels less than the 90th percentile for age and sex, high normal BP if average systolic and/or diastolic BP is between the 90th and 95th percentiles for age and sex, and high BP or *hypertension* if average systolic and/or diastolic BP is equal to or greater than the 95th percentile for age and sex on at least three occasions. It is important to emphasize that the finding of markedly elevated BP (severe hypertension) on examination of an individual patient should lead the physician to consider admitting the patient to a hospital for treatment and work-up, rather than waiting for repeated documentation by subsequent readings. The finding of high normal BP can be dealt with in an ambulatory setting.

Blood pressure standards

Blood pressure levels in the child and adolescent are dependent upon a multitude of factors, both genetic and environmental, many of which are unknown. Blood pressure increases with age during preadult years. This occurs in all populations studied, although the level and trend vary from population to population. Larger children (heavier and/or taller) have higher BPs than smaller children of the same age.

Height and weight change rapidly and continuously from infancy through adolescence and the rate of these changes makes important contributions to the BP level during growth. When the effects of changes in height and body mass during growth are taken into account, Voors and coworkers [4] found that blood pressure loses most of its positive association with age (i.e. BP does not increase with age *per se*). Blood pressure increases during puberty while marked changes in height and weight are also occurring. We do not, however, know to what degree the hormonal changes associated with sexual maturation affect BP.

Information about the relationship between BP and the maturational processes which occur at puberty has been gained with the use of skeletal aging techniques. Cornoni-Huntley and colleagues [5] reported that skeletal age is more consistently related to BP than chronologic age. Although sexual maturity ratings are useful, they are not as closely related to BP variation as skeletal age. Cornoni-Huntley and colleagues [5] found a significant relationship between degree of deviation in skeletal age from chronologic age and BP in both black and white children at ages 12–14 years (Fig. 9.1). Mean systolic BP was 8–10 mmHg higher in subjects with advanced skeletal maturity (>+2) than in subjects with similar skeletal and chronologic age (−1 to +1). The relationship between physiologic maturity and blood pressure was blunted in older adolescent females (Fig. 9.1). Obese children have higher BPs than lean children [3].

The level of BP in a given infant, child, or adolescent must be considered with respect to the individual's body size and sex as well as age. Height and weight should be used in assessing the medical significance of a BP recording judged to be high on age- or sex-specific distribution. Age- or sex-specific percentiles from infancy up to 18 years are shown in Figures 9.2 through 9.7. Phase V of the Korotkoff sounds (K5), characterized by the disappearance of all sounds, is often difficult to obtain in children and, for the most part, was not available in these data sets. K5 diastolic pressures are more easily obtainable in adolescence and were provided in the data sets. Therefore, Korotkoff phase IV (K4) diastolic BP (characterized by a low-pitched, muffled sound) was

used in the standards for infants and children 3–12 years of age and K5 diastolic BP was used for the standards for adolescents 13–18 years of age.

Hypertension in infancy (see Chapter 29)

There is an increasing recognition of hypertension in young infants managed in neonatal intensive care units, particularly those babies with indwelling umbilical artery catheters. Blood pressure rises rapidly in normal newborn infants during the first 48 h of life. Systolic readings by Doppler ultrasound correlate well with direct arterial pressure but diastolic readings do not. Blood pressure levels vary with state of agitation or alertness, are lower in sleeping than awake infants, and vary with body weight and postnatal age.

Devices using Doppler or oscillometric principles are now available for measuring BP and are more practical than other methods used in infants. They suffer from a number of problems:
1 hospital personnel are rarely trained adequately in their use;
2 frequently, only systolic BP can be measured accurately;

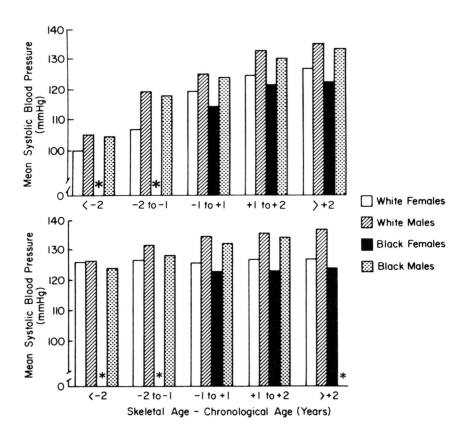

Fig. 9.1 Relationship between systolic blood pressure and physiologic maturity for youths 12–14 years of age (upper) and 15–17 years of age (lower). The difference between skeletal age is used as a surrogate measure of physiologic advancement. The asterisk indicates that only 1 (>2) or 2 (at −2 to −1) subjects were present in this class. From Cornoni-Huntley and coworkers [5], with permission.

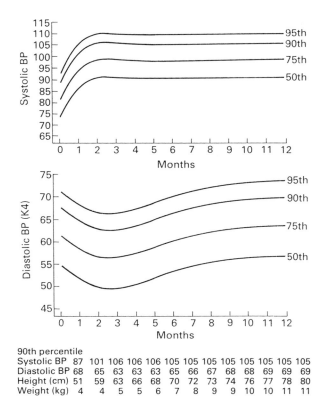

90th percentile
Systolic BP	87	101	106	106	106	105	105	105	105	105	105	105	105
Diastolic BP	68	65	63	63	63	65	66	67	68	68	69	69	69
Height (cm)	51	59	63	66	68	70	72	73	74	76	77	78	80
Weight (kg)	4	4	5	5	6	7	8	9	9	10	10	11	11

Fig. 9.2 Age-specific percentiles of blood pressure (BP) measurements in boys from birth to 12 months of age; Korotkoff phase IV (K4) is used for diastolic BP.

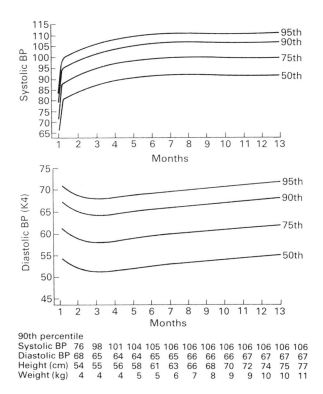

90th percentile
Systolic BP	76	98	101	104	105	106	106	106	106	106	106	106	106
Diastolic BP	68	65	64	64	65	65	66	66	66	67	67	67	67
Height (cm)	54	55	56	58	61	63	66	68	70	72	74	75	77
Weight (kg)	4	4	4	5	5	6	7	8	9	9	10	10	11

Fig. 9.3 Age-specific percentiles of blood pressure (BP) measurements in girls from birth to 12 months of age; Korotkoff phase IV (K4) is used for diastolic BP.

3 they are infrequently pretested for accuracy against intra-arterial pressure in the neonatal age group; and **4** they are expensive.

For practicing pediatricians outside the hospital setting, with limited resources for purchasing very expensive equipment, it may be difficult to measure routinely BP in infants and children 2–3 years of age. Infants with conditions that are currently known to put them at risk for hypertension are shown in Table 9.1. When such infants are encountered, and their BPs cannot be accurately measured, they should be sent to facilities capable of measuring BP in this age group.

Data on normal distribution of BP values in large samples of normal newborn infants of varying weights and ages are very limited. Criteria for what constitutes significant hypertension have, thus, been arbitrarily defined. A systolic BP of greater than 90 mmHg and diastolic BP greater than 60 mmHg in full-term newborn infants and systolic BP of greater than 80 mmHg and diastolic BP greater than 50 mmHg in premature infants is considered hypertensive by Adelman [6]. The Second Task Force report

Table 9.1 Conditions suggesting increased hypertension risk for infants

Abdominal bruit
Abdominal mass(es), e.g. Wilms' tumor, neuroblastoma
Certain acute clinical situations, e.g. burns, hemolytic–uremic syndrome
Coarctation of the aorta
Congenital adrenal hyperplasia
Neurofibromatosis
Failure to grow
Indwelling umbilical artery catheter
Administration of glucocorticoids and/or adrenocorticotrophic hormone
Orbital tumor
Suspected renal disease (hematuria, proteinuria)
Turner syndrome
Unexplained heart failure
Unexplained seizures

[3] defined significant hypertension as a systolic BP of equal to or greater than 96 mmHg in a newborn infant and equal to or greater than 104 mmHg at 7 days, and severe hypertension as systolic BP equal to or greater than 106 mmHg in the newborn infant

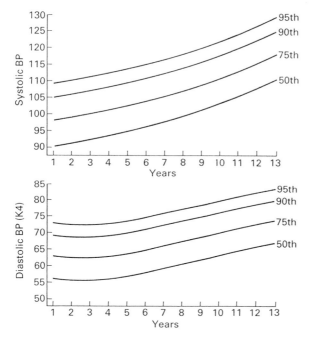

90th percentile
Systolic BP 105 106 107 108 109 111 112 114 115 117 119 121 124
Diastolic BP   69 68 68 69 69 70 71 73 74 75 76 77 79
Height (cm)   80 91 100 108 115 122 129 135 141 147 153 159 165
Weight (kg)   11 14 16 18 22 25 29 34 39 44 50 55 62

Fig. 9.4 Age-specific percentiles of blood pressure (BP) measurements in boys from 1 to 13 years of age; Korotkoff phase IV (K4) is used for diastolic BP.

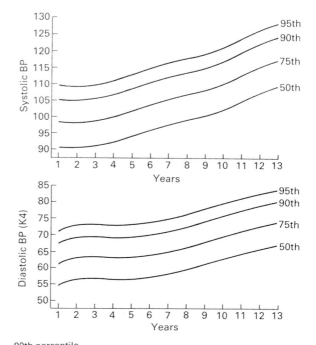

90th percentile
Systolic BP 105 105 106 107 109 111 112 114 115 117 119 122 124
Diastolic BP   67 69 69 69 69 70 71 72 74 75 77 78 80
Height (cm)   77 89 98 107 115 122 129 135 142 148 154 160 165
Weight (kg)   11 13 15 18 22 25 30 35 40 45 51 58 63

Fig. 9.5 Age-specific percentiles of blood pressure (BP) measurements in girls from 1 to 13 years of age; Korotkoff phase IV (K4) is used for diastolic BP.

and systolic BP equal to or greater than 110 mmHg at 7 days. Data for age-specific percentiles for male and female infants provided by the Second Task Force are shown in Figures 9.2 and 9.3.

Hypertension in school-aged children

The publication of the National Heart, Lung, and Blood Institute Task Force standards for the distribution of BP levels in children and adolescents has provided a basis for identification of subjects with elevated BP levels.

The recommendation of the Task Force was that children and adolescents who have BP levels above the 95th percentile on three or more separate examinations, even though they are asymptomatic, should be considered as having significant sustained elevation of BP, i.e. hypertension. Children who have lability in BP level on repeat examinations can be classified as having borderline hypertension if they have BP levels above the 90th but below the 95th percentile on more than two of three separate

occasions. This allows identification of subjects who might be at a higher risk of developing sustained hypertension later in life. Borderline hypertension in young adults is a predictor of future hypertension; these subjects have at least twice the frequency of developing established hypertension later than a similarly aged group of normotensive individuals [7]. We do not have similar data establishing the significance of boderline hypertension in children.

PREVALENCE OF HYPERTENSION IN CHILDHOOD

Primary (or essential) hypertension is a term used to describe hypertension for which no obvious cause is found. Secondary hypertension is the term used to describe elevated BP caused by a primary disease or abnormality in other organs, most frequently the kidney. Renal disease is the most common cause of severe hypertension in childhood.

The prevalence of essential hypertension in infancy

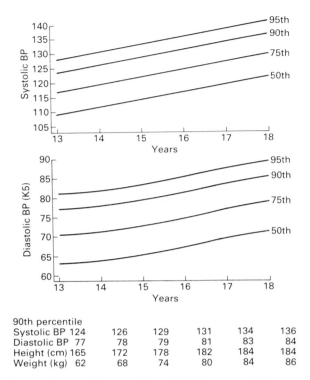

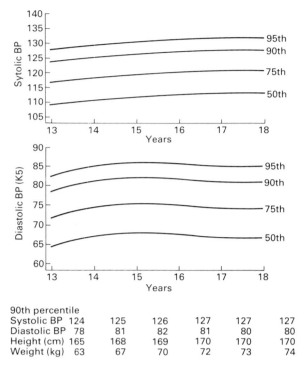

90th percentile						
Systolic BP	124	126	129	131	134	136
Diastolic BP	77	78	79	81	83	84
Height (cm)	165	172	178	182	184	184
Weight (kg)	62	68	74	80	84	86

Fig. 9.6 Age-specific percentiles of blood pressure (BP) measurements in boys from 13 to 18 years of age; Korotkoff phase V (K5) is used for diastolic BP.

90th percentile						
Systolic BP	124	125	126	127	127	127
Diastolic BP	78	81	82	81	80	80
Height (cm)	165	168	169	170	170	170
Weight (kg)	63	67	70	72	73	74

Fig. 9.7 Age-specific percentiles of blood pressure (BP) measurements in girls from 13 to 18 years of age; Korotkoff phase V is used for diastolic BP.

and the preschool period is unknown. Since the finding of a sustained elevation of BP in this age group is uncommon and is usually due to an underlying cause, the diagnosis of essential hypertension in these subjects is not practicable at this time.

The prevalence of primary (essential) hypertension in the childhood and adolescent population cannot be confidently defined on the basis of available data. The reports of prevalence of hypertension in children and adolescents vary considerably, depending on the criterion for hypertension, the population under study, the technique used for the measurement of BP, and the number of BP measurements obtained, etc. The classification of hypertension as mild, moderate, or severe is entirely arbitrary.

Surveys screening high-school students for hypertension identify a surprising number of them with elevated BP. Depending on the definition used for hypertension and the methodology, prevalence varies from 6 to 19% on initial screening [8–11]. When these same subjects are re-examined by the same personnel at a later time, however, there is a significant decrease in the number with hypertension on

retest. When three examinations are carried out only a small number of subjects (1–2.5%) are found to have sustained hypertension as defined by the Task Force [8–11]. This pattern of decreasing prevalence of hypertensive levels of BP in school populations subjected to retest examination has been invariably found in these studies. This pattern is in sharp contrast to the experience of health workers doing screening surveys in adults in the same community [9]. This experience emphasizes the need to be aware that BP changes continuously in children and adolescents and that there is a need for repeated BP measurements in order to identify subjects with sustained elevated BP.

Reichman and coworkers [11] found that race and sex differences consistent with those found with hypertension in adult populations in the USA, were evident. There were generally higher pressures among adolescent males than females and among blacks as compared to whites.

The predictive significance of sustained or labile hypertension (transient BP elevations) in childhood and adolescence with respect to the likelihood of developing sustained hypertension in adulthood however has not been established. Some data are of interest in this regard.

Higgins and colleagues [12] examined a group of students 13 years after they were initially seen when they were under 20 years of age. The accuracy of predicting high BP in later adulthood by BP rank as students was low: 44% for boys and 36% for girls in the two top deciles of risk.

Kuller and coworkers [13] examined 15–19-year-old high-school students 17 years later (mean age 34 years) and found 3 of 18 boys (17%) within the initially highest systolic BP percentile (>90%) were still in the highest percentile and 8 (44%) dropped below the 80th percentile. Weight gain was the major determinant of the subsequent finding of elevated BP in boys. The predictive values of finding elevated BP would need to be much higher to justify identifying subgroups for trials of preventive or therapeutic intervention in adolescents.

Heyden and co-authors [14] reported results of a follow-up examination in 30 young adults identified 7 years earlier in an epidemiologic study of a group of subjects 15–25 years of age, mean age 21 years. Initially 11 were labeled as hypertensive (37%; 2 of whom died from cerebral hemorrhage), 7 borderline (23%), and 12 (40%) had become normotensive. Four of 30 normotensive control subjects had developed borderline hypertension (13%). This study is frequently cited as evidence that hypertensive adolescents have considerable premature morbidity. However, it is difficult to extrapolate these findings to adolescents 12–18 years of age since this group (mean age 21 years initially) at the time of initial exam was composed of adolescents and young adults.

A subset of a group of children and adolescents initially studied at 9–18 years of age was re-evaluated at 30 years of age [15]. It was found that associations between the levels of blood pressure at 9 years of age and at 30 years of age were only significant for systolic BP in male subjects.

These data emphasize the need for more longitudinal studies of hypertensive children and adolescents into young adulthood in order to determine what the predictive value is of elevated BP detected in childhood or adolescence.

Secondary forms of hypertension

Elevated BP in children frequently has an underlying cause, e.g. parenchymal renal disease, renovascular or cardiovascular abnormalities, and various endocrinopathies. The probability that hypertension is secondary to such underlying factors is greater in younger children (<10 years of age) and when it is severe and symptomatic. There are few data on prevalence rates in the childhood population. Underlying organic disease is responsible for the majority of cases of severe symptomatic hypertension [16]. The prevalence of secondary forms of hypertension among asymptomatic children with hypertension detected by screening programs is so low (<0.5%) that their detection by mass screening studies of school populations is not cost-effective.

DISTRIBUTION OF CAUSES OF HYPERTENSION

The frequency of hypertension is variable and the rank of a particular type (i.e. essential) will depend on the definition used and the clinical setting of physicians reporting the data. The majority of severe persistent forms of hypertension in childhood leading to hospitalization have been found to be of secondary origin and renal disorders are the commonest cause found [16]. The major causes of sustained secondary hypertension in childhood are presented in Table 9.2. The distribution of types of hypertension found by chart review of cases hospitalized in two major metropolitan centers between 1970 and 1977 — New York (McCrory, unpublished observations) and London [17] — are given in Table 9.3. The majority of cases from both centers were found to have hypertension of renal origin. Within this category, renovascular disorders accounted for 8%. Cardiovascular diseases were second. In contrast to this distribution, Londe [16] found that only 5% of the patients found to have incidental hypertension (≥ the 90th percentile) in office practice had underlying disease of the urinary tract. There are clear limitations to extrapolating prevalence information from any of these studies.

The disorders of renal origin are particularly important because they include a number of forms of hypertension that are frequently curable. A recent report of surgically correctable hypertension of renal origin in childhood from a major hospital in Boston [18] found that slightly less than 10% of children attending the pediatric nephrology clinic had such a form of hypertension. The cases included children with renal artery narrowing (41%), atrophic scarred kidneys (41%), ureteropelvic junction obstruction

Table 9.2 Secondary hypertension in children

Renal origin	*Endocrine*
Parenchymal nephropathy	Obesity
Glomerulonephritides	Pheochromocytoma
Structural renal malformation	Hyperthyroidism (systolic
Polycystic disease	only)
Obstructive uropathy	Congenital adrenal
Ureteropelvic junction	hyperplasia
obstruction	17-hydroxylase deficiency
Reflux nephropathy	Primary hyperaldosteronism
Pyelonephritis	Cushing's syndrome
Segmental hypoplasia	
Renovascular	*Neurogenic tumors*
Wilms' tumor	Neurofibromatosis
Trauma	Neuroblastoma
Metabolic (cystinosis,	
oxalosis)	*Miscellaneous*
	Drug exposure
Cardiovascular	Sympathomimetic agents
Coarctation of the aorta	Glucocorticoids
Patent ductus arteriosus	Fracture immobilization
(systolic only)	Scoliosis repair
Arteriovenous fistula (systolic	Burns
only)	Heavy metal exposure
Aortic insufficiency	(lead, cadmium)
Polycythemia	Insect bites (scorpion)
Takayasu's arteritis	
	Central nervous system
	Increased intracranial
	pressure
	Dysautonomia

Table 9.3 Rank of causes of persistent hypertension in childhood. Children hospitalized for diagnostic work-up 1970–1977 in two metropolitan hospitals. Adapted from McCrory (unpublished observations) and Still and Cottom [17]

	London		New York	
Condition	No. of cases	%	No. of cases	%
Renal	78	78	62	61
Coarctation	15	15	13	13
Endocrine	—	—	6	6
Essential	1	1	7	7
Obesity	1	1	6	6
Miscellaneous	5	5	7	7
Total	100	101	101	100

(9%), and tumors (9%). The frequency of pyelonephritic atrophic renal disease, previously a major cause of hypertension, has been decreasing in the last two decades. This is a result of greatly improved methods of detection and treatment of children at risk because of the presence of recurrent urinary tract infection and upper tract obstruction or reflux nephropathy.

The management of renovascular hypertension in childhood is also undergoing continual improvement with new technologic advances (balloon angioplasty, partial nephrectomy) and the potential for relief of the associated hypertension is increasing.

The distribution of causes clearly varies with age. Coarctation was almost as common as renal disease in the 0–5-year age group in the New York City–London study. Obesity and essential hypertension are most commonly found in adolescence. Weight and obesity have been shown to be determinants of mean BP levels and prevalence of hypertension in children and adults [12]. While we do not understand the mechanisms involved in the relationships between weight, obesity, and BP, we do know that overweight children and young adults are at increased risk of being hypertensive and overweight at older ages. Obesity is an important potentially remediable risk factor for hypertension. While the highest incidence of essential hypertension in childhood is found in adolescents, the majority of these subjects have associated obesity [8,10,19]. Not all obese teenagers have hypertension, nor do fat adolescents necessarily become normotensive with weight loss. None the less, obesity-associated hypertension has important implications, both short-term (therapeutic) and long-term (risk factor for hypertensive cardiovascular disease).

Hormonal forms of juvenile hypertension are considered to be rare and as a result may sometimes be overlooked. The causes of hypertension in infancy differ significantly from those in children and adolescence.

Causes of hypertension in infancy (see Chapter 29)

Vascular accidents secondary to umbilical artery catheterizations performed in newborn infants are known to be one of the major causes of hypertension in early infancy [6]. Renovascular hypertension related to aortic and/or renal arterial thrombosis is the commonest type of hypertension seen but renal vein thrombosis or embolism secondary to such catheterizations has also been reported, as well as vessel aneurysm [6].

Coarctation of the aorta is the commonest cardiovascular disorder causing hypertension in infancy. Polycystic kidney disease is the major type of renal parenchymal disease causing hypertension in infants.

A variety of renal structural lesions can be associated with hypertension in infancy, including genitourinary abnormalities such as hydronephrosis, renal ectopia, renal arterial stenosis, and pelviureteral obstruction associated with hyperreninemia.

Cerebral thrombosis, central nervous system hemorrhage, and arteriovenous malformations may all be associated with hypertension. Hypertension commonly occurs during reconstructive surgery in newborn infants with abdominal wall defects and may persist for as long as 6 months [6]. Even though hypertension is rare in infancy any of the secondary forms of hypertension can occur.

The distribution of causes of childhood hypertension has a continuously changing pattern. The next decade should prove fruitful as new information accumulates concerning prevalence. We can also expect improvements in management from better understanding of mechanisms in the various forms of hypertension seen in the young.

REFERENCES

1 Beaglehole R, Eyles E. Salmond C et al. Blood pressure in Tokelaun children in two contrasting environments. *Am J Epidemiol* 1978;108:283−8.

2 Oliver WJ, Cohen El, Neel JV. Blood pressure, sodium intake and sodium related hormones in the Yanamamo Indians, a "no-salt" culture. *Circulation* 1975;52:146−51.

3 Report of the Second Task Force on blood pressure control in children−1987. *Pediatrics* 1987;79:1−25.

4 Voors AW, Webber LS, Fredricks RR, Berenson GS. Body weight and body mass as determinants of basal blood pressure in children−the Bogalusa heart study. *Am J Epidemiol* 1977;106:101−8.

5 Cornoni-Huntley J, Harlan WR, Leaverton PE. Blood pressure in adolescence. The United States health examination survey. *Hypertension* 1979;1:566−71.

6 Adelman RD. Neonatal hypertension. In: Loggie JM, Horan MJ, Gruskin AB et al., eds. *NHLBI Workshop on Juvenile Hypertension*. New York: Biomedical Information, 1984;267.

7 Julius S, Hansson L. Borderline hypertension: epidemiologic and clinical implications. In: Genest J, Kuchel O, Hamet P et al., eds. *Hypertension*. 2nd edn. New York: McGraw-Hill 1983:754.

8 Rames LK, Clarke WR, Connor WE et al. Normal blood pressures and the evaluation of sustained blood pressures in childhood: the Muscatine study. *Pediatrics* 1978;61:245−51.

9 Kilcoyne MM, Richter RW, Alsup PA. Adolescent hypertension 1. Detection and prevalence. *Circulation* 1974;50:758−64.

10 Loggie JMH, Rauh LW. Persistent systemic hypertension in the adolescent. *Med Clin North Am* 1975;59:1371−83.

11 Reichman LB, Cooper BM, Blumenthal S et al. Hypertension testing among high school students−I Surveillance procedures and results. *J Chron Dis* 1975;28:161−71.

12 Higgins MW, Keller JB, Metzner HL, Moore FE, Ostrander LD Jr. Studies of blood pressure in Tecumseh, Michigan II. Antecedents in children of high blood pressure in young adults. *Hypertension* 1980;2(suppl 1):1-117−123.

13 Kuller LH, Crook M, Almes MJ, Detre K, Reese G, Rutan G. Dormont high school (Pittsburgh, PA) blood pressure study. *Hypertension* 1980;2(suppl I):1-109−116.

14 Heyden S, Bartel AG, Hames CG, McDonough JR. Elevated blood pressure in adolescents, Evans County, GA. *JAMA* 1969;209:1683−9.

15 Woynarowska B, Mukherjee D, Roche AF et al. Blood pressure changes during adolescence and subsequent adult blood pressure levels. *Hypertension* 1985;7:695−701.

16 Londe S. Causes of hypertension in the young. *Pediatr Clin North Am* 1978;25:55−65.

17 Still JL, Cottom D. Severe hypertension in childhood. *Arch Dis Child* 1967;42:34−9.

18 Hendren WH, Kim SH, Herrin JT, Crawford JD. Surgically correctable hypertension of renal origin in childhood. *Am J Surg* 1982;143:432−42.

19 Levine LS, Lewy JE, New MI. Hypertension in high school students. *NY State J Med* 1976;76:40−4.

10 Evaluation of the Hypertensive Child and Adolescent

JENNIFER M. H. LOGGIE

When confronted by an infant, child, or adolescent with hypertension, the first question to be asked concerns the chronicity of the problem. This is important because the differential diagnosis is different for youngsters with acute rather than chronic hypertension. An acute transient rise in blood pressure is associated with a number of pediatric illnesses, and these are listed in Table 10.1. Also, in those genetically prone to hypertension, an acute transient rise in blood pressure may accompany many stressful situations such as anesthesia, fractures, lacerations, abdominal pain, etc. [1]. A good family history usually identifies these individuals and their blood pressure usually returns to a normal or high-normal range if they are followed over time. Diagnostic studies in this situation should be kept to a minimum, but long-term follow-up is important if stress-induced hypertension is indeed a marker for later hypertension. As an example, KL, a 5-year-old white female, presented to another hospital with abdominal pain and vomiting. She was rehydrated and sent home but returned within a week with similar symptoms. It was noted in retrospect that she had been hypertensive on both occasions with diastolic blood pressures as high as 110 mmHg. She was immediately evaluated with an abdominal angiogram, computerized tomography (CT) of the head, CT of the adrenal glands, and sundry other tests. All of these studies were normal and with time, the child's blood pressure returned to normal and has remained so over a 3-year period, except when she is stressed by an intercurrent illness when a transient rise occurs. Her mother has had hypertension since her late teenage years.

Clearly, the most helpful information to have when one is attempting to establish the chronicity of hypertension is past blood pressure readings. Unfortunately, these are by no means always available since routine blood pressure measurement in youngsters over 3 years of age is not yet uniformly obtained. In the absence of prior readings, one needs to look for evidence of target organ damage that may suggest chronicity. In children with even severe chronic hypertension or hypertensive encephalopathy, the optic fundi may show no more than retinal arteriolar nar-

Table 10.1 Conditions associated with acute transient hypertension or intermittent hypertension

Renal
Acute poststreptococcal glomerulonephritis
Hemolytic−uremic syndrome
Anaphylactoid purpura
Acute renal failure
Blood transfusion in patients with underlying renal disease

Metabolic
Hyperthyroidism (systolic)
Hypercalcemia
Hypernatremia
Hypovolemia (paradoxical hypertension)

Neurologic
Dysautonomia
Increased intracranial pressure (any cause)
Guillain−Barré syndrome

Drug-related
Steroid administration
Reserpine overdose
Amphetamine ingestion
Phencyclidine ingestion
Use of sympathomimetic agents (e.g. cold preparations, nosedrops)
Excessive ingestion of licorice (nonsynthetic)
Use of oral contraceptives

Miscellaneous
Burns
Stevens−Johnson syndrome
Cyclic vomiting
With orthopedic traction
Any form of stress in a hypertension-prone individual

rowing and arteriovenous nicking (Fig. 10.1). Hemorrhages and exudates are rarely found and papilledema may be absent even with encephalopathy. In acute severe hypertension, the fundi often have a very wet appearance associated with intense vasospasm of the retinal arterioles.

Just as there may be minimal funduscopic findings, there are infrequently cardiac findings that suggest chronicity. The heart is not often clinically enlarged and the electrocardiogram (ECG) and chest X-ray are usually unhelpful in detecting left ventricular hypertrophy, unless hypertension has been prolonged and severe. Therefore, if these studies are positive, they are helpful in determining chronicity; if negative, they tell one nothing about the duration of hypertension. The echocardiogram seems to be more sensitive for evaluating chamber size and wall thickness than the ECG and can be helpful [2]. If present, another helpful clue to the chronicity of hypertension is an elevated serum uric acid level. This may be present in both adults and children with chronic hypertension [3].

If one has established that a child or adolescent has acute hypertension in association with some underlying disease such as the hemolytic uremic syndrome, one treats the hypertension as a complication of that disease and extensive diagnostic studies to elucidate the etiology of the elevated blood pressure are unnecessary. Likewise, if one determines that a youth has hypertension transiently evoked by some form of stress, one may do little more diagnostically other than obtaining a urinalysis. However, faced with a child with chronic hypertension of unknown etiology, one's diagnostic evaluation is based to some degree on the level of blood pressure, the age, sex, and race of the patient, as well as the clinical findings and family history. The more severe the hypertension and the younger the child, the more probable that there is an underlying cause for the elevated pressure.

IMPORTANCE OF HISTORY

The importance of a careful personal and family history, as well as a careful physical examination, cannot be overemphasized. Tables 10.2 and 10.3 list the symptoms and signs that should be elicited. The family history is of particular importance since primary (essential) hypertension tends to be familial, as does pre-eclamptic toxemia. Likewise, there are some inherited renal disorders, such as polycystic kidney disease, and some hormonal disorders (multiple endocrine adenopathy II) that are familial.

When taking the family history it is not sufficient simply to ask which relatives have high blood pressure. One needs to know the age at detection of hypertension for parents, siblings, grandparents, aunts, uncles, and cousins. One also needs to know for these same individuals the age of occurrence of stroke, myocardial infarction, or other peripheral vascular disease. Furthermore, if parents and/or siblings

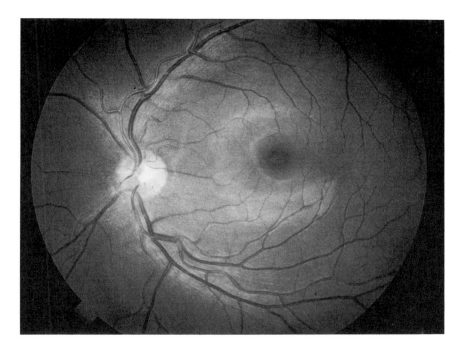

Fig. 10.1 Retinal photograph of an 18-year-old black male with essential hypertension showing retinal arteriolar narrowing, increased tortuosity, and arteriovenous nicking.

Table 10.2 Historical information that should be elicited

Information	Relevance
Family history of hypertension, pre-eclampsia, renal disease, tumors	Important in essential hypertension, inherited renal diseases, familial pheochromocytoma
Family history of early complications of hypertension and/or atherosclerosis	Suggests likely course of hypertension and/or presence of other coronary artery disease risk factors
Neonatal history	Use of umbilical artery catheter suggests need to evaluate renal vasculature and kidneys
Dietary history	Assessment of sodium and caloric consumption
Headaches, dizziness, epistaxis, visual problems	Nonspecific symptomatology
Abdominal pain, dysuria, frequency, nocturia, enuresis	May suggest underlying renal pathology
Joint pains or swelling, facial or peripheral edema	Suggestive of connective tissue disease and/or other forms of nephritis
Weight loss, failure to gain weight with good appetite, excess sweating, pallor, fevers, palpitations	In combination suggest pheochromocytoma
Muscle cramps, weakness, constipation	May suggest hyperaldosteronism with hypokalemia
Age of onset of menarche	May be helpful in suggesting hydroxylase deficiencies
Ingestion of prescription and over-the-counter drugs, contraceptives, illicit drugs	Drug-induced hypertension

have not had their blood pressure measured within a year, this should be done for all family members. It is not uncommon to find a parent or sibling of an index child with uncontrolled high blood pressure.

A unique condition, familial dexamethasone-suppressible hyperaldosteronism, which is an autosomal dominant disorder [4], may be suspected when there has been a striking amount of early-onset hypertension in a family. This is an important condition to diagnose, so that these families are not subjected to the conventional barrage of studies used in the evaluation of hypertension. In addition, at least in childhood, the blood pressure can be controlled with low doses of prednisone.

Presumably because of the frequent use of indwelling umbilical artery catheters in newborn infants, there have been increasing reports of renal artery thrombosis and embolism [5,6]. Therefore, a careful history of the neonatal course must be taken not only in the nursery, but also in the first 5 or 6 years of life when a child with hypertension is identified.

When taking a history it is useful to ask about the individual patient's diet and sodium consumption. Many of the youngsters in a hypertension clinic are overweight and few of them are aware of the hidden sodium in many of the foods that they eat. It is also important to try to determine the amount of exercise

they undertake, particularly if they are obese. Questions should also be asked about drug ingestion, including oral contraceptives and anabolic steroids, and about smoking and drinking habits in adolescents.

Since most hypertension is asymptomatic, it is unclear at what level of blood pressure headaches and dizziness do occur as symptoms of hypertension. The same is true for epistaxis and these complaints are all likely as common in the normotensive child and adolescent population as in the hypertensive one. However, severe headaches, particularly when they occur on awakening and are occipital in location, may be due to a markedly elevated blood pressure. The headaches may be reminiscent of those seen in children with brain tumors and they may be accompanied by vomiting and visual disturbances in the pre-encephalopathic state. Severe paroxysmal headaches accompanied by an acute rise in blood pressure should raise the suspicion of pheochromocytoma. However, youngsters with migraine headaches and hypertension may have exacerbations of the latter during one of their headaches. The character of the headache, as well as a family history of migraines, may help to differentiate between the two conditions. If not, appropriate biochemical testing may need to be done.

Table 10.3 Findings to look for on physical examination

Physical findings	Relevance
General	
Pale mucous membranes, facial, or pretibial edema	Renal disease
Pallor, evanescent flushing, increased sweating at rest	Pheochromocytoma versus hyperdynamic essential hypertension
Café-au-lait spots, neurofibromas	von Recklinghausen's disease
Moon face, hirsutism, buffalo hump, truncal obesity, striae	Cushing's syndrome
Webbing of the neck, low hairline, widely spaced nipples, wide carrying angle, etc.	Turner's syndrome
Elfin facies, usually some retardation	William's syndrome
Thyroid enlargement	Hyper- or hypothyroidism
Cardiovascular	
Absent or delayed femoral pulses, low leg pressure relative to arm pressure	Aortic coarctation
Heart murmur, rate, rhythm	Murmur-coarctation; tachycardia and/or arrhythmia; pheochromocytoma
Bruits over great vessels	Arteritis or arteriopathy
Sexual development	Delayed with hydroxylase deficiencies
Abdomen	
Epigastric bruit	Renovascular disease (isolated) or in association with William's or von Recklinghausen's disease
Unilateral or bilateral masses	Wilms' tumor, neuroblastoma, pheochromocytoma, polycystic kidneys, or other tumors
Bell's palsy	Chronic hypertension
Neurologic deficits (e.g. hemiparesis)	Chronic or severe acute hypertension with stroke
Hypertensive funduscopic changes	Chronic hypertension

Failure to grow or to gain weight may be seen in some children with underlying renal or renovascular hypertension [7]. When weight loss or failure to gain weight in association with a voracious appetite is accompanied by episodic flushing, pallor, sweating, palpitations, or unexplained fever, pheochromocytoma should be suspected. A past history of serious abdominal or back trauma may raise the suspicion that a renovascular lesion resulted and is causing hypertension.

IMPORTANCE OF PHYSICAL EXAMINATION

The physical examination, like the history, is geared to finding an underlying cause for hypertension. At a first visit, blood pressure should be measured in both arms and at least one leg. It should also be measured in one arm with the subject supine, sitting, and standing. The major arteries, like the brachials, carotids, and femorals, should all be palpated to detect inequalities or, in the case of the femoral artery, a lag between it and the radial artery. The heart and great vessels should be auscultated with care since bruits may be heard over one or another stenotic vessel. Epigastric bruits should be listened for routinely although in our experience only 30% of children with angiographically proven renal artery stenosis have had one [7]. Conversely, a number of children with epigastric bruits have had no angiographically demonstrable lesion.

Neurologic examination includes an assessment

for Bell's palsy, which may be the presenting finding in a child with hypertension, and a search for neurologic deficits that may be suggestive of a previous stroke. The fundi should also be routinely evaluated, for while hemorrhages and exudates are exceedingly rare, on occasion retinal arteriolar narrowing and arteriovenous nicking do occur, as does papilledema.

As mentioned earlier, one's diagnostic approach is to some degree influenced by the age of the child as well as the race and sex. Table 10.4 lists the commonest causes of sustained hypertension by age group. In newborn infants, there have been increasing reports of renal artery thrombosis and stenosis [5,6]. Coarctation of the aorta, commonest in infancy and in preschool children, usually manifests with much more severe systolic than diastolic hypertension. However, early in life, if there is a large shunt present or if the infant is in frank congestive heart failure, upper extremity hypertension may not be a feature [8]. Renal artery stenosis tends to present with rather severe hypertension, except perhaps in patients with neurofibromatosis or William's syndrome, when it may be milder [9]. Historically, most children with renal artery stenosis were said to present between the ages of 6 and 10 years [10]. However, now that blood pressure is measured earlier, especially in high-risk infants, many of these children are detected sooner. Males and females are equally affected, in contrast to the situation with hypoplasia of the kidney or bilateral chronic pyelonephritis or dysplasia. These conditions also may present with severe hypertension but occur more frequently in females.

Primary hypertension or hypertension of undetermined etiology has been described at all ages, from the newborn period onwards. The degree of elevation in blood pressure is generally mild-to-moderate and the greatest prevalence is seen in black teenagers of both sexes, as well as white male adolescents. This is not to say that white females never have essential hypertension. They do, but one should more assiduously pursue a secondary cause in them before labeling them as having primary hypertension. While essential hypertension likely consists of a number of subsets, clinically it is possible to identify two particular groups, those who are overweight and those who are thin and with evidence of a hyperdynamic cardiovascular state.

Hypertension secondary to an excess of endogenous hormones is uncommon but may present with severe hypertension. Pheochromocytoma, though relatively rare, is the commonest of the hormone-

Table 10.4 Commonest causes of chronic sustained hypertension by age group

Age group	Causes
Newborn infants	Renal artery thrombosis Renal artery stenosis Congenital renal malformations Coarctation of the aorta
Infancy to 6 years	Renal parenchymal diseases* Coarctation of the aorta Renal artery stenosis
6–10 years	Renal parenchymal diseases Renal artery stenosis Primary hypertension
Adolescence	Primary hypertension Renal parenchymal diseases

* Includes renal structural and inflammatory lesions, as well as tumors.

producing tumors. It usually, but not invariably, declares itself clinically by its signs and symptoms. The youngest reported case was in a 5-month-old child—an age when one might more likely suspect neuroblastoma, although these tumors infrequently present with cardiovascular complications. In boys, pheochromocytomas occur across the distribution of age while in girls, they tend to cluster around menarche.

Only a handful of cases of primary aldosteronism due to an adrenal adenoma have been reported in childhood, and these have all been in females [11]. Adrenal hyperplasia as a cause of aldosteronism in childhood is also rare and has been reported only in males [11]. Cushing's syndrome in childhood is usually due to the administration of exogenous steroids and much more rarely to an adrenal carcinoma.

After the clinical examination has been completed there are a few basic laboratory studies that should be ordered. These include a hemoglobin and hematocrit, urinalysis, urine culture in females, serum sodium, potassium, chloride, carbon dioxide content, a blood urea nitrogen, creatinine, and uric acid. Some believe that a first-morning urinary-specific gravity could replace other measures of renal function at a lesser cost. When primary hypertension is suspected on the basis of a negative physical examination, relatively mild hypertension, and a positive family history, the same basic investigations should be performed. At some time fasting cholesterol, triglycerides, high- and low-density lipoprotein cholesterol should also be measured. This is done in order to identify other coronary artery risk factors since these tend to cluster even in preadult life [12]. Some of the other diagnostic studies that are available are listed in Table 10.5. They need to be selected on a case-by-case basis, often after consultation with a radiologist or endocrinologist.

In the past, the traditional diagnostic evaluation of a hypertensive child followed a somewhat stereotyped format. After the basic studies noted above had been completed, there was a routine progression to excretory urography, and measurement of urinary catecholamines and their metabolites. Thereafter, particularly if the hypertension was moderate or severe, renal angiography was performed.

Since pheochromocytomas usually declare themselves clinically, it is unnecessary routinely to measure urinary catecholamines in all hypertensive youngsters. One must certainly keep the tumor in mind as it has been called the great mimic and, if there are subtle clinical clues to its presence, it may be necessary to measure plasma as well as urinary catecholamines. If plasma catecholamines are in the range seen with pheochromocytoma, it may also sometimes be necessary to perform a clonidine suppression test [13], which will be negative if a tumor is present. Thereafter CT of the abdomen should be undertaken in order to try to identify a tumor [14]. These occur anywhere that sympathetic tissue has existed, including the neck and chest, but are more common in the abdomen. Should the tumor prove to be malignant, the extent of its metastases may be better defined by an I^{131} metaiodobenzylguanidine scan than by an ordinary bone scan (see Chapter 25).

If the family history for hypertension is not striking; if the patient is not obese, and has moderate or severely elevated blood pressure without other symptoms suggesting pheochromocytoma, one should proceed to ultrasound of the kidneys or excretory urography since most relatively severe hypertension in childhood is renal or renovascular in origin. Any discrepancy in renal size usually suggests the need for renal angiography with sampling of blood for plasma renin activity (PRA) from each kidney. In our clinic we use the captopril renogram to screen patients who by the odds for age, race, or sex are unlikely to have renovascular hypertension but whose pressure is moderately elevated and not responding well to conventional drug therapy.

It is unclear in which children with hypertension, peripheral PRA, and serum aldosterone need to be measured. As already indicated, primary aldosteron-

Table 10.5 Diagnostic studies available for selected patients

Radiologic and radioisotope studies
Excretory urography
Renal ultrasonography
Renal radionuclide studies of flow and function
Renal angiography with measurement of renal vein renins
Computerized tomography of the kidneys*
Computerized tomography of the adrenal glands and/or abdomen
I^{131} metaiodobenzylguanidine scan

Hormonal studies
Quantitation of urine catecholamines and metabolites
Measurement of plasma catecholamines with or without clonidine suppression
Measurement of peripheral plasma renin activity and serum aldosterone
Quantitation of urinary aldosterone and electrolytes with and without salt-loading
Measurement of other hormones, e.g. free cortisol, 18 hydroxycorticosterone
Measurement of aldosterone and cortisol in adrenal venous effluent

* May be useful for detecting small tumors, e.g. hemangiopericytoma.

ism is rarely diagnosed in the young and other forms of mineralocorticoid excess are also uncommon but may be suspected if the peripheral PRA is low. If the family history of hypertension in young relatives is striking, the presence of a low PRA may suggest the need to study the family for familial dexamethasone-suppressible hyperaldosteronism.

Measurement of a high peripheral PRA may suggest a renal or renovascular cause for hypertension but it is not particularly useful since other studies, such as ultrasonography and angiography, need to be performed in order to delineate these lesions. It is our practice to measure peripheral PRA in patients with moderate or severe hypertension and without a strong family history of hypertension before drug therapy is initiated because in them a renal etiology for hypertension is likely. It is also our practice to measure PRA and aldosterone in children with any degree of hypertension when the family history for early onset of hypertension is very striking. For example, RW, aged 6 years, presented to us with a 1-year history of borderline blood pressures. The family history was remarkable in as much as his mother had had hypertension since the age of 7, and a maternal aunt and two cousins, aged 13 and 16, were all on medication for hypertension. The maternal grandfather died of a cerebral hemorrhage at age 42; a maternal uncle was hypertensive, as were both paternal grandparents. RW had low peripheral PRA and on being studied at the New York Hospital— Cornell Medical Center was found to have familial dexamethasone-suppressible hyperaldosteronism. Not all patients with aldosteronism have a low PRA, hypokalemia, and high serum aldosterone levels. When the condition is suspected it is advisable to quantitate urinary aldosterone and electrolytes before and after salt-loading.

Many of the patients seen in a hypertension clinic are obese and without evidence of Cushing's syndrome. Their diagnostic evaluation can usually be attenuated to include a hemoglobin and hematocrit, urinalysis, blood urea nitrogen, creatinine and uric acid, as well as fasting lipids. If hypertension is sustained over time, in this age range a renal ultrasound is indicated.

REFERENCES

1 Loggie JMH. The diagnostic evaluation of children and adolescents with hypertension. In: Hunt JC, Dreifus LS, Dustan HP *et al.*, eds. *Dialogues in Hypertension. Hypertension Update II*, vol 1. Lyndhurst, NJ: Health Learning Systems, 1984:43−56.

2 Devereux RB. Cardiovascular assessment of the hypertensive patient. In: Hunt JC, Dreifus LS, Dustan HP *et al.*, eds *Dialogues in Hypertension. Hypertension Update II*, vol 1. Lyndhurst, NJ: Health Learning Systems, 1984:27−42.

3 Prebis JW, Gruskin AB, Polinsky MS *et al.* Uric acid in childhood essential hypertension. *J Pediatr* 1981;98:702−7.

4 New MI, Oberfield SE, Levine LS *et al.* Demonstration of autosomal dominant transmission and absence of HLA linkage in dexamethasone suppressible hyperaldosteronism. *Lancet* 1980;i:550−1.

5 Goetzman BW, Stadalink RC, Bogren HG *et al.* Thrombotic complications of umbilical artery catheters: a clinical and radiographic study. *Pediatrics* 1975;56:374−9.

6 Fort KT, Teplick SK, Clark RE. Renal artery embolism causing neonatal hypertension. *Radiology* 1974;113:169−70.

7 Daniels SR, Loggie JMH, Towbin RB, McEnery PT. The clinical spectrum of juvenile renovascular hypertension. *Pediatrics* 1987;80:698−704.

8 Cottrill-Rolfes CM, Todd EP. Coarctation of the aorta. In: Kotchen TA, Kotchen JM, eds. *High Blood Pressure in the Young.* Bristol: John Wright 1983:175−207.

9 Daniels SR, Loggie JMH, Schwartz DE *et al.* Systemic hypertension secondary to peripheral vascular anomalies in patients with William's syndrome. *J Pediatr* 1985;106:249−51.

10 Ernst CB. Childhood renovascular hypertension. In: Kotchen TA, Kotchen JM, eds. *High Blood Pressure in the Young.* Bristol: John Wright, 1983;151−73.

11 Guthrie GP Jr. Adrenal disorders causing hypertension in children. In: Kotchen TA, Kotchen JM, eds. *High Blood Pressure in the Young.* Bristol: John Wright, 1983;209−26.

12 Occurrence of multiple risk factor variables for cardiovascular disease in children. In: Berenson GS ed. *Cardiovascular Risk Factors in Children.* Oxford: Oxford University Press, 1980:311−20.

13 Bravo EL, Tarazi RC, Fouad FM *et al.* Clonidine suppression test. A useful aid in the diagnosis of pheochromocytoma. *N Engl J Med* 1981;305:623−6.

14 Stewart BH, Bravo EL, Haaga J *et al.* Localization of pheochromocytoma by CT scan. *N Engl J Med* 1978;299:460−1.

11 General Considerations and Clinical Approach to the Management of Hypertension

ALAN R. SINAIKO

INTRODUCTION

Management of the hypertensive child traditionally has been patterned after strategies designed for treatment of hypertension in adults [1]. These strategies are based on a wealth of information gathered over the past few decades, showing that a reduction in hypertension-associated morbidity and mortality is correlated with reduction of blood pressure [2], particularly for individuals with severe disease. Although prevailing evidence and opinion suggest that drug treatment also is beneficial in adults with mild hypertension [1,3−6], antihypertensive intervention in this group is not universally accepted [7,8], and many questions remain unanswered. The superior effect of drug therapy on stroke compared to heart disease has not been explained; there are concerns about long-term drug therapy being associated with adverse effects that may potentiate, rather than relieve, hypertension-mediated organ disease; and there is evidence that overly aggressive therapy of mild hypertension may increase rather than decrease cardiovascular risk, because of excessive reduction in blood pressure [9]. Thus, there continues to be considerable controversy about the best clinical approach to mild hypertension in adults, and there is an acknowledged need for additional controlled clinical data [6].

In contrast to the situation in adults, questions about treatment of hypertension in children and adolescents have begun to be addressed only recently. Almost all would agree that antihypertensive drug therapy is indicated for children with severe hypertension (Table 11.1), defined by the 1987 Second Task Force on blood pressure control in children [10] as blood pressure greater than the 99th percentile of distribution. Failure adequately to treat this level of blood pressure ultimately results in the usual cardiovascular events associated with severe hypertension [11].

There is far less agreement about treatment of the child with significant (i.e. mild-to-moderate) hypertension (Table 11.2), defined as blood pressure between the 95th and 99th percentiles of distribution [10], and there are not any long- or short-term data to help clarify this issue. The recommended goal of treatment is reduction of blood pressure to a level below the 95th percentile. Treatment recommendations and goals are predicated on indirect evidence from epidemiologic studies of blood pressure tracking in which children at the higher distributions of blood pressure tend to maintain that distributional

Table 11.1 Definition of severe hypertension [10]

Age	Blood pressure (mmHg)	
	Systolic	Diastolic
Newborn	⩾106	−
7 days	⩾110	−
<2 years	⩾118	⩾82
3−5 years	⩾124	⩾84
6−9 years	⩾130	⩾86
10−12 years	⩾134	⩾90
13−15 years	⩾144	⩾92
16−18 years	⩾150	⩾98

Table 11.2 Definition of significant hypertension [10]

Age	Blood pressure (mmHg)	
	Systolic	Diastolic
Newborn	⩾96	−
7 days	⩾104	−
<2 years	⩾112	⩾74
3−5 years	⩾116	⩾76
6−9 years	⩾122	⩾78
10−12 years	⩾126	⩾82
13−15 years	⩾136	⩾86
16−18 years	⩾142	⩾92

position relative to their peer group as they age [12–14], and from cardiovascular studies showing a strong direct relationship between left ventricular size and blood pressure [15]. However, prospective data directly defining the relationship between childhood blood pressure and cardiovascular risk are not yet available, and there are justifiable concerns about the premature and overly aggressive use of antihypertensive drugs in the group with significant hypertension.

Antihypertensive intervention should begin with nonpharmacologic strategies that reduce blood pressure over a period of weeks or months in children and adolescents with mild hypertension. Because the immediate risk is low, rapid lowering of blood pressure is far less important than gradual, but steady, progress. There is no evidence that immediate reduction of blood pressure in the group with significant hypertension improves prognosis or well-being. Patience and firm reinforcement are particularly important for success, particularly when considering that these therapies may be necessary for many decades of life.

In this chapter, strategies for the clinical management of hypertension in children will be discussed. Drug therapy will be addressed only as it pertains to drug selection and therapeutic regimens, since each class of drugs is discussed in detail in other chapters of this book. It is hoped that the reader will use this information to develop his or her own rational and feasible approach to the blood pressure treatment of children and adolescents.

NONPHARMACOLOGIC THERAPY

Nonpharmacologic treatment should be introduced as initial therapy in patients with significant hypertension [10,16]; it should be emphasized as a component of general preventive health care delivery in children with high-normal blood pressure, i.e. blood pressure between the 90th and 95th percentiles of distribution [10], and should be included with drug therapy in patients with severe hypertension, in an attempt to reduce the number and dose of drugs required to control hypertension. Nonpharmacologic therapy includes weight reduction, exercise, and dietary modification.

Weight

Body size is the major factor accounting for blood pressure variability among children. This relationship is firmly established by age 6 years [17] and continues into later childhood [10,18,19]. Obviously, not all children with hypertension are overweight. However, there is a significant positive correlation between percentage overweight and systolic and diastolic blood pressure in adolescents [20], and the distribution curves of both systolic and diastolic blood pressure of obese adolescents are shifted significantly to the right when compared to the blood pressure distribution curves of normal-weight adolescents [21].

Weight loss is associated with a reduction in systolic and diastolic blood pressure [20,21], although not all children who lose weight will have a concomitant reduction in blood pressure. This may be a function of relative fatness, and the independent role of fatness in blood pressure regulation is poorly defined. Data from the Health Examination Survey suggest that blood pressure is influenced to a greater degree by components of body mass other than fat [22]. Obesity, of itself, has a major adverse effect on cardiovascular function [23], and weight reduction in adolescents has a positive effect on overall cardiovascular risk by reducing serum lipid and hormonal abnormalities that are prevalent in obese individuals [24,25]. Because hypertension in children and adolescents should be considered in the broader context of generalized cardiovascular risk, as is the case in adults, it seems reasonable that a primary goal of therapy should be the reduction of body weight to levels consistent with the patient's sex, age, and height [10].

Exercise

Most evidence suggests that physical fitness in children [26] and adolescents [27] is associated with lower blood pressure and other risk factors, although there are some exceptions [28]. Significant reductions in systolic and diastolic blood pressure occur after approximately 6 months of aerobic exercise training [19,29], and the added effect of exercise combined with weight reduction on blood pressure appears to be superior to weight reduction alone [21]. As might be expected, failure to maintain aerobic conditioning results in a return of blood pressure to pre-exercise levels [29]. Static exercise, such as weight training, may also cause a reduction in blood pressure [30], but its long-term effect on cardiovascular fitness needs to be evaluated before it can be broadly recommended.

The question about participation in sports by the hypertensive child inevitably arises, particularly in the adolescent age group. Blood pressure increases during exercise by an equivalent amount in children with moderate hypertension and those with normal blood pressure [31,32], so that the blood pressure of hypertensive children remains significantly higher regardless of degree of activity. The levels achieved during exercise do not appear great enough to warrant limitations on sports activities, without evidence of electrocardiographic or other cardiac abnormalities [32]. The best approach to the child with severe hypertension who wishes to participate in sports remains an issue. Because these children are likely to be at greater risk from strenuous exercise, sports activity should be restricted until blood pressure can be reduced below the 99th percentile of distribution. Even then, it is suggested that supervised testing should be conducted before approval is given to return to regular sports participation. Because the evidence, to date, strongly suggests that exercise has a beneficial effect on blood pressure, as well as other cardiovascular risk factors [33], it is contraindicated only in those children with persistent severe hypertension.

Diet

The role of dietary intervention in blood pressure management is still unsettled. The relationship between sodium intake and hypertension has been most widely studied, and a careful analysis of those data strongly suggests that dietary sodium reduction in sodium-sensitive individuals has a beneficial effect on blood pressure [34,35]. Adequate studies have not been performed in children, in part because methods used in humans to identify sodium-sensitive individuals are cumbersome and not absolutely reliable. The intake of sodium by virtually all individuals of all ages in industrialized countries far exceeds recommended daily allowances. Thus, sodium restriction can and should be attempted in hypertensive individuals without fear of adverse dietary consequences. Admittedly, reduction of sodium intake in free-living individuals is difficult, because of the pervasiveness of sodium in the contemporary diet (Table 11.3). Nevertheless, a significant impact can be made on sodium intake with proper education and reinforcement.

Dietary supplementation with potassium also may have an antihypertensive effect [36]. It has been

Table 11.3 Some foods with high sodium content

Breadcrumbs, seasoned
Most cold cereals
American cheese
Salad dressing
TV dinners
Pizza
Spaghetti sauce
Mexican-style foods
Bacon
Cured ham
Pork sausage
Canned soups
Almost all prepared foods at fast-food restaurants, e.g.
   McDonald's
   Burger King
   Wendy's
   Arby's
Dill pickles
Canned vegetables

suggested that the high prevalence of hypertension in accultured societies is a consequence of evolutionary change from the high-potassium—low-sodium dietary environment of prehistoric man to the high-sodium—low-potassium dietary environment of today [37]. Potassium has direct antihypertensive effects [38]. However, the relationship between dietary potassium intake and blood pressure in humans is not well understood, and in laboratory animals high-potassium diets protect against hypertension-mediated target organ disease independent of blood pressure response [39].

Increasing potassium intake as a nonpharmacologic dietary goal can be difficult. Potassium-rich foods are primarily fruits and vegetables (Table 11.4). Although encouraging an increased intake of these foods is dietarily sound, the relatively large quantity required on a daily basis to have a positive impact on blood pressure is very difficult for most patients to manage. Based on practical clinical considerations, the most prudent dietary approach, at the present time, is encouragement of an increase in potassium-containing foods and decrease in sodium-containing foods. This dual approach will increase the potassium:sodium ratio, which many believe to be the key element in cationic control of blood pressure.

The most recent dietary controversy involves the role of dietary calcium in blood pressure homeostasis [40]. Calcium is integral to the functioning of most physiological systems and, in particular, modulates

Table 11.4 Some foods with high potassium content

>10 mmol	
Avocado	$\frac{1}{2}$ fruit
Banana	1
Beans	$\frac{1}{2}$ cup
Orange juice	1 cup
Baked potato	1
Tomato juice	1 cup

7–10 mmol	
Cantaloupe	$\frac{1}{6}$ melon
Grapefruit juice	1 cup
Milk	1 cup
Orange, raw	1
Pineapple juice	1 cup
Raisins	$\frac{1}{4}$ cup
Tomato, raw	1
Yogurt	1 cup

stimulation–contraction coupling in vascular smooth muscle and stimulation–secretion coupling in adrenergic neurons. Because of these relationships, it seems paradoxical that an increase in calcium intake has been reported to have an antihypertensive effect [41]. Nevertheless, a convincing case for the use of dietary calcium in the treatment or prevention of hypertension has been made, based on epidemiological, clinical, and basic research studies [42,43].

The number of clinical studies of dietary calcium in normotensive and hypertensive humans is far too large to reference in this chapter. Despite strong support from some clinical trials for dietary calcium intervention, there are an equivalent number of reports that do not demonstrate any benefit from calcium supplementation. It is far from clear why this discrepancy exists. Additional information, currently being developed, should define the role of calcium in systemic hypertension, particularly in relationship to sodium and potassium. It would be premature to suggest modification of dietary calcium until these data are available.

Dietary caloric and lipid restrictions are important considerations as part of a general program of cardiovascular disease prevention. As noted above, weight reduction can be associated with a reduction in blood pressure, although its effect appears to be greatly enhanced when combined with an effective exercise program [24]. In adults, the independent risk from serum cholesterol and diastolic blood pressure follows almost identical patterns [16]. Although it is not clear whether serum lipid reduction *per se* affects blood pressure, serum lipid evaluation and dietary

counseling are recommended, using guidelines developed by the American Academy of Pediatrics [44].

ANTIHYPERTENSIVE DRUG THERAPY

Hypertensive emergencies (see Chapter 31)

Antihypertensive drug therapy should be started immediately in any patient presenting with symptomatic hypertension, i.e. severe hypertension with headache, eyeground changes, neurological findings, or malignant renal disease. The goal in treatment of hypertensive emergencies is reduction of blood pressure to levels that eliminate the risk of hypertension-related cardiovascular events, i.e. stroke, encephalopathy, or cardiac failure. It should be understood that the goal is *not* immediate reestablishment of normal blood pressure; this can be achieved more gradually as chronic drug therapy is incorporated into the therapeutic regimen. Precipitous drops in blood pressure should be avoided, because of the risk of hypotension-related adverse effects within the central nervous system, i.e. seizures or obtundation [45].

A number of drugs can be used to treat hypertensive emergencies, although the initial choice from among them depends on the severity of presentation (Table 11.5). For treatment of patients without neurological symptoms, the calcium channel blocking agent, nifedipine, may be the drug of choice, because of its effectiveness in children of all ages [46], ease of oral administration, rapid onset of action, and usual freedom from side-effects. Blood levels of nifedipine are detectable only 6 min after sublingual dosing [47], and this has been the preferred route of administration. However, nifedipine is also rapidly absorbed after oral administration [47], provided it is not taken with food [48], and blood levels are significantly higher than after sublingual dosing [47]. The highly variable duration of action and the fact that response seems to diminish with frequent repeated administration, regardless of dose, should be recognized as potential problems with nifedipine.

Hydralazine is also a useful drug, but may be less effective than nifedipine and must be used parenterally for a rapid effect. Repeated dosing with hydralazine is usually not tolerated because of flushing, tachycardia, headache, and nausea. Thus, if treatment is not successful with an initial dose followed by a second dose twice the amount of the first, it is best to select another drug.

Table 11.5 Acute antihypertensive drug therapy

Drug	Indication	Dose	Route
Nifedipine	Asymptomatic severe hypertension	0.25–0.5 mg/kg	Oral/sublingual
Hydralazine	Asymptomatic severe hypertension	0.2–0.4 mg/kg	i.v.
Labetalol	Symptomatic severe hypertension	1–3 mg/kg	i.v.
Diazoxide	Symptomatic severe hypertension	2–5 mg/kg	i.v.
Sodium nitroprusside	Symptomatic severe hypertension	0.5–8 µg/kg per min	i.v.

Patients with severe symptoms or who fail to respond to the above drugs should receive intravenous therapy with more effective agents. Labetalol is a newer β-adrenergic blocking agent which also has α-adrenergic blocking properties. Although clinical experience with this drug in children is limited at the present time, it is very effective in treating hypertensive emergencies in adults and allows a more gradual and controlled reduction of blood pressure. However, some patients have a paradoxical increase in blood pressure.

It is likely that, with the availability of labetalol, the use of diazoxide will decrease. Nevertheless, diazoxide remains a very effective antihypertensive agent because of its rapid clinical response. The use of a bolus injection may be associated with precipitous falls in blood pressure that can be avoided by using lower and slower infusion doses.

The most reliable of the drugs used for hypertensive emergencies continues to be sodium nitroprusside. It must be administered by continuous intravenous infusion, but its onset of action occurs within 30 s and its antihypertensive effect disappears almost as quickly, when the drug dose is reduced or discontinued. A potential limiting side-effect is tachycardia. Retention of thiocyanate or cyanide following nitroprusside metabolism is rarely a problem in patients with normal or moderately reduced renal function.

Chronic antihypertensive therapy

SEVERE HYPERTENSION

There is a general consensus that antihypertensive drugs are indicated for almost all patients with severe hypertension. Drug therapy can usually be withheld in the asymptomatic patient until a diagnostic evaluation has been completed and in patients with potentially curable lesions, i.e. renal artery stenosis or adrenal tumor, who will have corrective surgery within a short time.

SIGNIFICANT HYPERTENSION

Drug therapy can be delayed in patients with significant, i.e. mild-to-moderate, hypertension until attempts to control blood pressure with the non-pharmacologic intervention strategies described above have proven unsuccessful. Recommendations for drug therapy in children are based on the adult stepped-care model [1] in which therapy is started with a given drug and modified in a stepwise fashion depending on response. The stepped-care approach, as outlined in the Second Task Force Report [10], is still recommended for children and adolescents. However, the choice of drugs and the sequence in which they are used has been modified substantially in the brief period since the Report was published. This is the result of broader clinical experience with newer classes of antihypertensive drugs coupled with concerns about potentially important adverse effects recently recognized with the traditionally used agents.

In previous years, diuretics and β-adrenergic blocking drugs were recommended for first-line therapy. These drugs are currently undergoing careful review, because their use is associated with the development of serum lipid profiles known to be associated with high risk for atherosclerosis [49,50]. In addition, clinical intervention trials have shown that reductions in cerebrovascular events and congestive heart failure in diuretic-treated hypertensive adults have not been paralleled by similar reductions in cardiac mortality [2]. The effect of antihypertensive therapy on lipids has not been evaluated in children, and adverse cardiovascular outcomes in children will not be documented because of age and because the short-term adverse effects are clinically inconsequential. It seems foolish, however, to ignore these findings in choosing drugs for this age group, since long-term drug exposure is likely and will extend into adulthood.

Diuretic therapy is probably best reserved for patients with renal disease. Thiazide diuretics are effective until the glomerular filtration rate falls below 50% of normal, at which time a loop diuretic (furosemide or bumetanide) should be substituted. Aldactone may complement other diuretics in patients with diseases that increase aldosterone secretion — nephrotic syndrome, congestive heart failure, or liver failure — but has otherwise limited benefit in children. β-blocking drugs continue to be widely used. Choosing congeners with cardioselective or intrinsic sympathomimetic activity can minimize potential adverse effects, particularly increased serum lipids and hypoglycemia.

The major change taking place in antihypertensive drug therapy is the introduction of angiotensin converting enzyme (ACE) inhibitors and calcium channel blocking agents as first-line drugs. ACE inhibitors have been found to be very effective in children and adolescents and have a low incidence of side-effects. There are a few important caveats to their use:

1 the diagnosis of renal artery stenosis should be eliminated before these drugs are administered, because the kidney with renal artery stenosis is dependent on efferent arteriolar vasoconstriction, mediated via angiotensin II receptors, to maintain glomerular filtration. Inhibition of angiotensin II formation by ACE inhibitors will result in renal failure in patients with bilateral renal artery stenosis or renal artery stenosis in a solitary kidney;

2 although side-effects are uncommon with recommended doses, reduced drug clearance in patients with renal failure increases their incidence, and

3 because infants are more sensitive to ACE inhibitors, the starting dose should be 80–90% lower than the usual dose in older children [51].

The newest class of antihypertensive agents, the calcium channel blocking drugs, is likely to join the ACE inhibitors as the most commonly used antihypertensive drugs within the next few years. Although a large number of these molecules have been developed [52], only a few have been approved, or are on the verge of approval, for clinical use. Specific information about their use in children is sparse, with the exception of nifedipine. While nifedipine has become the most frequently used drug in acute hypertension in our institution, it is less effective in chronic therapy for children, primarily because of its short duration of action. Newer calcium channel blocking agents may be more useful. Our experience with nitrendipine, a new dihydropyridine compound, suggests that this drug is effective in children during short- and long-term therapy, has a longer duration of action, and is remarkably free of side-effects (Wells TG and Sinaiko AR, unpublished observations.)

Agents acting on the α-adrenergic nervous system, i.e. α_2-agonists clonidine and methyldopa, and the α_1-blocking agent prazosin, are generally considered to be second-line drugs. The very effective vasodilator minoxidil is usually reserved for patients who are refractory to other antihypertensive therapy. Its side effects of tachycardia and water retention always require concomitant therapy with a β-blocking agent and a loop diuretic, and the accompanying hypertrichosis, although not debilitating, has proven to be extremely unpleasant for patients and parents. It is the rare patient who will not respond to a regimen constructed from currently available antihypertensive drugs.

DRUGS PROMOTING HYPERTENSION

Certain drugs are known to cause hypertension or to cause a further increase in blood pressure when administered to a hypertensive individual. The most notorious of these are contraceptive pills. In the hypertensive female, these pills should be discontinued to determine whether an etiologic relationship can be identified, and in girls with established hypertension, even those well controlled by drugs or other interventions, they should not be started without a highly compelling reason. Glucocorticoids commonly cause hypertension after 3 or more weeks of daily therapy. Aminoglycosides, vancomycin, amphotericin, interferon, and cyclosporin are known to be nephrotoxic, and hypertension is frequently the initial clinical finding. Amphetamine-like drugs and a number of over-the-counter drugs containing decongestants can cause hypertension [53]. However, short-term use of these drugs in moderate dosage is rarely contraindicated, even in a hypertensive child.

COMPLIANCE

Compliance with antihypertensive regimens is dependent on age, motivation, and parental support. It is usually highest in younger children, because they rely on their parents for drug administration, and parents will usually be able and willing to accept this responsibility. As children progress into adolescence, compliance becomes a greater problem.

Nonpharmacologic strategies are particularly difficult for the adolescent and are rarely achieved without strong family support. It is virtually impossible to expect a change in eating behavior, i.e. reduction in sodium or saturated fat, without strong family support and agreement to participate in the dietary change. Weight reduction and exercise programs are difficult to maintain without regular reinforcement through group support, organized activities, and contact with the physician or other health care provider. Daily medication compliance is enhanced by using drugs requiring the lowest frequency of administration. Even then, strategies must be devised to provide daily reminders for the patient. While parents can be of great help in this regard, clear-cut contracts must be agreed upon between the parent and child to minimize the potential for conflict. With constructive support, pill-taking can be very successful. In a clinical trial currently in progress, we have found a compliance of 80–90% in 140 teenagers taking twice-daily capsules over a 2-year period.

ACKNOWLEDGMENT

Supported, in part, by *National Institutes of Health* grant HL-34659.

REFERENCES

1 The 1988 report of the joint national committee on detection, evaluation, and treatment of high blood pressure. *Arch Intern Med* 1988;148:1023–38.
2 Maxwell MH. Beyond blood pressure control: effect of antihypertensive therapy on cardiovascular risk factors. *Am J Hypertens* 1988;1:3665–715.
3 Hypertension Detection and Follow-up Program Cooperative Group. Effect of stepped care treatment on the incidence of myocardial infarction and angina pectoris. *Hypertension* 1984;6(suppl I):I-198–206.
4 Memorandum from the WHO/ISH. 1986 guidelines for the treatment of mild hypertension. *Hypertension* 1986;8:957–61.
5 Moser M, Gifford RW. Why less severe degrees of hypertension should be treated. *J Hypertens* 1985;3:437–47.
6 Grimm RH, Neaton JD, Prineas RJ. Primary prevention trials and the rationale for treating mild hypertension. *Clin Ther* 1987;9 (suppl D):20–30.
7 Ramsay LE. Mild hypertension: treat patients, not populations. *J Hypertens* 1985;3:449–55.
8 Kaplan NM. Critical comments on recent literature. The 1988 report of the joint national committee. *Am J Hypertens* 1989;2:72–4.
9 Kaplan NM. Critical comments on recent literature. The J curve and other problems with therapy. *Am J Hypertens* 1989;2:132–3.
10 Report of the Second Task Force on Blood Pressure Control in Children—1987. *Pediatrics* 1987;79:1–25.
11 Heyden S, Bartel AG, Harmes CG, McDonough JR. Elevated blood pressure levels in adolescents, Evans County, Georgia. *JAMA* 1969;209:1683–9.
12 Prineas RJ, Gomez-Marin O, Sinaiko AR. Electrolytes and blood pressure levels in childhood hypertension: measurement and change. *Clin Exp Hypertens* [A] 1986;8:583–604.
13 Sinaiko AR, Bass J, Gomez-Marin O, Prineas RJ. Cardiac status of adolescents tracking with high and low blood pressure since early childhood. *J Hypertens* 1987;4(suppl5):5378–80.
14 Munger RG, Prineas RJ, Gomez-Marin O. Persistent elevation of blood pressure among children with a family history of hypertension: the Minneapolis children's blood pressure study. *J Hypertens* 1988;6:647–53.
15 Mahoney LT, Schieken RM, Clarke WR, Lauer RM. Left ventricular mass and exercise responses predict future blood pressure: the Muscatine study. *Hypertension* 1988;12:206–13.
16 Stamler R, Stamler J, Grimm R et al. Nutritional therapy for high blood pressure. *JAMA* 1987;257:1484–91.
17 Prineas RJ, Gillum RF, Gomez-Marin O. The determinants of blood pressure levels in children: the Minneapolis children's blood pressure study. In: Loggie JMH, Horan MJ, Gruskin AB, Hohn AR, Dunbar JB, Havlik RJ, eds. *NHLBI Workshop on Juvenile Hypertension*. New York; Biomedical Information, 1984:21–35.
18 Prineas RJ, Gomez-Marin O, Gillum RF. Tracking of blood pressure in children and nonpharmacological approaches to the prevention of hypertension. *Ann Behav Med* 1985;7:25–9.
19 Clarke WR, Woolson RF, Lauer RM. Changes in ponderosity and blood pressure in childhood: the Muscatine study. *Am J Epidemiol* 1986;124:195–206.
20 Brownell KD, Kelman JH, Stunkard AJ. Treatment of obese children with and without their mothers: changes in weight and blood pressure. *Pediatrics* 1983;71:515–23.
21 Rocchini AP, Katch V, Anderson J et al. Blood pressure in obese adolescents: effect of weight loss. *Pediatrics* 1988;82:16–23.
22 Stallones L, Mueller WH, Christensen BL. Blood pressure, fatness, and fat patterning among USA adolescents from two ethnic groups. *Hypertension* 1982;4:483–6.
23 Messerli FH, Sundgaard-Riise K, Reisen E, Dreslinski G, Dunn FG, Frohlich E. Disparate cardiovascular effects of obesity and arterial hypertension. *Am J Med* 1983;74:808–12.
24 Becque MD, Katch VL, Rocchini AP, Marks CR, Moorehead C. Coronary risk incidence of obese adolescents: reduction by exercise plus diet intervention. *Pediatrics* 1988;81:605–12.
25 Rocchini AP, Katch V, Schork A, Kelch RP. Insulin and

blood pressure during weight loss in obese adolescents. *Hypertension* 1987;10:267–73.

26 Hofman A, Walter HJ, Connelly PA, Vaughan RD. Blood pressure and physical fitness in children. *Hypertension* 1987;9:188–91.

27 Fripp RR, Hodgson JL, Kwiterovich PO, Werner JC, Schuler HG, Whitman V. Aerobic capacity, obesity, and atherosclerotic risk factors in male adolescents. *Pediatrics* 1985;75:813–18.

28 Wilson SL, Gaffney FA, Laird WP, Fixler DE. Body size, composition, and fitness in adolescents with elevated blood pressures. *Hypertension* 1985;7:417–22.

29 Hagberg JM, Goldring D, Ehsani AA *et al*. Effect of exercise training on the blood pressure and hemodynamic features of hypertensive adolescents. *Am J Cardiol* 1983;52:763–8.

30 Hagberg JM, Ehsani AA, Goldring D, Hernandez A, Sinacore DR, Holloszy JO. Effect of weight training on blood pressure and hemodynamics in hypertensive adolescents. *J Pediatr* 1984;104:147–51.

31 Schieken RM, Clarke WR, Lauer RM. The cardiovascular responses to exercise in children across the blood pressure distribution. *Hypertension* 1983;5:71–8.

32 Fixler DE, Laird WP, Browne R, Fitzgerald V, Wilson S, Vance R. Response of hypertensive adolescents to dynamic and isometric exercise stress. *Pediatrics* 1979;64:579–83.

33 Fripp RR, Hodgson JL. Effect of resistive training on plasma lipid and lipoprotein levels in male adolescents. *J Pediatr* 1987;111:926–31.

34 Walczyk MH, McCarron DA. Electrolytes in hypertensive cardiovascular disease. *Am J Hypertens* 1988;1:3525–625.

35 Falkner B. Sodium sensitivity: a determinant of essential hypertension. *J Am Coll Nutr* 1988;7:35–41.

36 Luft FC, Weinberger MH. Potassium and blood pressure regulation. *Am J Clin Nutr* 1987;45:1289–94.

37 Meneely GR, Battarbee HD. High sodium–low potassium environment and hypertension. *Am J Cardiol* 1976;38:768–85.

38 Tannen RL. Effects of potassium on blood pressure control. *Ann Intern Med* 1983;98:773–80.

39 Tobian L, MacNeill D, Johnson MA, Ganguli MC, Iwai J. Potassium protection against lesions of the renal tubules, arteries, and glomeruli and nephron loss in salt-loaded hypertensive Dahl S rats. *Hypertension* 1984;6(Suppl I):I-170–6.

40 Symposium on calcium and hypertension. *Fed Proc* 1986;45:2732–62.

41 Van Breemen C, Canvin C, Johns A, Leizten P, Yamamoto H. Calcium regulation of vascular smooth muscle. *Fed Proc* 1986;45:2746–51.

42 McCarron DA, Morris CD. Metabolic considerations and cellular mechanism related to calcium's antihypertensive effects. *Fed Proc* 1986;45:2734–8.

43 Resnick LM, Nicholson JP, Laragh JH. Calcium metabolism in essential hypertension: relationship to altered renin system activity. *Fed Proc* 1986;45:2739–45.

44 Committee on Nutrition, American Academy of Pediatrics. Indications for cholesterol testing in children. *Pediatrics* 1989;83:141–42.

45 Perlman JM, Volpe JJ. Neurologic complications of captopril treatment of neonatal hypertension. *Pediatrics* 1989;83:47–52.

46 Siegler RL, Brewer ED. Effect of sublingual or oral nifedipine in the treatment of hypertension. *J Pediatr* 1988;112:811–13.

47 Reamsch KD, Sommer J. Pharmacokinetics and metabolism of nifedipine. *Hypertension* 1983;5(suppl II):II-18–24.

48 Reitberg DP, Love SJ, Quercie GT, Zinny MA. Effect of food on nifedipine pharmacokinetics. *Clin Pharmacol Ther* 1987;42:72–5.

49 Grimm RH. Thiazide diuretics and selective α blockers: comparison of use in antihypertensive therapy including possible differences in coronary heart disease risk reduction. *Am J Med* 1987;82(suppl 1A):26–30.

50 Stark RM. The atherogenic risk of antihypertensive therapy. *Am J Med* 1988;84(suppl 1B):86–8.

51 O'Dea RF, Mirkin BL, Alward CT, Sinaiko AR. Treatment of neonatal hypertension with captopril. *J Pediatr* 1988;113:403–6.

52 Abernethy DR, Schwartz JB. Pharmacokinetics of calcium antagonists under development. *Clin Pharmacokin* 1988;15:1–14.

53 Saken R, Kates GL, Miller K. Drug-induced hypertension in infancy. *J Pediatr* 1979;95:1077–9.

12 Diuretic Usage in Hypertensive Children

ALAN B. GRUSKIN, GARY R. LERNER,
AND LARRY E. FLEISCHMANN

Despite the wide use of diuretics to lower blood pressure in pediatric patients only a few systematic studies of the use of these agents to treat hypertensive disorders in children are available. This chapter has three objectives: to provide an overview of the mechanisms of action of diuretics as they relate to their blood pressure-lowering effect; to consider general guidelines for using diuretics as blood pressure-lowering agents, and intensively to consider available specific pediatric information on the role of diuretics in treating childhood hypertension in four general areas: acute and chronic renal disease, adrenal/renal tubular disorders, and essential hypertension. Most children with hypertension have one of these disorders. Data detailing the use of diuretics to treat other forms of childhood hypertension are not yet available and consequently will not be considered.

MECHANISM OF ACTION

The principal mechanism by which diuretics lower blood pressure is by enhancing sodium excretion, thereby reducing extracellular volume [1]. Some data exist suggesting that diuretics may act in part by a direct vasodilator effect on resistance vessels or by increasing the net production of vasodepressor substances. It has been suggested that diuretics directly affect resistance vessels by slowly altering smooth muscle content of sodium and/or calcium and improving their ability to relax. Four observations support the concept that the antihypertensive effect of diuretics is due solely to their impact on sodium balance:

1 no antihypertensive effect of diuretics can be demonstrated in anephric animals or in adults on chronic hemodialysis [2];
2 diuretics do not dilate vasculature in isolated smooth muscle preparations;

3 sodium loading prevents the hypotensive impact of diuretics [3];
4 finally, the lowering of systemic vascular resistance is a gradual effect. This reason is also compatible with a gradual change in smooth muscle tone.

Various combinations of changes in cardiac output and/or peripheral resistance are described as the physiologic reason for the decrease in blood pressure following acute and chronic administration of diuretics for periods of up to a few years [1]. In general acute usage of diuretics leads to a fall in blood volume and cardiac output with a rise in peripheral resistance insufficient to compensate for the reduced cardiac output. With prolonged diuretic administration, there is a fall in peripheral resistance toward normal with an increase in cardiac output. Chronic therapy with diuretics has been shown to maintain the initial reduction in plasma and extracellular volume and in total body exchangeable sodium. Chronic diuretic administration also leads to a reduction in the responsiveness of resistance vessels to sympathetic nervous system stimulation.

While diuretics can be used as single agents, they are also often needed to counteract the sodium retention associated with the use of nondiuretic antihypertensive agents. For example, the vasodilatory effect of hydralazine decreases effective arterial volume and leads to renal sodium retention. When diuretics are used in conjunction with other antihypertensive drugs, the dose of antihypertensive can often be significantly reduced. Diuretics which inhibit sodium reabsorption at each of the nephron sites where sodium and/or chloride moves across the luminal surface are now available (Table 12.1).

GENERAL GUIDELINES FOR USING DIURETICS

Data on the frequency with which diuretics satis-

Table 12.1 Sites of action of various types of diuretics currently used in managing high blood pressure in children

Site of action	Type	Agent
Proximal tubule	Thiazide	Metolazone
Ascending limb	Loop	Ethacrynic acid Furosemide
Cortical diluting segment	Thiazide	Chlorothiazide Chlorthalidone Hydrochlorothiazide Metolazone
Collecting tubule	Potassium-sparing	Spironolactone
Collecting duct	Potassium-sparing	Triamterene

factorily lower blood pressure for sustained periods of time in pediatric populations are limited (see below). In addition, criteria derived from the study of hypertensive children defining blood pressure as being mild, moderate, severe, and as constituting a potential hypertensive emergency are not available. It has been suggested that when diastolic pressure is increased by a factor of up to 1.15, 1.30, 1.50, and >1.50 above accepted 95% limits for age the child should be considered as having mild, moderate, severe, and a potential hypertensive emergency respectively [4]. These suggested values are based on somewhat arbitrary recommendations that have been used in adults. The Second Task Force guidelines which redefined the 95% confidence limits for blood pressure in children recommended that hypertension should be defined as significant when the average systolic and/or average diastolic blood pressure exceeds the 95th percentile but is less than the 99th percentile [5]. Severe hypertension was defined as levels of blood pressure persistently at or above the 99th percentile for age and sex [5]. However, the Task Force did not make any specific recommendations as to what levels of blood pressure in children constitute a hypertensive emergency. Because of the lack of specific pediatric information, it is difficult to transform to children blood pressure values developed in adults for use in treating defined increases in blood pressure. However, it appears that based on anecdotal and personal experience such transformations have practical value.

It has been suggested that thiazide diuretics will control blood pressure in up to 40% of adults with diastolic blood pressures up to 120 mmHg [1]. Although loop diuretics may be more effective [6], their side-effects argue against their use as initial agents. Indeed the usually recommended doses of thiazides to treat mild-to-moderate elevations of blood pressure may be too high; for example, adequate blood pressure control is possible in adults with a daily dose of hydrochlorothiazide of 12.5 mg 1–2 times a day rather than 25–50 mg/day [7]. Since many of the side-effects of thiazide diuretics are dose-dependent the potential benefit of using as low a dose as possible is obvious. There is no correlation between the antihypertensive effect of hydrochlorothiazide and its plasma concentration in either adults or children [8]. Data both supporting and refuting a relationship between pretreatment levels of plasma renin activity and the response to thiazide diuretics are available [9].

Combinations of thiazide diuretics and antihypertensive agents have been shown to be effective in treating adults with hypertension [10,11]. They offer the advantage of using lower doses of two drugs, limiting side-effects, and requiring less frequent administration of the drugs. Three available combinations in the USA are captopril and hydrochlorothiazide (Capozide), amiloride and hydrochlorothiazide (Moduretic), and chlorthalidone and atenolol (Tenoretic). Data reporting on the use of these drugs in children are not yet available.

A concern when thiazides are chronically used is their adverse effect on serum lipids [12,13]. An increase in serum triglyceride levels is a more constant feature than is increased cholesterol. Some investigators have not found elevations in serum cholesterol levels. The increase in triglyceride levels is also felt by some to be a transient phenomenon. The general feeling is that diuretic-related changes in lipid metabolism can be managed by dietary alterations. Weight reduction, avoidance of cigarette smoking, and regular physical activity will have a positive impact on high-density lipoprotein levels [14]. Periodic evaluations of serum lipids are indicated in patients being treated with diuretics.

Diuretics are used to lower blood pressure in patients with acute and chronic renal disease. Because they reduce the glomerular filtration rate (GFR) and have only a moderate effect on increasing sodium excretion, thiazides, exclusive of metolazone, are not effective in patients whose GFR is less than 30–40% of normal. Perhaps because of its action on proximal tubular reabsorption of sodium, metolazone lowered blood pressure in 78% of a group of 17 adults whose GFR ranged from 4 to 50 ml/min [15].

Because of their greater impact on the tubular reabsorption of solute, loop diuretics are more effective than thiazides in managing patients with chronic renal disease. Loop diuretics in large doses (up to 1−2 g of furosemide per day) in adults are able to increase sodium excretion in patients with severe renal insufficiency and may be helpful in treating hypertension associated with a low GFR [16]. No lowering of blood pressure should be expected when diuretics are given to patients with a GFR <5 ml/min [2]. The plasma half-life of furosemide is prolonged from 0.5 to 2−4 h in patients with renal failure [17]. Because of this prolongation of half-life, the recommended dose interval for furosemide administration for patients with renal failure is 3−4 times daily. The usual dose interval when using furosemide to treat an edematous state or essential hypertension is once or twice daily.

Furosemide does not lower GFR unless volume depletion occurs. Because of its association with non-reversible hearing loss, ethacrynic acid is usually reserved for patients in whom furosemide or metolazone fails. Noteworthy is the observation that thiazide diuretics have a flat-to-minimal dose−antihypertensive relationship at doses used clinically while loop diuretics do not. Thus, larger doses of loop diuretics are progressively more effective as saliuretic agents and blood pressure-lowering agents. Unfortunately larger doses of loop diuretics also lead to more side-effects including a worsening of blood pressure. This effect may be due to excessive renin release because of diuretic-induced volume depletion.

The potassium-sparing diuretics are of limited use as primary agents to treat hypertension; the single exception is the use of spironolactone to treat primary hyperaldosteronism [18]. These agents are used primarily in conjunction with other diuretics to control hypokalemia by preventing excessive renal potassium loss and to treat specific tubular transport defects associated with hypertension. Clinical usage of potassium-sparing agents can lead to hyperkalemia, especially in patients with a low GFR.

Some side-effects are common to all diuretics; others are agent-specific (Table 12.2). Most adverse reactions associated with the use of diuretics are due to their effect on renal tubular transport of solute and changes secondary to these effects. Extracellular volume depletion is generally due to the failure to replace excessive loss of sodium and water. Hyponatremia can occur because diuretics, especially thiazides, impair free water excretion. The administration of thiazides and loop diuretics can lead to metabolic alkalosis because the associated increase in potassium excretion and volume contraction increases the proximal tubular reabsorption of sodium and bicarbonate. Hyperuricemia occurs secondary to the effects of volume depletion on proximal tubule function. Increased amounts of urate are reabsorbed. Also, since thiazides and furosemide are weak acids, they compete with uric acid transport systems.

The diuretic response to a single oral dose of 1.0 mg/kg of furosemide differs between groups of hypertensive adolescents who are normouricemic or hyperuricemic. The 5 h excretory rates of water, sodium, and chloride in normouricemic and hyperuricemic hypertensive adolescents are summarized in Table 12.3. Not only did the total quantities differ, the fraction of the total amount excreted in each hour differed in the two groups. During the first 2 h after receiving furosemide, the hyperuricemic group excreted a higher fraction of the total amount of sodium, chloride, and water while lesser amounts were excreted during the ensuing 3 h [19]. Reasons for these differences are not clear but may in part be due to a slower rate of proximal tubular secretion of furosemide resulting in both a reduced rate of delivery of furosemide to the ascending limb of Henle and a lower intraluminal concentration of furosemide at its site of action. Furosemide and uric acid may share similar secretory pathways [20,21].

Thiazides reduce calcium excretion and occasionally lead to hypercalcemia. This effect is secondary to volume contraction and altered proximal tubule function. Conversely furosemide increases calcium excretion. A small increase in blood urea nitrogen (BUN) is a common finding in patients given diuretics, again secondary to an increased proximal tubule transport of urea because of extracellular volume depletion. Azotemia may be more common when more than one diuretic is used.

The use of thiazides or furosemide may be associated with impaired glucose homeostasis and nonketotic, hyperglycemic, hyperosmolar coma can develop in patients given thiazides [22]. Mechanisms affecting glucose regulation include the effects secondary to hypokalemia and suppression of the pan-

Table 12.2 Diuretics commonly used to treat hypertension in children

Diuretic	Chlorothiazide	Chlorthalidone	Ethacrynic acid
Dose: p.o.	10−20 mg/kg per day (hydrochlorothiazide 1−2 mg/kg)	1−2 mg/kg per day	2−3 mg/kg per day
Dose: i.v.	Not used	Not used	0.5−2 mg/kg
Time of maximal effect	3−4 h		p.o., i.v. 2 min
Duration of action	8−10 h	48−72 h	p.o. 6 h i.v. 2 h
Dose interval	q.d., b.i.d.	q.d., q.o.d.	p.o. q.d., b.i.d. i.v. q. 2−3 h
Fractional excretion of sodium	5−10%	5−10%	>15%
Adverse reactions	Hypokalemia Metabolic alkalosis Hyperuricemia Hyperglycemia Hyperlipemia Hypercalcemia Bone marrow suppression Hypersensitivity reactions GI symptoms Vomiting Diarrhea Constipation, etc. Interstitial nephritis	Hypokalemia Metabolic alkalosis Hyperuricemia Hyperglycemia Impotence GI symptoms Vomiting Diarrhea Constipation Bone marrow suppression Hypersensitivity reactions CNS symptoms Headache Dizziness	Dehydration Ototoxicity Metabolic alkalosis GI symptoms Heartburn Vomiting Diarrhea Constipation Hyperglycemia Agranulocytosis Hyponatremia Hypokalemia Hyperuricemia Hepatotoxicity ? Pancreatitis Hypersensitivity reactions CNS symptoms Vertigo Tinnitus Headache Confusion

GI= Gastrointestinal; CNS = central nervous system.

creatic secretion of insulin [23]. Diuretic-induced hyperglycemia may persist for over a year.

Should the biochemical consequences of diuretic therapy be actively treated? Some feel that therapy for diuretic-induced hypokalemia is not needed unless the serum potassium is less than 3 mmol/l. Others feel that even milder degrees of hypokalemia should be corrected because the extracellular concentration of potassium is a critical determinant of the cardiac action potential. The risk of experiencing a coronary artery death while receiving diuretics is increased 3.5-fold when the electrocardiogram is abnormal before starting thiazide diuretics [23]. In patients receiving digitalis, hypokalemia is associated with almost a doubling of arrhythmias. Ventricular ectopy in otherwise asymptomatic hypertensive adults can be reversed by giving potassium [23]. Reduction in sodium intake as part of an overall therapeutic plan in patients on thiazides minimizes the development of hypokalemia [24]. The con-

Table 12.2 (*Continued*)

Furosemide	Metolazone	Spironolactone	Triamterene
1−8 mg/kg per day	2−5 mg/1.73 m^2	1.5−3 mg/kg per day	0.7−4 mg/kg per day
1−4 mg/kg per day	Not used	Not used	Not used
p.o., i.v. 2 min	3−4 h	48−72 h	Several days
p.o. 6−9 h i.v. 2−3 h	18−24 h	12−24 h	7−9 h
p.o. q.d., b.i.d., t.i.d. i.v. q. 2−4 h	q.d.	b.i.d., q.i.d.	q.d., b.i.d.
>15%	5−10%	<5%	<5%

Dehydration
Ototoxicity
Metabolic alkalosis
GI symptoms
  Heartburn
  Vomiting
  Diarrhea
  Constipation
Hyperglycemia
Bone marrow
  suppression
Hyponatremia
Hypokalemia
Hyperuricemia
Intrahepatic cholestatic
  jaundice
Pancreatitis
CNS symptoms
  Tinnitus
  Vertigo
  Headache
  Blurred vision
Dermatologic
  hypersensitivity
Interstitial nephritis
Idiopathic edema
	Hypokalemia
	Metabolic alkalosis
	Hyponatremia
	Hyperuricemia
	Hyperglycemia
	Hypophosphatemia
	CNS symptoms
	  Vertigo
	  Headache
	  Parasthesias
	  Syncope
	GI symptoms
	  Constipation
	  Nausea
	  Vomiting
	  Diarrhea
	Hepatitis
	Leukopenia
	Aplastic anemia
	Dermatologic
	  hypersensitivity
	Chest pain, palpitations
		Hyperkalemia
		Metabolic acidosis
		Hyponatremia
		Gynecomastia
		GI symptoms
		  Cramps
		  Diarrhea
		Dermatologic
		  hypersensitivity
		Hirsutism
		Ataxia
		Amenorrhea
		Drug fever
			Hyper- and
			  hypokalemia
			GI symptoms
			  Nausea
			  Vomiting
			  Diarrhea
			Liver disease
			Anaphylaxis
			Blood dyscrasias
			  Megaloblastic
			  anemia
			  Thrombocytopenia
			CNS symptoms
			  Headache
			  Weakness
			  Dizziness
			Dry mouth
			Interstitial nephritis
			Photosensitivity
			Skin rash

comitant provision of potassium may be beneficial. Potassium supplementation should be considered in hypokalemic patients with arrhythmias (electrocardiogram changes), in patients on digitalis and in those scheduled to receive anesthesia and when serum potassium levels are below 3.0 mmol/l. Treatment strategies include the addition of a potassium-sparing diuretic, the use of potassium preparations, and an increase in the dietary intake of potassium. The alimentary addition of potassium without a concomitant reduction in sodium intake may not lead to

the anticipated increases in serum potassium levels. Symptomatic hyponatremia should be treated by acutely increasing serum sodium levels to values of 120−125 mmol/l. Asymptomatic hyponatremia should be corrected when serum levels of sodium are less than 125−130 mmol/l. Some suggest that asymptomatic hyperuricemia need not be routinely treated until serum levels exceed 10 mg/dl, at which time allopurinol therapy ought to be considered. Data supportive of treating diuretic-induced hyperuricemia are scanty.

Table 12.3 Total 5-h excretion of sodium, chloride, and water corrected to 1.73 m^2 in 28 adolescents with primary hypertension given 1.0 mg/kg of furosemide orally

Nature of hypertension	Sodium (mmol/5 h)	Chloride (mmol/5 h)	Water (ml/5 h)
Hyperuricemic (n = 13)	138	180	1300
Normouricemic (n = 15)	190	240	1700
p	0.03	0.02	0.01

Adapted from [19]

PEDIATRIC EXPERIENCE WITH DIURETICS

Acute renal disease

Diuretic agents reported as useful in treating hypertension associated with acute postinfectious nephritis include furosemide and thiazides given alone, in combination, or in conjunction with other antihypertensive agents such as hydralazine. In 5 children with acute glomerulonephritis and a blood pressure >130/90 mmHg given 1 mg/kg of furosemide intravenously, 3 experienced a slight reduction, but not to normal, in both systolic and diastolic blood pressure (numbers not provided) [25]. Blood pressure did not fall in the 2 children with the highest initial values. Despite the failure of furosemide adequately to lower blood pressure, weight decreased by 23% and mean urine volume, urinary sodium excretion, and osmolar clearance increased 8–12-fold ($p<0.01$). Tubular reabsorption of sodium decreased from 97.6 to 74.3%. Plasma volume, which was elevated prior to treatment (63.3 ± 3.6 ml/kg) did not change at 6 and 12 h after furosemide. It was suggested that the failure of the blood pressure to fall was related to the lack of change in plasma volume.

In another study of 25 children aged 3–15 years designed to evaluate the diuretic effect of furosemide in acute postinfectious glomerulonephritis, intravenously administered furosemide 1 mg/kg increased urine volume in all who received it; the diuretic response to a single dose of 1.0 mg/kg was minimal [26]. Oral doses of 2–5 mg/kg effectively increased urine output. The half-life for furosemide ranged from 2.3 to 4.4 h and did not correlate with BUN levels, which ranged from 11 to 93 mg/dl. Peak serum concentrations up to 4 h after administering

furosemide could not be correlated with urinary flow rates. Urine concentrations of furosemide as an indicator of diuretic effectiveness were also not reported. Unfortunately this study did not evaluate the impact of furosemide on lowering blood pressure.

In another study involving 24 children with poststreptococcal glomerulonephritis, it was shown that when furosemide was given, fewer doses of nondiuretic antihypertensive agents were needed to lower blood pressure [27]. Twelve children were treated with furosemide starting with a minimum of 40 mg b.i.d. which was increased daily as clinically indicated; 12 children were given placebo. The furosemide-treated group received a mean daily dose of 5.6 mg/kg with an approximate range of 1–13 mg/kg. Both groups received intramuscular hydralazine and reserpine every 12 h if any child's systolic blood pressure exceeded 140 mmHg. The diuretic or placebo was discontinued only after the child was normotensive, off parenteral antihypertensive drugs, and edema-free. Normal blood pressure without antihypertensive therapy was achieved in 4.5 and 7.7 days in the furosemide- and placebo-treated groups respectively. The furosemide- and placebo-treated groups became edema-free 4.5 and 7.9 days after starting treatment. Maximum creatinine levels were similar in both groups; the maximum BUN and BUN : creatinine ratios were higher in the furosemide-treated group.

Chronic renal disease

Chlorthalidone has been prospectively compared to propranolol in 12 children 3–15 years of age; of the 11 with chronic renal disease, 9 had creatinine clearances less than 80 ml/min per 1.73 m^2 [28]. The treatment design was that of a crossover study with each agent being given for 4–6 weeks. Diastolic hypertension was defined as blood pressure values >90 and >100 mmHg in children under and over 12 years of age respectively. Each agent was increased at 2-week intervals until an appropriate response was noted or a maximal dose was reached. Initial and maximal oral doses were propranolol 1–5 mg/kg per 24 h and chlorthalidone 0.5–1.7 mg/kg per 48 h. Blood pressure decreased in all 12 patients with both agents. Compared to initial values the blood pressure fell significantly ($p<0.01$) with both agents. Decreases in systolic, diastolic, and mean blood pressures with propranolol were 22.3, 21.5, and 22.3 mmHg and with chlorthalidone 17.2, 14.2, and 15 mmHg.

Even though both drugs were equally effective from a statistical perspective, fewer patients given chlorthalidone had acceptable responses. Diastolic blood pressure fell by at least 10 mmHg in 6 of 12 and 10 of 12 children receiving chlorthalidone and propranolol respectively. In 4 of 9 children with a reduced GFR chlorthalidone was more effective than propranolol. In 11 of 12 children receiving chlorthalidone serum potassium levels fell to 2.5−3.4 mmol/l and 4 were given supplemental potassium.

The combination of metolazone (0.2−0.4 mg/kg per day) and furosemide (2−4 mg/kg per day) effectively increased urinary sodium excretion in edematous children with chronic renal failure resistant to furosemide (4.0 mg/kg per day) alone. Data on the effect on blood pressure were not provided [29,30]. Children with serum albumin levels of <1.5 g/dl did not respond. In children with serum albumin levels <1.5 g/dl and edema resistant to furosemide at a dose of 3−4 mg/kg per day, we have observed improvement with the addition of metolazone. Others have found that children with nephrotic syndrome with creatinine clearances of 49 ± 40 ml/min per 1.73 m^2 who were previously unresponsive to 5 mg/kg per day of furosemide experienced a significant diuresis with somewhat lower doses of metolazone in combination with furosemide [31].

Diuretics are helpful in managing children with posttransplant hypertension [32]. In evaluating time-related blood pressure problems in 100 pediatric allografts, it was found that 62.5 and 26% of children with and without rejection did not require antihypertensive drugs. In 29% a diuretic, furosemide, alone or used in conjunction with an additional agent, usually a β-blocker (propranolol) or an oral vasodilator (hydralazine), controlled blood pressure. A diuretic plus three other agents was needed to control blood pressure in an additional 38%.

Primary hypertension

In 1977 the report of the National Heart, Lung, and Blood Institute Task Force o, blood pressure control in children recommended that those requiring chronic pharmacologic control of their blood pressure should be started on a stepped-care regimen beginning with a thiazide diuretic and adding other drugs if needed [33]. Since that time a number of other therapeutic regimens involving the use of non-diuretics as initial agents to treat primary hyper-

tension have been found to be equally, if not more, effective in adult populations. Classic stepped-care therapy has been modified. α- and β-blocking drugs, centrally acting antihypertensive agents, and renin-inhibiting agents have been suggested as alternative initial agents. The recommended use of these other drugs as initial therapy is based on the physician's concept of the pathophysiology of the hypertension in an individual patient and on the acute and chronic side-effects of the drug. However, should blood pressure fail to be lowered with a diuretic used alone initially, other antihypertensive agents can be added.

Prospective trials on the use of diuretic agents to treat primary hypertension in pediatric populations have become available since the initial Task Force report. A prospective clinical trial comparing clonidine to hydrochlorothiazide in 29 adolescents aged 13−19 years with primary hypertension reported significant decreases in both systolic and diastolic blood pressure with clonidine and systolic blood pressure with hydrochlorothiazide [34]. Following a placebo period lasting 4 weeks during which a pill count demonstrated a compliance rate of >79%, clonidine 0.1 mg or hydrochlorothiazide 25 mg was given for 12 weeks. All patients were then treated for another 12 weeks. In those whose blood pressure remained >140/90 mmHg, the dose of both drugs was doubled. Drug therapy was discontinued by tapering during week 25.

None of the adolescents given 25 mg/day of hydrochlorothiazide responded satisfactorily; the dose was then increased to 50 mg/day. This dose was associated with a lowering of blood pressure to normal values in 6 of 15; 9 failed to respond adequately. All 14 adolescents given clonidine experienced an acceptable lowering of blood pressure−4 and 10 on the lower and higher doses respectively. Changes in blood chemistries in the group given hydrochlorothiazide included decreases in serum potassium in 14 of 15 patients, decreases in serum chloride, and increases in serum carbon dioxide and uric acid.

Blood pressure response to a standardized mental stress test in these two groups differed [35,36]. Neither clonidine nor hydrochlorothiazide altered the systolic blood pressure response to mental stress. Compared to clonidine, those on hydrochlorothiazide developed higher diastolic blood pressures and less of a fall in heart rate in response to mental stress. Mean norepinephrine levels were similar in both groups prior to therapy and were also similar after mental stress in the drug-free period. During drug treatment, levels of plasma norepinephrine fell from 223 to 166 pg/ml with clonidine and increased from 225 to 282 pg/ml with hydrochlorothiazide. While still on treatment and following mental stress, norepinephrine levels increased in the clonidine group from 166 to 204 pg/ml while increasing in the hydrochlorothiazide group from 282 to 313 pg/ml.

In summary, regulation of catecholamine release improved to a greater degree following treatment with clonidine when compared to hydrochlorothiazide.

Another study reported on a prospective trial comparing no treatment to a combination of hygienic interventions as well as the administration of propranolol and chlorthalidone to treat children whose blood pressures were at or above the 90th percentile, [37,38]. The treated group were given propranolol 20 or 40 mg/day for children with weight under and over 40 kg, respectively and chlorthalidone 6.25 or 12.5 mg/day for children with weight under and over 40 kg, respectively. Treatment was continued for at least 6 months and follow-up was continued for a total duration of 18 months. The treated group experienced a 5 mmHg fall in both systolic and diastolic blood pressure; the control group had a 3 mmHg drop [37,38]. After stopping active treatment, blood pressures in the treated group remained in the 60−70% range for the remainder of the 18-month trial. Noteworthy is the low dose of both drugs compared to the doses usually recommended for children.

Tubular disorders associated with hypertension

Hypertension associated with primary hyperaldosteronism (increased aldosterone, suppressed renin activity, hypokalemia, and metabolic alkalosis) can be successfully treated in most patients by giving spironolactone [18,39]. However, not all patients, including children (personal experience with one case), with primary hyperaldosteronism will respond to this agent.

Patients with Gordon syndrome — hyperkalemia, hyperchloremic acidosis, hyporeninemia, normal GFR, and hypertension — respond to thiazide diuretics by lowering their blood pressure [40]. Patients with similar biochemical findings but without hypertension — the Spitzer−Weinstein syndrome — do not need antihypertensive therapy. It has been suggested that the pathogenesis of the Gordon syndrome is related to a deficiency of some natriuretic and/or chloriuretic factor.

Liddle syndrome (hypertension, hypokalemia secondary to renal potassium-wasting, metabolic alkalosis, and suppressed renin and aldosterone) can be successfully controlled by the chronic administration of triamterene or amiloride [41,42]. The etiology of this disorder has been postulated to be a renal tubular defect leading to a hyperabsorption of sodium.

Miscellaneous studies involving diuretics in childhood hypertension

The additional effect of nondiuretic antihypertensive agents to hydrochlorothiazide has been evaluated in a group of 9 children ages 1 month to 16 years in whom adequate blood pressure control had not occurred despite polypharmacy [43]. Six of 9 children had primary intrinsic renal disorders; 1 had renal artery stenosis and 2 had essential hypertension. Blood pressure values while off therapy were not provided. Each child completed the following protocol. Initially, each patient received hydrochlorothiazide 2−4 mg/kg per day (1 was given 8 mg/kg per day) for 4 weeks. This was followed by the addition to hydrochlorothiazide of successive 6-week courses of methyldopa 10−60 mg/kg per day, propranolol 1−2 (up to 8 in 1 case) mg/kg per day, and propranolol with minoxidil 0.1−0.5 up to a maximum of 20 mg/day in combination with propranolol. Two weeks of hydrochlorothiazide treatment was given between each course of therapy. In comparison to blood pressure values obtained with hydrochlorothiazide alone, mean diastolic blood pressures were significantly lower with the addition of the other drugs (Table 12.4). Significant changes in systolic blood pressure occurred only in the group given minoxidil and propranolol. This regimen was also the most effective in lowering diastolic blood pressure.

Diuretic usage in newborn babies and infants

The effectiveness of diuretics as antihypertensive agents in newborn babies and infants is unclear. Although widely used in conjunction with nondiuretic antihypertensive agents as part of an overall therapeutic plan, age-specific data are unavailable. Diuretics are widely used as saliuretic agents in this age group to treat congestive heart failure, respiratory

Table 12.4 Blood pressure-lowering effect in children of antihypertensive agents added to hydrochlorothiazide (HCTZ)

	HCTZ	HCTZ plus methyldopa	HCTZ plus propranolol	HCTZ plus propranolol plus minoxidil
Systolic pressure (mmHg)				
Mean	148	142	141	128*
SEM	8	8	6	4
Diastolic pressure (mmHg)				
Mean	98	88*	85*	75*
SEM	4	4	2	2

Adapted from [43].
*Significantly different from HCTZ; $p < 0.05$.

distress syndrome, renal-related edema, and nephrogenic diabetes insipidus. Newborn infants given furosemide at a dose of >2 (up to 16) mg/kg per day for more than 12 days have developed nephrocalcinosis, renal calculi, hyperparathyroidism, gallstones, and possibly osteopenia secondary to furosemide-related hypercalciuria [44,45]. Follow-up studies report that improvement in renal calcification occurs. However, levels of serum creatinine may remain abnormally high and calculated GFR low in the majority [46].

In a group of 30 premature infants, usage of furosemide, chlorothiazide, and spironolactone was associated with hypercalciuria [47]. Covariant analysis demonstrated a positive correlation between urinary calcium excretion and the intake of vitamin D, calcium, and sodium.

The response of 16 normal males aged 6−47 days to oral doses of chlorothiazide 75 mg q.d., triamterene 20 mg q.d., and spironolactone 25 mg b.i.d. has been reported [48]. Chlorothiazide produced increases in excretory rates of sodium, chloride, potassium, and water; spironolactone of water and sodium, and triamterene of only sodium. A 10-month-old child being treated with chlorothiazide for nephrogenic diabetes insipidus developed reversible neutropenia [49].

Thus, the newborn baby and infant can respond to diuretics. Additional data are needed to better understand the relationship between diuretic administration and the following: the newborn baby's normally low GFR which influences the filtered load of sodium as well as the diuretic agent; developmentally related tubular transport mechanisms for diuretics; nonrenal metabolism of diuretics and the pharmacokinetics of diuretics. More information is also needed on the practical issues of dose, clinical effects, adverse reactions, and whether diuretics adversely affect growth in the young.

CONCLUSIONS

Our impression of the effectiveness of diuretics as blood pressure-lowering agents is that they are useful as single drugs in treating mild-to-moderate elevations in blood pressure. Their clinical usefulness is considerably extended when used in combination with other antihypertensive agents. Side-effects are similar to those experienced by adults.

REFERENCES

1 Prichard BNC, Owens CWI. Drug treatment of hypertension. In: Genest J, Kuchel O, Hamet P, Cantin M, eds. *Hypertension — Physiopathology and Treatment*. 2nd edn. 1983:1171−1210, McGraw Hill, N.Y.

2 Bennett WM, McDonald WJ, Hartnett MN et al. Do diuretics have antihypertensive properties independent of natriuresis? *Clin Pharmacol Exp Ther* 1977;22:499−504.

3 Winer BM. Antihypertensive mechanisms of salt depletion induced by hydrochlorothiazide. *Circulation* 1961;24:788−96.

4 Gruskin AB. Primary hypertension in the adolescent: facts and unresolved issues. In: Loggie J, Horan MJ, Gruskin AB et al. eds. *NHLBI Workshop on Juvenile Hypertension: The Child at Risk for Hypertension*. New York: Biomedical Information, 1984;305−34.

5 National Heart, Lung, and Blood Institute, Bethesda, Maryland. Report of the Second Task Force on blood pressure control in children − 1987. *Pediatrics* 1987;79:1−25.

6 Davidov M, Kakaviatos N, Finnerty FA. Antihypertensive properties of furosemide. *Circulation* 1967;36:125−135.

7 Beermann B, Groschinsky-Grind M. Antihypertensive effect of various doses of hydrochlorothiazide and its relation to the plasma level of the drug. *Eur J Clin Pharmacol* 1978;13:195−201.

8 Mirkin B, Sinaiko A, Cooper M *et al.* Hydrochlorothiazide therapy in hypertensive and renal insufficient children: elimination kinetics and metabolic effects. *Pediatr Res* 1972;11:418 (abstract).

9 Wyndham RN, Gimenez L, Walker WG *et al.* Influence of renin levels on the treatment of essential hypertension with thiazide diuretics. *Arch Intern Med* 1987;147:1021−25.

10 Clementy J, Schwebig A, Mazaud C *et al.* Comparative study of the efficacy and tolerance of capozide and moduretic administered in a single daily dose for the treatment of chronic moderate arterial hypertension. *Postgrad Med J* 1986;62(suppl 1):132−34.

11 Shand DG. On the rationale for diuretic/β-blocker combinations in the treatment of hypertension. *Evaluation of Tenoretic: A Symposium, A Special Report, Postgraduate Medicine*: Custom Communications, August 1984.

12 Grimm RH, Leon AS, Hunninghake DB *et al.* Effects of thiazide diuretics on plasma lipids and lipoproteins in mildly hypertensive patients. A double-blind controlled trial. *Ann Intern Med* 1981;94:7−11.

13 Gruskin AB. Antihypertensive drug usage in children with primary hypertension. In: *88th Ross Conference on Pediatric Research. Childhood Hypertension.* 1984, Columbus, Ohio.

14 Grimm RH Jr, Hunninghake DB. Lipids and hypertension: implications of new guidelines for cholesterol management in the treatment of hypertension. *Am J Med* 80 (suppl 2A) 1986;80:56−63.

15 Bennett WM, Porter GA. Efficacy and safety of metolazone in renal failure and the nephrotic syndrome. *J Clin Pharmacol* 1973;13:357−64.

16 Allison MEM, Kennedy AC. Diuretics in chronic renal disease: a study of high dosage furosemide. *Clin Sci* 1971;41:171−87.

17 Huang CM, Atkinson AJ, Levin M *et al.* Pharmacokinetics of furosemide in renal failure. *Clin Pharmacol Ther* 1974;16:659−66.

18 Battle DC, Kurtzman NA. Clinical disorders of aldosterone metabolism. *Dis Mon* 1984;8:1−55.

19 Prebis JW, Gruskin AB, Baluarte HJ *et al.* Dual response to furosemide (F) in hypertensive children and its relationship to hyperuricemia. *Circulation* 1979;(suppl 2):207 (abstract).

20 Prebis JW, Gruskin AB, Polinsky MS *et al.* Uric acid in childhood essential hypertension. In: Gruskin AB, Norman ME, eds. *Developments in Nephrology.* Boston: Martinus Nijhoff, 1980:122−6.

21 Prebis JW, Gruskin AB, Polinsky MS *et al.* Uric acid in childhood essential hypertension. *J Pediatr* 1981;98:702−7.

22 Curtis JC, Horrigan F, Ahearn D *et al.* Chlorthalidone-induced hyperosmolar hyperglycemic nonketotic coma. *JAMA* 1972;220:1592−3.

23 Weinberger MH. Diuretics and their side effects. Dilemma in the treatment of hypertension. *Hypertension* 1988;11 (suppl II):II-16-II-20.

24 Ram CVS, Garrett BN, Kaplan NM. Moderate sodium restriction and various diuretics in the treatment of hypertension. Effects of potassium wastage and blood pressure control. *Arch Intern Med* 1981;141:1015−19.

25 Repetto HA, Lewy JE, Brando JL, Metcoff J. The renal functional response to furosemide in children with acute glomerulonephritis. *J Pediatr* 1972;80:660−6.

26 Pruitt AW, Boles A. Diuretic effect of furosemide in acute glomerulonephritis. *J Pediatr* 1976;89:306−9.

27 Retan JW, Dillon HC. Furosemide in the treatment of acute post-streptococcal glomerulonephritis. *South Med J* 1969;62:157−60.

28 Bachmann H. Propranolol versus chlorthalidone—a prospective therapeutic trial in children with chronic hypertension. *Helv Paediatr Acta* 1984;39:55−61.

29 Arnold WC. Efficacy of metolazone and furosemide in children with furosemide-resistant edema. *Pediatrics* 1984;74:872−5.

30 Arnold WC. Reply to a letter to the Editor: Garin EH, Richard GA: Reply to Editor—Metolazone and furosemide therapy for edema. *Pediatrics* 1986;77:130−1.

31 Garin EH, Richard GA. Edema resistant to furosemide therapy in nephrotic syndrome: treatment with furosemide and metolazone. *Int J Pediatr Nephrol* 1981;2:181−4.

32 Ingelfinger JR. Hypertension in end-stage renal disease and renal transplantation. In: Ingelfinger JR, ed. *Pediatric Hypertension.* Philadelphia: W B Saunders, 1982;252−68.

33 Report of the Task Force on blood pressure control in children. *Pediatrics* 1977;58:797−819.

34 Falkner B, Onesti G, Lowenthal DT, Affrime MB. Effectiveness of centrally acting drugs and diuretics in adolescent hypertension. *Clin Pharmacol Ther* 1982;32:577−83.

35 Falkner B, Onesti G, Affrime MB, Lowenthal DT. Effects of clonidine and hydrochlorothiazide on the cardiovascular response to mental stress in adolescent hypertension. *Clin Sci* 1982;63:455s−8s.

36 Falkner B. Cardiovascular reactivity and psychogenic stress in juveniles. In: Loggie J, Horan MJ, Gruskin AB *et al.*, eds. *NHLBI Workshop on Juvenile Hypertension: The Child at Risk for Hypertension.* New York, Biomedical Information, 1984;161−72.

37 Berenson GS, Voors AW, Webber LS *et al.* A model of intervention for prevention of early essential hypertension in the 1980's. *Hypertension* 1983;5:41−54.

38 Berenson GS. Management of the mildly hypertensive youth: can adult hypertensive disease be prevented? In: Loggie J, Horan MJ, Gruskin AB *et al.*, eds. *NHLBI Workshop on Juvenile Hypertension: The Child at Risk for Hypertension.* New York: Biomedical Information, 1984;387−410.

39 Spark RF, Melby JC. Aldosteronism in hypertension. The spironolactone response test. *Ann Intern Med* 1968;69: 685−91.

40 Gordon RD. Syndrome of hypertension and hyperkalemia with normal glomerular filtration rate. *Hypertension* 1986;8:93−102.

41 Liddle GW, Bledsoe T, Coppage WS Jr. A familial renal disorder simulating primary aldosteronism but with negligible aldosterone secretion. *Trans Assoc Am Phys* 1963;76:199−213.

42 Wang C, Chang TK, Yeung RTT *et al.* The effect of triamterene and sodium intake on renin, aldosterone, and erythrocyte sodium transport in Liddle's syndrome. *J Clin Endocrinol Metab* 1981;52:1027.

43 Sinaiko AR, Mirkin BL. Management of severe childhood hypertension with minoxidil: a controlled clinical study. *J Pediatr* 1977;91:138−42.

44 Hufnagle KG, Khan SN, Penn D, Cacciarelli A, Williams P.

Renal calcifications: a complication of long-term furosemide therapy in preterm infants. *Pediatrics* 1982;70:360−3.

45 Venkataraman PS, Han BK, Tsang RC, Daugherty CC. Secondary hyperparathyroidism and bone disease in infants receiving long-term furosemide therapy. *Am J Dis Child* 1983;137:1157−61.

46 Ezzedeen F, Adelman RD, Ahlfors CE. Renal calcification in preterm infants: pathophysiology and long-term sequelae. *J Pediatr* 1988;113:532−9.

47 Atkinson SA, Shah JK, McGee C, Steele BT. Mineral excretion in premature infants receiving various diuretic therapies. *J Pediatr* 1988;113:540−5.

48 Walker RD, Cumming GR. Response of the infant kidney to diuretic drugs. *Can Med Assoc J* 1964;91:1149−53.

49 Schotland MG, Grumbach MM. Neutropenia in an infant secondary to hydrochlorothiazide therapy: with a review of hematologic reactions to "thiazide" drugs. *Pediatrics* 1963;31:754−7.

13 Drugs Affecting the Adrenergic Nervous System

ALAN R. SINAIKO

INTRODUCTION

The adrenergic (or sympathetic) nervous system has been a focus for therapeutic intervention in patients with elevated blood pressure since the earliest days of antihypertensive therapy. Prior to the introduction of pharmacotherapy 30–35 years ago, surgical sympathectomy was utilized as a primary intervention strategy in severe hypertension, based on the well recognized relationship between adrenergic function and blood pressure homeostasis. Thus, it is not surprising that the introduction of effective antihypertensive agents corresponded with an intensive investigative effort to develop drugs that could influence adrenergic regulation of blood pressure. The outcome of this effort has been so striking that drugs affecting the adrenergic nervous system currently comprise the largest class of antihypertensive medications.

The anti-adrenergic drugs form a diverse group with a variety of pharmacologic actions. The ongoing anatomic, physiologic, and biochemical dissection of the adrenergic nervous system has led, in recent years, to the design of new drugs directed at specific sites along the adrenergic neurotransmission pathway. This is in contrast to earlier agents which elicited nonspecific anti-adrenergic effects through diffuse reductions in neuronal stores of the adrenergic neurotransmitter norepinephrine.

To appreciate the mechanisms of action and clinical pharmacology of drugs that modify adrenergic activity, it is essential to begin with a brief discussion of the adrenergic nervous system. The following summary is provided with the acknowledgment that more detailed reviews are available elsewhere [1,2].

THE ADRENERGIC NERVOUS SYSTEM

Adrenergic neurons are found within the central and peripheral nervous systems. They comprise a proximal cell body, a distal nerve terminal, and an axon connecting the two. Each nerve terminal has multiple branches, so that adrenergic innervation of any given tissue involves countless cellular activation sites.

The primary adrenergic neurotransmitter is the catecholamine norepinephrine (Fig. 13.1). Biosynthesis of norepinephrine begins in the cytoplasm of the nerve terminal following uptake of the circulating amino acid tyrosine. Tyrosine undergoes conversion by tyrosine hydroxylase to L-dopa (3,4-dihydroxyphenylalanine) which is subsequently converted to dopamine (3,4-dihydroxyphenylethylamine) by the L-aromatic amino acid decarboxylase. Dopamine is then taken up by vesicles located within the nerve terminal where it is converted by dopamine-hydroxylase to norepinephrine. Norepinephrine is stored within these vesicles until it is released from the nerve terminal.

The formation of norepinephrine also takes place within the adrenal medulla. However, the adrenal biosynthetic pathway contains an additional step in which norepinephrine is converted to epinephrine through enzymatic methylation by phenylethanolamine-N-methyltransferase. Epinephrine functions

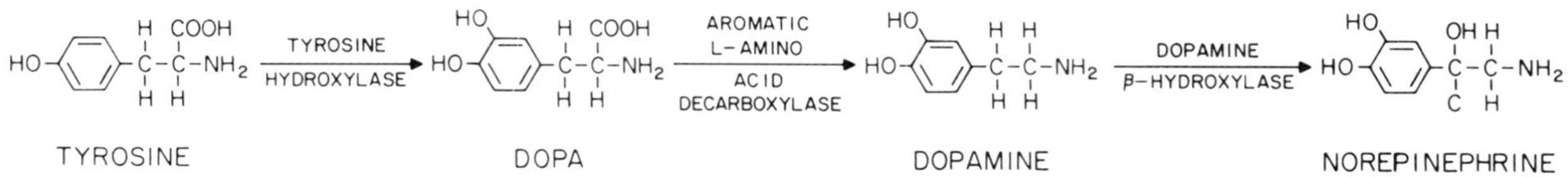

Fig. 13.1 Biosynthetic pathway of norepinephrine.

138

as a neurohormone after its release into the circulation from the adrenal.

Upon stimulation of the adrenergic neuron, norepinephrine is released by a process of exocytosis from the nerve ending into the synaptic cleft, the space between the nerve ending and receptor sites on the effector tissue (Fig. 13.2). Following its release, norepinephrine may follow any one of the following pathways:

1 a portion is bound to post- or presynaptic receptor sites;

2 the majority of norepinephrine is taken up by the nerve terminal where it is either stored in the neuronal vesicles for release at a later time or undergoes metabolism to inactive products by the enzyme monoamine oxidase (MAO);

3 a lesser amount of norepinephrine is taken up by other tissues and metabolized by MAO and a second enzyme, catechol-O-methyltransferase (COMT);

4 the smallest amount of norepinephrine escapes the synaptic cleft, neuronal re-uptake, and tissue uptake to find its way into the circulation where it is ultimately metabolized in the liver by MAO and COMT or is excreted unchanged in the urine.

Norepinephrine interacts with adrenergic receptors located on either side of the synaptic cleft (Fig. 13.2). The initial classic division of adrenergic receptors by Ahlquist [3] into α and β components has been expanded to include α_1- and α_2-receptors and β_1- and β_2-receptors [4]. Receptor classification is based on the degree of response to specific α- and β-adrenergic agonists and antagonists and is the sole determinant of receptor type. Typing and subtyping of adrenergic receptors is totally distinct from any qualitative or quantitative assessment of adrenergic elicited tissue function, which varies within receptor type and depends on tissue location. Table 13.1 lists some tissue receptor types and responses.

In addition to the presence of adrenergic receptors at postsynaptic sites on effector tissues, both α- and β-receptors have been identified at presynaptic sites located on the nerve endings themselves. It is believed that α_2-receptors modulate neurotransmitter activity through a negative feedback mechanism that inhibits catecholamine release from the nerve ending when these receptors are occupied by norepinephrine. In contrast, activation of presynaptic β_2-receptors appears to enhance norepinephrine secretion, and there is some evidence that this positive feedback action is controlled through the circulating catecholamine, epinephrine [2].

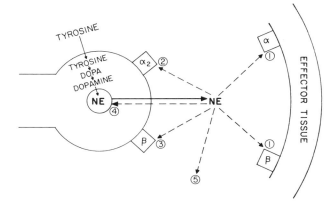

Fig. 13.2 Neuronal processing and release of norepinephrine. After release of norepinephrine from the nerve endings into the synaptic cleft, it follows a combination of the following pathways:

1 activation of postsynaptic α_1-β_1- or β_2-receptors or α_2-receptors located outside the synaptic cleft;

2 activation of presynaptic α_2-receptors which inhibit neuronal norepinephrine release;

3 activation of presynaptic β_2-receptors which enhance norepinephrine release (although there is evidence that these receptors are activated primarily by circulating epinephrine);

4 re-uptake by the neuron and restorage in vesicles or metabolism by monoamine oxidase;

5 escape from the synaptic cleft into the circulation and metabolism by tissue monoamine oxidase and catechol-O-methyltransferase or excretion unchanged in the urine.

β-ADRENERGIC BLOCKING DRUGS

β-Adrenergic blocking drugs rival the diuretics as the most frequently used class of antihypertensive agents and are currently recommended as first-line therapy for hypertension in adults and children. Although, worldwide, the number of β-blockers available for clinical use has increased rapidly since their introduction 20 years ago, in the USA the choice is relatively limited (Tables 13.2 and 13.3). Nevertheless, the selection currently marketed in this country offers all of the pharmacologic characteristics intrinsic to the β-blockers, so that it is possible to tailor therapy to individual patient needs while attempting to minimize potential adverse responses.

Pharmacologic characteristics of β-blockers

β-Adrenergic blocking drugs can be categorized according to a series of pharmacologic properties that are possessed in varying degrees by each member within the group (Table 13.2) [5].

Table 13.1 Tissue innervation according to adrenergic receptor type

Receptor type	Tissue	Response
α_1	Arteriole	Constriction
	Veins	Constriction
	Kidney	Natriuresis and diuresis
α_2	Neuronal (presynaptic)	↓ Norepinephrine release
	Central nervous system	↓ Efferent activity
	Arteriole	Constriction
	Fat cells	↓ Lipolysis
	Pancreas	↓ Insulin release
	Kidney	↑ Diuresis
β_1	Cardiac	↑ Inotropic and chronotropic effect
	Fat cells	↑ Lipolysis
β_2	Neuronal (presynaptic)	↑ Norepinephrine
	Arteriole	Dilatation
	Bronchi	Dilatation
	Liver	↑ Glycogenolysis
		↑ Gluconeogenesis
	Pancreas	↑ Insulin release
	Kidney	↑ Renin release

↑ = Stimulatory;
↓ = inhibitory.

Table 13.2 Pharmacologic properties of β-adrenergic blocking drugs

Drug	Cardioselectivity	Intrinsic sympathomimetic activity	Membrane stabilizing	Lipid solubility	Potency
Propranolol	o	o	+	High	1.0
Acebutolol	+	+	+	Weak	0.3
Atenolol	+	o	o	Weak	1.0
Metoprolol	+	o	o	Moderate	1.0
Nadolol	o	o	o	Weak	1.0
Pindolol	o	+	o	Moderate	6.0
Timolol	o	o	o	Weak	6.0
Carteolol	o	+	o	Weak	20.0
Penbutalol	o	+	o	High	4.0

CARDIOSELECTIVITY

Selectivity of a β-adrenergic blocking drug refers to its capacity to block β_1- or β_2-adrenergic receptors. Because cardiac β-adrenergic innervation is β_1 in type, drugs such as metoprolol, atenolol, and acebutolol, which are specific β_1-blockers, have been termed "cardioselective." Propranolol and all other currently available β-blockers are "non-selective" and act at both β_1- and β_2-receptor sites.

Selectivity is relevant only when low-to-moderate drug doses are used. At higher drug doses, such as those commonly used to treat systemic hypertension, a crossover effect is seen, as inhibition of β_2 in addition to β_1 responses occurs. Thus, the potential for adverse clinical reactions, such as bronchoconstriction, in patients treated with β_1-blockers cannot be neglected with cardioselective β-blockers.

LIPID SOLUBILITY

The degree of partitioning of a drug between a mixture of water and an organic solvent determines its partition coefficient, the measure of lipid solubility. Drugs with reduced lipid solubility, such as atenolol and nadolol, have low partition coefficients, i.e. are found primarily in the water phase, whereas the remaining β-blockers have high partition coefficients and are highly lipid-soluble.

Lipid solubility is important because it describes the capacity of a drug to penetrate the central nervous system. Patients with well controlled hypertension but experiencing symptoms of central nervous system disorder while receiving propranolol may continue to obtain the antihypertensive benefit from β-blocker therapy by substituting a less lipid-soluble agent, such as atenolol.

INTRINSIC SYMPATHOMIMETIC ACTIVITY [6]

The primary effect of all of the β-adrenergic blocking drugs is to inhibit response in β-adrenergic innervated tissues by occupying receptor sites and preventing access to β-adrenergic agonists. However, the molecular configuration of some of the β-blockers is such that, in addition to the inhibitory effect, they elicit a small but none the less significant agonist response, known as intrinsic sympathomimetic activity, in the effector tissue.

The partial agonist effect of these agents is of a significantly lower degree than that observed with pure agonists such as isoproterenol, and the effect on receptor blockade and antihypertensive response does not appear to be compromised. While the clinical relevance of intrinsic sympathomimetic activity has not been established, preliminary evidence suggests that this effect may partially neutralize the impact of β-adrenergic blockade on responses unrelated to blood pressure control, thereby reducing the intensity of potential adverse reactions such as hypoglycemia or Raynaud's disease.

MEMBRANE-STABILIZING EFFECT

Some β-adrenergic blocking drugs possess a quinidine-like activity expressed as an alteration in myocardial electrochemical conduction [7]. This property appears to be an *in vitro* phenomenon since it requires drug concentrations many times in excess of those observed in humans.

POTENCY

β-Adrenergic blocking potency is defined as the capacity of a drug to inhibit the tachycardic response to isoproterenol compared to inhibition by the reference β-blocker, propranolol. Although potency affects the amount of drug required to achieve an equivalent clinical response, it has had little clinical significance, since less potent drugs can generally be administered in higher doses without increasing the incidence of adverse reactions.

Proposed mechanisms for antihypertensive effect

It is not at all clear how the β-adrenergic blocking drugs decrease blood pressure or which of the properties described above are operative in producing that response. The following physiologic systems are thought to govern the antihypertensive mechanism(s) of the β-blockers. Although any one of these could predominate, it seems more likely that a combination of factors determines the ultimate outcome.

CARDIOVASCULAR SYSTEM [8]

Immediately after the administration of β-blocking drugs, cardiac output and rate decrease but blood pressure remains unchanged. Peripheral vascular resistance increases as β-receptor-mediated peripheral vasodilation is inhibited, leaving the α-adrenergic vasoconstrictor response unopposed. This response has been observed with both selective (β_1) and nonselective (β_1, β_2) β-blockers.

As β-blocker therapy is continued, cardiac output and heart rate remain low and blood pressure also decreases, despite the persistence of peripheral vascular resistance at levels equal to or slightly above baseline levels. When a β-blocker with intrinsic sympathomimetic activity is administered, the reduction in blood pressure is equivalent to that noted when using a β-blocker without this property, but the reduction in cardiac output and heart rate is attenuated. Thus, because of the delay in antihypertensive response, despite an immediate cardiac effect, and because of a lack of correlation between the reduction in cardiac output and blood pressure, it is unlikely that the influence of β-blockers on systemic blood pressure is mediated only via an effect on cardiac function.

RENIN—ANGIOTENSIN SYSTEM

Renin secretion from the kidney is regulated, in part, by β-adrenergic mechanisms and is inhibited by propranolol [9]. Using the high, low, and normal renin classification system of Laragh's group [10], early clinical studies suggested the hypotensive response to propranolol was dependent on suppression of renin—angiotensin system activity and that only patients with high or normal levels of plasma renin activity could be expected to respond to β-adrenergic blocking drugs [11]. On further examination, however, it has become clear that plasma renin activity is not the sole predictor of therapeutic success. While patients with high levels of plasma renin activity can be expected to respond to low or moderate doses of a β-blocker, even patients with low plasma renin activity can exhibit a reduction in blood pressure with β-blocker therapy [12].

It has also been suggested that β-blockers are not likely to be effective in blacks because of the prevalence of a volume-dependent low-renin type of hypertension [13]. However, it appears that this distinction also is not as clear as predicted and that these drugs may be equally effective in blacks as in whites [14]. Thus, it seems that plasma renin activity serves as a physiologic marker relating dosage requirements to ease of blood pressure control rather than as an absolute predictor of degree of success with β-blocker therapy.

CENTRAL NERVOUS SYSTEM

Propranolol penetrates the blood—brain barrier to become highly concentrated in brain tissue [15]. This fact, coupled with evidence of a direct central antihypertensive effect for propranolol, has led to consideration of the central nervous system as its primary site of antihypertensive action [16,17]. The role of central β-adrenergic receptors in control of blood pressure is poorly defined and the central antihypertensive effect of propranolol may not be related to either its β-blocking or membrane-stabilizing properties [18]. With the development of newer β-adrenergic blocking drugs, such as atenolol and nadolol, possessing extremely low lipid solubility but with an equivalent capacity of other β-blockers to reduce blood pressure, it seems less likely that access to central adrenoceptors is critical for β-adrenergic blocker effectiveness.

Drug disposition (Table 13.3)

The factors influencing overall drug disposition vary between the β-blockers and between patients receiving the same β-blocker [19]. Because the therapeutic index of these drugs (i.e. the ratio between the drug concentration causing adverse effects and the drug concentration resulting in the desired therapeutic response) is high enough that interpatient variability is not a major issue, population-based recommended dosing regimens can be used without great concern about side-effects and with the understanding that doses can be titrated upward in an attempt to achieve a satisfactory therapeutic response.

The β-blockers are well absorbed from the gastro-intestinal tract after oral administration. However, bioavailability of certain drugs, such as propranolol, may be severely limited by the first-pass phenomenon, in which a larger percentage of drug is avidly extracted from the portal blood immediately after absorption and prior to reaching the systemic circulation. The result is a reduction of circulating plasma drug concentrations when compared to levels observed after intravenous administration. With continued oral dosing, hepatic extraction becomes saturated, leading to higher steady-state blood levels and a slightly prolonged half-life [20].

A relationship between plasma drug concentration and pharmacologic effect has not been established for the β-blockers, with the exception of the inhibitory response to isoproterenol and exercise-induced tachycardia [21]. For this reason, and because of the wide variability in drug disposition between patients, levels of β-blocking drugs are rarely measured today. Older data describing levels as high as 700 ng/ml in children attest to the safety of these drugs and the limited need to obtain drug levels [22]. Although absolute dosing requirements have not been established in children, a starting dose equivalent to 0.5—1 mg/kg twice daily of propranolol is tolerated by almost all pediatric patients, and restricting maximal doses to 8 mg/kg per 24 h will prevent excessive drug concentrations.

The β-blockers are either excreted by the kidney or metabolized by the liver. Propranolol is the only β-blocker to form an active metabolite (4-hydroxy-propranolol), but this appears to be of little clinical importance. The plasma half-life varies between drugs from the shorter-acting preparations (propranolol and metoprolol) to the longer-acting ones (atenolol and nadolol). The antihypertensive

Table 13.3 Disposition of β-adrenergic blocking drugs

	First-pass effect	Plasma half-life (h)	Clearance	Adjustment in renal failure
Propranolol	Yes	3–4	Hepatic	No
Acebutolol	No	3–4	Renal	Yes
Atenolol	No	6–9	Renal	Yes
Metoprolol	No	3–4	Hepatic	No
Nadolol	No	14–24	Renal	Yes
Pindolol	No	3–4	Both	Severe
Timolol	No	4–5	Hepatic	No
Carteolol	No	5–7	Renal	Yes
Penbutalol	Yes	5–6	Hepatic	No

effect has not been related to plasma concentration and exceeds the expected duration of drug action based on plasma half-life. Thus, even preparations with short half-lives can be administered on a twice-daily basis and may be effective when given only once a day.

Adverse effects (Table 13.4)

The diffuse tissue distribution of β-adrenergic receptors suggests that the potential for adverse reactions with the β-adrenergic blocking drugs is substantial. The reported incidence of side-effects with these drugs in children is exceptionally low and of doubtful clinical significance, with the exception of patients with underlying cardiovascular, pulmonary, renal, or metabolic diseases.

CARDIOVASCULAR

β-adrenergic blocking agents are contraindicated in patients with overt congestive heart failure in whom sympathetic input is critical for maintaining chronotropic and inotropic reserve. Electrocardiographic, echocardiographic, or X-ray evidence of hypertension-induced left ventricular hypertrophy, in the absence of cardiac failure, should not of itself influence the selection of β-blocker therapy, since the antihypertensive effect of these drugs will often reverse this ventricular response to elevated systemic pressure.

Resting bradycardia of varying degrees will be noted in children of all ages during β-blocker administration but it is rarely severe enough to warrant withdrawal of therapy. Because these drugs act as competitive antagonists to norepinephrine, their effect can be overcome by an increase in endogenous

Table 13.4 Adverse effects of β-adrenergic blocking drugs

Bradycardia
Cardiac failure
Raynaud's disease
Bronchoconstriction
Reduction of glomerular filtration rate
Central nervous system effects
  Nightmares
  Confusion
  Agitation
  Depression
  Sleep disturbances
Hypoglycemia
Inhibition of symptoms of hypoglycemia
Altered serum lipoprotein concentrations

sympathetic activity; while exercise-induced tachycardia is reduced, it is not entirely prevented and patients retain the capacity to respond under conditions of stress [23]. Peak cardiac exercise conditioning may be less than maximal, and we have recently observed a teenage swimmer complain of reduced stamina, requiring a reconditioning period immediately after propranolol was discontinued.

An increase in peripheral vascular resistance occurs during β-blocker therapy and can uncover or exacerbate Raynaud's disease in patients with collagen-vascular disease. Peripheral vasoconstriction is the result of reflex sympathetic activation secondary to a reduction in heart rate and cardiac output, and β-adrenergic blockade of peripheral β-receptor-mediated vasodilatation, thus leaving α-receptor-mediated vasoconstriction unopposed. Use of β-blockers with intrinsic sympathomimetic activity may modify this response by maintaining a degree of the vasodilatory effect.

PULMONARY

Bronchial dilatation is mediated via activation of β_2-adrenergic receptors. Therefore, the use of β-adrenergic blocking drugs is likely to be associated with an exacerbation of symptoms in asthmatic patients and may aggravate pulmonary insufficiency in patients with chronic lung disease.

The use of cardioselective (or β_1) preparations to treat patients with a history of bronchospasm may prevent pulmonary complications at low drug doses. However, even the cardioselective drugs may be active at β_2 sites when higher doses are used, so that administration of any of the β-blocking drugs to patients with obstructive forms of lung disease should be discouraged.

RENAL

The chronic use of propranolol in adults has been associated with a reduction in glomerular filtration rate [24,25]. This effect is not observed in all treated patients and appears to be related to an increased sympathetic tone found in patients demonstrating a poor antihypertensive response to β-blocker therapy. It is not clear whether this is a problem with all β-blockers, since maintenance of renal blood flow and glomerular filtration rate and a decrease in renal vascular resistance have been reported with administration of nadolol [26]. Despite the common association of childhood hypertension with renal disease, it would be premature to suggest that β-blocker therapy should be withheld from these patients, and it seems unlikely, based on broad clinical experience, that it is an important clinical problem in this age group.

CENTRAL NERVOUS SYSTEM

The concentration of β-adrenergic blocking drugs within the central nervous system is determined by their lipid solubility. Drugs with high lipid solubility, such as propranolol, are highly concentrated in brain tissue, whereas access of drugs with low lipid solubility, such as atenolol is limited.

Propranolol has been associated with a number of central nervous system side-effects in adults, including nightmares, dreams, confusion, agitation, and depression. Similar findings are infrequent in children and are more likely to present in the form of sleep disturbances. In patients with a good anti-

hypertensive response to β-adrenergic blockade but central nervous system side-effects, changing to atenolol may permit the continued use of a β-blocker.

METABOLIC

β-Adrenergic blocking drugs adversely affect glucose [27] and lipid metabolism [28,29]. Regulation of glucose homeostasis is mediated, in part, through β-adrenergic receptor activation of glycogenolysis and gluconeogenesis and inhibition of insulin secretion. Consequently, β-blocker therapy retards the usual homeostatic response to hypoglycemia.

Hypoglycemia has not been a problem with β-blocker therapy in patients with normal pancreatic function. In contrast, patients with diabetes mellitus may have an exaggerated hypoglycemic response with a reduction in the rate of rise of blood glucose after insulin administration. This is compounded by the concomitant inhibition of the systemic response to hypoglycemia, i.e. tachycardia, palpitations, and hunger, thus eliminating the warning signs crucial to the diabetic in preventing severe hypoglycemia and its systemic complications.

The recognition that β-adrenergic blocking drugs have an adverse effect on lipoprotein metabolism is relatively recent. A large number of independent studies are now available for review and suggest that a specific increase in total and very low density lipoprotein triglyceride and decrease in high density lipoprotein (HDL-C) fractions occur, to the exclusion of changes in either total or low density lipoprotein cholesterol (LDL-C) levels [28]. These changes persist during long-term β-blocker therapy and appear to be dependent on the pharmacologic characteristics of the β-blocker. The changes in triglyceride and HDL-C concentrations are less severe when cardioselective drugs are used and even less affected by drugs with intrinsic sympathomimetic activity.

It seems reasonable to assume that these changes are mediated via alterations in adrenergic activity, particularly since changes in lipoprotein metabolism in the opposite direction from those observed with the β-blockers occur with α-adrenergic blocking drugs. Lipoprotein metabolism may be influenced by a number of adrenergically mediated functions, including alterations in blood flow to adipose tissue or skeletal muscle, direct effects on adipocyte-related triglyceride hydrolysis, and modulation of insulin release from the pancreas.

α-ADRENERGIC AGENTS

During the past decade there has been a renewal of interest in the α-adrenergic component of the sympathetic nervous system. While the primary direction in β-adrenergic investigation has been refinement of molecular drug structure in an attempt to produce newer and clinically attractive therapeutic agents, α-adrenergic investigation has been more basic in nature. The result has been an expanding definition of the role of the α-adrenergic receptor in sympathetically mediated cardiovascular control, particularly with regard to blood pressure homeostasis [30,31].

In contrast to β-adrenergic directed drug therapy, which is limited to agents possessing receptor antagonist properties, α-adrenergic agonists as well as antagonists have successfully been used to treat hypertension. At the present time, the number of drugs in each group for which there is a reasonable amount of clinical experience is small. Therefore, this section will be devoted to a discussion of these drugs as reference drugs for specific classes of α-adrenergic agents, with the understanding that additional molecules are being developed or, in some cases, are already in an early marketing stage (Table 13.5).

α-Adrenergic blocking drugs

The earliest α-adrenergic blocking drugs, phenoxybenzamine and phentolamine, were nonselective in nature, possessing both α₁- and α₂-blocking properties. Despite expectations of therapeutic efficacy, their promise was never fulfilled because of a relative ineffectiveness in reducing systemic blood pressure coupled with a high incidence of side-effects such as tachycardia and orthostatic hypotension.

The use of α-blocking drugs to treat hypertension became a practical consideration with the development of prazosin, a selective α_1-blocker [32]. Because α_1-receptors are located at postsynaptic sites and primarily within peripheral vascular resistance vessels, the antihypertensive action of prazosin is mediated through vascular smooth muscle relaxation, similar in effect to that observed with vasodilators such as hydralazine. However, the reflex increase in sympathetic activity, expressed as an increase in heart rate, cardiac output, and renin secretion, does not occur.

It has been suggested that effectiveness and relative absence of side-effects with prazosin, in contrast to the nonselective α-blockers, is related to its α_1 selectivity. As noted earlier in this chapter, α_2-blocking drugs inhibit the negative feedback action of neuronally released norepinephrine at presynaptic sites. The outcome of presynaptic α_2 inhibition is an increased release of norepinephrine to compete with the antagonist at α-adrenergic post-synaptic sites as well as an enhanced and unopposed effect at the cardiac postsynpatic β-adrenoceptor. It seems unlikely that the effectiveness of prazosin and absence of side-effects are totally related to the drug's lack of activity at α_2-presynaptic sites, since vasodilators, which also lack α_2-blocking capacity, cause highly significant reflex sympathetic changes in cardiac activity. It is possible that the modifying effect on cardiac and other reflexly stimulated events during prazosin therapy results from the concomitant dilatation of venous capacitance vessels which are also richly innervated with α_1-adrenergic receptors, or that prazosin directly inhibits baroreceptor function.

Prazosin is well absorbed after oral administration. It is metabolized by the liver, and dosing adjustments in patients with renal failure or on dialysis are not

Table 13.5 α-Adrenergic drugs

Drug	Receptor type	Action	Starting dose	Frequency
Prazosin	α_1	Antagonist	0.25−0.5 mg	b.i.d−t.i.d.
Clonidine	α_2	Agonist	0.05−0.1 mg	b.i.d.
Methyldopa	α_2	Agonist	5−10 mg/kg	b.i.d.
Guanabenz	α_2	Agonist	0.07−0.17 mg/kg*	b.i.d.
Urapidil*	α_1	Antagonist		
Guanfacine*	α_2	Agonist		
Trimazosin*	α_1	Antagonist		
Indoramin*	α_1	Antagonist		

* Not yet released for use in the USA.

necessary. Despite a relatively short plasma half-life, its biologic effect is such that in most cases it can be administered on a twice-daily schedule (see also Chapter 14).

Side-effects with prazosin are minimal and rarely a problem in children. Of particular note is the so-called first-dose effect in which severe orthostasis may occur in conjunction with the initial prazosin dose. This effect appears to be dependent on fluid balance so that patients receiving aggressive diuretic therapy at the time when prazosin is started may be at particular risk.

The orthostatic effect almost always remits with ongoing prazosin therapy. This appears to be the result of an increase in density of arteriolar post-synaptic α_2-receptors. Under usual circumstances, these receptors are located outside the synaptic cleft [33] and, although activated by circulating norepine-phrine, play a seemingly secondary role to the α_1-receptor in vascular reactivity. During α_1-receptor blockade with prazosin orthostasis diminishes as the number of α_2-receptors increases [34], without inter-fering with the antihypertensive effect.

A unique feature of prazosin is its capacity to alter lipoprotein metabolism so as to establish lipid pro-files in treated patients that are less atherogenic than those found in patients receiving other anti-hypertensive agents. In direct comparison with thiazide diuretics and β-adrenergic blockers, it has been shown in a number of studies that prazosin decreases total cholesterol and LDL-C and increases HDL-C [35–37]. Thus, despite the acknowledgment that prazosin does not offer any major anti-hypertensive advantage over other agents, its low incidence of adverse clinical effects — in particular on lipid metabolism — may ultimately result in its selection as a first-order drug in the design of antihypertensive regimens.

α-Adrenergic agonists

All α-adrenergic agonists used to treat hypertension act specifically at the α_2-receptor. A preponderance of experimental data has established that the major antihypertensive effect of these drugs is mediated via direct activation of postsynaptic adrenoceptors within the central nervous system, resulting in a reduction of electric outflow activity along the sym-pathetic tract. This is in marked contrast to the situation in the peripheral sympathetic system where postsynaptic α-adrenoceptor activation is charac-teristically associated with arteriolar vasoconstriction and hypertension.

The antihypertensive effect of α_2-agonists is potentiated peripherally by activation of neuronal presynaptic α_2-receptors so as to reduce further nor-epinephrine release in the arteriolar resistance vessels. Although α_2 presynaptic receptors are also found in the central nervous system, their role in blood pressure control has not been established.

Clonidine

Clonidine is the principal α_2-agonist available for clinical use and is currently considered the reference drug for this class of centrally acting agents. It is metabolized primarily by the liver, with approxi-mately one-third of a daily dose excreted by the kidney [38]. Its moderately long half-life of 8 h permits twice-daily dosing.

The clinical response to clonidine reflects its α_2-adrenoceptor activity. Shortly after administration, there is a rise in systemic blood pressure resulting from the stimulation of α_2 postsynaptic adrenoceptors innervating peripheral arteriolar resistance vessels. However, within a short time there is a fall in blood pressure accompanied by suppression of cardiac activity and renin secretion, as the central inhibitory effects of clonidine on neuronal transmission become predominant.

Clonidine therapy is associated with a high inci-dence of dry mouth and sedation. It seems reason-able to suggest that, in addition to suppression of adrenergic electric neuronal traffic to the periphery, clonidine also suppresses adrenergic activity within the central nervous system itself, as has been noted with adrenergic agents such as reserpine that reduce adrenergic neurotransmission by depleting neuronal catecholamine stores.

A critical adverse reaction observed with clonidine has been rebound hypertension occurring after the drug is abruptly withdrawn from patients on chronic therapy. This sudden increase in blood press-ure to potentially malignant levels is apparently the result of a surge of adrenergic activity as central suppression of adrenergic nerve conduction remits [39]. In addition to the severe elevations of blood pressure, cardiac arrhythmias have also been de-scribed as a complication of clonidine withdrawal [40]. When it becomes medically indicated to dis-continue clonidine, gradual withdrawal with careful observation can prevent this syndrome.

Clonidine overdose can cause central nervous system effects, bradycardia, and hypotension—similar to findings with other α_2-agonists [41]. Symptomatic treatment in the form of atropine, norepinephrine, and naloxone has been reported to be effective.

Methyldopa

Methyldopa is the oldest of the α_2-adrenergic agonists and was one of the most widely used antihypertensive drugs until the early 1970s. As newer antihypertensive agents, in particular the β-blockers, became available, the popularity of methyldopa declined. With the resurgence of interest in α_2-agonists, attention has again turned to methyldopa [42].

Methyldopa possesses the same basic molecular structure, with the exception of the addition of a methyl group, as the naturally occurring catecholamine, dopa and consequently gains easy access to the catecholamine metabolic pathway (Fig. 13.1). The result is production of methylnorepinephrine which displaces norepinephrine from its storage site in the nerve ending.

It had been assumed that the effectiveness of methyldopa was mediated via the production of methylnorepinephrine, which was termed a "false transmitter," because it was generally considered to be of lesser potency than norepinephrine as an adrenergic agonist. However, these two catecholamines are approximately equipotent in producing a pressor response [43]. It was not until after the mechanism of action of clonidine was understood and the importance of central α_2-adrenoceptors was recognized that the role of methylnorepinephrine as an α_2-agonist became clear.

The pharmacology of methyldopa has previously been described [44]. In particular, only a small proportion of absorbed drug enters the catecholamine metabolic pathway to form methylnorepinephrine, with the majority of methyldopa being excreted unchanged by the kidney. Consequently, in patients with renal failure, side-effects occur rapidly unless the dose is reduced. The major side-effect with methyldopa is sedation, which occurs in almost every patient after therapy is initiated or during the course of therapy when the daily dose is increased. This effect usually seems to remit within 7–10 days, despite continued therapy. Other serious but less frequent side-effects are development of a positive direct Coombs test, a lupus erythematosus-like syndrome, hepatitis, and colitis.

Guanabenz [45]

Disposition data from studies in adults [46] show that guanabenz is well absorbed from the gastrointestinal tract but undergoes substantial first-pass hepatic metabolism. Its duration of antihypertensive action and elimination half-life are approximately 12 h, permitting twice-daily dosing. It is cleared almost entirely by hepatic metabolism. Dosing recommendations have been established for adolescents in whom 3–12 mg/day (0.07–0.17 mg/kg per day) administered on a twice-daily schedule has been shown to be safe and effective [47].

DRUGS ACTING AT BOTH THE α- AND β-ADRENERGIC RECEPTOR

One of the more interesting developments in antihypertensive pharmacology is labetalol, a drug that acts at both α- and β-adrenoceptors [48]. It is generally referred to as a primary β-adrenergic blocking agent with α-adrenergic blocking properties because it is approximately eight times more potent in blocking β-than α-receptors. In addition to its adrenergic blocking properties, labetalol is also a selective β_2-agonist in the peripheral vasculature [49].

The pharmacologic and pharmacokinetic properties of labetalol represent a combination of the other β-blockers. The drug is well absorbed after oral administration but is extensively metabolized by the first-pass phenomenon, reducing its bioavailability to a level similar to propranolol. It is cleared from the body almost entirely by hepatic metabolism, with only 5% excreted unchanged in the urine. The plasma half-life of labetalol is approximately 4 h.

Labetalol is less potent than either the α-adrenergic antagonists or propranolol. It does not have intrinsic sympathomimetic or membrane-stabilizing activity and is weakly lipid-soluble, so that negligible amounts of labetalol gain access to brain tissue.

Because of its lower molar potency in comparison to other adrenergic blocking drugs, high drug doses of labetalol are required to achieve an equivalent antihypertensive response. The antihypertensive effectiveness of labetalol is not greater than other commonly used agents, but side-effects appear to be fewer because of its pharmacologic properties. Nevertheless, side-effects observed during treatment with the other β-blockers must be considered during labetalol therapy.

A potential therapeutic indication for labetalol is

treatment of hypertensive crisis [50]. Because the drug dose can be titrated during intravenous administration, blood pressure may be brought under control more gradually without the dramatic reductions in blood pressure that can occur with administration of vasodilators.

ACKNOWLEDGMENT

This study was supported, in part, by *National Institutes of Health grant HL-34659.*

REFERENCES

1 Axelrod J, Weinshilbaum R. Catecholamines. *N Engl J Med* 1972;287:237−42.

2 Langer SZ, Cavero I, Massingham R. Recent developments in noradrenergic neurotransmission and its relevance to the mechanisms of action of certain antihypertensive agents. *Hypertension* 1980;2:372−82.

3 Ahlquist RP. A study of the adrenotropic receptors. *Am J Physiol* 1948;153:556−600.

4 Lefkowitz RJ, Carm MG, Stiles GL. Mechanisms of membrane-receptor regulation. *N Engl J Med* 1984;310:1570−9.

5 Frishman WH, ed. *Clinical Pharmacology of the β-Adrenoceptor Blocking Drugs*. 2nd edn. Norwalk, CT: Appleton-Century-Crofts, 1984;27−49.

6 Taylor SH. Intrinsic sympathomimetic activity: clinical fact or fiction? *Am J Cardiol* 1983;52:160−260.

7 Williams EMV. Mode of action of β receptor antagonists on cardiac muscle. *Am J Cardiol* 1966;18:399−405.

8 Frohlich ED, Dunn FG, Messerli FH. Pharmacologic and physiologic considerations of adrenoceptor blockade. *Am J Med* 1983;17:9−14.

9 Sinaiko AR. Influence of adrenergic nervous system on vasodilator-induced renin release in the conscious rat. *Proc Soc Exp Biol Med* 1981;167:25−9.

10 Brunner HR, Laragh JH, Baer L. Essential hypertension: renin and aldosterone, heart attack and stroke. *N Engl J Med* 1972;286:441−9.

11 Buhler FR, Laragh JH, Baer L, Vaughan ED, Brunner HR. Propranolol inhibition of renin secretion. *N Engl J Med* 1972;287:1209−14.

12 Hollifield JW, Sherman K, Vander Zwagg R, Shand DG. Proposed mechanisms of propranolol's antihypertensive effect in essential hypertension. *N Engl J Med* 1976;295:68−73.

13 Friedman B, Gray JM, Gross S, Levit S. United States experience with oxprenolol in hypertension. *Am J Cardiol* 1983;52:430−80.

14 Veterans Administration cooperative study group on antihypertensive drugs. Comparison of propranolol and hydrochlorothiazide for the initial treatment of hypertension. *JAMA* 1982;248:1996−2003.

15 Myers MG, Lewis PJ, Reid JL, Dollery CT. Brain concentration of propranolol in relation to hypotensive effect in the rabbit with observations on brain propranolol levels in man. *J Pharmacol Exp Ther* 1975;192:327−35.

16 Day MD, Roach AG. Central adrenoceptors and the control of arterial blood pressure. *Clin Exp Pharmacol Physiol* 1974;1:342−60.

17 Reid JL, Lewis PJ, Myers MG. Cardiovascular effects of intracerebrovascular d-l-dl-propranolol in conscious rabbit. *J Pharmacol Exp Ther* 1974;188:394−9.

18 Privitera PJ, Webb JG, Walle T. Effects of centrally administered propranolol on plasma renin activity, plasma norepinephrine and arterial pressure. *Eur J Pharmacol* 1979;54:51−60.

19 Thadani U. β-Blockers in hypertension. *Am J Cardiol* 1983;52:100−50.

20 Evans GH, Shand DG. Disposition of propranolol. *Clin Pharmacol Ther* 1973;14:487−93.

21 McDevitt DG, Shand DG. Plasma concentrations and the time-course of β blockade due to propranolol. *Clin Pharmacol Ther* 1975;18:708−13.

22 Mirkin BL, Sinaiko AR. Clinical pharmacology and therapeutic utilization of antihypertensive agents in children. In: New MI, Levine LS, eds. *Juvenile Hypertension*. New York: Raven Press, 1977;195−217.

23 Colfort DJ, Shand DG. Plasma propranolol levels in the quantitative assessment of β-adrenergic blockade in man. *Br Med J* 1970;3:731−4.

24 Bauer JH, Brooks CS. The long-term effect of propranolol therapy on renal function. *Am J Med* 1979;66:405−10.

25 De Leeuw PW, Birkenhager WH. Renal response to propranolol treatment in hypertensive humans. *Hypertension* 1982;4:125−31.

26 Textor SC, Fouad FM, Bravo EL, Tarazi RC, Vidt RG, Gifford RW. Redistribution of cardiac output to the kidneys during oral nadalol administration. *N Engl J Med* 1982;307:601−4.

27 Laper J, Blohme G, Smith U. Effect of cardioselective blockade in the hypoglycemic response in insulin-dependent diabetes. *Lancet* 1979;i:458−62.

28 Weidmann P, Uehlinger DE, Gerber A. Antihypertensive treatment and serum lipoproteins. *J Hypertens* 1985;3:297−306.

29 Weinberger MH. Antihypertensive therapy and lipids. Paradoxical influences on cardiovascular disease risk. *Am J Med* 1986;80(suppl 2A):64−70.

30 van Zwieten PA, Timmermans PBMWM, Brummelen PV. Role of adrenoceptors in hypertension and in antihypertensive drug therapy. *Am J Med* 1984;77:17−25.

31 van Zwieten PA, Timmermans PBMWM. Cardiovascular β-receptors. *J Mol Cell Cardiol* 1983;15:717−33.

32 Colucci WS. α-Adrenergic receptor blockade with prazosin. *Ann Intern Med* 1982;97:67−77.

33 Wilffert B, Timmermans PBMWM, van Zwieten PA. Extrasynaptic location of α-2 and non-innervated β-2 adrenoceptors in the vascular system of the pithed normotensive rat. *J Pharmacol Exp Ther* 1982;221:762−8.

34 Pettinger WA, Smyth DD, Umemura S. Renal α-adrenoceptors, their locations and effects on sodium excretion. *J Cardiovasc Pharmacol* 1985;7(suppl 8):524−7.

35 Rouffy J, Jaillard J. Effects of two antihypertensive agents on lipids, lipoproteins and apoproteins A and B. *Am J Med* 1986;80:100.

36 Velasco M, Hurt E, Silva H *et al.* Effects of prazosin and propranolol on blood lipids and lipoproteins in hypertensive patients. *Am J Med* 1986;80:109−13.

37 Lithell H, Aberg H, Selinus I. Metabolic effects of a change in antihypertensive treatment. *Am J Med* 1986;80:114−19.

38 Keranen A, Nykanen S, Taskinen J. Pharmacokinetics and side-effects of clonidine. *Eur J Clin Pharmacol* 1978;13: 97−101.

39 Hansson L, Hunyor SN, Julius S, Hoobler SW. Blood pressure crisis following withdrawal of clonidine (Catapres, Catapresan), with special reference to arterial and urinary catecholamine levels, and suggestions for acute management. *Am Heart J* 1973;85:605−10.

40 Peters RW, Hamilton BP, Hamilton J, Kuzbida G, Paulis R. Cardiac arrhythmias after abrupt clonidine withdrawal. *Clin Pharmacol Ther* 1983;34:435−9.

41 Hall AH, Smolinska SC, Kulig KW, Reinack BH. Guanabenz overdose. *Ann Intern Med* 1985;102:787−8.

42 van Zwiten PA, Theolen MJMC, Timmermans PBMWM. The hypotensive activity and side effects of methyldopa, clonidine and guanficine. *Hypertension* 1984;6(suppl II):II-28−33.

43 Altura BM. Peripheral vascular actions of α-methyldopa and its mode of action on arterioles. *Proc Soc Exp Biol Med* 1974;145:129−34.

44 Sinaiko AR, Mirkin BL. Clinical pharmacology of antihypertensive drugs in children. *Pediatr Clin North Am* 1978;25: 137−57.

45 Baum T, Shropshire AT, Rowles G *et al.* General pharmacologic actions of the antihypertensive agent 2,6-dichlorobenzylidine aminoguanidine acetate (Wy-8678). *J Pharmacol Exp Ther* 1970;171:276−87.

46 Meacham RH, Emmett M, Kyrakopoulos AA *et al.* Disposition of C-guanabenz in patients with essential hypertension. *Clin Pharmacol Ther* 1980;27:44−52.

47 Walsur PO, Rath A, Kilbourne K, Deitch MW. Guanabenz for adolescent hypertension. *Pediatr Pharmacol* 1984;4:1−6.

48 Proceedings of a symposium on labetalol. *Br J Clin Pharmacol* 1976;3(suppl 3):627−824.

49 Baum T, Sybertz EJ. Pharmacology of labetalol in experimental animals. *Am J Med* 1983;75:15−23.

50 Vlachakis ND, Marmde RF, Maloy SW, Medakovic M, Kasseur N. Pharmacodynamics of intravenous labetalol and follow-up therapy with oral labetalol. *Clin Pharmacol Ther* 1985;38:503−8.

14 The Vasodilators

THOMAS R. WELCH AND C. FREDERIC STRIFE

INTRODUCTION

The vasodilators include some of the oldest and most effective antihypertensives. These drugs act on vascular smooth muscle, decreasing peripheral resistance and thus lowering systemic blood pressure. The agents differ both in their modes of action and in their relative effects on the arterial and venous systems.

In the therapy of hypertension, these medications find their widest use in two clinical situations. The parenteral vasodilators (principally diazoxide and nitroprusside) are first-line drugs for the control of acute severe hypertension and hypertensive encephalopathy. Neither of these agents provides practical chronic management of hypertension, so that their use will usually need to be followed by the institution of a regimen of oral antihypertensives.

The second context in which vasodilators have a role is in the chronic oral therapy of moderate-to-severe hypertension. The drugs most often used in this situation are hydralazine and prazosin. Vasodilators, when used alone, almost invariably result in sodium retention and tachycardia. Thus, these drugs are inappropriate as single agents. Most often, they are introduced after adequate control of blood pressure has not been achieved with a diuretic and a β-blocker.

A third oral agent, minoxidil, occupies an intermediate therapeutic niche. This drug usually provides predictably rapid control of acute blood pressure elevations in children who are already under chronic treatment with other agents. The drug, however, is inappropriate for the treatment of hypertensive encephalopathy and its side-effects preclude chronic administration in childhood.

The past decade has witnessed an explosion of clinical and laboratory investigation on the pharmacology of these agents. Much of this work has been stimulated by the observation that vasodilator-induced alterations in the vascular tone may be of great benefit to patients with congestive heart failure [1]. This discussion, however, will be limited to the vasodilator management of hypertension in childhood. We will review the pharmacology and clinical use of oral and parenteral vasodilators for acute and chronic management of hypertension (Table 14.1).

ORAL VASODILATORS

Hydralazine

PHARMACOLOGY

Hydralazine has been used in the therapy of hypertension for over 30 years. The drug acts directly on the vascular smooth muscle to produce relaxation and vasodilatation; it has a more pronounced effect on the arteriolar than on the venous system [2–4].

Studies of hydralazine pharmacokinetics have been complicated by difficulties in defining its active forms [5]. Following oral administration, the drug is nearly completely absorbed with peak serum concentrations achieved at 1–2 h [4]. The agent undergoes first-pass metabolism in the liver, primarily by acetylation. Acetylation phenotype may thus influence the plasma hydralazine concentration, with "slow" acetylators achieving higher levels. The $t_{\frac{1}{2}}$ of hydralazine has been reported to range from less than 1 h to 8 h [5,6]. Apparently, however, the drug is rapidly bound to vascular smooth muscle with high affinity, and its loss from these sites proceeds more slowly than its clearance from plasma [4,7]. Although only about 15% of the drug is excreted unchanged in the urine, renal excretion of metabolites is important and dosage adjustments must be made for patients with renal insufficiency [8].

Table 14.1 Vasodilator drugs useful in childhood hypertension

| Drug | Dosage | | | Onset of action | How supplied* |
	Starting	Maximum	Interval		
Hydralazine (oral) (Apresoline®)	1 mg/kg per day up to 40 mg/day	4 mg/kg per day (300 mg)	q. 6–12 h	1–2 h	10, 25, 50, 100 mg tablets
Hydralazine (i.v.)	0.15 mg/kg per dose	0.5 mg/kg (40 mg)	q. 4–6 h	10–20 min	20 mg ampoules
Prazosin (oral) (Minipress®)	0.5–1 mg/dose	20 mg/day	q. 8–12 h	30–90 min	1, 2, 5 mg capsules
Minoxidil (oral) (Loniten®)	0.2 mg/kg per dose up to 20 mg/kg per dose	1 mg/kg (50 mg)	q. 12–24 h	1–2 h	2.5, 10 mg tablets
Diazoxide (i.v.) (Hyperstat®)	0.25 mg/kg per min	5 mg/kg (300 mg)	Continuous	Immediate	300 mg ampoules
Nitroprusside (i.v.)	0.5 µg/kg per min	10 µg/kg per min	Continuous	Immediate	2 mg (2000 µg) ampoules

*In the U.S.A.

CLINICAL USE

Oral hydralazine is most useful in moderate-to-severe hypertension. In general, the drug should only be started if the patient is already receiving a diuretic and β-blocking agents. Although hydralazine is most often used on an every 6-h basis, there is good evidence that it is nearly equally effective when used every 12 h [7]. Such a regimen may improve compliance and apparently is possible because of the strong affinity of the drug for vascular smooth muscle. In patients with end-stage renal disease, the drug may be given once daily, and additional doses after dialysis are not required [8].

We usually begin oral hydralazine in a dosage of 1 mg/kg per day, increasing if necessary to a maximum of 4 mg/kg per day (maximum 300 mg/day). The side-effects of hydralazine seem to be less noticeable when the drug is increased slowly.

ADVERSE EFFECTS AND IMPORTANT INTERACTIONS

Hydralazine has a number of bothersome effects which may limit its use. A hyperdynamic cardiovascular state with tachycardia and palpitations is the reflex response to the unopposed vasodilator action of the drug. These effects are minimized by adequate β-blockade [4,9]. In many patients, especially teenagers, headache is a common and unacceptable accompaniment of therapy. More severe side-effects, including drug fever and pancytopenia, are exceedingly uncommon but require discontinuation of the drug.

A lupus-like syndrome, usually characterized by synovitis, elevated antinuclear antibody titers, and normocomplementemia, has been associated with this drug. The syndrome is multifactorial, with risk factors including sex (female), race (white), heredity (human leukocyte antigen DR4+), drug dose (high), and acetylation phenotype (slow) [10]. The syndrome is exceedingly rare in the pediatric age group, and is reversible upon discontinuation of the drug. Idiopathic (i.e. not drug-related) systemic lupus erythematosus is not a contraindication to the use of hydralazine.

The concomitant use of hydralazine and other vasodilators may precipitate severe hypotension. This occurs most often when a patient being treated with hydralazine receives diazoxide for acute severe hypertension, and may be avoided by careful titration of the diazoxide dose. The combination of hydralazine and prazosin (in addition to a diuretic and β-blocker) has been reported to be safe and effective for severe hypertension uncontrolled by either agent alone [11]. Hydralazine has been reported to decrease the first-pass liver clearance of propranolol, resulting in higher levels of the latter drug, especially if the two are given together [12]. Thus, a downward adjustment in propranolol dosage may occasionally be necessary when hydralazine is begun.

Prazosin (see also Chapter 13)

PHARMACOLOGY

Prazosin was the first member of a new class of antihypertensive agents which antagonize peripheral α_1-adrenergic receptors. Prazosin is rapidly and almost completely absorbed after oral administration. Peak plasma concentrations are achieved within 2—3 h. The half-life is 2—3 h, with the drug being eliminated according to first-order kinetics. The antihypertensive effect persists for much longer than expected (up to 10—12 h), presumably because of the persistence of active metabolites [13]. Although the drug is extensively metabolized by the liver and excreted via the biliary system, patients with chronic renal or cardiac failure may exhibit prolonged plasma half-lives [14,15].

Prazosin exerts its hypotensive effect by competitively blocking the vascular postsynaptic α_1-adrenergic receptors [13,16—18]. The drug has relative affinity for α_1-receptors when compared to α_2-receptors [19], thus preventing the vascular smooth muscle contractile response to norepinephrine without interfering with its activity at α_2 sites [16].

Therapeutic doses of prazosin result in a decrease in peripheral arterial resistance, venous tone, and mean arterial pressure without a significant increase in heart rate. The explanation for the relative lack of tachycardia and renin release observed after prazosin administration may in part be due to the combined actions of the drug in decreasing vascular tone in both arterioles and venules, preventing the marked increase in venous return and cardiac output observed with agents that reduce arteriolar vascular tone only. In this respect, prazosin resembles nitroprusside [20]. Terazasin, another α_1 blocking agent, has a longer duration of action.

CLINICAL USE

Prazosin appears most beneficial for treatment of patients with essential hypertension or hypertension resulting from primary renal disease. Prazosin may also aid in controlling hypertension resulting from catecholamine-producing tumors. Prazosin is most effective when given with a diuretic and β-blocking agent [20] for treatment of moderate-to-severe hypertension. Occasionally prazosin is used as a single agent for treatment of mild-to-moderate hypertension in patients who cannot tolerate diuretics or β-adrenergic blockers. However, when used as a single agent, fluid retention and the resulting increase in plasma volume may limit its antihypertensive effect.

Treatment with prazosin should be started with 1 mg (less in young children) given at bedtime to avoid the marked postural change in mean arterial pressure occasionally seen as a complication of the first dose. The drug can subsequently be given 2 or 3 times per day and the dose raised slowly until the desired lowering of blood pressure is achieved. It has been suggested that patients who experience a marked decrease in blood pressure after the first dose with no associated tachycardia usually thereafter require only a small dose to maintain adequate reduction of blood pressure [21]. In contrast, patients who exhibit only a minimal decrease in blood pressure after the first dose usually have significant tachycardia and require higher doses of prazosin to maintain blood pressure control. A total dose of more than 20 mg/day usually does not result in further blood pressure reduction.

ADVERSE EFFECTS AND IMPORTANT INTERACTIONS

In general the side-effects associated with prazosin treatment are mild and rarely necessitate withdrawal of the drug. The major acute side-effect, termed "first-dose effect," is a syndrome characterized by transient faintness, dizziness, palpitation, and rarely syncope occurring soon after the first dose or as a response to subsequent dose increments. This syndrome is exaggerated by exercise, pre-existing sodium restriction, or diuretic-induced sodium depletion [22], and appears to be dose-related [23].

Side-effects associated with chronic use are uncommon and include headache, drowsiness, nausea, dry mouth, fluid retention, depression, rashes, urinary incontinence, and polyarthralgia.

Minoxidil

PHARMACOLOGY

Minoxidil is an extremely effective oral vasodilator reserved for use in patients with severe hypertension resistant to conventional anti-hypertensive therapy. After oral administration minoxidil is rapidly and almost completely absorbed from the gastrointestinal tract [24]. The peak plasma concentration occurs in approximately 1 h and the half-life is about 4 h [25].

Kinetic studies in adult patients have shown that a single oral dose has an onset of antihypertensive action within 2 h, a maximal effect at about 4 h, and a total duration of action which may exceed 24 h [26,27].

Minoxidil is rapidly metabolized by the liver. The metabolites and a small amount of unchanged minoxidil are completely cleared from the plasma and excreted in the urine within 12 h of oral administration. The disparity between the duration of plasma levels and the antihypertensive effects is best explained by binding of minoxidil to vascular smooth muscle receptors [27]. Minoxidil is not bound to plasma proteins and the drug can be removed from plasma by hemodialysis.

Minoxidil acts directly to relax arteriolar smooth muscle. The resulting vasodilatation is accompanied by decreased peripheral vascular resistance and lowered systolic and diastolic blood pressures [26,27]. The hypotensive effect is accompanied by activation of the peripheral sympathetic nervous system with resulting increases in heart rate, cardiac index, renin, aldosterone secretion, and plasma norepinephrine concentration. Sodium and water retention also occur. These adverse effects can be blunted with concurrent administration of β-adrenergic blocking and diuretic agents [24,27]. In some patients with renal parenchymal disease there may be a decline in renal function. However, in patients with previously uncontrolled malignant hypertension renal function often improves [28] after an initial period of deterioration.

CLINICAL USE

Minoxidil is generally reserved as adjunctive therapy for adults [27,28] and children [29,30] with severe hypertension refractory to a multiple drug treatment schedule. The effectiveness of minoxidil is generally independent of the underlying cause of the hypertension. However, the drug has been shown to be especially useful in severe hypertension secondary to renal parenchymal disease [30]. It may be contraindicated in patients with pheochromocytoma, in whom it may stimulate secretion of catecholamines.

The starting dose of minoxidil is 0.1−0.2 mg/kg per dose [30] or up to 5−10 mg for an adult. The dose can be increased by 50−100% until optimum blood pressure control is achieved. When chronic therapy is anticipated the dose, given once or twice per day, should be raised every 1−3 days. A β-blocking agent and diuretic should always be used in conjunction with minoxidil to diminish stimulation of the sympathetic nervous system and sodium and water retention. Congestive heart failure can be a serious problem in some patients, particularly those with renal disease and pre-existing cardiac dilatation. Aggressive diuretic therapy and occasionally even hemodialysis may be necessary to control volume overload.

In patients hospitalized for acute hypertensive control, minoxidil, in combination with diuretic and β-adrenergic blocking agents, has been shown to effect a rapid smooth decrease in blood pressure over several hours in adults. In children, with chronic hypertension secondary to renal disease, we have found that a single oral dose of 0.2 mg/kg of minoxidil lowered systolic and diastolic blood pressure to ≤95% for age within 4 h in 8 of 11 patients. Currently the most common use for minoxidil in our center is for acute control of severe hypertension in patients with chronic hypertension, such as the children mentioned above. With the advent of newer antihypertensive agents it is rare indeed for children to be treated chronically for hypertension with minoxidil.

ADVERSE EFFECTS AND IMPORTANT INTERACTIONS

The most common side-effects associated with chronic use of minoxidil are hypertrichosis, sympathetic overactivity (increased heart rate, increased stroke volume), and elevation of plasma renin activity resulting in fluid and salt retention. The increased sympathetic activity, fluid, and sodium retention can usually be alleviated by simultaneous administration of β-adrenergic blocking agents and diuretics. Hypertrichosis is an unpleasant side-effect, especially in women and children, and occurs in virtually all patients. Hair growth, most prominent on the forehead, trunk, and upper arms, usually appears during the first 3−4 weeks of therapy. It is not permanent and disappears 2−4 months after stopping minoxidil [29,30]. Pericardial effusion has also been seen in patients treated with minoxidil but this is usually in association with predisposing factors such as uremia, collagen vascular disease, cardiac failure, or infections [31]. Rebound hypertension following rapid withdrawal of minoxidil has been reported in a few patients [32].

Minoxidil can be used in conjuction with most

antihypertensive agents. However, administration of Minoxidil with α-adrenergic blocking agents (phenoxybenzamine and guanethidine), β-adrenergic blocking agents or clonidine has been associated with postural hypotension. Long-acting drugs, such as guanethidine, are best stopped several days prior to initiating therapy with minoxidil.

PARENTERAL VASODILATORS

Hydralazine

Parenteral hydralazine, while not as effective as diazoxide or nitroprusside, still has an important place in the treatment of hypertension. We use this agent most often to control mild-to-moderate hypertension in the patient unable to use an oral drug. A child with established hypertension who must temporarily discontinue oral medications for surgery, for example, can often be treated safely and effectively with intravenous hydralazine. The dose must be titrated to the child's response; 0.15 mg/kg per dose is a reasonable starting amount, but intravenous dosages as high as 3.7 mg/kg per day can be used. The intravenous route is preferred over intramuscular administration.

Diazoxide

PHARMACOLOGY

Diazoxide is an agent with strong structural similarity to the thiazide diuretics, although it has no diuretic properties. The drug is a powerful arteriolar dilator, with minimal effects on the venous system. Administration of this agent produces marked decreases in peripheral vascular resistance and systemic blood pressure. Reflex increases in heart rate and cardiac output occur, as with all vasodilators, but these changes are not of sufficient magnitude to blunt the drug's hypotensive effects [33].

Diazoxide is strongly protein-bound, with about 90% of the drug in serum bound to albumin. Since the agent appears to be excreted predominantly through the kidneys, this protein-binding results in one of the longest half-lives (20−30 h) of any antihypertensive drug. The therapeutic effectiveness of diazoxide, however, appears to be a function of the immediate binding of free drug to vascular muscle. Thus, there is no close correlation between serum diazoxide concentrations and antihypertensive effect. Furthermore, although decreased clearance may cause drug levels to be higher in patients with renal insufficiency, these patients rarely require dosage modification [8,33].

CLINICAL USE

Although oral diazoxide is reported to have some antihypertensive effect, the drug's clinical usefulness is restricted to the parenteral therapy of severe hypertension and hypertensive encephalopathy. Experience with the use of this drug in children goes back at least to 1966 [34], and the first extensive report of its pediatric use was published in 1971 [35]. The agent has a long reputation for safety, and can be considered the drug of choice for hypertensive crises in children in whom pheochromocytoma is either excluded or considered unlikely.

Because of the protein-binding of diazoxide, it is often suggested that the drug should be given by very rapid (30 s or less) bolus injection into a high-flow peripheral vein. Dosages of 3−5 mg/kg (maximum 300 mg) are usually recommended for such bolus therapy [36]. For several years, however, it has been recognized that slow infusion of diazoxide is an equally effective mode of therapy [37,38]. More importantly, such an approach to using the drug may obviate the profound hypotension that sometimes complicates treatment with a bolus of diazoxide. This consideration is especially important in patients who have already received other antihypertensive drugs and who are thus at greater risk for diazoxide "overshoot." "Minibolus" injections of drug have also been recommended, but we see no advantage to this approach over slow infusion [39].

An appropriate infusion rate for diazoxide is 0.25 mg/kg per min, with a maximum total dose of 5 mg/kg or 300 mg over 20 min. Blood pressure should be monitored continuously during this infusion, and administration of the drug may be discontinued when the target pressure is reached. Occasional patients who do not respond to the initial infusion may benefit from an additional 20 min (5 mg/kg) of therapy, but failure to obtain acceptable blood pressure control after this is an indication to begin nitroprusside.

The duration of effect of diazoxide is variable, but control for 12 or more hours is common. Repeat infusions may be given as necessary to maintain acceptable blood pressure. Diazoxide produces avid renal sodium retention, and concurrent administration of a diuretic is mandatory unless renal function is severely compromised.

ADVERSE EFFECTS AND IMPORTANT INTERACTIONS

In large studies, diazoxide has been remarkably free of major adverse effects when used for the treatment of childhood hypertension [35,36]. Profound hypotension occasionally develops, but this appears most often in patients who have already received antihypertensive drugs (especially other vasodilators) [40]. Slow infusion therapy may prevent the occurrence of this problem.

Evidence of impaired organ perfusion (especially myocardial and cerebral) has been seen in some adults treated with diazoxide. In some cases, this has resulted in myocardial ischemia and infarction [41]. These complications are unlikely to occur in children who have a more normal myocardium and vascular bed.

Diazoxide interferes with pancreatic insulin release, an effect which has led to its use in some hypoglycemic states. Hyperglycemia may develop in patients receiving diazoxide for hypertension, but this rarely presents a management problem. None the less, monitoring of blood sugar in patients receiving the drug over several days is prudent, as nonketotic hyperglycemic coma has developed on occasion [42]. Patients with underlying defects in carbohydrate tolerance are more at risk for diazoxide hyperglycemia. We have recognized elevated blood sugars most often in children receiving the drug in the immediate postrenal transplant period, where the stresses of chronic renal failure and pharmacologic dosages of corticosteroids and β-blocking agents are operative. Patients continuing to require diazoxide in these circumstances may need concurrent insulin therapy.

Like the related thiazide diuretics, diazoxide can inhibit tubular uric acid excretion. This is rarely a problem in children. Hypersensitivity reactions (fever, rash, thrombocytopenia) are also rare; individuals with hypersensitivity to thiazides will usually display similar reactions with diazoxide. Reduction in dosage of coumadin anticoagulants may be needed because of displacement of bound drug from serum proteins by diazoxide [33].

Nitroprusside

PHARMACOLOGY

Sodium nitroprusside is pharmacologically related to the organic nitrates such as amyl nitrate and nitroglycerin, whose hemodynamic properties have been recognized since the middle of the 19th century. The drug is a primary relaxor of vascular smooth muscle, with negligible effects on nonvascular smooth muscle. Nearly equivalent dilatation of both the arteriolar and venous circulation is achieved with this agent. This results in reduction of both cardiac pre- and after-load, a combination of properties not shared with the other parenteral vasodilators [43].

The antihypertensive usefulness of this drug is exclusively achieved by continuous infusion. The onset of action is within minutes, and therapeutic effect is lost almost as rapidly upon interruption of the infusion.

The sodium nitroprusside molecule is rapidly broken down *in vivo*. This breakdown releases 5 cyanide ions and a nitroso group; the latter is most probably responsible for the drug's antihypertensive effects [2]. Cyanide ions undergo conversion to thiocyanate, a process dependent both upon the enzyme rhodanase and upon availability of thiosulfate or other sulfur-containing substrates [44]. Thiocyanate is considerably less toxic than cyanide, and is excreted in the urine.

CLINICAL USE

Although published experience with nitroprusside in children is scant [45–48], it is the drug of choice in hypertensive crises unresponsive to diazoxide, or when the latter drug is contraindicated. In particular, the drug might be selected for the initial therapy of severe hypertension in a child with cardiac insufficiency that might benefit from the preload reduction that nitroprusside, in contrast to diazoxide, provides.

Because of the dramatic changes in blood pressure that this drug can cause, it must be given in the controlled environment of an intensive care unit. Capability for the continuous monitoring of blood pressure must be available, which usually means the use of an indwelling arterial catheter. Administration of nitroprusside must be carefully controlled by an infusion pump. Nitroprusside may be given via a central or peripheral vein, but in either case it is advisable to have additional venous access available to avoid any interruption of the infusion if the original access becomes compromised. Nitroprusside undergoes a photodegradation, and the diluted drug must be protected from ambient light by an opaque cover such as a paper bag or aluminum foil.

Infusion of nitroprusside is usually begun at a rate of 0.5 µg/kg per min, with increases of 0.5–1.0 µg/kg per min made at 10-min intervals until acceptable blood pressures are achieved. Infusion rates of 2–3 µg/kg per min are usually effective, but the dose can be increased to 10 µg/kg per min if necessary [48]. Higher infusion rates are associated with a greater likelihood of toxicity, and nitroprusside should be discontinued or another drug added if an infusion rate of 10 µg/kg per min does not prove adequate.

Using the example of a 10-kg child in whom nitroprusside is to be begun, the contents of one vial of Nipride (50 mg sodium nitroprusside) are diluted in 500 ml of 5% dextrose solution. This results in a solution containing 0.1 mg (or 100 µg) per ml. An initial infusion rate of 0.5 µg/ml per min would thus be achieved at a flow rate of 0.05 ml/min (3 ml/h). This could be raised in 0.05–0.1 ml/min (3–6 ml/h) increments to a maximum of 1 ml/min (60 ml/h). If such a high infusion rate is required, then dilution of sodium nitroprusside in a smaller volume of 5% dextrose would be advisable.

There are reports of children receiving nitroprusside infusions for as long as a month, although the need for such prolonged use is now most unusual [46,47]. As soon as the patient is able to take oral antihypertensive drugs, they should be begun and the infusion of nitroprusside decreased accordingly.

ADVERSE EFFECTS AND IMPORTANT INTERACTIONS

The major acute complications of the use of nitroprusside in hypertension are associated with overtreatment and hypotension. Beginning the infusion at a slow rate and increasing it judiciously will usually prevent this problem. Hypotension generally responds quickly to discontinuation of the infusion; pressors are rarely necessary.

Patients whose hypertension is associated with volume depletion may display a complex hemodynamic picture after nitroprusside infusion, associated with a severe drop in cardiac output in the face of normotension. Hemodynamic monitoring and careful volume replacement are necessary under these conditions [49].

Abrupt discontinuation of nitroprusside occasionally precipitates acute pulmonary edema. This presumably results from the autotransfusion effect of a decrease in venous capacitance. When it occurs, reinitiation of nitroprusside is necessary.

Problems related to cyanide release from nitroprusside are a major cause for concern in the use of this agent. Thiocyanate, the product of hepatic detoxification of cyanide, is potentially toxic. Thiocyanate toxicity begins with anorexia, fatigue, and nausea, progressing to such major central nervous system manifestations as psychosis and coma [43]. Toxicity is related to concentrations of thiocyanate in blood, with symptoms beginning at 5–10 mg/dl and fatalities reported at 20 mg/dl. Thiocyanate serum concentrations, thus, should be kept under 10 mg/dl. Because thiocyanate is excreted by the kidneys, blood levels may approach toxicity in patients with renal insufficiency. Hemodialysis has been reported to permit continued nitroprusside administration with safe thiocyanate blood levels [47]. We have also used peritoneal dialysis successfully.

Impaired thiocyanate production may lead to accumulation of cyanide in patients receiving nitroprusside. This may occur with hepatic insufficiency (because of deficient rhodanase activity) [50] or with thiosulfate substrate unavailability [44] (as with chronic malnutrition). Some reports suggest that even otherwise normal subjects may accumulate potentially harmful amounts of cyanide with nitroprusside infusions in the range of 2–3 µg/kg per min [44]. Obviously, following thiocyanate levels will not suffice in the identification of this problem. Patients requiring more than 3 days of therapy, especially with doses over 3–5 µg/kg per min, must have cyanide levels followed closely. A metabolic acidosis may be the earliest sign of cyanide toxicity and, if otherwise unexplained, should lead to discontinuation of the drug until cyanide blood levels can be obtained.

REFERENCES

1 Franciosa JA, Cohn JW. Hemodynamic responsiveness to short- and long-acting vasodilators in left ventricular failure. *Am J Med* 1978;65:126–33.
2 Kreye VAW. Direct vasodilators with unknown modes of action: the nitro-compounds and hydralazine. *J Cardiovasc Pharmacol* 1984;6:S646–55.
3 Lipe S, Moulds RFW. *In vitro* differences between human

arteries and veins in their responses to hydralazine. *J Pharmacol Exp Ther* 1980;217:204−17.

4 Koch-Weser J. Hydralazine. *N Engl J Med* 1976;295:320−3.

5 Ludden TM, Shepherd AMM, McNay JL, Lin M-S. Hydralazine kinetics in hypertensive patients after intravenous administration. *Clin Pharmacol Ther* 1980;28:736−42.

6 Shepherd AMM, McNay JL, Ludden TM, Lin M-S, Musgrave GE. Plasma concentration and acetylator phenotype determine response to oral hydralazine. *Hypertension* 1981;3:580−5.

7 Wulff K, Lenz K, Krogsgaard AR, Holst B. Hydralazine in arterial hypertension. *Acta Med Scand* 1980;208:49−54.

8 Bennett WM, Aronoff GR, Morrison G *et al*. Drug prescribing in renal failure: dosing guidelines for adults. *Am J Kidney Dis* 1983;3:155−93.

9 Steens JD, Binstok G, Mullane JF *et al*. Propranolol−hydralazine combination in essential hypertension. *Clin Ther* 1983;5:525−39.

10 Batchelor JR, Welsh KI, Tinoco RM *et al*. Hydralazine-induced systemic lupus erythematosus: influence of HLA-DR and sex on susceptibility. *Lancet* 1980;i:1107−9.

11 Russell GI, Swart S, Bing RF, Thurston H, Swales JD. Combined prazosin and hydralazine in resistant hypertension. *Lancet* 1980;i:543.

12 McLean AJ, Skews H, Bobik A, Dudley FJ. Interaction between oral propranolol and hydralazine. *Clin Pharmacol Ther* 1980;27:726−32.

13 Stanaszek WF, Kellerman D, Brogden RN, Romankiewicz JA. Prazosin update: a review of its pharmacological properties and therapeutic use in hypertension. *Drugs* 1983;25:339−84.

14 Baughman RA, Arnold S, Benet LZ. Altered prazosin pharmacokinetics in congestive heart failure. *Eur J Clin Pharmacol* 1980;17:425−8.

15 Rubin P, Blaschke T. Prazosin protein binding in health and disease. *Br J Clin Pharmacol* 1980;9:177−82.

16 Graham RM, Oates HF, Stoker LM, Stokes GM. α blocking action of the antihypertensive agent, prazosin. *J Pharmacol Exp Ther* 1977;201:747−52.

17 Cavero I, Lefevre F. Cardiovascular effects of prazosin in spontaneously hypertensive rats (SHR). *Clin Exp Pharmacol Physiol* 1977;4(suppl 3):61−4.

18 Oates HF, Graham RM, Stoker LM, Stokes GS. Haemodynamic effects of prazosin. *Arch Int Pharmacodyn Ther* 1976;224:239−47.

19 Davey MJ. Aspects of the pharmacology of prazosin. *Med J Aust* 1980;2(suppl):4−8.

20 Graham RM, Pettinger WA. Prazosin. *N Engl J Med* 1979;300:232−5.

21 Larochelle P, DuSouich P, Hamet P, Larocque P, Armstrong J. Prazosin plasma concentration and blood pressure reduction. *Hypertension* 1982;4:93−101.

22 Stokes GS, Graham RM, Gain JM, Davis PR. Influence of dosage and dietary sodium on the first-dose effects of prazosin. *Br Med J* 1977;1:1507−15.

23 Rosendorff C. Prazosin: severe side effects are dose-dependent. *Br Med J* 1976;2:508.

24 DuCharmi DW, Fryburger WA, Graham BE, Carlson RG. Pharmacologic properties of minoxidil: a new hypotensive agent. *J Pharmacol Exp Ther* 1973; 184:662−70.

25 Lowenthal DT, Affrime MB. Pharmacology and pharmacokinetics of minoxidil. *J Cardiovasc Pharmacol* 1980;2(suppl 2):S93−106.

26 Gottlieb TB, Katz FH, Chidsey CA. Combined therapy with vasodilator drugs and β-adrenergic blockage in hypertension. A comparative study of minoxidil and hydralazine. *Circulation* 1972;45:571.

27 Campese VM. Minoxidil: a review of its pharmacological properties and therapeutic use. *Drugs* 1981;22:257−78.

28 Rudd P, Blaschke TF. Antihypertensive agents and the drug therapy of hypertension. In: Gilman AG, Goodman LS, Rall TW, Murad F, eds. *Goodman and Gilmans The Pharmacological Basis of Therapeutics*. New York: Macmillan, 1985:784−805.

29 Sinaiko AR, Mirkin BL. Management of severe childhood hypertension with minoxidil: a controlled clinical study. *J Pediatr* 1977;91:138−42.

30 Pennisi AJ, Takahashi M, Bernstein BH *et al*. Minoxidil therapy in children with severe hypertension. *J Pediatr* 1977;90:813−19.

31 Martin WB, Spodick DH, Zins GR. Pericardial disorder occurring during open-label study of 1869 severely hypertensive patients treated with minoxidil. *J Cardiovasc Pharmacol* 1980;2(suppl):S217−27.

32 Makker SP, Moorthy B. Rebound hypertension following minoxidil withdrawal. *J Pediatr* 1980;96:762−6.

33 Koch-Weser J. Diazoxide. *N Engl J Med* 1976;294:1271−4.

34 Dunea G, Gantt CL. Diazoxide in hypertensive crisis. *Lancet* 1966;i:638.

35 McLaine PN, Drummond KN. Intravenous diazoxide for severe hypertension in childhood. *J Pediatr* 1971;79:829−32.

36 McCrory WW, Kohaut EC, Lewy JE, Lieberman E, Travis LB. Safety of intravenous diazoxide in children with severe hypertension. *Clin Pediatr* 1979;18:661−71.

37 Garrett BN, Kaplan NM. Efficacy of slow infusion of diazoxide in the treatment of severe hypertension without organ hypoperfusion. *Am Heart J* 1982;103:390−4.

38 Huysmans FTM, Thien T, Koene RA. Acute treatment of hypertension with slow infusion of diazoxide. *Arch Intern Med* 1983;143:882−4.

39 McNair A, Andreasen F, Nielsen PE. Antihypertensive effect of diazoxide given intravenously in small repeated doses. *Eur J Clin Pharmacol* 1983;24:151−6.

40 Davey M, Moodley J, Soutter P. Adverse effects of a combination of diazoxide and hydralazine therapy. *South Afr Med J* 1981;59:496−7.

41 Kumar GK, Dastoor FC, Robayo JR, Razzaque MA. Side effects of diazoxide. *JAMA* 1976;3:275−6.

42 Charles MA, Danforth E. Nonketotic hyperglycemia and coma during intravenous diazoxide therapy in uremia. *Diabetes* 1971;20:501−7.

43 Palmer RF, Lasseter KC. Sodium nitroprusside. *N Engl J Med* 1975;292:294−7.

44 Pasch T, Schulz V, Hoppelshauser G. Nitroprusside-induced formation of cyanide and its detoxication with thiosulfate during deliberate hypotension. *J Cardiovasc Pharmacol* 1983;5:77−85.

45 Elberg AJ, Gorman HM, Baker R, Strauss J. Use of sodium nitroprusside during kidney biopsy in a 9-year-old boy. *Clin Nephrol* 1980;14:104−5.

46 Luderer JR, Hayer HH, Dubynsky O, Berlin CM. Long term

administration of sodium nitroprusside in childhood. *J Pediatr* 1977;91:490—1.

47 Elberg AJ, Gorman HM, Baker R, Wenger AJ, Strauss J. Prolonged nitroprusside and intermittent hemodialysis as therapy for intractable hypertension. *Am J Dis Child* 1978;132:988—9.

48 Gordillo-Paniagua G, Valosquez-Jones L, Martini R, Valdez-Bolanos E. Sodium nitroprusside treatment of severe arterial hypertension in children. *J Pediatr* 1975;87:799—802.

49 Domenighetti G, Perret C. Variable hemodynamic response to sodium nitroprusside in hypertensive crisis. *Intensive Care Med* 1982;8:187—91.

50 Kim YH, Foo M, Terry RD. Cyanide encephalopathy following therapy with sodium nitroprusside. *Arch Pathol Lab Med* 1982;106:392—3.

15 Calcium Channel Antagonists and ACE Inhibitors

GARY R. LERNER AND ALAN B. GRUSKIN

CALCIUM CHANNEL ANTAGONISTS

Role of calcium in smooth muscle contraction

Intracellular calcium binds to a protein, calmodulin. This complex then activates a number of enzymes. One of these is myosin light chain kinase (MLCK) which causes phosphorylation of the 20 000 Da light chain of myosin and activates magnesium adenosine triphosphatase (MgATPase) which in turn activates actin. Unless myosin is phosphorylated there will not be any muscle contraction, since unphosphorylated myosin is unable to be activated by actin [1]. However it has been shown that the MgATPase activity of unphosphorylated myosin can be activated by actin if the actin concentration is high enough [2].

Although initiation of muscle contraction requires phosphorylation of MLCK, other factors are involved in maintaining tension [3,4]. Caldesmon is bound to thin filaments in smooth muscle and is a calmodulin-binding protein. This binding to actin which inhibits MgATPase activity *in vitro* can be reversed by the presence of calcium and calmodulin. The calcium-calmodulin complex can cause caldesmon dissociation and relieve the inhibition [5]. Others have not shown that this reversal is dependent upon caldesmon dissociation [6]. Another mechanism for modulating smooth muscle contraction involves the direct binding of calcium to myosin which leads to a further increase in the activity of actin-activated MgATPase activity [7].

Smooth muscle relaxation has been correlated with dephosphorylation of the 20 000 Da light chain myosin [8]. Another factor controlling MLCK activity is a cyclic adenosine monophosphate (cAMP)-dependent kinase. Two moles of phosphate are incorporated into the enzyme when calmodulin is not present. This decreases the ability of MLCK to bind and be activated by calmodulin, and reduces the ability of smooth muscle to contract [9]. Decreases in intracellular Ca^{++}, possibly mediated by increases in cAMP, can cause smooth muscle relaxation [10].

In vitro evidence supports a role for protein kinase C in muscle relaxation. This calcium-dependent enzyme, which is activated by phospholipid, can phosphorylate a number of substrates including smooth muscle myosin and platelet myosin [11]. It incorporates 1 mol of phosphate into the 20 000 Da light chain at a site different from that used by MLCK [12]. Contrary to the actions of MLCK, protein kinase C decreases actin-activated MgATPase activity of myosin if myosin has been previously phosphorylated and activated by MLCK [13]. This leads to a lowered affinity of actin for myosin. Protein kinase C can also phosphorylate myosin in the absence of MLCK and can therefore decrease the affinity of myosin for MLCK. Both actions of protein kinase C lead to a down-regulation of actin-activated MgATPase and a down-regulation of contractile activity [9] (Fig. 15.1).

How does this calcium-mediated system relate to patients with hypertension? The concentration of intracellular calcium is a principal determinant of the contractile state of the muscle cell. Intracellular calcium levels are increased by a number of cellular processes including mobilization of cellular stores and increased permeability of the cell membrane. The permeability changes are secondary to opening of specific channels within the membrane. Channel opening can be induced by changes in membrane potential, by binding of neurohumoral mediators to receptors, or by binding to receptors followed by membrane depolarization. Cellular stores of calcium can be mobilized by neurohumoral mediators [14].

Cytoplasmic levels of calcium decrease when pumps such as sodium—potassium (Na^+-K^+)-ATPase, calcium (Ca)-ATPase, or Na^+,Ca^{++} exchange systems are activated. This process is also accelerated by

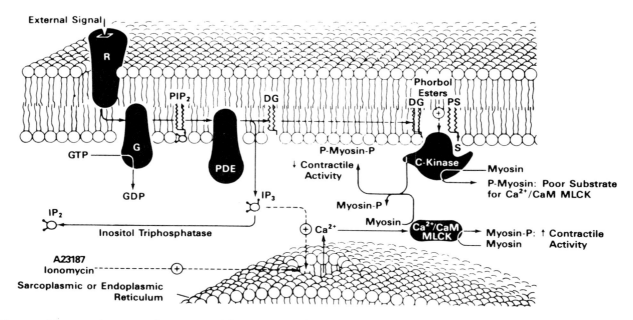

Fig. 15.1 Schematic diagram to illustrate two different myosin phosphorylation pathways activated by calcium in smooth muscle and nonmuscle cells. For protein kinase C (C-kinase) activation the external signal binds to a receptor (R), which interacts with G protein to activate phosphatidylinositol 4,5-biphosphate (PIP_2) phosphodiesterase (PDE). PIP_2 is hydrolyzed to inositol triphosphate (IP_3) and diacylglycerol (DG). Inositol triphosphate can release calcium from the sarcoplasmic reticulum of smooth muscle cells or the endoplasmic reticulum of nonmuscle cells. In these circumstances calcium can activate a number of kinases including myosin light chain kinase. Calcium activates protein kinase C using phosphatidyl serine (PS) as a cofactor. This phosphorylation occurs at a different amino acid residue in the 20 000 Da light chain of myosin (see text). From [9], with permission.

production of cAMP, and/or the hyperpolarization of the membrane [15,16] (Fig. 15.2).

The vascular response to norepinephrine and the activation of calcium transport into the cell varies among vascular smooth muscles. Consequently, the response of certain groups of vessels to calcium channel blockade varies in their ability to inhibit sympathetic induced contraction [17]. Calcium entry blocking agents can also inhibit constriction of arteries induced by substances such as serotonin and prostaglandin $F2_\alpha$. Inhibition of cyclooxygenase leads to a greater entry of calcium and vascular constriction.

In summary, a rise in intracellular calcium predisposes the smooth muscle cell to contract. Some report that dietary supplements of calcium lower blood pressure [18,19]. The pathophysiology has not been fully elucidated. One scheme proposes that in patients with elevated blood pressure intracellular calcium can be increased in association with a low serum ionized calcium, a high parathyroid hormone (PTH), and an increased urinary calcium excretion [20,21]. The elevated PTH causes an increase in intracellular calcium and increases blood pressure. In such cases calcium supplementation would raise serum

calcium, decrease PTH secretion, and lower blood pressure. Clinical trials with calcium supplementation have not been conclusive; however, a significant fall in blood pressure has been observed in patients with decreased ionized calcium and increased PTH compared to other hypertensive individuals whose levels of calcium and PTH were not so altered [22,23].

Clinical applications of calcium channel blocking agents

CLASSIFICATION (Table 15.1; Fig. 15.3)

Calcium channel blocking agents are compounds that alter the cellular function of calcium in three ways: first, they inhibit its entry; second, they inhibit its release; and third, they interfere with one of its intracellular actions [24]. Calcium channel entry blocking agents include drugs that specifically inhibit calcium entry into the cells secondary to tissue excitation. This inhibition of calcium entry is due to the interaction of the drug with the calcium channels which would have been activated either by mem-

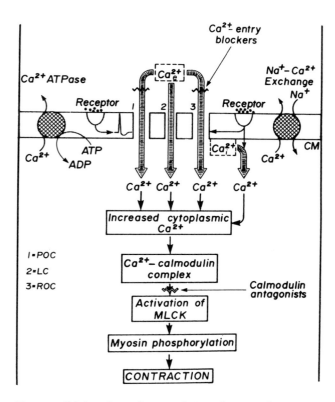

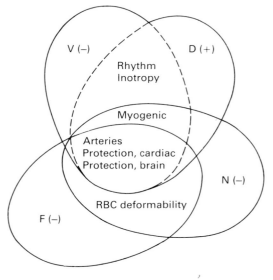

Fig. 15.3 Differentiation of specific calcium entry blockers on the basis of functional criteria and of binding data.
V = verapamil-like; D = diltiazem-like; N = nifedipine-like; F = flunarizine-like. (+) and (−) refer to stimulation and inhibition of (^{3}H)-dihydropyridine binding, respectively. Rhythm and inotropy refer to cardiac effects as observed *in vivo*, which are more pronounced with verapamil and diltiazem than with nifedipine. From [24], with permission.

Fig. 15.2 Calcium-dependent regulation of contractile activity in vascular smooth muscle. Cytoplasmic calcium (Ca^{2+}) levels are increased by calcium influx through cell membrane (CM) potential-operated calcium channels (1 = POC), passive calcium "leak" pathway (2 = LC; calcium entry that occurs under resting conditions), and receptor-operated calcium channels (3 = ROC). Receptor occupation by a specific agonist (closed circles) may also induce release of calcium from intracellular storage sites or may depolarize cell membrane and activate potential-operated channel. Calcium activates myosin light chain kinase (MLCK) by binding to calmodulin. Activated MLCK catalyzes phosphorylation of myosin, which increases actin−myosin interactions, resulting in contraction. Cytoplasmic calcium levels are reduced through operation of cell membrane pumps, including Ca^{2+}-ATPase (far left) and Na^{+}/Ca^{2+} countertransport (far right), that promote calcium efflux. Closed wavy lines, inhibited by calcium-entry blockers; open wavy lines, inhibited by hydrophobic compounds including pimozide and trifluoperazine. From [14], with permission.

brane depolarization or receptor stimulation. Blockade of the "slow" channels is achieved by drugs such as nifedipine, verapamil, and diltiazem. These drugs represent three subclasses of calcium blocking agents: dihydropyridines, phenylalkylamines, and benzothiazepines, respectively. They are representative of the calcium channel blocking agents used to treat

hypertension. Each class has varying potencies and side-effects.

PHARMACOKINETICS

The calcium channel blocking agents mentioned in this chapter are metabolized by the liver. The metabolites formed after hepatic metabolism are inactive [25]. The dihydropyridines—nifedipine, nitrendipine, and nicardipine—even though chemically similar, have different pharmacokinetic properties [26]. Nifedipine has the lowest volume of distribution of the group. It also has the highest plasma levels in relation to the dose, and thus the highest bioavailability: 40−60% (the ratio of the amount of drug available at sites of action after an oral dose compared to that available after an intravenous dose). Nifedipine, which is 90% protein-bound, has a mean half-life of 2.5 ± 2.4 h ranging from 2.5 to 3.4 ± 10.4 h after parenteral administration [27]. After an oral dose absorption was fast and the maximum plasma concentration was noted as early as 0.33−0.52 h.

Verapamil has a similar half-life after a single oral or intravenous dose: 3.5 versus 3.7 h and 4.5 versus 4.8 h in two studies [28,29]. Elimination is solely by

Table 15.1 Calcium modulators: agents affecting Ca^{2+} movements (calcium antagonists)

Agents acting at the plasma membrane
Calcium entry blockers
   Group I: Selective calcium entry blockers
          Group IA: Agents selective for slow calcium
                 channels in myocardium (slow
                 channel blockers)
            Phenylalkylamines: verapamil, gallopamil (D600)
            Dihydropyridines: nifedipine, nicardipine,
            niludipine, nimodipine, nisoldipine,
            nitrendipine, ryosidine
            Benzothiazepines: diltiazem; fostedil (KB-944)
   Group II: Nonselective calcium entry blockers
          Group IIA: Agents acting at similar concentrations
                 on calcium channels and fast sodium
                 channels
            Bencyclane, bepridil, caroverine,
            etafenone, fendiline, lidoflazine,
            perhexiline, prenylamine, SKF 525A,
            terodiline, tiapamil
          Group IIB: Agents interacting with calcium
                 channels while having another
                 primary site of action
            They include, among others, agents acting on:
            1 sodium channels (local anesthetics, phenytoin);
            2 catecholamine receptors (benextramine,
              nicergoline, phenoxybenzamine,
              phenothiazines, pimozide, propranolol,
              WB-4101, yohimbine derivatives);
            3 benzodiazepine receptors (diazepam,
              flurazepam);
            4 opiate receptors (loperamide,
              fluperamide);
            5 cyclic nucleotide phosphodiesterases
              (amrinone, cromoglycate, papaverine).
            Barbiturates
            Cyproheptadine
            Indomethacin
            Reserpine
Sodium−calcium exchange inhibitors
   Amiloride and derivatives

Agents acting within the cell
Acting on sarcoplasmic reticulum
   Dantrolene, TMB-8
Acting on mitochondria
   Ruthenlum red
Calmodulin antagonists
   Phenothiazines: trifluoperazine, chlorpromazine
   Naphthalene derivatives: W7
   Local anesthestics: dibucaine
   Dopamine antagonists: pimozide, haloperidol
   Calmidazolium (R24571)

From [24], with permission.

liver metabolism, utilizing the cytochrome P450 system [30]. Its metabolites lack activity except for the N-demethylated compound which exhibits 20% of the activity of the parent drug. There is extensive first-pass elimination such that the oral bioavailability is only 20% [27]. Because of the high first-pass extraction, plasma concentrations after an oral dose can vary by as much as 10-fold in different subjects [27].

Diltiazem is metabolized via deacetylation in the liver and undergoes enterohepatic recirculation. Bioavailability increases after long-term oral administration from 38 to 90%.

SYSTEMIC EFFECTS

Vasodilatation is the primary antihypertensive action of the calcium channel blocking agents. Nifedipine has the greatest vasodilating effect of the three; vasodilatation is progressively less with verapamil and ditiazem (Table 15.2). In isolated human vessels there is a concentration-dependent vascular relaxation of sympathetically constricted arteries and veins [32]. Nifedipine administration, in addition to lowering blood pressure, causes an increase in heart rate and cardiac contractility secondary to β-adrenergic stimulation [33]. Verapamil also has a vasodilatory effect on the peripheral resistance vessels, but does not cause the reflex tachycardia or increase in cardiac output seen with nifedipine [32]. This blunting of the sympathetic response to vasodilatation is due to the direct negative inotropic and chronotropic effects of the drug. Diltiazem also does not produce a change in heart rate and cardiac output in response to peripheral dilatation [34]. The effects and side-effects of these drugs are a continuum, with those giving the most vasodilatation also causing the most headaches, tachycardia, and flushing. Those drugs, such as verapamil and diltiazem, which have less vasodilation but more negative inotropy, cause more conduction disturbances as side-effects (Table 15.3).

Nifedipine has been used singly in hypertensive emergencies; it has been used alone or in combination with other antihypertensive drugs for chronic therapy. In a group of adults given nifedipine alone (10 mg four times/day orally) and subsequently followed by the addition of methyldopa (250 mg four times/day orally), blood pressure decreased from an average of 210/126 to 170/101 mgHg on nifedipine alone and to 145/87 mmHg during combination therapy [36]. During combination therapy the heart rate was noted to be reduced significantly and cardiac index increased slightly when compared to single

Table 15.2 Pharmacologic effects of calcium antagonists

	Vascular smooth muscle tone	Formation and conduction of cardiac electric impulses	Inotropic state
Nifedipine	↓ ↓ ↓	o/ ↓	o/ ↓
Verapamil	↓	↓ ↓	↓ ↓
Diltiazem	↓	↓ ↓	↓

From [31], with permission.

Table 15.3 Ranking of adverse effects of calcium antagonists

Adverse effect	Ranking
Vasodilatation	N > D > V
Negative inotropic effects	V > D > N
Conduction disturbances	V > D > N
Gastrointestinal effects	V > D > N
Impaired glucose tolerance	N > V > D
Interaction with cardiac glycosides	V > N > D
Interaction with β-blockers	V > N > D

N = nifedipine; D = diltiazem; V = verapamil.
From [35], with permission.

therapy with nifedipine. Thus the use of methyldopa can ameliorate the reflex tachycardia noted with the use of nifedipine as well as potentiating its antihypertensive effect. Aoki and coworkers [37] in a study of 24 hypertensive adults investigated the combination of nifedipine and propranolol: the addition of the β-blocker potentiated the antihypertensive effect of nifedipine, prolonged its effect, and suppressed nifedipine-induced tachycardia and other nifedipine-induced side-effects. This effect of β-blocking agents has been confirmed by others [38].

When nifedipine and captopril are used together an additive effect on the fall in blood pressure occurs [39]. The vasodilatory effects of these two drugs are achieved by different mechanisms and can thus augment the other's effect on the fall in blood pressure. Nifedipine induces a sympathetic response which can increase the secretion of renin and the production of angiotensin II; captopril blocks the conversion of angiotensin I to angiotensin II. When captopril was given to patients receiving nifedipine, the heart rate, which had increased significantly in response to nifedipine use alone, returned to baseline. This is brought about by the decrease in symp-

athetic nervous system activity due to the decreased production of angiotensin II [39,40]. The mean arterial pressure decreased an additional 8.9% [39].

Both nitrendipine and nicardipine are similar in their properties to nifedipine, with the advantage that they are both longer-acting. However a new sustained-release preparation of nifedipine is now available.

OTHER EFFECTS OF CALCIUM CHANNEL BLOCKING AGENTS

Cardiac conduction

The major nonvascular effects of the calcium channel blocking agents are those affecting cardiac conduction. Both verapamil and diltiazem have greater effects than nifedipine on the cardiac conduction system (Table 15.2). The major clinical use for verapamil has been to treat conduction abnormalities such as paroxysmal supraventricular tachycardia, atrial fibrillation, and flutter [41]. Because of its negative effect on contractility, it has also been used to treat hypertrophic obstructive cardiomyopathy [42]. Contraindications to using verapamil in the young include sick sinus syndrome; severe congestive heart failure not caused by supraventricular tachycardia; second- or third-degree heart block; severe hypotension or cardiogenic shock, and concurrent therapy with β-adrenergic antagonists [41].

Central nervous system effects

There are reports of the use of some calcium channel antagonists in the treatment of seizures. Nifedipine, verapamil, and diltiazem are not amongst the drugs used for this purpose since they are not selective for the central nervous system [43,44]. Calcium channel blocking agents such as lidoflazine and nimodipine have been used to treat seizures. They affect the central nervous system without causing systemic hypotension or negative inotropic effects. By increasing cerebral blood flow nifedipine may reduce serious central nervous system sequelae, such as seizures, secondary to acute hypoxia that may occur after a sudden reduction in blood pressure [45].

Renal function

In adults with essential hypertension treated for 4 weeks with only nifedipine, significant increases in glomerular filtration rate and effective renal plasma flow occurred independently of any changes in blood pressure [46]. Others have described a nifedipine-related diuresis and natriuresis [47,48].

Miscellaneous

The calcium channel blocking agents have been found to have neither a favorable nor an unfavorable effect upon plasma lipid levels [49]. While black patients have been shown to have a limited response to antihypertensive agents such as β-blockers and possibly angiotensin converting enzyme (ACE) inhibitors, calcium blocking agents do appear to be effective in black adults [49].

Side/adverse effects

The side-effects observed when using calcium channel blocking agents, in addition to their primary action as vasodilators, are related to other effects such as negative inotropism, conduction disturbances, gastrointestinal disturbances, metabolic effects, and drug interactions [35] (Tables 15.3 and 15.4). Because the indications as well as the expected pharmacologic effects of individual drugs differ, the incidence of adverse effects varies from report to report and drug to drug. Reactions related to vasodilatation are most common with nifedipine (headache, flushing, tachycardia, dizziness). The headache and flushing appear to be dose-related and are also related to the rate of absorption [31]. The adverse reactions caused by vasodilatation appear to decrease in severity with continued treatment and respond to a decrease in dose [50]. There are few data that directly compare the adverse effects of these three calcium channel blocking agents in patients with essential hypertension [35]. Much of the data compiled for nifedipine has been in patients treated for coronary insufficiency. Nitrendipine, another dihydropyridine, has been studied in patients with essential hypertension and elicited the same adverse effects as nifedipine.

Reactions related to a negative inotropic effect are more common with the use of verapamil, since for the same degree of vasodilatation the negative inotropic effect is greatest for verapamil, less for diltiazem, and least for nifedipine [51] (Table 15.3). When used in patients with compromised left ventricular function, dyspnea and heart failure were more frequently reported with verapamil [52]. Adverse reactions related to conduction disturbances such as third-degree arteriovenous block are seen more frequently with verapamil than diltiazem. Nifedipine has not been reported to cause cardiac arrhythmias in therapeutic doses [31]. The most common side-effect of verapamil is constipation, with the incidence exceeding 30% [53].

NIFEDIPINE

This agent is discussed in detail because of its utility in the management of severe hypertension and because it is the agent which has been in longest use in the treatment of hypertension. Most studies aimed at evaluating nifedipine as an antihypertensive agent have been done in adults. All have shown efficacy in the treatment of hypertensive crises. Nifedipine is also effective for long-term therapy. In a study of 27 hypertensive patients, a single oral dose of 10 mg reduced the mean arterial blood pressure by 21% [36]. After an additional 3 weeks of therapy with a dose of 10 mg every 6 h, the mean reduction in blood pressure was similar to that following the initial dose [54]. When given for 12 weeks to 22 hypertensive patients, a progressive decrease was found in supine

Table 15.4 Adverse reactions related to vasodilatation induced by calcium antagonists

	Nifedipine	Verapamil	Diltiazem
Flushing	+ +	+	+
Headache	+ +	+	+
Hypotensive reactions	+	+	+
Ankle edema	+ +	+	+
Symptomatic tachycardia (adrenergic-mediated)	+ +	+	+
Precordalgia (?)	+	+	+

From [31], with permission. + = Medium reaction, + + = severe reaction.

and standing blood pressures without any effect on heart rate [55]. When nifedipine was given for 12 months, no deterioration in blood pressure control occurred [56].

The usefulness of nifedipine in hypertensive emergencies has been dramatic. When given sublingually, its onset of action occurs within 1–5 min. Sublingual administration produces a more rapid fall in blood pressure than that observed following an oral dose (onset <20 min) [38]. After a 10 mg sublingual dose of nifedipine was given to 30 patients whose mean systolic and diastolic blood pressure was 224/125 mmHg, a fall in blood pressure occurred within 5 min and a peak effect was seen in 30–60 min [57]. At 60 min the diastolic blood pressure had decreased to less than 110 mmHg in 93% of patients and to less than 100 mmHg in 67%. Those individuals receiving 20 mg had an even greater decline in their blood pressure. Farine and Arbus observed that nifedipine administered in children by biting then swallowing the capsule has a quick onset of action and has peak levels higher than those observed for sublingual use [58].

In another study, oral nifedipine was given to 25 adult patients with a mean blood pressure greater than 130 mmHg [59]. Blood pressure fell from 221/126 (±22/14) to 152/89 (±20/12) mmHg after 30 min (p<0.001). An effect was first observed after 10 min and a peak effect after 30–40 min. The study also evaluated cerebral blood flow and found that it increased after nifedipine and decreased after clonidine. The fall in blood pressure is directly related to the severity of the initial pretreatment systolic and diastolic blood pressures. Available data indicate no or minimal effect on blood pressure-lowering in normotensive people. Hypotension after therapy in hypertensive patients is rarely observed [38,54, 59,60]. Toxic ingestions of calcium channel blocking agents, however, have been associated with severe hypotension.

Pediatric use

Data on the use of nifedipine in hypertensive emergencies for the pediatric population are available (see also Chapter 31). A single dose of 0.25–0.5 mg/kg was given sublingually to 21 children, age 8–16 years, whose pretreatment blood pressure was 183/137 (±19/21) mmHg [61]. Within 30 min blood pressure fell to 132/98 (±21/17) mmHg (p<0.001). The maximal decrease in blood pressure was observed

30 min after the dose, with the duration of action being 6 h [blood pressure 134/100 (±14/15) mmHg].

Similar to the adult experience, there was a significant increase in heart rate from 108 to 117 beats/min (p<0.01). Another study reported the successful use of a single sublingual dose of nifedipine in 16 children, aged 6 weeks to 14 years, in treating 20 episodes of hypertensive crisis, defined as a sudden increase in systolic and/or diastolic pressure, exceeding the age-dependent 95th percentiles by at least 20 mmHg [62]. The dose ranged from 0.05 to 0.86 (mean 0.33) mg/kg. Within 90 min of administration of nifedipine, systolic blood pressure fell a mean of 29% (initial 182 mmHg) and diastolic blood pressure fell a mean of 27% (initial 111 mmHg). The drug had its onset of action within 10–20 min; its peak action was noted in 60–90 min and the duration of action was between 4 and 12 h. A positive correlation was noted between the percentage decrease in blood pressure and the initial systolic blood pressure. After nifedipine, blood pressure was not satisfactorily lowered in an additional 4 patients who were markedly volume-expanded.

In another study, nifedipine was given sublingually (median dose 0.37 mg/kg) to 12 infants and children (median age 0.1–17 years) for acute hypertension, defined as a blood pressure more than 20% above the 95th percentile for age [63]. Within 1 h the blood pressure fell to normal levels for age. Others have also reported and recommended the use of sublingual and/or oral nifedipine in both hypertensive emergencies and long-term treatment of moderate-to-severe hypertension in children [64,65]. For emergencies, a dose of 0.3–0.5 mg/kg can be repeated as often as every 30–60 min; up to 1 mg/kg per day in divided doses, every 4–6 h, can be used for chronic therapy.

ANGIOTENSIN CONVERTING ENZYME INHIBITORS

Physiology

Renin was first noted to have a hypertensive effect in 1898 when Tigerstadt and Bergmann [66] showed that an extract of rabbit kidney raised blood pressure. It is secreted from the juxtaglomerular cells of the afferent renal arteriole, which are in contact with the macula densa from the distal tubule of the same nephron. The position of these specialized vascular-like cells (juxtaglomerular) places them near structures that carry and transmit different signals for the release of renin. These structures include the baroreceptor mechanism, macula densa, and sympathetic nervous system. Serum potassium, and other hormonal inputs are also involved.

The renin—angiotensin—aldosterone system participates in three homeostatic systems: volume status, blood pressure control, and electrolyte balance. A reduction in systemic blood pressure increases renin release by the juxtaglomerular cells by decreasing stretch and transmural tension. This mechanism accounts for renin release in response to either systemic hypotension or local hypotension within the kidney, as occurs with renal artery narrowing. The other components of the renin—angiotensin—aldosterone system are then triggered to maintain volume and blood pressure. Angiotensin II(AII), which is generated from angiotensin I (AI) by angiotensin converting enzyme (ACE), then causes vasoconstriction as well as release by the adrenal gland of aldosterone. Aldosterone increases the renal tubular reabsorption of sodium, thereby increasing intravascular volume.

Because of the anatomic position of the macula densa it plays a role in signaling for renin release based on compositional changes in the distal tubular fluid. Studies have shown that an increased delivery of sodium chloride to the distal tubule increases renin release [67,68]. It has also been shown that renin release and increased plasma renin activity are stimulated by decreased sodium chloride delivery and inhibited in situations such as volume overload, which increases the distal delivery of sodium chloride [69—71].

The sympathetic nervous system directly innervates components of the juxtaglomerular apparatus [72]. Renin release is stimulated via the β-adrenergic system, while α-adrenergic stimulation is associated with a decrease in renin secretion. Because of the direct effect of the β-adrenergic system upon renin release, β-blockade has been used alone and more recently in combination with ACE inhibition to treat hypertension. The sympathetic nervous system is not absolutely required for renin secretion to be accomplished, as evidenced in the case of renal transplantation. Its effect on renin secretion can be separated from the baroreceptor and macula densa mechanisms. Sympathetic stimulation is involved in renin release in response to such conditions as exercise, stress, and upright posture [73—76].

Prostaglandins such as prostacyclin and prosta-

glandin E_2 have a direct effect on renin release from the juxtaglomerular cells [77]. They are not required for release secondary to renal nerve stimulation or baroreceptor stimulation. Prostaglandins, however, are necessary for renin release associated with renal hypoperfusion in the autoregulatory range and for renin release related to changes in macula densa activity [78,79]. Nonsteroidal anti-inflammatory drugs (NSAIDS] are able partially to suppress renin release [80,81]. The mechanism is related to the decreased production of vasodilatory prostaglandins (prostacyclin and prostaglandin E_2).

Other stimuli, such as an increased intracellular concentration of calcium in juxtaglomerular cells, have an inhibitory effect on renin release [82] while increased levels of intracellular cAMP can cause an elevation in renin secretion [83] (Table 15.5).

RENIN—ANGIOTENSIN SYSTEM, PROSTAGLANDINS AND BRADYKININ

Renin is a proteolytic enzyme which cleaves AI from renin substrate (angiotensinogen). Because of the large amounts of circulating ACE, AI undergoes rapid conversion to the octapeptide AII. The half-life of AII is brief—approximately one circulation time [84].

The response to AII by sensitive cells requires the presence of calcium in the surrounding medium and can be blocked by calcium channel blocking agents [85,86]. Cytosolic calcium, which increases after the cell's stimulation by AII, may be the second messenger mediating the response to AII [87,88]. Angiotensin II also releases arachidonic acid from cell membranes, leading to the formation of prostaglandin E_2 and prostacyclin [89,90]. These prostaglandins antagonize the vasoconstrictive actions of AII on glomerular capillaries. Angiotensin II decreases glomerular plasma flow and the ultrafiltration coefficient (Kf) [91] but preserves single nephron glomerular filtration rate by increasing transcapillary pressure and increasing the production of vasodilatory prostaglandins. In clinical conditions such as congestive heart failure, liver disease, and hypovolemia there are increased levels of renin, AII, and prostaglandin synthesis. NSAIDS given in these circumstances cause a noticeable decrease in glomerular filtration rate and renal plasma flow. If captopril is then given glomerular filtration rate and renal plasma flow are restored. Under conditions where AII, catecholamines, and vasopressin are increased, renal hemodynamics become prostaglandin-dependent,

Table 15.5 Factors influencing renal renin release

	Stimulatory	Inhibitory
Baroreceptor mechanism	↓ Juxtaglomerular cell stretch	
Sympathetic control	β-Adrenoceptor agonists	β-Adrenoceptor antagonists β-Adrenoceptor agonists
Macula densa	↑ Loop NaCl transport Prostaglandins	
Prostaglandins	Prostaglandin E_2 Prostacyclin	Nonsteroidal anti-inflammatory agents
Hormones	Histamine, glucagon Parathyroid hormone	Angiotensin II Vasopressin
Extracellular ions	↓ $[Ca^{++}]$	↑ $[K^+]$, ↑ $[Ca^{++}]$
Other factors	Kallikrein	

From [71], with permission.

and prostaglandin inhibition potentiates the constrictive effects of these agents [91].

Other vasodilating agents are indirectly involved in the balance exhibited in counteracting the vasoconstrictive actions of AII. Bradykinin, a product of the kallikrein—kinin system, is degraded to inactive compounds by kininase II, which is ACE (Fig. 15.4). Thus the vasodilatory effect of ACE inhibitors is due to the decreased degradation of bradykinin as well as the decreased production of AII. Bradykinin also stimulates the production of prostaglandin E_2 and prostacyclin [93]. The precise role of this kallikrein—kinin system remains controversial because changes in the blood levels of these compounds do not occur and because the physiologic effects of bradykinin occur at the tissue level [92].

ACTIONS OF ANGIOTENSIN II

Angiotensin II has a number of physiologic effects. It is a powerful vasoconstrictor of arterioles. It increases peripheral vascular resistance, especially in the hypovolemic state. There are regional differences in vascular responsiveness to AII; the renal vasculature is the most responsive [71,94]. The renal effects of AII include efferent arteriolar vasoconstriction greater than afferent; increased tubular sodium reabsorption, especially at the proximal tubule; glomerular mesangial constriction resulting in a decrease in ultrafiltration coefficient (Kf), and a negative feedback for renin release [95]. Nonrenal effects of AII include stimulation of the secretion of antidiuretic hormone,

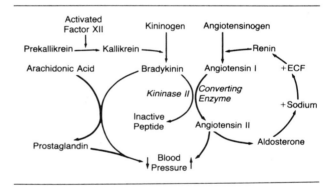

Fig. 15.4 The relation of the renin—angiotensin—aldosterone system to bradykinin and prostaglandin production. These interactions may occur in the circulation but are more likely to occur in tissue, except for the effect of angiotensin II on aldosterone secretion (see text). ECF = extracellular fluid. From [92], with permission.

mineralocorticoids, and catecholamines; increased myocardial contraction at both atrial and ventricular levels; increased thirst; inhibition of the vagus nerve; release of neurotransmitters in the central nervous system; catecholamine release from peripheral sympathetic nerves, and reduced salt and water absorption from the gut [71,95].

In summary, the ultimate effect of AII production is to maintain blood pressure and circulating volume. This is accomplished by the many aforementioned mechanisms which result in the adjustment of vascular resistance and renal sodium excretion.

ANGIOTENSIN CONVERTING ENZYME

Angiotensin converting enzyme, which is found in high concentrations in the vascular endothelium of the lungs [96], is also found in the kidney and brain [97−99]. In the kidney the enzyme has been identified in afferent arterioles, glomeruli, and proximal tubules and provides support for a localized renal action of ACE and AII [100,101]. The enzyme has a molecular weight of 130 000−160 000 Da [102]. Because ACE cleaves dipeptides from a variety of substrates, it is a nonspecific carboxypeptidase [95,103]. The enzyme contains zinc which is involved in the steric configuration of the substrate−enzyme-binding site and permits cleavage of dipeptides from the carboxyterminal end [104,105]. The first available synthetic ACE inhibitor, captopril, has a sulfhydryl group near the carboxyterminal end. The sulfhydryl group acts as a zinc ligand and is the presumed mechanism for its inhibitory effect [106]. Enalapril, a newer ACE inhibitor, contains a carboxyl group that functions as a zinc ligand [107].

Class action

The class contains drugs that differ in ligand binding to ACE's zinc (sulfhydryl for captopril; carboxyl for enalapril and lisinopril; phosphinic acid for fosinopril; Table 15.6). Additionally various ACE inhibitors differ in the form in which they are given, i.e. active versus prodrug. The prodrugs—enalapril was the first described—which are converted by the liver to the active form have an increased duration of action because it takes longer for their blood levels to peak [108,109].

The ACE inhibitors lower peripheral vascular resistance without significantly changing heart rate or cardiac output [108,110]. Explanations for the lack of reflex tachycardia include a down-regulation in baroreceptor reflex sensitivity [111], venodilation caused by ACE inhibition, and parasympathetic modification [112]. While it would be expected that patients with high plasma renin activity should respond with a more dramatic fall in blood pressure, such a correlation is not always noted [113]. This observation provides support for the theory that nonrenin-mediated mechanisms are also involved in the blood pressure reduction caused by ACE inhibitors. The duration of the hypotensive effect after ACE inhibitor administration is longer than can be explained by ACE inhibition alone. The fall in diastolic pressure is greater than the systolic fall. The drugs also increase

Table 15.6 Classification of angiotensin converting enzyme inhibitors

Natural
Peptides
   Snake (e.g. teprotide, $BPP_{5\alpha}$)
   Human (e.g. [des-pro³] bradykinin, enkephalins, substance P etc.)
   Microbial (e.g. muracein, ancovenin, talopectin)
Nonpeptides (e.g. bicyclic lactams, phenacein)

Synthetic
Peptides (e.g. val-trp, phe-ala-pro)
Peptide analogs (di- or tripeptide, etc.)
   Sulfur as zinc ligand (e.g. captopril, alacepril)
   Carboxyl as zinc ligand (e.g. enalapril, ramipril, lisinopril, cilazapril*)
   Phosphinyl as zinc ligand (e.g. fosinopril)
Peptide surrogates (tri- or pentapeptides, etc.) (ester or ketomethyl, $-COSCH_2-$, etc.), as substitutes for peptide bond [-CONH-]

* Conformationally restricted.
From [95], with permission.

blood flow to the kidneys, brain, and heart [114,115]. The increase in renal blood flow, which is accomplished without a change in glomerular filtration rate, is due to the preferential dilation of efferent as opposed to afferent glomerular arterioles [113]. The drugs do not promote retention of salt and water as seen with other vasodilators. This is due in part to decreases in aldosterone production and the natriuretic effect related to an increased renal blood flow [116]. Clinically significant potassium retention does not occur unless renal insufficiency is present or potassium-sparing diuretics or potassium supplements are also being ingested. Due to the inhibition of AII production by ACE inhibitors, there is a decreased activity of the sympathetic nervous system and other systems whose hormonal release is partly dependent upon the action of AII [40].

Regression of left ventricular hypertrophy in hypertensive patients whose blood pressure was controlled with ACE inhibitors has been observed [117]. It is not yet clear whether this is due to the effect of a lowered blood pressure (although drugs such as hydralazine and minoxidil do not elicit such a response) or to the effect on a local-tissue renin−angiotensin system which has been identified in the myocardium [118].

In summary, ACE inhibitors elicit a fall in blood pressure secondary to decreased peripheral vasoconstriction. Additionally, they cause an increase in cardiac output [113,119], an increase in regional blood flow to the kidneys, brain, and coronary arteries, and an increased excretion of sodium and fluid with some retention of potassium. Also, decreases in pre-existing proteinuria in parenchymal renal diseases and diabetes mellitus have been described. This observation has been attributed to changes in intra-renal hemodynamics and the preservation of glome-rular filtration rate [120−122].

Captopril

The onset of action of captopril is within 15 to 30 min and its peak action is noted at 1−2 h after ingestion (Table 15.7). Its duration of action is dose-dependent (<6 h at 6.25 mg and up to 12 h for 75 mg in adults). In order to achieve maximum absorption it is rec-ommended that the drug be taken 1 h before or 2 h after meals [108,110]. It was originally suggested that ACE inhibitors should be used only when other therapy failed or if patients experienced unacceptable side-effects from their antihypertensive regimen [110]. Also, their use was reserved for patients thought to have renin-mediated hypertension. Currently, ACE inhibitors are recommended as first-step therapy in adults with essential hypertension, much like diuretics and β-blocking agents [123] and even as the preferred drug for hypertension control because of their salutary effect on quality of life [124]. A review of the literature reveals that 35−70% of adults with essential hypertension had a good re-sponse (diastolic blood pressure <90 mmHg) when ACE inhibitors were used as monotherapy [93]. When used in combination with a diuretic an additional 20−25% had their blood pressure normalized. In another review, 50−60% of hypertensive subjects did not respond to monotherapy with ACE inhibitors [113].

Black adult patients with essential hypertension show a smaller response to ACE inhibitors, partly due to the lower plasma renin levels found in this race. The racial difference in response to ACE in-hibitors is abolished if diuretics are added to the therapeutic regimen [125]. The combination of ACE inhibitors with calcium channel blocking agents is more effective than administering ACE inhibitors together with nonspecific vasodilators such as hydrala-zine, or with β-blocking agents [93,113].

Besides hypertension, another indication for capto-pril is its use to treat congestive heart failure [126,127]. There are varying reports of its efficacy in children

Table 15.7 Pharmacologic effects of single doses of converting enzyme inhibitors*

Agent	Prodrug	Time of onset (min)		Time of peak effect (h)		Duration of effect (h)			Metabolism	Elimination	Dose (mg)
		Presence detected in blood	BP levels affected	Presence detected in blood	BP levels affected	Presence detected in blood	Biologic systems affected	BP levels affected			
Captopril	No	5−10	15−30	0.5−1.5	1−2	4−5	5−10	6−10	Extensive metabolism to disulfides	Mainly in urine; $\frac{1}{3}$ unchanged; 95% within 24 h	100
Enalapril	Yes	60	60−120	3−4	4−8	48−72	18−48	18−30	None after enalaprilat formed; 60% conversion rate	60−75% in urine within 72 h	20
Lisinopril	No	60	60	6−10	2−4	48−96	24−48	18−30	None	30% in urine after 24 h; 70% in feces	10

* The duration of the therapeutic effect is dependent on the dose as well as the half-life.
BP = Blood pressure.
Adapted from [92].

with this condition [128,129].

Patients with a solitary kidney, such as a renal transplant, with a stenotic artery, may experience decreases in renal function after receiving ACE inhibitors [130]. The mechanism for the decreased renal function is thought to be related to the increased efferent arteriolar dilatation in addition to the state of maximal afferent dilatation induced by the response to the stenosis. This results in decreased glomerular filtration pressure, decreased filtration fraction, and a decrease in glomerular filtration rate [131]. In patients with hypertension without renal artery stenosis, the use of captopril may increase renal blood flow and glomerular filtration rate [132]. Angiotensin converting enzyme inhibitors should not be used for chronic therapy when hypertension is secondary to bilateral renal artery stenosis or unilateral stenosis in a solitary kidney (see Chapter 22).

In adults, an initial starting dose of 25 mg twice a day, increasing at 2−4-week intervals to a maximum of 150 mg/day is recommended [92]. It has been recommended that dosage changes should be done gradually, as slowly as every 4−6 weeks; this slower course, as well as using much lower total daily doses than were initially employed, can help contribute to a lower incidence of adverse or side-effects [92,133,134]. Even though the onset of action of captopril is relatively fast, it is felt that there are long-term effects on blood pressure, occurring over weeks. Drug dosing needs to be adjusted for renal insufficiency and renal failure. If the creatinine clearance is less than 30 ml/min, the initial dose should be reduced by 50−70% [92]. This is consistent with data obtained in children [135]. Captopril clearance fell by 50% (14−18 versus 27 ml/min per kg) in a pediatric patient whose glomerular filtration rate decreased from 59 to 10−21 ml/min per 1.73 m². In children other than newborn infants the recommended initial dose of captopril is 0.3 mg/kg up to a daily dose of 5−6 mg/kg in divided doses [64,136,137]. The lowest effective dose should be continued and adjusted in accordance with changes in blood pressure [137].

PEDIATRIC USES

An early report of the use of ACE inhibitors involved a 10-year-old 31 kg hypertensive boy who was refractory to standard antihypertensive therapy including sodium nitroprusside [138]. He was suffering from hypertensive encephalopathy and was treated with captopril. The child responded to an oral dose of

12.5 mg, with a drop in blood pressure from 160/130 to 140/105 mmHg 30 min after administration. The patient experienced a continued fall in blood pressure to 130/90 mmHg by day 2, a gradual rise by day 5 to 150/104 mmHg, and a further decline to 130/85 mmHg by day 10 after incrementally increasing the dose of captopril to 223 mg/day in four divided doses. The "triphasic" response following the administration of captopril has been reported in adults and children and should be sought [138−140]. Careful titration of the dose is indicated until a steady blood pressure is attained. This dose titration should be individualized for each patient and should be done over several weeks in patients whose hypertension is nonemergent in order to reduce significant adverse effects. In 9 patients, age 6−18 years, treated with captopril for a variety of underlying causes for hypertension, all responded to therapy with their blood pressure either controlled by captopril alone or by captopril and other drugs whose dose had been significantly reduced [140,141]. The protocol was such that the final dose of captopril did not exceed 2 mg/kg per dose, every 8 h.

The hypertension associated with coarctation of the aorta is responsive to captopril therapy. Coarctation may present with hypertension, heart failure, and elevated plasma renin activity. In a 2-day-old child with coarctation, an improved ejection fraction (32 to 45%) and lowered blood pressure (170/80−90 to 110/70 mmHg) were observed after captopril 0.3 mg/kg per dose T.I.D. [128]. Higher doses may be required in older patients (see below). Postcoarctectomy hypertension can often be severe and is responsive to captopril with or without β-blockade [128].

While many of the initial experiences with captopril therapy in hypertensive children reported good short-term success, the data obtained by an international collaborative study group showed that good long-term control of blood pressure also occurred with captopril [137]. The report summarized the experience of using captopril to treat hypertension for 3−12 months in 73 children aged 15 years or younger. The etiologies for hypertension included: renal parenchymal disease (19), renal vascular disease (16), hemolytic−uremic syndrome (13), renal transplant (13), vasculitis syndromes (6), essential, malignant, or "renin-induced" hypertension (5), and hypertension following repair of coarctation and ventricular septal defect (1). In 63 subjects, baseline systolic and diastolic blood pressure were greater than the 95th percentile; in 7 only the diastolic blood pressure was elevated, and 2 showed elevation of systolic blood pressure alone. Systolic blood pressure was normalized in 62 and 53%, and diastolic blood pressure in 56 and 45%, after the second and sixth months of therapy. For both systolic and diastolic pressures, approximately 75% of patients experienced either a normalization of blood pressure (<95th percentile) or partial response (blood pressure decreased by at least 10% from baseline, but not to normal levels). The antihypertensive response was relatively constant over the 12-month period but a smaller percentage of patients had their blood pressure normalized during the first month than during succeeding months (systolic: 42 versus 53−62%; diastolic: 34 versus 45−56%). No difference in long-term response was noted in the children with high compared to low initial pretreatment levels of plasma renin activity. Others have confirmed this observation in long-term response [115,142], although the initial blood pressure response correlated to the pretreatment level of plasma renin activity [143].

The combination of increased monitoring of blood pressure in the Neonatal Intensive Care Unit and the development of normal blood pressure data for newborn infants of all gestational ages has resulted in hypertension—particularly severe hypertension—being recognized more frequently. The use of umbilical arterial lines is one of the major causes for renovascular hypertension in the newborn infant (144). Elevated plasma renin activity would be expected and ACE inhibitors are a good choice to treat this problem.

Newborn infants may be more sensitive to captopril than older children and adults [145]. Satisfactory blood pressure control was accomplished in hypertensive newborn infants with a lower captopril dose (initial dose 0.01 mg/kg; peak dose 0.85 ± 0.3 mg/kg per day at day 4; subsequent maintenance dose 0.48 ± 0.19 mg/kg per day) than that recommended for older children and adults [146]. A number of studies have confirmed a marked hypotensive response sometimes leading to oliguria and/or acute renal failure in newborn infants treated with initial doses of captopril of 0.3 mg/kg per dose or more [145,146].

Renal parenchymal disease as well as obstructive uropathy can be treated with ACE inhibition in the newborn period. Captopril has been successfully used to treat hypertension (systolic blood pressure >90 mmHg) in sick, hypertensive, hyperreninemic newborn babies undergoing extracorporeal membrane oxygenation therapy. Adequate blood pressure control was accomplished with a dose of 0.3 mg/kg per dose. Blood pressure control was associated with a significant decrease in the incidence of intraventricular hemorrhage compared to that observed in historically untreated infants undergoing extracorporeal membrane oxygenation [147].

Enalapril

Enalapril is an ACE inhibitor that differs from captopril in the form that it is given (prodrug versus active) and by its mechanism of inhibition. Enalapril, as well as other second-generation ACE inhibitors, differs from captopril in that it competes with renin substrate for ACE binding sites, instead of chelating wih the ACE zinc atom [40]. The drug is rapidly absorbed from the gastrointestinal tract whether or not food is present. It is converted by the liver to its active diacid form, enalaprilat. In patients with liver disease, adjustments in dosage need to be made since biotransformation to the active drug is delayed and the duration of action is increased in such patients [148,149]. In people with normal liver function, the onset of action is 1−2 h (compared to 15−30 min for captopril), peak effect is at 4−8 h (1−2 h for captopril), and the duration of action is 18−30 h (6−10 h for captopril; Table 15.7). Because of its longer onset of action, enalapril and other ACE prodrug inhibitors are not suitable for the initial treatment of hypertensive emergencies. Enalaprilat is excreted by the kidney by tubular secretion, without further modification [150,151].

Except for differences in the onset and duration of action, the ACE inhibitors currently available for clinical use have similar effects on blood pressure. Enalapril at a dose of 2.5−30 mg/day was reported to control hypertension in 15 pediatric patients (ages 6 weeks to 18.5 years) with underlying renal lesions. In this study the drug was substituted for captopril as follows: 1 mg enalapril for each 7−10 mg captopril, and 20 mg propranolol, respectively. All children experienced good control of blood pressure after 5 to more than 12 months of treatment. At the end of the follow-up period, 6 were on lower doses of enalapril, 6 were on the same dose, and 1 was on a higher dose than that initially given during the study. Treatment was able to be discontinued in 2. The 4 patients who were on other antihypertensive drugs in addition to captopril were able to be maintained on enalapril alone [152].

Recommended doses for enalapril in children and adults, range from 2.5 to 40 mg/day, given either once or twice daily [92,113,152,153]. To prevent hypotension, the lower dose is recommended for patients already taking diuretics since they already have a stimulated renin−angiotensin system. As with captopril, a lower dose is needed in patients with renal failure (glomerular filtration rate <30 ml/min).

Side/adverse effects of captopril and enalapril
(Table 15.8)

Adverse effects of ACE inhibitors can be divided into those related to the class of drug or to individual drugs within the class. The more important side-effects include hypotension, renal dysfunction, coughing, and angioedema. Hypotension can occur with any ACE inhibitor, and tends to occur at the time of peak onset of action of the drug (2 h with captopril; 4−6 h with enalapril) [154]. The effect is dose-related, seen more often as a first-dose effect, and is exaggerated by the use of diuretics, low-sodium diets, and high pretreatment plasma renin activity [92, 154]. It is also seen more frequently with the shorter-acting captopril than with the slower-onset, longer-acting enalapril which produces a more gradual decrease but also a more protracted hypotension [40].

Renal insufficiency occurs with ACE inhibitors, especially in patients suffering from bilateral renal vascular disease or in patients with a solitary kidney with renal artery stenosis (see above). In 9 premature, hypertensive infants treated with captopril, 17 episodes of a decrease in systolic blood pressure of more than 40% from baseline occurred. These hypotensive episodes were unpredictable in their onset and occurred 1−54 days after the initiation of therapy. In 4 infants there were 7 episodes of severe decreases in blood pressure (57 $\pm$ 10%), sustained for 17 $\pm$ 6 h and accompanied by oliguria (<1 ml/kg per h) for 18 $\pm$ 12 h. The hypotension was unresponsive to volume expansion and inotropic therapy. Changes in neurologic status occurred within 18 $\pm$ 6 h of the onset of oliguria. When the duration of decrease in blood pressure was only 2.8 $\pm$ 2 h, there were no significant renal or central nervous system abnormalities noted, except for one seizure in 1 infant immediately after captopril administration. It is possible that the renal autoregulatory mechanism may have been reset due to chronic hypertension or renovascular disease.

Table 15.8 Class-specific side-effects of angiotensin converting enzyme inhibitors

---

Hypotension — especially first dose in patients who are sodium-depleted or who have been previously treated with diuretics or who have congestive heart failure and borderline hypotension; also appears in severe renovascular hypertension
Reversible elevation of blood urea nitrogen or creatinine
Acute renal failure in renal artery stenosis or severe congestive heart failure
Hyperkalemia with potassium supplements, or potassium-sparing diuretics
Cough
Angioedema

From [113], with permission.

The initial doses used were 0.3 mg/kg, which were later decreased to 0.15 mg/kg, in line with other recommendations for neonatal dosing [137,146]. Even though the lower blood pressure values were still within the normal range for age, oliguria developed, suggesting that a decrease in renal perfusion had occurred. When the blood pressure was restored, renal function returned to normal, even while captopril was continued. These data indicate that close monitoring of renal function must be done when patients, especially newborn infants, undergo therapy with ACE inhibitors.

Hyperkalemia should be an expected side-effect of treatment with ACE inhibitors because of a decreased production of aldosterone. However the adrenal gland can still respond directly to other stimuli by producing aldosterone. Consequently, hyperkalemia only develops in those patients who remain on potassium-sparing diuretics or potassium supplements, have congestive heart failure, or renal failure [40,92,113,154].

Coughing is an increasingly recognized side-effect of ACE inhibitors [40,113]. It is dry in nature, sometimes with a tickling quality. The incidence increases with longer duration of action of the drug [92]. The reported incidence in patients receiving captopril and enalapril is 0.5 and 1.3%, respectively [92]. Incidences as high as 10−15% have been reported in adult patients [155].

Angioedema, which is a rare effect, can lead to respiratory arrest and death. Its occurrence is usually within the first month of therapy and is more frequent with the longer-acting agents (0.2 versus 0.1%, enalapril versus captopril) [92,156].

The ACE inhibitors have been associated with increased fetal wastage in laboratory animals and are contraindicated in pregnancy [92]. Many of these reports are specific to captopril [157,158]. One report has documented acute renal failure in a newborn infant whose mother had been treated with enalapril 20 mg/day for 17 days prior to delivery [159]. Complete suppression of ACE was found in the infant, while plasma renin activity was increased 8- and 10-fold above values for normal and premature infants, respectively. The AII levels were also suppressed. The active drug, enaprilat, was found in the infant's plasma corresponding to the mother's expected level and was successfully removed by peritoneal dialysis. It is speculated that because renal perfusion pressure is low and the control of glomerular filtration rate appears to depend upon AII levels immediately after birth, the newborn child may be more sensitive to ACE inhibition during postnatal life.

Other side-effects seem to be drug-specific and related to the chemical structure of the drug. Captopril has a mercapto group that appears to contribute to a number of its side-effects. Other drugs that are different pharmacologically but share a mercapto group, such as penicillamine, also share the same side-effects [160]. Allergic rashes occur with both captopril and enalapril, but their incidence is higher in patients receiving captopril (2.5–10 versus 1.3%, captopril versus enalapril [92,155,161,162]. The rash is usually mild, maculopapular, and pruritic, is self-limited, and occurs within the first 3 months of therapy. It appears to be dose-related. Because there does not appear to be significant crossreactivity between captopril and enalapril, a reaction to one does not preclude the use of the other in the same patient [163].

Neutropenia and agranulocytosis are worrisome side-effects of captopril that are usually reversible upon withdrawal of the drug [40]. The reported incidence ranges from 0.02 up to 7.2%, depending upon whether the patient has received a high dose, has renal insufficiency, has collagen vascular disease, and is concurrently receiving immunosuppressive drugs [164]. A lower incidence of blood dyscrasias has been reported with the use of enalapril at the usual daily doses of 5–20 mg, even in patients with renal failure [165].

Taste disturbances are more common with captopril than with enalapril—1–2 versus 0.5%, respectively [92]. They occur within the first 3 months of therapy and are more common in patients with renal insufficiency [110]. Nephrotic syndrome with the appearance of membranous nephropathy on biopsy has been reported with the use of captopril [166,167], while others have failed to observe an increased incidence of this pathologic change in hypertensive individuals treated with captopril [168,169].

REFERENCES

1 Sellers JR. Mechanism of the phosphorylation-dependent regulation of smooth muscle heavy meromysin. *J Biol Chem* 1985;260:15815–19.

2 Wagner PD, Vu N-D. Regulation of the actin-activated ATPase of aorta smooth muscle myosin. *J Biol Chem* 1986;261:7778–83.

3 Aksoy MO, Mras S, Kamm KE, Murphy RA. Calcium, cAMP, and changes in myosin phosphorylation during contraction of smooth muscle. *Am J Physiol* 1983;245:C255–70.

4 Kamm KE, Stull JT. The function of myosin and myosin light chain kinase phosphorylation in smooth muscle. *Annu Rev Pharmacol Toxicol* 1985;25:593–620.

5 Sobue K, Takahashi K, Wakabayashi I. Caldesmon 150 regulates the tropomyosin-enhanced actin-myosin interaction in gizzard smooth muscle. *Biochem Biophys Res Commun* 1985;132:645–51.

6 Lash JA, Sellers JR, Hathaway DR. The effects of caldesmon on smooth muscle octo-HMM ATPase activity and binding of HMM to actin. *J Biol Chem* 1986;261:16155–60.

7 Chacko S, Rosenfeld A. Regulation of actin-activated ATP hydrolysis by arterial myosin. *Proc Natl Acad Sci USA* 1982;79:292–6.

8 Haeberle JR, Hathaway DR, De Paoli-Roach AA. Dephosphorylation of myosin by the catalytic subunit of a type-2 phosphatase produces relaxation of chemically skinned uterine smooth muscle. *J Biol Chem* 1985;260:9965–8.

9 Adelstein RS, Sellers JR. Effects of calcium on vascular smooth muscle contraction. *Am J Cardiol* 1987;59:4B–10B.

10 Jones AW, Bylund DB, Forte LR. cAMP-dependent reduction in membrane fluxes during relaxation of arterial smooth muscle. *Am J Physiol* 1984;246:H306–11.

11 Naka M, Nishikawa M, Adelstein RS, Hidaka H. Phorbol ester-induced activation of human platelets is associated with protein kinase C phosphorylation of myosin light chains. *Nature* 1983;306:490–2.

12 Nishikawa M, Sellers JR, Adelstein RS, Hidaka H. Protein kinase C modulates *in vitro* phosphorylation of the smooth muscle heavy meromysin by myosin light chain kinase. *J Biol Chem* 1984;259:8808–14.

13 Nishikawa M, Hidaka H, Adelstein RS. Phosphorylation of smooth muscle heavy meromysin by calcium-activated, phospholipid-dependent protein kinase. *J Biol Chem* 1983;258:14069–72.

14 Vanhoutte PM. Calcium-entry blockers, vascular smooth muscle, and systemic hypertension. *Am J Cardiol* 1985;55:17B–23B.

15 Bohr DF, Webb RC. Lowering of activator calcium concentration in the relaxation of vascular smooth muscle. In: Vanhoutte PM, Leusen I, eds. *Mechanisms of Vasodilation*. Basel: S. Karger, 1978:37–47.

16 Vanhoutte PM. Differential effects of calcium entry blockers on vascular smooth muscle. In: Weiss GB, ed. *New Perspectives on Calcium Antagonists*. Washington, DC: American Physiological Society, 1981:109−21.

17 Vanhoutte PM. Heterogeneity of postjunctional vascular α adrenoceptors and handling of calcium. *J Cardiovasc Pharmacol* 1982;4:S91−6.

18 McCarron DA, Morris CD, Henry HJ et al. Blood pressure and nutrient intake in the United States. *Science* 1984; 223:1392−7.

19 Sempos C, Cooper R, Kovar MG et al. Dietary calcium and blood pressure in National Health and Nutrition Examination Surveys I and II. *Hypertension* 1986;8:1067−74.

20 Pak CYC. Calcium and hypertension. In: Horan MJ, Blaustein M, Dunbar JB et al. eds. *NIH Workshop on Nutrition and Hypertension: Proceedings from a Symposium*. New York: Biomedical Information, 1985:155−65.

21 McCarron DA. Calcium metabolism and hypertension. *Kidney Int* 1989;35:717−36.

22 McCarron DA, Morris CD. Blood pressure response to oral calcium in persons with mild to moderate hypertension. *Ann Intern Med* 1985;103:828−31.

23 Meese RB, Gonzalez DG, Casparian JM et al. The inconsistent effects of calcium supplements upon blood pressure in primary hypertension. *Am J Med Sci* 1987;294:219−24.

24 Godfraind T. Classification of calcium antagonists. *Am J Cardiol* 1987;59:11B−23B.

25 Raemsch KD, Sommer J. Pharmacokinetics and metabolism of nifedipine. *Hypertension* 1983;5(suppl II):18−24.

26 Raemsch KD, Graefe KH, Scherling D, Sommer J, Ziegler R. Pharmacokinetics and metabolism of calcium-blocking agents nifedipine, nitrendipine, and nimodipine. *Am J Nephrol* 1986;6(suppl I):73080.

27 McAllister RG, Hamann SR, Blovin RA. Pharmacokinetics of calcium-entry blockers. *Am J Cardiol* 1985;55:30B−40B.

28 Eichelbaum M, Somogyi A, von Unruh GE, Dengler HJ. Simultaneous determination of the intravenous and oral pharmacokinetic parameters of D, L-verapamil using stable isotope-labelled verapamil. *Eur J Clin Pharmacol* 1981; 19:133−137.

29 McAllister RG, Kirsten EB. The pharmacology of verapamil. IV. Pharmacokinetics and drug effects after single intravenous and oral doses in normal subjects. *Clin Pharmacol Ther* 1982;31:418−426.

30 Eichelbaum M, Endo M, Remberg G, Schomerus M, Dengler HJ. The metabolism of D, L-14C-verapamil in man. *Drug Metab Dispos* 1979;7:145−8.

31 Ohnmeiss H, Nazzari M. Side effects of calcium antagonists. *Am J Nephrol* 1986;6(suppl 1):81−6.

32 Mikkelsen K, Andersson KE, Pedersen OL. The effect of nifedipine on isolated human peripheral vessels. *Acta Pharmacol Toxicol* 1978;43:291−8.

33 Stone PG, Antman EM, Mueller JE, Braunwald E. Calcium channel blocking agents in the treatment of cardiovascular disorders. II. Hemodynamic effects and clinical applications. *Ann Intern Med* 1980;93:886−904.

34 Bourassa MG, Cote P, Theroux P, Tubau JF, Genain C, Waters DD. Hemodynamics and coronary flow following diltiazem administration in anesthetized dogs and in humans. *Chest* 1980;78:225−7.

35 Russell RP. Side effects of calcium channel blockers. *Hypertension* 1988;11(suppl II):II42−8.

36 Guazzi MD, Fiorentini C, Oliveri MT, Bartorelli A, Necchi G, Polese A. Short and long term efficacy of a calcium antagonist (nifedipine) combined with methyldopa in the treatment of severe hypertension. *Circulation* 1980;61: 913−19.

37 Aoki K, Kondo S, Mochizaki A et al. Antihypertensive effect of a cardiovascular calcium antagonist in hypertensive patients in the absence and presence of β-adrenergic blockade. *Am Heart J* 1978;96:218−26.

38 Frishman WH. Calcium channel blockers in systemic hypertension. *Am J Nephrol* 1987;7(suppl 1):57−66.

39 Pieri R, Nardecchia A, Pirrell A. Combined nifedipine and captopril treatment in moderately severe primary hypertension. *Am J Nephrol* 1986;6(suppl 1):111−14.

40 Gavras H, Gavras I. Angiotensin converting enzyme inhibitors: properties and side effects. *Hypertension* 1988; II (suppl II):II37−41.

41 Cho C, Pruitt AW. Therapeutic uses of calcium channel blocking drugs in the young. *Am J Dis Child* 1986;140: 360−6.

42 Spicer RL, Rocchini AP, Crowley DC et al. Hemodynamic effects of verapamil in children and adolescents with hypertrophic cardiomyopathy. *Circulation* 1983;67:413−19.

43 Waquier A, Fransen J, Clincke G et al. Calcium entry blockers as cerebral protecting agents. In: Godfraind T, ed. *Calcium Entry Blockers and Tissue Protection*. New York: Raven Press, 1985:163−72.

44 Wellens D. Twenty-seven calcium entry blockers in development: a new chapter in pharmacology. In: Godfraind T, ed. *Calcium Entry Blockers in Cardiovascular and Cerebral Dysfunctions*. The Hague: Martinus Nijoff, 1984:25−42.

45 White BC, Winegar CD, Wilson RF et al. Possible role of calcium blockers in cerebral resuscitation: a review of the literature and synthesis for future studies. *Crit Care Med* 1983;11:202−7.

46 Reems GP, Hamery A, Lau A, Bauer JH. Effect of nifedipine on renal function in patients with essential hypertension. *Hypertension* 1988;11:452−6.

47 Luft FC, Aronoff GR, Sloan RS, Fineberg NS, Weinberger MH. Calcium channel blockage with nitrendipine: effects on sodium homeostasis, the renin−angiotensin system, and the sympathetic nervous system in humans. *Hypertension* 1985;7:438−42.

48 MacGregor GA, Pevahouse JB, Cappuccio FP, Markandu ND. Nifedipine, sodium intake, diuretics, and sodium balance. *Am J Nephrol* 1987;7(suppl 1):44−8.

49 Man in't Veld AJ. Calcium antagonists in hypertension. *Am J Med* 1989;86(suppl 4A):6−14.

50 Ekelund LG. Calcium channel blocking drugs for chronic stable angina−nifedipine. *Int J Cardiol* 1982;2:13−17.

51 Abate G, Ficic F, Paddu P, Marmo E. Farmaci bluccanti i cannali del calcio i diltiazem. *Eur Rev Med Pharmacol Sci* 1983;5(suppl 5):5−45.

52 Hutchinson R, Lorimar AR, Lakear A, McAlpine SG. β-blocker and verapamil, a cautionary tale. *Br Med J* 1984; 289:659−60.

53 Lewis JG. Adverse reactions to calcium antagonists. *Drugs* 1983;25:196−222.

54 Murakami M, Murakami E, Takekoshi N et al. Antihypertensive effect of (4-2 nitrophenyl)-2,6-dimethyl-1,4-dihydropyridine-3,5-dicarbonic acid demethlyester (nifedipine, BAY-A 1040), a new coronary vasodilator. J Heart J 1972;13:128−35.

55 Guintolli F, Guidi G, Scalabrino A et al. Nifedipine as single drug therapy in hypertension. Curr Ther Res 1981; 30:447−52.

56 Oliveri MT, Barturelli C, Pulese A, Fiorentini C, Moruzzi P, Guazzi MD. Treatment of hypertension with nifedipine, a calcium antagonistic agent. Circulation 1979;59:1056.

57 Ellrodt AG, Ault M, Riedinger MS, Murata GH. Efficacy of sublingual nifedipine in hypertensive emergencies. Am J Med 1985;79:19−25.

58 Farine M, Arbus GS. Management of hypertensive emergencies in children. Pediatr Emer Care 1989;5:51−5.

59 Bertel O, Conen D, Radu EW, Muller J, Lang C, Dubach UC. Nifedipine in hypertensive emergencies. Br Med J 1983;286:19−21.

60 Guazzi M, Olivari MT, Polese A, Giorentini C, Magrini F, Muruzzi P. Nifedipine, a new antihypertensive with rapid action. Clin Pharmacol Ther 1977;22:528−32.

61 Dilmen U, Caglar MK, Senses A, Kinik E. Nifedipine in hypertensive emergencies of children. Am J Dis Child 1983; 137:1162−5.

62 Roth B, Herkenrath P, Krebber J, Abu-Chaaban M. Nifedipine in hypertensive crises of infants and children. Clin Ex Hyperten Pract 1986;8:871−7.

63 Rascher W, Bonzel KE, Ruder H, Muller-Wiefel DE, Scharer K. Blood pressure and hormonal responses to sublingual nifedipine in acute childhood hypertension. Clin Exp Hyperten Theory Pract 1986;8:859−69.

64 Scharer K. Hypertension in children and adolescents−1986. Pediatr Nephrol 1987;1:50−8.

65 Dillon MJ. Investigation and management of hypertension in children, a personal perspective. Pediatr Nephrol 1987; 1:59−68.

66 Tigerstadt R, Bergmann PG. Nieve und Krieslauf. Scand Arch Physiol 1988;8:233.

67 Thurau K, Mason J. The internal function of the juxtaglomerular apparatus. In: Thurau K, Kidney and Urinary Tract Physiology. London: Butterworth, 1974:357.

68 Thurau K, Gruner A, Mason J, Dahlerm H. Tubular signal for the renin activity in the juxtaglomerular apparatus. Kidney Int 1982;22(suppl 12):555.

69 Vander AJ. Control of renin release. Physiol Rev 1967; 47:359.

70 Brown JJ, Davies DI, Lever AF, Robertson JIS. Influence of sodium loading and sodium depletion on plasma renin in man. Lancet 1963;ii:278.

71 Bellerman BJ, Levenson DJ, Brenner BM. Renin, angiotensin, kinins, prostaglandins, and leukotrienes. In: Brenner BM, Rector FC Jr, eds. The Kidney. Philadelphia: WB Saunders, 1986:281−340.

72 Barajas L. The innervation of the juxtaglomerular apparatus. An electron microscopic study of the innervation of the glomerular arterioles. Lab Invest 1964;13:916.

73 Benelli J, Waldhausl W, Magomettchnigg D, Schwarzmeir J, Korn A, Hitzenberger G. Effect of exercise and of prolonged oral administration of propranolol on hemodynamic variables, plasma renin concentration, plasma aldosterone and cAMP. Eur J Clin Invest 1977;7:337.

74 Dampney R, Stella AL, Golin R, Zanclotti A. Vagal and sinoaortic reflexes in postural control of circulation and renin release. Am J Physiol 1979;237:H146.

75 Michelakis AM, McAllister RG. The effect of chronic adrenergic receptor blockade on plasma renin activity in man. J Clin Endocrinol Metab 1972;34:386.

76 Kaplan NM. The renin−angiotensin system. In: Kaplan NM, ed. Clinical Hypertension. Baltimore: Williams & Wilkins, 1978:178.

77 Data JL, Gerber JG, Crump WJ, Frohlich JG, Hollofield JW, Nies AS. The prostaglandin system. A role in canine baroreceptor control of renin release. Circ Res 1978;42:454.

78 Fremman RH, Davis JO, Villareal R. Role of renal prostaglandins in the control of renin release. Circ Res 1984;54:1.

79 Francesco LL, Osborn JL, DiBona GF. Prostaglandins in renin release during sodium deprivation. Am J Physiol 1982;243:F537.

80 Keeton TK, Campbell WB. The pharmacologic alteration of renin release. Pharmacol Rev 1981;32:81.

81 DeForrest JM, Davis JO, Freeman RH et al. Effects of indomethacin and meclofenemate on renin release and renal hemodynamic function during chronic renal sodium depletion in conscious dogs. Circ Res 1980;47:99.

82 Park CS, Malvin RL. Calcium in the control of renin release. Am J Physiol 1978;235:F22.

83 Stadel JM, DeLean A, Lefkowitz RJ. Molecular mechanisms of coupling in hormone receptor adenylate cyclase systems. Adv Enzymol Relat Areas Mol Biol 1982;53:2.

84 Hodge RL, Ng KKF, Vane JR. Disappearance of angiotensin from the circulation of the dog. Nature 1967;215:138.

85 Ichikawa I, Miele JF, Brenner BF. Reversal of renal cortical actions of angiotensin II by verapamil and manganese. Kidney Int 1979;16:137.

86 Churchill PC. Calcium channel antagonists and renin release. Am J Nephrol 1987;7(suppl 1):32−8.

87 Peach MJ. Molecular actions of angiotensin. Biochem Pharmacol 1981;30:2745.

88 Elliot ME, Alexander RC, Goodfriend TL. Aspects for angiotensin action in the adrenal. Key roles for calcium and phosphotidyl inositol. Hypertension 1982;4(suppl II):1152.

89 Buonassisi V, Venter JC. Hormone and neurotransmitter receptors in an established vascular endothelial cell. Proc Natl Acad Sci (USA) 1976;3:1612.

90 Alexander RW, Gimbrone MA Jr. Stimulation of prostaglandin E synthesis in cultured human umbilical vein smooth muscle cells. Proc Natl Acad Sci (USA) 1976;73:1617.

91 Dunn MJ, Scharschmidt LA. Prostaglandins modulate glomerular actions of angiotensin II. Kidney Int 1987; 31(suppl 20):S95−101.

92 Williams GH. Converting enzyme inhibitors in the treatment of hypertension. N Engl J Med 1988;319:1517−25.

93 McGiff JC, Terragno NA, Malik KU, Lenigro AJ. Release of a prostaglandin E-like substance from canine kidney by bradykinin. Circ Res 1972;31:36−43.

94 Reid IA. Actions of angiotensin II on the brain: mechanism and physiologic role. Am J Physiol 1984; 246:F533−43.

95 Kostis JB. Angiotensin converting enzyme inhibitors. I:

Pharmacology. *Am Heart J* 1988;116(part I):1580−91.

96 Ody C, Junod AF. Converting enzyme activity in endothelial cells from pig pulmonary artery and aorta. *Am J Physiol* 1977;232:C95.

97 Kokobu T, Takada Y. Biochemistry of human converting enzyme. *Clin Exp Hypertens (A)* 1987;A9:217−28.

98 Caldwell PRB, Segal BC, Hsu KC, Das M, Soffer RL. Angiotensin converting enzyme: vascular endothelial localization. *Science* 1976;191:1050.

99 Phillips MI. New evidence for brain angiotensin and for its role in hypertension. *Fed Proc* 1983;42:2667.

100 Ledingham JGG. Overview: physiology I. *Kidney Int* 1987; 31(suppl 20):S49−50.

101 Kriz W. A periarterial pathway for intrarenal distribution of renin. *Kidney Int* 1987;31(suppl 20):S51−6.

102 Lee H-J, Larue JN, Wilson IB. Human plasma converting enzyme. *Arch Biochem Biophys* 1971;142:548.

103 Skidgel RA, Erdos EG. The broad substrate specificity of human angiotensin I converting enzyme. *Clin Exp Hypertens (A)* 1987;9:243−60.

104 Kostis JB, Raia JJ Jr, DeFelice EA, Barone JA, Deeter RG. Comparative clinical pharmacology of ACE inhibitors. In: Kostis JB, DeFelice EA, eds. *Angiotensin Converting Enzyme Inhibitors*. New York: Allan R. Liss, 1987.

105 Shapiro R, Riordan JF. Inhibition of angiotensin converting enzyme: mechanism and substrate dependence. *Biochemistry* 1984;23:5225−33.

106 Ondetti MA, Cushman DW. Enzymes of the renin−angiotensin system and their inhibitors. *Annu Rev Biochem* 1982; 51:283−308.

107 Patchett A, Harris E, Tristram E. A new class of angiotensin-converting enzyme inhibitors. *Nature* 1980;288:280−83.

108 Todd PA, Heel RC. Enalapril: a review of its pharmacodynamic and pharmacokinetic properties, and therapeutic use in hypertension and congestive heart failure. *Drugs* 1986;31:198−248.

109 Brunner HR, Nussberger J, Waeber B. The present molecules of converting enzyme inhibitors. *J Cardiovasc Pharmacol* 1985;7(suppl 1):S2−11.

110 Vidt DG, Bravo EL, Fouad FM. Captopril. *N Engl J Med* 1982;306:214−19.

111 Guidicelli JF, Berdeaux A, Edouard A, Richer C, Jacolot D. The effect of enalapril on baroreceptor mediated reflex function in normotensive subjects. *Br J Clin Pharmacol* 1985;20:211−18.

112 Ajayi AA, Campbell BC, Meredith PA, Kelman AW, Reid JL. The effect of captopril on the reflex control of heart rate: possible mechanisms. *Br J Clin Pharmacol* 1985;20:17−25.

113 Kostis JB. Angiotensin converting enzyme inhibitors. II Clinical use. *Am Heart J* 1988;116(part 1):1591−1605.

114 Zachariah PK, Bonnet G, Chrysant G *et al*. Evaluation of antihypertensive efficacy of lisinopril compared to metaprolol in moderate to severe hypertension. *J Cardiovasc Pharmacol* 1987;9(suppl 3):S53−8.

115 Gavras H, Brunner HR, Turini GA *et al*. Antihypertensive effect of the oral angiotensin-converting enzyme inhibitor SQ 14225 in man. *N Engl J Med* 1978;298:991−5.

116 Hollenberg NK, Meggs LG, Williams GH *et al*. Sodium intake and renal responses to captopril in normal man and essential hypertension. *Kidney Int* 1981;20:240.

117 Dunn FG, Oigman W, Ventura HO, Messerli FH, Koterin I, Frohlich ED. Enalapril improves systemic and renal hemodynamics and allows regression of left ventricular mass in essential hypertension. *Am J Cardiol* 1984;53:105−8.

118 Dzau VJ, Re RN. Evidence for the existence of renin in the heart. *Circulation* 1987;75(suppl 1):I134−6.

119 Gavras H, Liang C, Brunner HR. Redistribution of regional blood flow after inhibition of the angiotensin-converting enzyme. *Circ Res* 1978;43(suppl 1):159−63.

120 Blythe WB. Captopril and renal autoregulation. *N Engl J Med* 1983;308:390−1.

121 DeVenuto G, Andretti C, Mattarei M, Pegoretti G. Long term captopril therapy at low doses reduces albumin excretion in patients with essential hypertension and no sign of renal impairment. *J Hypertens* 1985;3(suppl I):S143−5.

122 Trachtman H, Gauthier B. Effect of angiotensin-converting enzyme inhibitor therapy on proteinuria in children with renal disease. *J Pediatr* 1988;112:295−7.

123 The 1988 report of the Joint National Committee on Detection, Evaluation and Treatment of High Blood Pressure. *Arch Intern Med* 1988;148:1023−38.

124 Sassano P, Chatellier G, Billaud E, Alhenc-Gelas F, Corvol P, Menard J. Treatment of mild to moderate hypertension with or without the converting enzyme inhibitor enalapril: results of a 6-month double-blind trial. *Am J Med* 1987; 83:227−35.

125 Vidt DG. A controlled multi-clinic study to compare the antihypertensive effects of MK-421, hydrochlorothiazide, and MK-421 combined with hydrochlorothiazide in patients with mild to moderate hypertension. *J Hypertens* 1984;2(suppl 2):81−8.

126 Gavras H, Faxon DP, Berkoben J, Brunner HR, Ryan TJ. Angiotensin converting enzyme inhibition in patients with congestive heart failure. *Circulation* 1978;58:770−76.

127 Romankiewicz JA, Brogden RN, Heel RC, Speight TM, Avery GS. Captopril: an update review of its pharmacological properties and therapeutic efficacy in congestive heart failure. *Drugs* 1983;25:6−40.

128 Schneeweiss A. Cardiovascular drugs in children: angiotensin-converting enzyme inhibitors. *Pediatr Cardiol* 1988; 9:109−15.

129 Shaw NJ, Wilson N, Dickinson DF. Captopril in heart failure secondary to a left to right shunt. *Arch Dis Child* 1988;63:360−3.

130 Curtis JJ, Luke RG, Whelchel JD, Diethelm AG, Jones P, Dusten HP. Inhibition of angiotensin-converting enzyme in renal transplant recipients with hypertension. *N Engl J Med* 1983;308:377−81.

131 Zusman RM. Renin- and non-renin mediated antihypertensive actions of converting enzyme inhibitors. *Kidney Int* 1984;25:969−83.

132 Gavras H, Brunner HR, Gavras I. Captopril in the treatment of hypertension. *Ann Intern Med* 1981;95:505−6.

133 Irvin JD, Viau JM. Safety profiles of the angiotensin converting enzyme inhibitors captopril and enalapril. *Am J Med* 1986;81(suppl 4C):46−50.

134 Edwards IR, Coulter DM, Beesley DM, MacIntosh D. Captopril: 4 years of post marketing surveillance of all patients in New Zealand. *Br J Clin Pharmacol* 1987;23:529−36.

135 Sinaiko AR, Mirkin BL, Hendrick DA, Green TP, O'Dea RF. Antihypertensive effect and elimination of captopril in

hypertensive children with renal disease. *J Pediatr* 1983; 103:799−805.

136 Hymes LC, Warshaw BL. Captopril: long-term treatment of hypertension in a preterm infant and in older children. *Am J Dis Child* 1983;137:263−6.

137 Mirkin BL, Newman TJ. Efficacy and safety of captopril in the treatment of severe childhood hypertension: report of the international collaborative study group. *Pediatrics* 1985; 75:1091−100.

138 Oberfield SE, Case DB, Levine LS, Rappaport R, Rauh W, New MI. Use of the oral angiotensin I-converting enzyme inhibitor (captopril) in childhood malignant hypertension. *J Pediatr* 1979;95:641−4.

139 Case DB, Atlas SA, Laragh JH, Sealey JE, Sullivan PA, McKinstry D. Clinical experience with blockage of the renin−angiotensin aldosterone system by an oral converting-enzyme inhibitor SQ 14225 (captopril) in hypertensive patients. *Prog Cardiovasc Dis* 1978;21:195.

140 Friedman A, Chesney RW, Ball D, Goodfriend T. Effective use of captopril (angiotensin I-converting enzyme inhibitor) in severe childhood hypertension. *J Pediatr* 1980; 97:664−7.

141 Friedman AI, Chesney RW. Effect of captopril on the renin−angiotensin system in hypertensive children. *J Pediatr* 1983;103:806−9.

142 Sullivan JM, Ginsburg BA, Ratts TE *et al.* Hemodynamic and antihypertensive effects of captopril, an orally active angiotensin converting enzyme inhibitor. *Hypertension* 1979;1:397−401.

143 Hodsman GP, Isles CG, Murray GD *et al.* Factors related to first dose hypotensive effect of captopril: prediction and treatment. *Br Med J* 1983;286:832−4.

144 Hypertension in the first year of life. In: Ingelfinger JR, ed. *Pediatric Hypertension.* Philadelphia: WB Saunders, 1982: 229−40.

145 Tack ED, Perlman JM. Renal failure in sick hypertensive premature infants receiving captopril therapy. *J Pediatr* 1988;112:805−10.

146 O'Dea RF, Mirkin BL, Alward CT, Sinaiko AR. Treatment of neonatal hypertension with captopril. *J Pediatr* 1988; 113:403−6.

147 Sell LL, Cullen MC, Lerner GR, Whittlesey GC, Shanley CJ, Klein MD. Hypertension during extra corporeal membrane oxygenation: cause, effect, and management. *Surgery* 1987; 102:724−30.

148 Becker RH, Scholkens B. Ramipril: review of pharmacology. *Am J Cardiol* 1987;59:3D−11D.

149 Dzau VJ, Colucci WS, Williams GH, Curfman G, Meggs L, Hollenberg NK. Sustained effectiveness of converting-enzyme inhibition in patients with severe congestive heart failure. *N Engl J Med* 1980;302:1373−9.

150 Kubo SH, Cody RJ. Clinical pharmacokinetics of the angiotensin converting enzyme inhibitors. *Clin Pharmacokinet* 1985;10:377−91.

151 Sinhvi SM, Duchin KL, Willard DH *et al.* Renal handling of captopril: effect of probenecid. *Clin Pharmacol Ther* 1982; 32:182−9.

152 Miller K, Atkin B, Rodel PV Jr, Walker JF. Enalapril: a well-tolerated and efficacious agent for the pediatric hypertensive patient. *J Cardiovasc Pharmacol* 1987;10(suppl 7): S154−6.

153 Enalapril for hypertension. *Med Let* 1986;28:53−4.

154 DiBianco R. Adverse reactions with angiotensin converting enzyme (ACE) inhibitors. *Med Toxicol* 1986;1:122−41.

155 Hood S, Nicholls MG, Gilchrist NL. Cough wih angiotensin converting enzyme inhibitors. *NZ Med J* 1987;100:6−7.

156 Davies RO, Irvin JD, Kramsch DK, Walker JF, Moncloa F. Enalapril worldwide experience. *Am J Med* 1984;77:23−35.

157 Rothberg AD, Lorenz R. Can captopril cause fetal and neonatal renal failure? *Pediatr Pharmacol* 1984;4:189−192.

158 Guignard JP, Burgener F, Calame A. Persistent anuria in a neonate: a side effect of captopril? *Int J Pediatr Nephrol* 1981;2:133.

159 Schubiger G, Flury G, Nussberger J. Enalapril for pregnancy induced hypertension: acute renal failure in a neonate. *Ann Intern Med* 1988;108:215−16.

160 Captopril: benefits and risks in severe hypertension *Lancet* 1980;ii:129−30.

161 Frohlich ED, Cooper RA, Lewis EJ. Review of the overall experience of captopril in hypertension. *Arch Intern Med* 1984;144:1441−4.

162 Hollenberg NK. Angiotensin-converting enzyme inhibition: renal aspect. *J Cardiovasc Pharmacol* 1985;7(suppl I):S40−4.

163 Barnes JN, Davies ES, Gent CB. Rash, eosinophilia, and hyperkalemia associated with enalapril. *Lancet* 1983;ii: 41−2.

164 Cooper RA. Captopril-associated neutropenia: who is at risk? *Arch Intern Med* 1983;143:659−60.

165 Moncloa F, Sromousky JA, Walker JF, Davies RO. Enalapril in hypertension and congestive heart failure. Overall review of efficacy and safety. *Drugs* 1985;30(suppl I):82−9.

166 Hoorntje SJ, Weening JJ, The TH, Kallenberg CGM, Donker JM, Hoedemacher PJ. Immune-complex glomerulopathy in patients treated with captopril. *Lancet* 1980;i:1212−15.

167 Textor SC, Gephardt GN, Bravo EL *et al.* Membranous glomerulopathy associated with captopril therapy. *Am J Med* 1983;74:705−12.

168 Captopril Collaborative Study Group. Does captopril cause renal damage in hypertensive patients? *Lancet* 1982; i: 988−90.

169 Lewis EJ. Captopril Collaborative Study Group. Proteinuria and abnormalities of the renal glomerulus in patients with hypertension. *Clin Exp Pharmacol Physiol* 1982;7(suppl): 105−15.

16 Heterogeneity of Essential Hypertension

HARRIET P. DUSTAN

Essential hypertension is the diagnosis used when no cause is found to explain elevated arterial pressure. Such a diagnosis, in contrast to "hypertension of undefined cause," implies a cause—an implication that is strengthened by frequent reference to the spontaneously hypertensive rat of the Aoki–Okomoto strain as the experimental model of essential hypertension. However, essential hypertension presents such a heterogeneity of findings that it is difficult to conclude that it is monocausal; in fact, the heterogeneity is so great as to suggest that what we now call essential hypertension is a collection of hypertensions of several causes. This is not surprising considering the number of factors known to control arterial pressure.

Cardiac contraction creates the arterial pressure and this provides the energy for the flow of blood. What blood flow accomplishes is so vital to life that it is not surprising that there are many factors that regulate pressure (Table 16.1) and that these factors are all interrelated. Arterial pressure itself is a function of cardiac output (CO) and vascular resistance and each of these is influenced by the indirect determinants of pressure. The striking feature of these indirect determinants is their interrelationship. The renal pressor system is an excellent example of this interrelatedness: angiotensin II, the functional component of this system, is directly vasoconstrictor, affects both central and peripheral sympathetic nervous activity, increases aldosterone production leading to a positive sodium balance, and, in its own right, diminishes the renal excretion of salt and water.

Hypertension is now considered a disease of dysregulation and when one looks at the determinants of arterial pressure it is obvious that hypertension could have many causes. Not only could it result from an excess of any of the indirect determinants in Table 16.1 but also from altered relationships among them. The possibilities seem legion and added to these are factors that have only recently been found (e.g. atrial natriuretic peptides and aldosterone-stimulating factor), those that may play a role but not a dominant one (e.g. prostaglandins, kinins, and vasopressin), and those yet to be described. In addition, age and race are compounding variables because both affect the known determinants of arterial pressure as well as affecting responsiveness to antihypertensive drugs.

It is the purpose of this chapter to summarize the heterogeneity of essential hypertension and to point out those subgroups which seem to have special characteristics relevant to etiology and to therapy.

HEMODYNAMICS OF HYPERTENSION

Hemodynamic studies were the first to show the heterogeneity of essential hypertension. This came as a surprise because the early hemodynamic investigations of hypertension had shown a normal CO and elevated vascular resistance. Thus, it was conventional wisdom for 25 years that the hemodynamic fault of essential hypertension was raised total peripheral resistance (TPR). However, in the 1950s reports began to emerge that some hypertensive individuals had elevated CO and normal vascular

Table 16.1 Determinants of arterial pressure

Direct
    Cardiac output
    Vascular resistance

Indirect
    Activity of the autonomic nervous system
    Sodium stores and/or extracellular
        fluid volume
    The renal pressor system
    Salt active hormones

resistance and by 1970 it was clear that essential hypertension presented a variety of patterns.

The hemodynamic heterogeneity of essential hypertension became evident when large numbers of patients were studied who presented a wide range of blood pressure values. Dividing hypertensive patients into classes as labile, moderate, and severe allowed Frohlich and colleagues [1] to see different hemodynamic patterns of essential hypertension (Table 16.2). Subjects with labile hypertension were those with some normal diastolic pressures (i.e. <90 mmHg) and some elevated. Most of these patients had modest elevations of CO (Fig. 16.1), normal or only slightly elevated TPR, a slightly elevated heart rate, and an increased rate of left ventricular ejection. Although these were group characteristics they were not universally present in all patients since a few had normal output, elevated TPR, and normal left ventricular ejection rate.

In the groups with progressively higher arterial pressure levels different hemodynamic changes were found. As pressure rose, CO tended to fall but the decrease was statistically significant only in the severely hypertensive patients in whom markedly elevated TPR was the hemodynamic hallmark. They also had a significantly depressed mean rate of left ventricular ejection. Patients with mild and moderate hypertension had low normal CO, elevated TPR, and low normal left ventricular ejection rate; only the TPR was significantly different from normal.

There are three ways to increase CO: (a) increased total blood volume; (b) redistribution of blood from the peripheral capacitance vessels to the central circulation; and (c) increased cardiac performance (Fig. 16.2). Increased blood volume is not a characteristic of hypertension although it does occur rarely (see below). Thus, the increased CO of labile or borderline hypertension has been found to be associated with either a relative increase in central blood volume [2−4] or increased myocardial contractility [1,2]; the relative increase in central blood volume by an increased ratio of cardiopulmonary blood volume (CPBV) to total blood volume (TBV). This ratio is often elevated in labile or borderline hypertension and usually normal in patients with higher pressures.

From these hemodynamic studies has come the conclusion that labile hypertension represents a hyperkinetic circulation characterized by increased CO, stroke volume, and mean rate of left ventricular ejection. This overactivity is lacking in more advanced stages of hypertensive vascular disease. Furthermore,

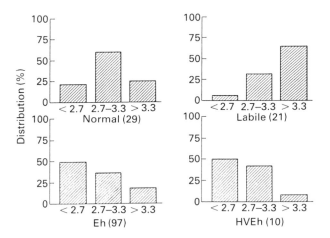

Fig. 16.1 Percentile distribution of cardiac index in normotensive control subjects and subjects with essential hypertension — established (EH), labile, and hypervolemic (HVEH). Cardiac index is expressed in litres/min per m² of body surface area. Numbers in parentheses are the numbers of subjects in that group. From [1], with permission.

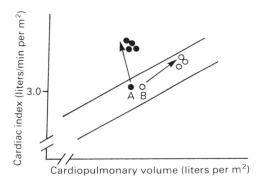

Fig. 16.2 Determinants of cardiac output in high output states. Although cardiac output is directly related to cardiopulmonary blood volume it can also be increased by increasing the ejection fraction without changing central blood volume. From *Clinical Hypertension*, Searle and Co. 1973, with permission.

in such patients hemodynamic functions are influenced not only by the height of the arterial pressure but also by the presence or absence of cardiac hypertrophy, as reported by Frohlich and coworkers [5] and Fouad and colleagues [6]. Those with normal-sized hearts have normal CO and left ventricular ejection rate and elevated TPR. In contrast, those with cardiac hypertrophy have significantly reduced CO and left ventricular ejection, along with a more marked elevation of TPR.

Does this heterogeneity of hemodynamic findings in essential hypertension represent a continuum or does each group go through the natural lifespan of

Table 16.2 Hemodynamic characteristics in essential hypertension

		Hypertensive vascular disease				Hypertensive heart disease		
	Control	Labile	Mild	Moderate	Severe	Normal sized heart	Left atrial abnormality	Left ventricular hypertrophy
Number of subjects	25	30	30	30	16	54	20	23
Age (years)	34	31	43	48	52	39	49	48
Sex: M/F ratio	20:5	23:7	23:7	23:7	12:4	37:17	14:6	20:3
Body surface area (m^2)	1.87	1.86	1.89	1.83	1.94	1.84	1.89	1.92
Mean arterial pressure (mmHg)	92	106	123	134	149	117	131	148
Heart rate (beats/min)	68	75	77	75	76	75	79	74
Cardiac index (l/min per m^2)	3.1	3.4	2.8	2.8	2.5	3.1	2.9	2.5
Total peripheral resistance (PRU) mmHg/l	17	18	25	27	32	21	24	31
Intravenous ejection rate (ml/s per m^2)	152	165	140	142	129	149	135	129
Stroke volume (ml/beat)	84	84	67	71	66	77	71	67

From [2], with permission.

its hypertension retaining the same hemodynamic characteristics from beginning to end? The answer is probably both. In support of this conclusion are the longitudinal studies of Julius and co-authors [7], Birkenhager and associates [8], and Lund-Johansen [9] which showed a small decrease in CO and rise in TPR over several years with little change in blood pressure, and the report of Ibrahim and coworkers [10] which described elevated CO and hyperkinetic circulation in some patients with severe hypertension of more than 10 years duration. In this regard it is instructive to recall the experience with metyrapone hypertension in dogs [11]. Of 9 dogs, hypertension throughout the entire study was explained in 5 by elevated CO with slightly increased TPR, in 3 by elevated TPR, and in 1 by autoregulation, i.e. an elevated CO at first with decreased resistance, followed by a fall in CO to control levels and rising resistance.

These experiences with clinical and experimental hypertension indicate that there are several ways in which elevated arterial pressure is expressed hemodynamically and that there is no surely predictable pattern. However generalities can be drawn that have relevance for the care of hypertensive patients. Young

people, those with labile or borderline hypertension, and those with tachycardia and/or cardiac awareness are likely to have an elevated CO and normal or only slightly elevated vascular resistance. In these patients, measures to "quiet" the hyperkinetic circulation are indicated. In contrast, almost every patient with severe hypertension will have a markedly elevated peripheral vascular resistance and elimination or reduction of this abnormality should be a therapeutic goal. This is probably best done with a vasodilator.

ACTIVITY OF THE AUTONOMIC NERVOUS SYSTEM

Physiologic correlates

Frohlich and coworkers [12] were the first to report heterogeneity in response to orthostatic stress depending upon the severity of the hypertension. They studied hemodynamic changes evoked by a 50° head-up tilt in 52 untreated hypertensive patients and compared the results with those obtained in normotensive subjects. In normal subjects the mean blood pressure response to tilt was a ±10 mmHg change and a similar result was obtained in 24 hypertensive subjects. However, abnormalities were found in 28 of the individuals with hypertension: 18 had orthostatic hypertension and 10 orthostatic hypotension. Those with orthostatic hypertension tended to be younger than the other groups and to have milder hypertension. Those who had previously been treated had responded well to drugs that act through neural mechanisms. Of the three groups, they had the highest CO at rest and a markedly increased vascular resistance in response to head-up tilt (Fig. 16.3). Blood pressure increases in response to the Valsalva maneuver were also statistically significantly greater in the subjects with orthostatic hypertension. The authors concluded that head-up tilt could be used to test for a neurogenic component in hypertensive patients.

Since that time there have been repeated demonstrations that this subgroup of patients with essential hypertension has physiologic characteristics indicating increased activity of the sympathetic nervous system. The modest elevation of CO that often occurs in borderline or mild hypertension has been found to have a neurogenic basis: it can be reduced to normal with autonomic blockade using propranolol and atropine [13] and it is directly related to a central redistribution of blood volume (increased CPBV:TBV ratio) that is neurogenically mediated [4]. The elevated heart rate has clearly been shown to have a neurogenic basis which has two components, sympathetic and parasympathetic. The work of Julius and Hansson using autonomic blockade found that not only is there increased sympathetic drive to the heart but also a withdrawal of parasympathetic inhibition [13].

There is growing evidence that inheritance may play a role in the neurogenic abnormalities that characterize early hypertension. Falkner and colleagues found that when adolescents performed mental arithmetic those with labile hypertension and those at risk of becoming hypertensive because of a positive family history had exaggerated pressure and heart rate responses when compared to normotensive adolescents without a familial predisposition [14]. That this may represent the beginning of essential hypertension is suggested by their finding that over half the adolescents who had borderline hypertension when first seen, later developed sustained hypertension and had exaggerated pressure and heart rate responses to mental stress in the early stages when their hypertension was still borderline [15].

Plasma catecholamines

There is much heterogeneity found in the reports of plasma catecholamines in hypertensive patients [16]. Generally speaking, plasma norepinephrine is higher in hypertensive than in normotensive people, but usually not significantly so. However, within the hypertensive groups abnormalities have emerged. In normotensive subjects plasma norepinephrine levels rise with age and there is a significant correlation with age. This is not so in the hypertensive subjects because levels tend to be higher in younger age groups. Since borderline hypertension is more often found in young people and since this condition is often characterized by increased activity of the sympathetic nervous system, it is likely that the higher

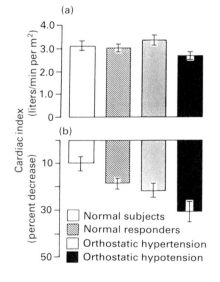

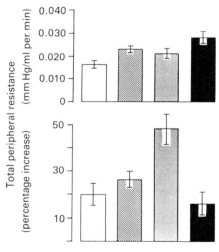

Fig. 16.3 Hemodynamics of normotensive control and hypertensive subjects classified according to mean arterial pressure (MAP) responses to head-up tilt: normal responders (MAP ±10 mmHg), orthostatic hypertensives (MAP increase >10 mmHg), and orthostatic hypotensives (MAP decrease >10 mmHg). Section (A) shows supine cardiac index and total peripheral resistance of the four groups and (B) percentile changes in these functions following a 5-min 50° head-up tilt. Adapted from [12], with permission.

plasma catecholamines in younger people with hypertension is a reflection of increased sympathetic activity.

Another heterogeneity concerns catecholamine responses to exercise stress. Goldstein found that exercise significantly increased the mean hypertensive–normotensive differences in plasma norepinephrine although there was marked variability within the hypertensive group [17]. A study by Duncan and co-authors reported the effects of exercise on plasma catecholamine levels and arterial pressure in white men with mild hypertension (diastolic pressure 90–104 mmHg) [18]. Sixteen weeks of an aerobic exercise program significantly reduced pressure, heart rate, and plasma norepinephrine levels in patients who had elevated plasma norepinephrine concentrations before the exercise program began. Thus it may be that this represents a subgroup of hypertensive individuals whose hypertension will specifically respond to exercise.

SODIUM STORES AND SODIUM BALANCE

Salt excess has long been implicated as a factor in essential hypertension. Since sodium is the chief determinant of extracellular fluid volume one would expect that hypertension would be characterized by abnormalities in plasma volume, extracellular fluid volume, or sodium stores. However, this is not the case. Tarazi and colleagues found that when diastolic blood pressure was greater than 105 mmHg, plasma volume was reduced modestly but significantly [19]. Patients with lower pressures had normal plasma volume and a small number of mild-to-moderately hypertensive individuals had expanded plasma volume. The diminished plasma volume seemed likely to represent a decreased venous capacity since Ulrych and coworkers found that even with diminished plasma volume there was central redistribution of blood that accounted for modest elevation of CO [3], and Safar and colleagues have stressed the importance of decreased venous compliance as an accompaniment (and probably the explanation) of reduced plasma volume [4].

Extracellular fluid volumes have been found to be normal in essential hypertension [20]. This means that patients with reduced plasma volume have a reduced ratio of plasma to interstitial fluid volume (Fig. 16.4). Also, total exchangeable sodium has been found to be normal [21].

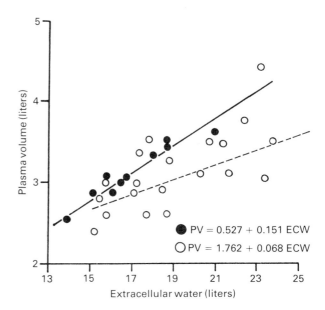

Fig.16.4 The relationship between plasma volume and extracellular fluid volume in normotensive and hypertensive men. Note that for any given extracellular fluid volume, plasma volume tended to be lower in hypertensive than normotensive individuals. From [20], with permission.

Thus, although there is some heterogeneity within the body sodium stores or extracellular fluid volumes of essential hypertension, this occurs only in the plasma volume. The predominant characteristic is modest hypovolemia. Some patients however are normovolemic while a small subset has hypervolemia. Hypertension in this last group may be particularly responsive to diuretic therapy [19].

Given the relative normality of exchangeable sodium and extracellular fluid volumes in essential hypertension, one would expect that sodium excretion in response to a salt load would follow a fairly homogeneous pattern. This is not the case, however, and the picture is one of considerable complexity because sodium handling by the kidney following a salt load is in part determined by the prior sodium intake. For example, when an intravenous salt load was given daily for 3 days to patients who had previously eaten a 150 mmol/l sodium diet for 3 days, 20% of hypertensive subjects had a negative sodium balance while the rest retained from 0.5 to 3.5 mmol/l per kg [22]. In contrast, when the salt loading had been preceded by 4 days of rigid sodium restriction (9 mmol/l per day plus furosemide 1 mg/kg given the first day) each patient retained sodium. The distribution of values was not unimodal because about 25% retained 3–4 mmol/l sodium per kg and 30% retained between 7 and 8 mmol/l per kg. No relationship was found between these sodium balance data and arterial pressure changes in response to variations in salt intake. This lack of relationship raises questions as to the actual value of population-based sodium-restricted diets, as currently recommended.

THE RENIN–ANGIOTENSIN SYSTEM

Among people with essential hypertension there is marked heterogeneity of plasma renin activity (PRA) and levels can be low, normal, or high [23]. Procedures for making the classification vary but mostly are based on PRA responsiveness to one or more stimuli that increase renin release. However, Laragh classifies his patients by referencing PRA to 24-h urinary sodium excretion. Using this technique he found that 30% of patients with essential hypertension had low renin, 55% normal, and 15% high renin activity [24].

There has been much interest in low-renin essential hypertension because it was thought at one time to result from mineralocorticoid excess. Accordingly, many studies have been done and experience gained in a large number of patients. To stimulate renin release most of these studies have used a negative sodium balance with or without orthostatic stress; however some have used blood pressure reduction with a vasodilator. Using these procedures, the frequency of low-renin hypertension has ranged from 17 to 46% of patients studied [25].

The heterogeneity of the renin–angiotensin system in essential hypertension is further contributed to by age and race. Plasma renin activity falls with advancing age regardless of race. Low PRA occurs more frequently in black than in white patients and is found in normotensive as well as hypertensive blacks.

A point of interest in the heterogeneity of the renal pressor system in essential hypertension is the focus on the low-renin state; this is in contrast to the other systems controlling arterial pressure where excesses rather than deficiencies are emphasized. This stress given low-renin hypertension seems inappropriate because elevated pressure should depress renin release. Thus it is possible that normal- and high-renin hypertension represent the abnormalities, not low-renin.

Although provocative measures to stimulate renin release have been used to classify hypertensive patients according to renin status, responses to sodium loading, which suppresses renin release, have

been found to designate a group of individuals with normal- or high-renin hypertension that appear to be an important subgroup. Williams and Hollenberg report that as many as 50% of patients with normal–high-renin hypertension are what they call "nonmodulators," patients who do not have an increase in renal blood flow with sodium loading and who have a delayed suppression of PRA (Fig. 16.5) [26]. They also have abnormal plasma aldosterone responses to sodium restriction and angiotensin II infusion, as will be detailed below. Of practical interest is the fact that all the abnormalities are reversed by treatment with a converting enzyme inhibitor.

SALT ACTIVE HORMONES

Aldosterone is one of the major hormones influencing sodium excretion. Because of this, one would expect considerable heterogeneity of plasma levels in essential hypertension but this apparently is not so; basal plasma aldosterone levels are normal and show no impressive heterogeneity. It is in the aldosterone–renin relationships and in the response of aldosterone to various stimuli that the heterogeneity appears. In low-renin hypertension aldosterone is normal whereas it should be low in the sodium-replete state, the plasma aldosterone response to infused angiotensin II is exaggerated, yet during sodium depletion that response is less than normal [21]. Also, the rise in plasma aldosterone that occurs with salt deprivation is blunted in essential hypertension [21].

Williams and Hollenberg have examined a number of aspects of these deranged aldosterone responses of essential hypertension and from these studies has come a description of a subgroup of patients in whom the abnormalities can be explained by an excess of or increased responsiveness to angiotensin II [26]. These are the "nonmodulators" referred to in the previous section as having no rise in renal blood flow and a delayed suppression of PRA with salt loading. Their aldosterone abnormalities are a diminished production in response to infused angiotensin II and to sodium depletion (Fig. 16.5). These abnormal aldosterone responses are eliminated by a few days' treatment with a converting enzyme inhibitor.

Natriuretic hormones

For several years investigators have searched for a circulating hormone that increases sodium excretion through direct action on the kidney [27,28].

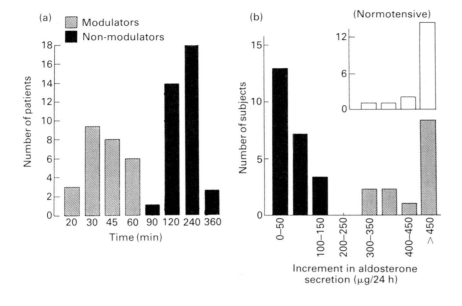

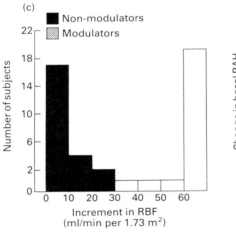

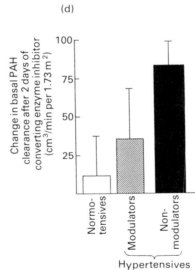

Fig. 16.5 Plasma renin activity (PRA), aldosterone, and renal blood flow characteristics of patients with nonmodulating and modulating hypertension (see text for definitions). (A) Time for occurrence of a 30% suppression of PRA in response to an infusion of 0.9% saline. Note that all modulators had experienced this degree of suppression by 60 min whereas in nonmodulators suppression was delayed. (B) Diminished response of aldosterone secretion in nonmodulators with acute volume depletion. (C) Increments of renal blood flow (RBF) with salt loading after salt depletion. Note that nonmodulators did not increase RBF as modulators did. (D) Response of RBF (change in PAH clearance) to salt loading after salt depletion when a converting enzyme inhibitor has been given for 2 days. Note that the sluggish response of the nonmodulators was normalized by the treatment. Adapted from [25], with permission.

More recently interest has focused on an inhibitor sodium–potassium adenosine triphosphatase (Na^+-K^+-ATPase) [29]. The hypothesis is that sodium homeostasis during high-salt feeding is maintained by generation of a hormone that inhibits renal Na^+-K^+-ATPase and allows an appropriate natriuresis. In addition, it inhibits the enzyme in vascular smooth muscle, leading to a derangement in intracellular electrolyte concentrations, and a decrease in membrane potential thereby increasing excitability, thus causing vasoconstriction.

More recently a number of other membrane cation transport systems have been implicated as having relevance to hypertension [30]. Since they are present in blood cells, both red and white cells have been studied in the possibility that abnormalities in this accessible tissue would reflect similar abnormalities in renal tubular cells and vascular smooth muscle. The sodium and potassium transport systems that have been studied are:

1 the ouabain-sensitive Na^+-K^+-ATPase (the sodium pump) which mostly determines the membrane potential;

2 furosemide-sensitive, sodium–potassium cotransport which moves these two cations together either in or out;

3 a ouabain-resistant, phloretin-sensitive, one-for-one sodium–sodium exchange, called countertransport, that can be detected with lithium; and

4 a transport of sodium as $NaCO_3$ which represents only a small leak.

In addition to these transport systems, there has been study of blood cell sodium content which is taken as an indicator of the state of the transport systems.

De Wardener and MacGregor [28] have reported that leukocytes of patients with essential hypertension had higher sodium concentration than cells from normotensive people and that plasma of patients contained a factor that inhibited ouabain-sensitive sodium efflux from leukocytes of normotensive control subjects. This they interpreted as evidence for a circulating hormone that inhibits Na^+-K^+-ATPase. Cole [31] did not find such evidence. He measured sodium efflux in red blood cells of untreated patients with essential hypertension, the children of hypertensive parents, and control subjects without a family history of hypertension. In the untreated hypertensive individuals, both ouabain-sensitive and insensitive efflux was increased; however, red cell Na^+-K^+-ATPase was normal. He interpreted these findings as indicative of a change in pump control mechanisms rather than a change in enzyme activity. Also, he could not show abnormalities of sodium efflux in normotensive offspring of hypertensive parents. This finding is different from results of others because, for example, using lithium efflux to study countertransport, Clegg and co-authors found abnormalities in subjects with a positive family history [32], in confirmation of the original report of Canessa and colleagues [33].

When abnormalities of cotransport [34] and countertransport [33] were reported in 1980 it was expected that blood cell membrane abnormalities would allow quick recognition of specific groups of hypertensive patients and new insights into etiology. These expectations have not been fulfilled completely, but progress is being made. A review of this research area has been published [35]. The work summarized indicates that many of the transport systems are genetically linked [36,37], that there seems to be some relationship to blood pressure [38], and that there are clear racial differences [38].

SUMMARY

As detailed in this review, inadequate control of peripheral vascular resistance is not the only hallmark of essential hypertension; the other is heterogeneity of physiologic and biochemical characteristics.

It seems likely that careful study of subgroups with homogeneous characteristics will provide new diagnostic groupings with specific therapeutic implications for that large number of people now considered to have essential hypertension.

REFERENCES

1 Frohlich ED, Tarazi RC, Dustan HP. Re-examination of the hemodynamics of hypertension. *Am J Med Sci* 1969;257:9−23.

2 Tarazi RC. The hemodynamics of hypertension. In: Genest J, Kuchel O, Hamet P, Cantin M, eds. *Hypertension: Physiopathology and Treatment*. 2nd edn. New York: McGraw-Hill, 1983:15−42.

3 Ulrych M, Frohlich ED, Tarazi RC, Dustan HP, Page IH. Cardiac output and distribution of blood volume in central and peripheral circulations in hypertensive and normotensive man. *Br Heart J* 1969;31:570−4.

4 Safar ME, Weiss YA, London GM, Frackowiak RF, Milliez PL. Cardiopulmonary blood volume in borderline hypertension. *Clin Sci Mol Med* 1974;47:153−64.

5 Frohlich ED, Kozul VJ, Tarazi RC, Dustan HP. Physiological comparison of labile and essential hypertension. *Circ Res* 1970;26,27(suppl I):55−69.

6 Fouad FM, Tarazi RC, Gallagher JH, MacIntyre WJ, Cook SA. Abnormal left ventricular relaxation in hypertensive patients. *Clin Sci* 1980;59(suppl):411s−14s.

7 Julius S, Quadir H, Gajendragadkar S. Hyperkinetic stage: a precursor of hypertension? A longitudinal study of borderline hypertension. In: Gross F, Strasser T, eds. *Mild Hypertension: Natural History and Management*. Bath: Pitman Medical, 1979:116−26.

8 Birkenhager WH, Schalekamp MADH, Krauss XH, Kolsters G, Zaal GA. Consecutive hemodynamic patterns in essential hypertension. *Lancet* 1972;i:560−4.

9 Lund-Johansen P. Hemodynamic alterations in hypertension—spontaneous changes and effects of drug therapy. *Acta Med Scand* 1977;(suppl 603):1−14.

10 Ibrahim MM, Tarazi RC, Dustan HP, Bravo EL. Cardioadrenergic factor in essential hypertension. *Am Heart J* 1974;88:724−32.

11 Bravo EL, Tarazi RC, Dustan HP. Multifactorial analysis of chronic hypertension induced by electrolyte-active steroids in trained, unanesthetized dogs. *Circ Res* 1977;(suppl I):140−5.

12 Frohlich ED, Tarazi RC, Ulrych M, Dustan HP, Page IH. Tilt test for investigating a neural component in hypertension. Its correlation with clinical characteristics. *Circulation* 1967;36:387−93.

13 Julius S, Hansson H. Borderline hypertension: epidemiologic and clinical implications. In: Genest J, Kuchel O, Hamet P, Cantin M, eds. *Hypertension. Physiopathology and Treatment*. 2nd edn. New York: McGraw-Hill, 1983:753−64.

14 Falkner B, Onesti G, Angelakos ET, Fernandez M, Longman C. Cardiovascular response to mental stress in normal adolescents with hypertensive parents. *Hypertension* 1979;1:23−30.

15 Falkner B, Onesti G, Angelakos ET. Cardiovascular response to stress in adolescents. In: Onesti G, Kim KE, eds. *Hyperten-*

sion in the Young and the Old. New York: Grune & Stratton, 1981:11−17.

16 Goldstein DS. Plasma norepinephrine in essential hypertension. A study of the studies. *Hypertension* 1981;3:48−52.

17 Goldstein DS. Plasma norepinephrine during stress in essential hypertension. *Hypertension* 1981;3:551−6.

18 Duncan JJ, Farr JE, Upton SJ, Hagan RD, Oglesby ME, Blair SN. The effects of aerobic exercise on plasma catecholamines and blood pressure in patients with mild essential hypertension. *JAMA* 1985;254:2609−13.

19 Tarazi RC, Dustan HP, Frohlich ED, Gifford RW, Hoffman GC. Plasma volume and chronic hypertension. *Arch Intern Med* 1970;125:835−42.

20 Tarazi RC, Dustan HP, Frohlich ED. Relation of plasma to interstitial fluid volume in essential hypertension. *Circulation* 1969;40:357−65.

21 Fraser R, Brown JJ, Lever AF, Robertson JIS. Control of aldosterone in hypertension. In: Genest J, Kuchel O, Hamet P, Cantin M, eds. *Hypertension: Physiopathology and Treatment.* 2nd edn. New York: McGraw-Hill, 1983:338−48.

22 Dustan HP, Kirk KA. Relationship of sodium balance to arterial pressure in black hypertensive patients. *Am J Med Sci* 1988;31:378−83.

23 Dustan HP, Tarazi RC, Frohlich ED. Functional correlates of plasma renin activity in hypertensive patients. *Circulation* 1970;41:555−67.

24 Laragh J. The renin−angiotensin−aldosterone system for blood pressure regulation and for subdividing patients to reveal and analyze different forms of hypertension. In: Laragh JH, Buhler FR, Seldin DW, eds. *Frontiers of Hypertension Research.* New York: Springer-Verlag, 1981:183−203.

25 Dunn MJ, Tannen RL. Low renin hypertension. *Kidney Int* 1974;5:317−24.

26 Williams GH, Hollenberg NK. Are non-modulating patients with essential hypertension a distinct subgroup? *Am J Med* 1985;79(suppl 3C):3−9.

27 Dahl LK, Knudsen KD, Iwai J. Humoral transmission of hypertension: evidence from parabiosis. *Circ Res* 1969;24−25(suppl I):I-21−33.

28 de Wardener HE, MacGregor GA. The natriuretic hormone and its possible relationship to hypertension. In: Genest J, Kuchel O, Hamet P, Cantin M, eds. *Hypertension: Physiopathology and Treatment.* 2nd edn. New York: McGraw-Hill, 1983:84−95.

29 Overbeck HW, Derifield RS, Pamnami MB, Sozen T. Attenuated vasodilator responses to K^+ in essential hypertensive man. *J Clin Invest* 1974;53:678−86.

30 Meyer P, Garay RP, De Mendonca M. Ion transport systems in hypertension. In: Genest J, Kuchel O, Hamet P, Cantin M, eds. *Hypertension.* 2nd edn. New York: McGraw-Hill, 1983:108−16.

31 Cole CH. Erythrocyte membrane sodium transport in patients with treated and untreated essential hypertension. *Circulation* 1983;68:17−22.

32 Clegg G, Morgan DB, Davidson C. The heterogeneity of essential hypertension. Relation between lithium efflux and sodium content of erythrocytes and a family history of hypertension. *Lancet* 1982;ii:891−4.

33 Canessa M, Adragna N, Solomon HS, Connolly TM, Tosteson DC. Increased sodium−lithium countertransport in red cells of patients with essential hypertension. *N Engl J Med* 1980;302:772−6.

34 Garay RP, Elghozi JL, Dagher G, Meyer P. Laboratory distinction between essential and secondary hypertension by measurement of erythrocyte cation fluxes. *N Engl J Med* 1980;302:769−71.

35 Horan MJ, Dzau VJ, Canessa M, eds. Workshop on cation transport and natriuretic factors. *Hypertension* 1987;10(suppl I):I-1−130.

36 Canessa M, Brugnara C, Escobales N. The Li^+-Na^+ exchange and Na^+-K^+-Cl^- cotransport systems in essential hypertension. *Hypertension* 1987;10:I-4−10.

37 Williams RR, Hasstedt SJ, Hunt SC, Wu LL, Ash KO. Genetic studies of cation tests and hypertension. *Hypertension* 1987;10:I-37−41.

38 McDonald A, Trevisan M, Cooper R *et al.* Epidemiological studies of sodium transport and hypertension. *Hypertension* 1987;10:I-41−47.

17 Etiologic Factors in Essential Hypertension

BONITA FALKNER

It is now generally accepted that the aberrant regulatory mechanisms which progress to the condition of essential hypertension have their onset in the young [1−4]. In discussing the etiology of this condition, it is necessary to consider the potential contributing effects of both genetic factors [5,6] and environmental conditions [7]. As proposed by Folkow [8], a genetic constellation of predisposing physiologic elements may be characteristic of certain populations. While no specific genetic pattern or reliable genetic marker has emerged to account for essential hypertension, it is believed that genetic factors place an individual at a certain risk level. Other factors are necessary to modulate onset and intensity of hypertension. These include environmental factors such as dietary patterns and stress which function as precipitating factors and enhance the underlying predisposing elements. The role of genetic factors is discussed elsewhere (see Chapter 7). This chapter will focus primarily on environmental factors.

POPULATION STUDIES

One epidemiologic approach to study the interaction of heredity and environment has been some classic investigations in adult migrant populations which have evaluated the effects of acculturation on Polynesians, Melanesians, and South African Zulus. When groups from relatively primitive cultures develop greater cultural contact, they develop higher blood pressures and a greater tendency for blood pressure to rise with age [9]. Investigations of migrant populations including US blacks [10], Africans [11], and Eastern Island Polynesians [12] have shown a rising blood pressure in the migrant group. Typically, in such shifts from a rural to a more urban environment, there are changes in dietary intakes of sodium, potassium, and calories. Body weight increases and levels of activity are altered. Such differences alone have not been found to be sufficient to account for the blood pressure rise [9].

Similar studies in children have been carried out in the Polynesian population from Tokelau Island and the New Zealand Maoris. Both have a common genetic origin. The Tokelauan society, at the time of study in 1971, still largely followed the traditional social patterns, whereas the Maoris in New Zealand were urbanized with environmental characteristics of New Zealand and other western countries. Blood pressures for both boys and girls were higher in the New Zealand Maoris than in the Tokelauans. This difference could be explained by greater body mass in the Maoris in adolescence but not in younger children [13]. Similarly, blood pressure levels of urbanized Filipino children living in Manila were significantly higher than in children of the same age living in rural communities in Luzon [14].

Environmental factors appear to affect blood pressure regulation at a young age. A study involving a group of families in a west London suburb covered a range of social and environmental conditions. The results indicated that the child's weight, pulse rate, and level of blood pressure of parents influence the blood pressure level in children [15]. The investigators suggested that within a given environment the children who warranted greater surveillance for potential hypertension were those whose parents had a greater blood pressure. This proposal is consistent with the concept proposed by Folkow [8] in which environmental factors function as precipitating factors to enhance a genetic predisposition to the development of high blood pressure.

OBESITY

Epidemiologic investigations have related blood pressure in children to body weight, height, and degree of sexual maturation [16−20]. Body weight and increases in body weight have consistently correlated with blood pressure in both children and adults [21,22]. In the Muscatine study, Lauer and coworkers demonstrated that children with consistently higher blood pressure values and those with upward-tracking blood pressure had significantly greater levels of height, weight, relative weight, and triceps skinfold thickness than those with lower levels of blood pressure [23].

Obesity acts as a significant risk factor for the development of essential hypertension in adults [24]. In addition, weight reduction lowers blood pressure in some obese hypertensive patients [25]. The mechanism linking obesity to hypertension is unclear. It is known that obesity adversely affects cardiac function by adding volume to an already increased peripheral vascular resistance, thereby accentuating left ventricular work [26]. However, obesity is determined by a mixture of genetic, environmental, and behavioral factors. There is suggestive evidence that body fat distribution may be determined by variations in adrenal androgen function which in turn have a regulatory effect on blood pressure [27]. Thus, there may be a neuroendocrine link to obesity-related hypertension. At present, for clinical purposes, childhood obesity should be considered a risk factor for cardiovascular disease [28] even though the mechanism is not delineated.

STRESS

Environmental stress has been demonstrated to have a significant effect on the prevalence and onset of essential hypertension in adults [7]. Plasma catecholamines are generally higher in essential hypertension, indicating elevated sympathetic neural activity [29,30]. In humans under experimental conditions, centrally mediated stress elicits a spectrum of neurogenic-cardiovascular responses including elevation of systolic blood pressure [31,32]. Adults with borderline essential hypertension and those with a family history of essential hypertension have greater increases of blood pressure [33,34] and increased levels of plasma and urinary catecholamines [35,36] when exposed to stress.

Children with hypertensive parents react to mental stress with greater heart rate and blood pressure response than do those with normotensive parents [37,38]. Adolescents from families with or without essential hypertension were exposed to a standardized alerting stimulus of forced mental arithmetic.

Offspring of hypertensive parents showed high basal heart rates, and a heart rate response to stress which was both greater and more prolonged than that observed in the genetically normotensive control population. This increased responsiveness, as well as higher plasma catecholamine levels, was present in adolescents already displaying marginal hypertension and also in some normotensive offspring of hypertensive parents [37]. Collins and associates compared 8−13-year-old children with either hypertensive or normotensive fathers. In response to auditory stimuli, children of hypertensive fathers showed a more sustained heart rate increase, faster pulse transit time, and larger skin resistance response [39].

McCrory and colleagues [40], demonstrated higher plasma norepinephrine levels in adolescents with essential hypertension and borderline hypertension when at rest. With standing, the increases in norepinephrine levels and blood pressure were blunted in the hypertensive subjects. However, individuals with borderline hypertension and normotensive siblings of hypertensive adolescents had values which correlated with resting values. Another observation was reported by Katz and coworkers, who found that adolescents with blood pressure in the upper 15th percentile of the population demonstrated a blunted pressor response to the change from supine to seated posture [41]. Thus, there is evidence for altered sympathetic activity and baroreceptor sensitivity in the young with higher blood pressure. In early hypertension, cardiac output is increased and peripheral resistance is normal, which is consistent with increased adrenergic drive. It has been proposed that these responses reflect an autonomic nervous system imbalance which may play a causal role in the pathogenesis of essential hypertension [42]. However, whether these experimental responses reflect a normal process occurring in childhood and progressing to essential hypertension remains to be proven.

SODIUM

Among populations, the correlation of chronic dietary sodium intake with the prevalence of hypertension has resulted in the concept that sodium plays an etiologic role in the development of essential hypertension. In addition, extensive experimental animal studies have contributed to an understanding of the role of sodium in hypertension. Crosscultural studies comparing sodium intake to the prevalence of hypertension in the population support this concept [43–45]. However, the association of sodium intake with blood pressure among individuals within a given population has been difficult to demonstrate [46,47]. Studies in children on the effect of high sodium concentrations in drinking water have yielded conflicting results [48–52]. Cooper and co-authors [53] were able to demonstrate a quantitatively weak but significant linear relationship between blood pressure and sodium excretion in children aged 11–14 years. However, these observations required seven consecutive 24-h urine collections per subject to adjust for intra-individual variation. A recent epidemiologic investigation in young infants has provided evidence for a small but significant effect of sodium intake on blood pressure in the first 6 months of life [54]. In established hypertension, a reduction in dietary sodium may reduce blood pressure [55]. In addition, dietary maneuvers to lower sodium intake in young adults may lower blood pressure [56]. However, as yet there have been no reports which have demonstrated such an effect in children.

While the role of sodium in the pathogenesis of essential hypertension in humans is poorly delineated, in studies of experimental animals the effects of sodium intake are more striking [57]. There is evidence in both humans and in experimental animals that blood pressure response to altered sodium intake varies. This has resulted in the concept of sodium sensitivity or sodium resistance. This response to salt intake may be genetically determined. Thus, it is unlikely that a high sodium intake functions as an isolated etiologic factor. More recent studies have pursued the interaction of sodium intake with other physiologic parameters.

The interrelationship between neurogenic activity and blood volume modified by sodium intake has been studied in adults. Luft and associates studied the effects of a wide range of sodium intake on norepinephrine values in normal men and demonstrated a decrease in sympathetic activity with an increasing sodium load [58]. They also found that black subjects excreted less sodium and potassium than white subjects with greater suppression of plasma renin activity [59]. In another study, higher levels of plasma norepinephrine were present in hypertensive individuals than in normal control subjects at each level of dietary sodium intake [60].

Young adults with borderline hypertension respond to increased dietary sodium with echocardiographic measurements of a disproportionate rise in cardiac index and an inadequate fall in total peripheral resistance [61]. Also it has been observed that hypertensive subjects exhibit greater changes than normotensive individuals in plasma catecholamines and plasma renin activity in response to sodium deprivation and treadmill exercise [62]. These studies suggest a relationship of sympathetic activity and sodium balance.

Falkner and coworkers [63] investigated the interaction of stress and sodium intake on blood pressure regulation in adolescents who varied in their genetic risk for essential hypertension. Normotensive offspring of hypertensive (FH+) and normotensive parents (FH−) were compared. The cardiovascular response to the stress of mental arithmetic was compared before and after 14 days of sodium loading with 10 g/day sodium chloride in addition to their usual diet. The baseline blood pressures were significantly higher in the FH+ but not the FH− subjects after sodium loading. This study indicated that normotensive children with a low genetic risk for hypertension were resistant to the effect of sodium loading, while the FH+ subjects were sensitive to sodium loading.

The effect of a higher sodium intake in sodium-sensitive or resistant individuals appears to depend on a volume–vascular interrelationship. In studies of vascular hemodynamics, forearm vascular resistance (FVR) of normal subjects falls as dietary sodium is increased [64]. A high sodium intake in individuals with borderline hypertension results in a decrease in forearm blood flow (FBF) and an increase in FVR. These changes are augmented by norepinephrine infusion or sympathetic stimulation [65]. Koolen and Van Brummelen [66] studied plasma norepinephrine and FBF at high and low sodium intake in patients with essential hypertension. Patients with hypertension who were salt-sensitive had higher norepinephrine levels during the control period, and norepinephrine release increased with the high-salt period. While on a high-salt diet, the FBF decreased in salt-sensitive subjects while it increased in salt-insensitive subjects. These studies suggest that the sodium-sensitive blood pressure response is related both to adrenergic activity and to vascular resistance.

POTASSIUM

While the evidence supporting a significant role of dietary sodium in the development of essential hypertension is substantial, there has been a recent resurgence of interest in the level of dietary potassium as a factor in hypertension. Epidemiologic studies indicate an inverse relationship between potassium intake and blood pressure. Other studies indicate that a reduction in the dietary sodium: potassium ratio reduces blood pressure [67]. Tobian and co-authors found that potassium added to the diets of salt-loaded hypertensive Dahl S rats protected the animals from developing arteriolar and renal lesions without decreasing the blood pressure [68]. In dogs made hypertensive by avoidance, conditioning, and saline infusions, subsequent potassium infusion decreased the blood pressure [69,70].

In children, Berenson and colleagues found a lower urinary potassium excretion in black subjects, and in response to oral potassium (80 mmol/day) there was a natriuresis and a reduction in blood pressure [71]. The observations by Sullivan and coworkers of higher serum and urinary potassium levels in young individuals with borderline hypertension resistant to a dietary sodium load suggested that potassium blunted the effect of the high sodium intake [61]. Hypertensive patients given potassium chloride supplementation with a high-salt diet gained less weight, and had less increase in plasma volume and cardiac output than those without potassium chloride. Plasma norepinephrine levels were lower in those supplemented with potassium chloride, indicating a reduction in adrenergic activity [72]. Skrabal and colleagues studied the effect of a low-sodium/high-potassium diet on 20 young normotensive adults, 10 of whom had a family history of hypertension. The higher-potassium diet reduced the diastolic blood pressure by an average of 5 mmHg in 10 of 20 subjects, of whom 7 had a family history of essential hypertension. In all subjects, the low-sodium/high-potassium diet reduced the blood pressure rise produced by a norepinephrine infusion or by mental stress [73].

These studies indicate that potassium has a natriuretic effect, can modify the activity of the central and peripheral nervous system, may alter the renin–angiotensin system, and affect vascular tone [67]. The role of dietary potassium or the sodium: potassium ratio as a regulator of blood pressure in the young has not been investigated.

In addition to sodium and potassium, other ions may contribute significantly to blood pressure regulation. Blaustein hypothesized that a sodium–calcium exchange mechanism is one of the mechanisms controlling intracellular calcium activity, and as such

controls vascular tone [74]. Epidemiologic studies report variable associations with blood pressure and calcium intake [75–77]. A more specific association of calcium was reported by Resnick and coworkers, who found a significantly positive correlation of serum calcium with plasma renin activity in essential hypertension and a negative correlation of serum magnesium with renin activity in essential hypertension [78]. While it is plausible that calcium may play a significant role in blood pressure regulation, further study is necessary to clarify this.

GLUCOSE-INSULIN

An association of plasma insulin with blood pressure in children (9–12 years) was first reported by Florey and colleagues [79]. They found a weak relationship of insulin with blood pressure and a stronger relationship between plasma glucose and blood pressure in childhood. Voors and associates compared childhood blood pressure strata with an index of peripheral insulin resistance. The product of the 1-h glucose and insulin level following a glucose load was greatest in white males in the highest blood pressure stratum. They also found a correlation of 1-h insulin with body weight in all blood pressure strata for blacks and whites [80]. In children, Smoak and co-authors [81] reported a relationship of obesity to the clustering of systolic blood pressure, fasting insulin, and plasma lipids in children. In another report from the Bogalusa Heart Study, fasting insulin levels track in older children (9–14 years), correlate with blood pressure and ponderosity, and are significantly higher in black children [82]. Rocchini and colleagues [83] studied the effect of diet, exercise, and weight loss on blood pressure and plasma insulin levels in obese adolescents. While weight loss resulted in a decrease in plasma insulin and blood pressure, they also found, in the group with added exercise, that the decrease in blood pressure was related to the decrease in fasting insulin independent of the changes in body weight or body fat. This report suggests that the effect of insulin on blood pressure may be mediated by factors other than adiposity.

Experimental studies in Sprague–Dawley rats have demonstrated that a diet high in refined sugars results in an increase in plasma insulin and a concurrent increase in blood pressure [84]. The addition of exercise training to the sugar-loaded animals attenuated the increase in both plasma insulin and blood pressure [85]. The link between insulin-stimulated glucose metabolism and high blood pressure remains to be determined. Until the mechanisms underlying this phenomenon are clarified, it is reasonable to modify children's diets to replace refined sugar with complex carbohydrates.

RENAL

Manipulations of blood volume, by altering sodium and potassium intake in essential hypertension, appear to unmask an aberrant relationship between sympathetic tone and vascular sensitivity. Guyton and colleagues have proposed that the kidney functions as the final common pathway of blood pressure regulation by its control of salt and water excretion in both essential hypertension and in the normotensive state [86]. Changes in renal blood flow have been identified in early mild hypertension [87] and in normotensive offspring of hypertensive parents [88,89]. Bianchi and co-authors [88] demonstrated that normotensive children of hypertensive parents have a significantly raised renal plasma flow and a tendency toward lower plasma renin activity. These observations indicate that these children have a slightly raised extracellular fluid volume. On the other hand, Hollenberg and coworkers demonstrated that during psychologic stimulation renal blood flow decreases and plasma renin activity increases in patients with essential hypertension and also in the normotensive offspring of hypertensive individuals [90,91]. These investigations have demonstrated variations in renal regulation of volume by sodium excretion in the young. This function is related not only to sodium load, but also appears to be associated with neurogenic activity and a genetic predisposition for essential hypertension.

Light and associates [92] have provided some evidence to link variations in sympathetic nervous system function to changes in blood volume via renal regulation of sodium excretion. In young adult men under the stress of intense competitive tasks, sodium excretion decreased in the high-risk group for hypertension and increased in the low-risk group [92]. Skrabal and colleagues studied salt-sensitive young men with a positive family history of hypertension. The greater sympathetic responsiveness in the salt-sensitive offspring of hypertensive individuals was linked to enhanced proximal tubular sodium reabsorption [93]. These studies indicate that the tendency to retain sodium during neurogenic stress may be genetically mediated and may also contribute to the development of essential hypertension.

CARDIAC

The predisposition to essential hypertension, or the prehypertensive state in childhood, is regulated through genetic factors. Culpepper and co-authors [94] proposed that the genetic predisposition in the young may facilitate the development of cardio-vascular changes at pressure loads which are mildly elevated and of relatively short duration. These investigators and others have demonstrated that adolescents with blood pressure in the highest quartile have greater left ventricular mass and myocardial posterior wall thickness [95−97]. Schieken and coworkers [98] demonstrated that adolescents in the upper blood pressure quartile had increasing vascular resistance after adjusting for body size. These data concur with a study by Mahoney and associates [99], who demonstrated greater FVR at maximal vasodilatation in adolescents at the upper blood pressure quartile, suggesting the presence of changes in vascular structure in the high blood pressure group.

A biracial study of echocardiographic function and blood pressure in children of young adults in Bogalusa demonstrated a correlation of cardiac output with body size, and an increase in cardiac output with age and blood pressure quartile. Following adjustment for body size, white males had greater cardiac output than black males. Black males had higher peripheral vascular resistance than whites. Of further interest was the finding that peripheral vascular resistance was greater in black males than white males, even at lower blood pressure quartiles [100].

Echocardiography with Doppler measurements is beginning to provide new insights to cardiovascular structure and hemodynamics in the young. In a study by Schieken and coworkers [101] on aortic stiffness, the maximal frequency shift in the descending aorta divided by the Doppler acceleration time was investigated in 11-year-old children. These investigators found that aortic stiffness, after adjustment for height and weight, correlated significantly with systolic but not with diastolic blood pressure. In another report, Graettinger and colleagues [102] investigated diastolic blood pressure as a determinant of Doppler left ventricular filling indices in normotensive adolescents. In their study, systolic blood pressure did not correlate with any of the Doppler filling indices, although systolic pressure was related to echocardiographic left ventricular mass. Diastolic pressure did not correlate with left ventricular mass in these normotensive adolescents. However, there was a significant inverse relationship of diastolic blood pressure with parameters of left ventricular filling indices. The authors suggest that these changes may be very early manifestations of prehypertensive alterations in left ventricular diastolic function.

Echocardiography provides a noninvasive technology to study cardiovascular development in children and has sufficient sensitivity to detect early deviations in both structure and function. Its limitations at present are related to the predictability of present findings to the development of future hypertension for given individuals. This issue will be resolved by extended longitudinal studies or correlation of echocardiographic measures with other markers that strongly relate to the prehypertensive condition. An example of other potential markers, which have been investigated, is the cell membrane transport rate of electrolytes. However, to date these techniques do not clearly identify prehypertensive people.

Another issue regarding the application of echocardiographic technology to the detection of prehypertensive children is the available data for normal limits. Further data are needed to determine the relationship of left ventricular mass to height across age groups before the upper normal limits of left ventricular mass can be defined and criteria for left ventricular hypertrophy in childhood determined [103].

CATION TRANSPORT

Clearly, the etiologic factors in essential hypertension cannot be assessed for their isolated effects. One factor affects the function of other factors or systems. A unifying etiologic mechanism in essential hypertension may be some genetically mediated factor operating at a molecular or cellular level. Such a biologic element may be related to cell membrane function. Basic studies have demonstrated the presence of a plasma factor which effects a prolonged diuresis [104]. Volume expansion may enhance release of this natriuretic hormone. This substance then exerts a generalized effect in dampening the electrogenic sodium–potassium membrane pumps. In the kidney, this effect would reduce sodium reabsorption. However, this interference with sodium pump mechanisms on other cells such as vascular smooth muscle cells or tonically active autonomic

neurons would enhance sensitivity to neurogenic stimuli [8].

Variations in sodium transport mechanisms have been described in essential hypertension. Canessa and coworkers [105] demonstrated an increase in the maximum rate of sodium–lithium countertransport in hypertensive subjects, while Garay and Meyer, [106] reported a relative deficiency in the sodium–potassium cotransport system. Both investigators have also found similar changes in first-degree relatives of hypertensive individuals.

Studies by Canessa and colleagues have provided evidence that the functional role of sodium–potassium cotransport is to perform net sodium extrusion under physiologic ionic conditions. The "second sodium pump" might be present in the late proximal tubule, the loop of Henle, and in the distal tubule as well as in vascular smooth muscle or arterial endothelium [105]. It is suggested that these membrane transport mechanisms are linked to sodium–potassium adenosine triphosphatase (Na^+-K^+-ATPase), which generated the sodium and potassium gradients utilized by sodium–potassium transport. The Na^+-K^+-ATPase will be specifically important if the sodium pump is modulated by plasma factors (hormonal).

It has been proposed that the natriuretic hormone alters the sodium pump. The net effect of inhibition of Na^+-K^+-ATP would be natriuresis, decrease in sodium pump, and increased vascular smooth muscle contractility. The genetic result is an altered vascular response to neurogenic stimuli [8].

SUMMARY

Blood pressure is the response to a variety of interacting mechanisms. A single etiologic factor for essential hypertension has not been isolated. In the young, while the aberrant mechanisms leading to hypertension are probably operative, their effect on blood pressure is small. However, the effect of these dysregulatory patterns on other parameters may be greater. For example, the effect of a sodium load on the renal excretory capacity may result in a greater effect on the extracellular volume than on blood pressure in the young. Similarly, in the young, cardiovascular reactivity to certain stimuli may be quite different among various risk groups, while little difference is present in resting blood pressure.

Much is yet to be determined about the pathogenetic mechanisms for essential hypertension which are operating in the young. However, what is currently relevant is the ability to identify those individuals who would benefit from greater surveillance. As suggested by Holland and Beresford [15], children of parents having elevated blood pressure are a logical group to observe and in whom possibly to institute preventive measures.

REFERENCES

1 Londe S, Bourgoignie JJ, Robson AM, Goldring D. Hypertension in apparently normal children. *J Pediatr* 1971;78:569−77.

2 Report of the Task Force on blood pressure control in children. *Pediatrics* 1977;58(suppl):797−820.

3 Zinner SA, Levy PS, Kass EH. Familial aggregation of blood pressure in childhood. *N Engl J Med* 1971;284:401.

4 Berenson GS, Cresanta JL, Weber LS. High blood pressure in the young. *Annu Rev Med* 1984;35:535−60.

5 Paffenbarger RS Jr, Thorne MC, Wing AL. Chronic disease in former college students. VIII. Characteristics in youth predisposing to hypertension in later years. *Am J Epidemiol* 1968;88:25−32.

6 Such AF, Mendlowitz M, Wolf RL, Gitlow SR, Naftchi NE. Identification of essential hypertension in patients with labile blood pressure. *Chest* 1971;59:402−6.

7 Gutmann MC, Benson H. Interaction of environmental factors in the systemic arterial blood pressure. *Medicine* 1971;50:543−53.

8 Folkow B. Physiological aspects of primary hypertension. *Physiol Rev* 1982;62(2):347−504.

9 Cassel J. Studies of hypertension in migrants. In: Oglesby P, ed. *Epidemiology and Control of Hypertension*. New York: Stratton International, 1975:41−5.

10 Stamler J, Berkson DM, Lindberg HA. Socioeconomic factors in the epidemiology of hypertensive disease. In: Stamler J, Stamler F, Pullman TN, eds. *The Epidemiology of Hypertension*. New York: Grune & Stratton, 1967.

11 Shaper AG. Cardiovascular disease in the tropics. III Blood pressure and hypertension. *Br Med J* 1972;3:805−7.

12 Cruz-Coke R, Etcheverry R, Nagel R. Influence of migration on blood pressure of Eastern Islanders. *Lancet* 1964;i:697−9.

13 Beaglehole R, Salmond CE, Prior IAM. Blood pressure studies in Polynesian children. In: Oglesby P, ed. *Epidemiology and Control of Hypertension*. New York: Stratton International, 1975:407−17.

14 Cabral EI, Lopez WL, Guzman SV, Abesamis BY, De la Paz A. Blood pressure in infants and children from Luzon. In: Onesti G, Kim K, eds. *Hypertension in the Young and the Old* New York: Grune & Stratton, 1981:149−53.

15 Holland WW, Beresford SAA. Factors influencing blood pressure in children. In: Oglesby P, ed. *Epidemiology and Control of Hypertension*. New York: Stratton International, 1975;375−83.

16 Harlan WR, Cornoni-Huntley J, Leaverton PE. Blood pressure in childhood. National Health Examination Survey. *Hypertension* 1979;1:559−65.

17 Cornoni-Huntley J, Harlan WR, Leaverton PE. Blood pressure in adolescents. US Health Examination Survey. *Hypertension* 1979;1:566−71.

18 Prineas RJ, Gillum RS, Horibe H, Hannan PF. Minneapolis Children's Blood Pressure Study. Part II: Multiple determinants of blood pressure. *Hypertension* 1980;2(suppl): I 24−8.

19 Katz SH, Hediger MC, Schall JI et al. Blood pressure, growth and maturation from childhood to adolescence. *Hypertension* 1980;2(suppl I):55−69.

20 Voors AW, Webber LS, Harsha DH, Berenson GS. Racial differences in cardiovascular risk factors of youth. Bogalusa Heart Study. In: *Abstracts of 18th Annual Conference on Cardiovascular Disease, Epidemiology*. Dallas, TX: American Heart Association 1978.

21 Report of the Hypertension Task Force. *Current Research and Recommendations from the Task Force Reports on Therapy, Pregnancy, Obesity*, vol 9. Publication (NIH) 79−1631. US Department of Health, Education and Welfare, Washington, DC. 1979.

22 Havlik RD, Hubert HB, Fabsity RR, Feinleib M. Weight and hypertension. *Ann Intern Med* 1983;98:855−9.

23 Lauer RM, Clarke WR, Beaglehole R. Level, trend, and variability of blood pressure during childhood. The Muscatine Study. *Circulation* 1984;69:242−9.

24 Dustan HP. Mechanisms of hypertension associated with obesity. *Ann Intern Med* 1983;98:860−4.

25 Reisin E, Abel R, Modan M, Silverberg DS, Eliahou HE, Modan B. The effect of weight loss without salt restriction on the reduction of blood pressure in overweight hypertensive patients. *N Engl J Med* 1978;298:1−6.

26 Frohlich ED, Messerli FD, Reisin E, Dunn FG. The problem of obesity and hypertension. *Hypertension* 1983;5(suppl III):III 71−8.

27 Katz SH, Hediger ML, Zemel BS, Parks IS. Blood pressure, body fat, and dehydroepiandrosterone sulfate variation in adolescence. *Hypertension* (in press).

28 Report of the Second Task Force on Blood Pressure Control in Children. *Pediatrics* 1987;79(1):1−25.

29 Goldstein DS. Plasma catecholamines in essential hypertension: an analytical review. *Hypertension* 1983;5:86−99.

30 Goldstein DS, Labe CR, Chernow B et al. Age dependence of hypertensive−normotensive differences in plasma norepinephrine. *Hypertension* 1983;5(1):108−4.

31 Brod J, Fencl V, Higi A, Jirka J. Circulatory change underlying blood pressure elevation during acute emotional distress (mental arithmetic) in normotensive and hypertensive subjects. *Clin Sci* 1959;18:269−75.

32 Light KC. Cardiovascular responses to effortful coping: implications for the role of stress in hypertension development. *Psychophysiology* 1981;18:261−70.

33 Light KC, Obrist PA. Cardiovascular reactivity to behavioral stress in young males with and without marginally elevated casual systolic pressure: a comparison of clinic, home, and laboratory measures. *Hypertension* 1980;2:802−8.

34 Manuck SB, Proietti JM. Parental hypertension and cardiovascular response to cognitive and isometric challenge. *Psychophysiology* 1982;19(5):481−9.

35 Bauman R, Ziprian H, Godicke W, Hartrodt W, Naumman E, Lauter J. The influence of acute psychic stress situations and vegetative parameters of essential hypertension at the early stage of the disease. *Psychother Psycosom* 1973;22:131−40.

36 Nestle PJ. Blood pressure and catecholamine excretion after mental stress in labile hypertension. *Lancet* 1969;i:692−5.

37 Falkner B, Onesti G, Angelakos ET, Fernandez M, Langman C. Cardiovascular response to mental stress in normal adolescents with hypertensive parents. *Hypertension* 1979;1:23.

38 Lawler KA, Allen NT. Risk factors for hypertension in children: their relationship to psychophysiologic responses. *J Psychosom Res* 1981;23:199−204.

39 Collins FH, Baer PE, Bourianoof GG. Orienting behavior of children with hypertensive fathers. Paper presented at the Annual Meeting of the Society for Psychophysiologic Research. Vancouver BC, 1980.

40 McCrory WW, Klein AA, Rosenthal RA. Blood pressure, heart rate, and plasma catecholamines in normal and hypertensive children and their siblings at rest and after standing. *Hypertension* 1982;4(4):507−13.

41 Katz SH, Zemel B, Hediger ML *et al*. Resting, seated and supine blood pressure interrelationship in adolescents. In: Gruskin AB, Norman ME, eds. *Proceedings of the International Pediatric Nephrology Symposium*. The Hague: Martinus Nijhoff, 1980.

42 Julius S, Randall OS, Esler MD, Kashima T, Ellis C, Bennett J. Altered cardiac responsiveness and regulation in the normal cardiac output type of borderline hypertension. *Circ Res* 1975;36,37(suppl I):I−199.

43 Stamler J, Katz LN, Pick R, Rodbard S. Dietary and hormonal factors in experimental atherogenesis and blood pressure regulation. In: Pincus G, ed. *Recent Progress in Hormone Research*. New York: Academic Press, 1955: 401−52.

44 Dahl LK. Evidence for an increased intake of sodium in hypertension based on urinary excretion of sodium. *Proc Soc Exp Biol Med* 1957;94:23.

45 Freis ED. Salt, volume and the prevention of hypertension. *Circulation* 1976;53:589−95.

46 Swaye PS, Gifford RW, Berrenttoni JN. Dietary salt and essential hypertension. *Am J Cardiol* 1972;29:33−8.

47 Dawber TR, Kannel WB, Kogan A, Donabedian RK, McNamara PM, Pearson G. Environmental factors in hypertension. In: Stamler J, Stamler R, Pullman TN, eds. *The Epidemiology of Hypertension*. New York: Grave & Stratton, 1967:255.

48 Tuthill RW, Calabrese EJ. Elevated sodium levels in the public drinking water as a contributor to elevated blood pressure levels in the community. *Arch Environ Health* 1979;34:197−204.

49 Hofman A, Valhenburg HA, Vaandroger GJ. Increased blood pressure in school children related to high sodium levels in drinking water. *J Epidemiol Commun Health* 1980; 34:179−81.

50 Hallenbeck WH, Brenninmon GR, Anderson RJ. High sodium in drinking water and its effect on blood pressure. *Am J Epidemiol* 1981;114:817−26.

51 Pomrehn PR, Clarke WR, Sowers MF, Wallace RB, Lauer RM. Community differences in blood pressure levels and drinking water sodium. *Am J Epidemiol* 1983;118:60−71.

52 Folson AR, Prineas RJ. Drinking water composition and blood pressure: a review of the epidemiology. *Am J Epidemiol* 1982;115:818−32.

53 Cooper R, Soltero I, Liu K, Berkson D, Levinson S, Stamler J. The association between urinary sodium excretion and blood pressure in children. *Circulation* 1980;62:97−104.

54 Hofman A, Hazelbrock A, Valkenburg HA. A randomized trial of sodium intake and blood pressure in newborn infants. *JAMA* 1983;250:370−3.

55 MacGregor GA, Best F, Cam J. Double-blind randomized crossover trial of moderate sodium restriction in essential hypertension. *Lancet* 1982;i:351−5.

56 Costa FV, Ambrosioni E, Montebugnoli L, Paccaloni L, Basconi L, Magnani B. Effect of a low salt diet and of acute salt loading and blood pressure and intralymphocytic sodium concentration in young subjects with borderline hypertension. *Clin Sci* 1981;51:21−3.

57 Dahl LK, Heine M, Tassinari L. Effects of chronic excess salt ingestion: evidence that genetic factors play an important role in susceptibility to experimental hypertension. *J Exp Med* 1962;15:1173−90.

58 Luft FC, Rankin LI, Henry DP *et al*. Plasma and urinary norepinephrine values at extremes of sodium intake in normal men. *Hypertension* 1979;1:261−6.

59 Luft FC, Grim CE, Higgins JT Jr, Weinberger MH. Difference in response to sodium administration in normotensive white and black subjects. *J Lab Clin Med* 1977;90: 555−62.

60 Masuo K, Ogihara T, Kumahara Y, Yamatodani A, Wada H. Increased plasma norepinephrine in young patients with essential hypertension under three sodium intakes. *Hypertension* 1984;6:315−21.

61 Sullivan JM, Ratts TE, Taylor JC *et al*. Hemodynamic effects of dietary sodium in man. *Hypertension* 1980;2:506−14.

62 Robertson D, Shand DG, Hollinfield JW, Nies AS, Frolich JC, Oates JA. Alterations in the responses of the sympathetic nervous system and renin in borderline hypertension. *Hypertension* 1979;1:118−24.

63 Falkner B, Onesti G, Angelakos E. Effect of salt loading on the cardiovascular response to stress in adolescents. *Hypertension* 1981;3(suppl II):II 195−9.

64 Kirkendall WM, Connor WE, Abboud F, Rastogi SP, Anderson TA, Fry M. The effect of dietary sodium on blood pressure of normotensive men. In: Genesti J, ed. *International Symposium on Renin−Angiotensin. Adolescence-Sodium in Hypertension*. Berlin: Springer-Verlag, 1972; 360−73.

65 Mark AL, Lawton J, Abboud FM, Fitz AE, Connor WE, Heistad DD. Effects of high and low sodium intake on arterial pressure and forearm vascular resistance in borderline hypertension. *Circulation* 1975;36,37(suppl):I-194.

66 Koolen MI, Van Brummelen P. Adrenergic activity and peripheral hemodynamics in relation to sodium sensitivity in patients with essential hypertension. *Hypertension* 1984; 6:820−5.

67 Treasure J, Ploth D. Role of dietary potassium in the treatment of hypertension. *Hypertension* 1983;5:864−72.

68 Tobian L, MacNeil D, Johnson MA, Ganguli MC, Iwai J. Potassium protection against lesions of the renal tubules, arteries, and glomeruli and nephron loss in salt-loaded hypertensive Dahl S. rats. *Hypertension* 1984;6(suppl I):I-170−6.

69 Anderson DE, Kearns WD, Better WE. Progressive hypertension in dogs by avoidance conditioning and saline infusion. *Hypertension* 1983;5:286−91.

70 Anderson DE, Kearns WD, Worden TJ. Potassium infusion attenuates avoidance-saline hypertension in dogs. *Hypertension* 1983;5:415—420.

71 Berenson GS, Webber LS, Srinivasan SR, Cresanta JL, Frank GC, Farris R. Black—white contrasts as determinants of cardiovascular risk in childhood. Precursors of coronary artery and primary hypertensive diseases. *Am Heart J* 1984;108:672—83.

72 Fujito Tan Ando K. Hemodynamic and endocrine changes associated with potassium supplementation in sodium-loaded hypertensives. *Hypertension* 1984;6:184—92.

73 Skrabal F, Aubock J, Hortnagi H. Low sodium—high potassium diet for prevention of hypertension: probable mechanisms of action. *Lancet* 1981;2(8252)895—900.

74 Blaustein M. Sodium ions, calcium ions, blood pressure regulation and hypertension, a reassessment and a hypothesis. *Am J Physiol* 1977;232:C165—73.

75 Stanton JL, Braitman LE, Riley AM, Koo CS, Smith JL. Demographic, dietary, life style and anthropometric correlates of blood pressure. *Hypertension* 1982;4(SUPPL III):III-136—42.

76 Connor SL, Connor WE, Henry H, Sexton G, Keenan EJ. The effects of familial relationships, age, body weight and diet on blood pressure and the 24-hour urinary excretion of sodium, potassium and creatinine in men, women, and children of randomly selected families. *Circulation* 1984;70:76—85.

77 Garcia-Palmieri MR, Costas R, Cruz-Vidal M, Sorlie PD, Tillotson J, Havlik R. Milk consumption, calcium intake and decreased hypertension in Puerto Rico. *Hypertension* 1984;6:322—8.

78 Resnick LM, Laragh JH, Sealey JE, Alderman MH. Divalent cations in essential hypertension. Relations between serum ionized calcium, magnesium, and plasma renin activity. *N Engl J Med* 1983;309:888—91.

79 Florey CV, Uppal S, Lowy S. Relation between blood pressure, weight, and plasma sugar and serum insulin levels in school children aged 9—12 years in Westward Holland. *Br Med J* 1976;1:1368—71.

80 Voors AW, Radhakrishnamurthy B, Srinivasan SR, Webber LS, Berenson GS. Plasma glucose level related to blood pressure in 272 children ages 7—15 years sampled from a total biracial population. *Am J Hygiene* 1981;113:347—56.

81 Smoak CG, Burke GL, Webber LS, Harsha DW, Srinivasan SR, Berenson GS. Relation of obesity to clustering of cardiovascular disease risk factors in children and young adults. *Am J Epidemiol* 1987;125:364—72.

82 Burke GL, Webber LS, Srinivasan SR, Radhakrishnamurthy B, Freedman DS, Berenson GS. Fasting plasma glucose and insulin levels and their relationship to cardiovascular risk factors in children: the Bogalusa heart study. *Metabolism* 1986;35:441—6.

83 Rocchini AP, Katch V, Schork A, Kelch RP. Insulin and blood pressure during weight loss in obese adolescents. *Hypertension* 1987;10:367—73.

84 Hwang I-S, Ho H, Hoffman B, Reaven G. Fructose-induced insulin resistance and hypertension in rats. *Hypertension* 1987;10:512—16.

85 Reaven GM, Ho H, Hoffman BB. Attenuation of fructose-induced hypertension in rats by exercise training. *Hypertension* 1988;12:129—32.

86 Guyton AC, Coleman TG, Crowley AW, Schell KW, Manning RD, Norman RA. Arterial pressure regulation. *Am J Med* 1972;52:584—94.

87 Hollenberg NK, Adams DF. Renal circulation in hypertensive disease. *Am J Med* 1976;60:773—84.

88 Bianchi G, Picotti GB, Bratchi G *et al*. Familial hypertension and hormonal profile, renal hemodynamics, and body fluids of young normotensive subjects. *Clin Sci Mol Med* 1978;4:3675—715.

89 Hollenberg NK, Adams DF, Solomon H, Chenitz WR, Burger BM, Abrams HL. Renal vascular tone in essential hypertension and secondary hypertension: hemodynamics and angiographic responses to vasodilators. *Medicine* 1975;54:29—44.

90 Hollenberg NK, Williams GH, Adams DF. Essential hypertension: abnormal renal vascular and endocrine response to mild psychogenic stimulus. *Hypertension* 1981;3(1):11—17.

91 Hollenberg NK, Sandor T. Vasomotion of renal blood flow in essential hypertension. Oscillations in xenon transit. *Hypertension* 1984;6:579—85.

92 Light KC, Koepke JP, Obrist PA, Willis PW. Psychological stress induces sodium and fluid retention in men at risk for hypertension. *Science* 1983;220:429—31.

93 Skrabal F, Herholz H, Newymar M *et al*. Salt sensitivity in humans is linked to enhanced sympathetic responsiveness to enhanced proximal tubular reabsorption. *Hypertension* 1984;6:152—8.

94 Culpepper WS, Sodt PC, Messerli FH, Ruschhaupt DC, Arcilla RA. Cardiac status in juvenile borderline hypertension. *Ann Intern Med* 1983;98(1):1—7.

95 Laird WP, Fixler DE. Left ventricular hypertrophy in adolescents with elevated blood pressure: assessment by chest roentgenography, electrocardiography, and echocardiography. *Pediatrics* 1981;67:255.

96 Goldring D, Hernandez A, Choi S *et al*. Blood pressure in a high school population. II *Clin J Pediatr* 1979;95:298—304.

97 Zahka KG, Neill CA, Kidd L, Cutilletta MA, Cutilletta AF. Cardiac involvement in adolescent hypertension. *Hypertension* 1981;3:664—8.

98 Schieken RM, Clarke WR, Lauer RM. Left ventricular hypertrophy in children with blood pressure in the upper quartiles of distribution. The Muscatine study. *Hypertension* 1981;3:669—75.

99 Mahoney LT, Clarke WR, Mark AL, Lauer RM. Forearm vascular resistance in the upper and lower quartiles of blood pressure in adolescent boys. *Pediatr Res* 1982;16:163—5.

100 Soto LF, Kitcuchi DA, Arcilla RA, Savage DD, Berenson SG. Echocardiographic functions and blood pressure levels in children and young adults from a biracial population. The Bogalusa heart study. *Am J Med Sci* 1989;297(5):271—9.

101 Schieken RM, Moskowitz WB, Bodurtha J, Mosteller M, Eaves L, Nance W. Aortic stiffness: A new Doppler echocardiographic measure predictive of systolic blood pressure in children. *J Am Coll Cardiol* 1988;11:1297—1300.

102 Graettinger WF, Weber MA, Gardin JM, Knoll ML. Diastolic blood pressure as a determinant of Doppler left ventricular filling indexes in normotensive adolescents. *J Am Coll Cardiol* 1987;10:1280—5.

103 Daniels SR, Meyer RA, Liang Y, Bove KE. Echocardiographically determined left ventricular mass index in normal children, adolescents, and young adults. *J Am Coll*

Cardiol 1988;12:703−8.

104 DeWardener HE. Natriuretic hormone. *Clin Sci Mol Med* 1977;53:1−8.

105 Canessa M, Adragna N, Solomon HS, Conolly TM, Tosteson DC. Increased sodium lithium counter transport in red cells of patients with essential hypertension. *N Engl J Med* 1980;302:772.

106 Garay RP, Meyer P. A new test showing abnormal net Na^+ and K^+ fluxes in erythrocytes of essential hypertensive patients. *Lancet* 1979;i:349.

107 Canessa M, Spalvins A, Falkner B. Red cell Na^+ counter transport and cotransport in normotensive and hypertensive blacks and their juvenile offspring. *Hypertension* 1984; 6:344−51.

18 Management of Patients with Essential Hypertension

STEPHEN R. DANIELS

INTRODUCTION

Over the last decade there has been an increasing interest in hypertension in children. The publication of standards of normality for blood pressure in infants, children, and adolescents has led to an increase in the frequency with which it is measured in these age groups. Moreover, the question of which children to treat and when, if they have essential hypertension, has come to the forefront. The drug treatment of secondary hypertension in youngsters is widely accepted by pediatricians, even when it is in the range seen with primary hypertension. The benefits of pharmacologic therapy in youths with severe hypertension have been established clinically [1–3]. The goal of therapy for these patients is to lower blood pressure to a normal or near-normal level for age without causing unpleasant side-effects. If there is an underlying cause that is surgically correctable, this can then be addressed. Both pharmacologic and non-pharmacologic methods have been used to lower blood pressure in patients with secondary hypertension but rarely can they be managed by the latter alone. Since blood pressure is often markedly elevated in these patients, they often require two or three different drugs in order to achieve normotension.

The treatment of primary hypertension in childhood is more controversial. Much of the difficulty lies in the lack of definitive knowledge about the relationship between childhood and adult blood pressure levels, and the absence of documentation of the association between hypertension in childhood and the subsequent development of morbidity and mortality (see Chapter 31). This means that, given the current state of knowledge, it is not possible to predict which children are at risk for future problems as they grow into adulthood, and if they are at risk, how great the risk may be. Further, with respect to morbidity, no clinical trials have been performed in which the natural history of essential hypertension in children has been compared to the drug-treated history.

STUDIES ON ADULTS

A number of clinical trials have been done in hypertensive adults. It may be helpful to extrapolate from the results of these studies on the question of the efficacy of treatment because more definitive studies have been done which make the guidelines for the treatment of essential hypertension clearer for adults, particularly when they have moderate or severe hypertension.

A number of studies have established that elevated systolic and diastolic blood pressure increases the risk of cardiovascular disease in adults [3–5]. The Society of Actuaries has shown that there is no threshold pressure at which the risk suddenly increases, but rather there is a smooth gradation of rising risk with increasing blood pressure [6]. Data from the Framingham study also support the concept of a continuous risk function [7].

The protection against the increased risk of cardiovascular disease which is provided by antihypertensive drug therapy has also been definitely demonstrated for adults. The Veterans Administration Cooperative Study followed male veterans with diastolic blood pressures between 90 and 129 mmHg [8,9]. Subjects who were randomly allocated to the treatment group were given a diuretic, reserpine, and a vasodilator. The study showed that, exclusive of myocardial infarction, morbidity and mortality were markedly diminished in the drug-treated group with diastolic blood pressure greater than 104 mmHg. In the group with blood pressure between 90 and 104 mmHg treatment also improved outcome, but the improvement was less than that for the group with higher blood pressure [8,9].

Other studies have since expanded on these find-ings. The Hypertension Detection and Follow-up Program was a large-scale, community-based, ran-domized controlled clinical trial of antihypertensive therapy [10−13]. Blood pressure was screened in 158 906 adults between the ages of 30 and 69. The 10 940 individuals found to have persistently elevated blood pressure were included in the study. In all, 71% had diastolic blood pressure 90−104 mmHg, 19% had diastolic pressures between 105 and 114 mmHg, and 10% were over 115 mmHg. The subjects were randomized to a group who were referred to the usual health care resources in the community (referred-care) or to an experimental group who received aggressive stepped-care antihypertensive therapy (stepped-care). Subjects in both groups were followed over a 5-year period. The stepped-care group had a 20% lower overall mortality than the referred-care group. This decreased mortality was associated with a 5 mmHg lower average diastolic blood pressure in the stepped-care group. It is important to re-member, however, that the 20% reduction in mor-tality represents an actual difference in survival of 1.5% between the two groups. In the stepped-care group, 94% of the subjects were alive at the end of 5 years compared to 92.5% in the referred-care subjects [10,11]. Also for the youngest group in the study (ages 30−49) there were no differences in mortality between the stepped-care and referred-care groups [11].

The Australian trial is another clinical trial of anti-hypertensive drug therapy in adults [14]. The subjects in this trial were free of identifiable cardiovascular damage at the time of entry. The trial was stopped after 6 years with an average follow-up of 4 years, when it was noted that the drug-treated group had 30% less morbidity and mortality than did the group treated with placebo. This decrease was associated with an average diastolic blood pressure 6 mmHg lower in the treatment group. However, closer analy-sis of the study reveals that the 30% excess morbidity occurred in placebo-treated subjects whose diastolic blood pressure averaged above 100 mmHg. For those with diastolic blood pressure below 100 mmHg there were fewer complications for those on placebo than those on drug therapy [15]. There are several possible explanations for this result, but one is that for adult patients with diastolic blood pressure below 100 mmHg the risk of drug therapy may begin to outweigh the benefits of blood pressure reduction over the short term. The experience of the Multiple

Risk Factor Intervention Trial (MRFIT) may support this conclusion. The MRFIT study showed increased mortality in the retrospectively identified group of subjects with electrocardiogram abnormalities at entry, including ventricular premature beats, incom-plete right bundle branch block, first-degree atrio-ventricular block, and ST depression or elevation; this group then received drug treatment with thiazide diuretics during the study [16].

The interpretation of the results from each of these large clinical trials has been somewhat contro-versial. This has led to much discussion about what level of blood pressure gives a favorable risk:benefit ratio for pharmacologic treatment of hypertension in adults, [17−19]. A Lancet editorial suggests that within the population of adults with mild hyperten-sion there are probably subsets of individuals who are at increased risk for developing specific compli-cations of hypertension [20]. If further research can better define these subsets it may help to resolve the dilemma of when to treat patients with mild hypertension.

WHEN TO LOWER BLOOD PRESSURE IN CHILDREN

This is a complicated subject for which no clear answer is available. From the preceding discussion it should be evident that even for adults there is contro-versy about whether or not mild hypertension should be treated. For children, some have suggested that essential hypertension should be treated with phar-macologic agents only when the blood pressure is very high, while others have suggested more ag-gressive treatment guidelines similar to those used for adults [21]. Oliver has pointed out that there is an important difference between removing a risk fac-tor such as smoking and adding a new, perhaps unknown, risk by prescribing a drug to lower blood pressure [22]. He has also said that the aggressive-ness in drug prescription for hypertension should be inversely proportional to age [22]. Nevertheless, antihypertensive therapy is necessary for children in hypertensive emergencies or with chronic blood pressure elevation which cannot be ameliorated by nonpharmacologic means.

Berenson and coworkers [23] have shown that blood pressure can be lowered in pediatric patients using a combination of pharmacologic and nonphar-macologic therapy. They studied 1604 children, who constituted 89% of all children aged 8−18 years in the biracial community of Franklinton, LA. After an initial blood pressure screening, those children in the upper decile for mean blood pressure were re-examined on three occasions. Children who remained consistently in the top decile were then randomly assigned to a treatment or a comparison group. The treatment consisted of: (a) dietary counseling and alteration to reduce sodium and calories; (b) encouragement to increase aerobic exercise; and (c) drug treatment with low-dose propranolol and chlorthalidone. It was found that during the 6 months of observation the average systolic and diastolic blood pressure of the children in the treatment group remained 5 and 3 mmHg lower respectively than the control group.

The study of Berenson and co-authors [23] may answer the question of whether blood pressure can be lowered in children—this was never in doubt, based on extensive clinical experience. However, it does not begin to answer the question of whether this is good for children. No outcome measures other than blood pressure levels were studied and the subjects were only followed over a 6-month period. Further research is needed better to delineate when the pharmacologic treatment of essential hypertension in children is advantageous.

The risk for cardiovascular disease is based on a number of factors, including the level of blood pressure. Other important risk factors include a positive family history of cardiovascular disease, abnormal plasma lipids and lipoproteins, glucose intolerance, smoking, and the presence of early target-organ damage such as the presence of left ventricular hypertrophy. All of these factors should be considered in the decision to treat children with essential hyper-

tension with antihypertensive drugs.

Despite all of the difficulties involved in the decision of when to treat hypertension in children, the Second Task Force on blood pressure control in children has published guidelines for making this decision [24]. The Task Force suggests that with the increasing recognition of mild forms of hypertension in children, the problem should be approached with an emphasis on general counseling about cardiovascular risk factors.

Children with blood pressures persistently above the 95th percentile for age and gender should be candidates for blood pressure-lowering interventions [24]. Nonpharmacologic treatment strategies, such as dietary modification, should be introduced as the initial treatment for primary hypertension at most levels of blood pressure elevation and should be tailored to meet the needs of the individual patients. The nutritional-hygienic measures that should be used are discussed in detail in Chapter 11. The Task Force defined levels of blood pressure indicative of significant and severe hypertension based on the new distribution of blood pressure by age (Table 18.1). Pharmacologic forms of antihypertensive therapy should be reserved for two instances: (a) for patients with severe hypertension; or (b) when blood pressure remains significantly elevated after several weeks to months of nonpharmacologic therapy.

Other factors to be considered in the decision-making process include the risk factors discussed previously, especially the presence of symptoms or signs related to an elevated blood pressure, and evidence of target-organ injury. It is also recommended that nonpharmacologic therapy be continued even after pharmacologic therapy is instituted as it may

Table 18.1 Classification of hypertension by age group to aid in making therapeutic decisions

Age group (years)	Significant hypertension	Severe hypertension
Newborn		
7 days	Systolic BP ≥100 mmHg	Systolic BP ≥100 mmHg
8–30 days	Systolic BP ≥100 mmHg	Systolic BP ≥120 mmHg
Infants (≤2 years)	Systolic BP ≥124 mmHg	Systolic BP ≥134 mmHg
	Diastolic BP ≥74 mmHg	Diastolic BP ≥90 mmHg
Children (3–12 years)	Systolic BP ≥130 mmHg	Systolic BP ≥144 mmHg
	Diastolic BP ≥86 mmHg	Diastolic BP ≥96 mmHg
Adolescents (13–18 years)	Systolic BP ≥144 mmHg	Systolic BP ≥160 mmHg
	Diastolic BP ≥90 mmHg	Diastolic BP ≥104 mmHg

BP = Blood pressure.

still be beneficial for the patient and may decrease his or her medication requirements. The Task Force has estimated that if nonpharmacologic treatment strategies are maximized, less than 1% of children will require drug therapy to control essential hypertension [24].

The goals of antihypertensive therapy should be: **1** to reduce the diastolic blood pressure to less than the 90th percentile for the child's age and gender; **2** to have minimal side-effects from treatment; and **3** to achieve a high degree of patient compliance. When pharmacologic therapy is necessary, the lowest dose of drug necessary to reduce blood pressure effectively should be used. It should be remembered that it may be possible to reduce or withdraw antihypertensive medication once an extended course of effective blood pressure control has been established. The continued use of nonpharmacologic measures will improve the chance of success of this process. The patient should be closely monitored during an attempt to reduce or withdraw medications in order to detect the return of blood pressure to hypertensive levels [24].

Despite the increase in knowledge on hypertension in children over the past decade, many questions remain unanswered. Loggie [25] has outlined those questions which need to be answered about the natural and drug-treated histories of primary hypertension in the young (Table 18.2). Hopefully answers to these questions will be forthcoming in the next decade. In the meantime the timing of the introduction of drug treatment for primary hypertension in pediatric patients remains an empiric decision.

Table 18.2 Questions about natural and drug-treated histories of primary hypertension in the young

---

Natural history of primary hypertension
Who develops sustained hypertension either in later childhood or in adult life?
Who is at risk to develop target-organ damage?
Why do some youths develop one complication of hypertension while others develop different complications at the same levels of pressure?
Is left ventricular hypertrophy really evidence of target-organ damage or part of the "disease"?
What is the significance of the hyperuricemia seen in some youths with early hypertension? Does it reflect subtle renal damage?
What is the time course of development of funduscopic changes in youngsters with primary hypertension?

History of treated primary hypertension
Can blood pressure be lowered to normal with nonpharmacologic interventions such as weight loss, salt restriction, and stress reduction?
Can blood pressure be lowered to normal with low doses of antihypertensive drugs?
Can target-organ damage be prevented or reversed?
Can the later risk of coronary heart disease and/or stroke be reduced by interventions?
What are the risks of drug therapy (physiologic, psychologic, biochemical, hormonal)?
Is drug therapy, once initiated, needed for the rest of life?

REFERENCES

1 Caliguri LA, Shapiro AP, Holliday MA. Clinical improvement in chronic renal hypertension in children. *Pediatrics* 1963;31:758–66.
2 Still JL, Cottom DG. Severe hypertension in childhood. *Arch Dis Child* 1967;42:34–9.
3 Gill DG, Mendes da Costa B, Cameron JS, Joseph MC, Ogg CS, Chantler C. Analysis of 100 children with severe and persistent hypertension. *Arch Dis Child* 1976;51:951–6.
4 Roberts WL. The hypertensive diseases. Evidence that systemic hypertension is a greater risk factor to the development of other cardiovascular diseases than previously suspected. *Am J Med* 1975;59:523–32.
5 Dawber TR. *The Framingham Study. The Epidemiology of Atherosclerotic Disease.* Cambridge, MA: Harvard University Press, 1980.
6 Societies of Actuaries and Association of Life Insurance Medical Directors of America. *Blood Pressure Study, 1979.* Chicago, IL: Recording and Statistical Corp., 1980.
7 Kannel WB, Dawber TR, Sorlie P, Wolf PA. Components of blood pressure and risk of atherothrombotic brain infarction: the Framingham study. *Stork* 1976;7:327–31.
8 Veterans Administration Cooperative Study Group on Antihypertensive Agents. Effects of treatment on morbidity in hypertension. Results in patients with diastolic blood pressures averaging 115 through 129 mmHg. *JAMA* 1967;202:116–22.
9 Veterans Administration Cooperative Study Group on Antihypertensive Agents. Effects of treatment on morbidity in hypertension. II. Results in patients with diastolic blood pressure averaging 90 through 114 mmHg. *JAMA* 1970;213:1143–52.
10 Hypertension Detection and Follow-Up Program Cooperative Group. Five year findings of the hypertension detection and follow-up program. I. Reduction in mortality of persons with high blood pressures, including mild hypertension. *JAMA* 1979;242:2562–71.
11 Hypertension Detection and Follow-Up Program Cooperative Group: Five year findings of the hypertension detection and follow-up program. II. Mortality by race, sex and age. *JAMA* 1979;242:2572–7.
12 Hypertension Detection and Follow-Up Program Cooperative Group: Five year findings of the hypertension detection and follow-up program. III. Reduction in stroke incidence among persons with high blood pressure. *JAMA* 1982;247:633–8.
13 Hypertension Detection and Follow-Up Program Cooperative Group: The effect of treatment on mortality in "mild"

hypertension: results of the hypertension detection and follow-up program cooperative group. *N Engl J Med* 1982; 307:976−80.

14 Report on the Management Committee. The Australian therapeutic trial in mild hypertension. *Lancet* 1980;i:1261−7.

15 Kaplan NM. Systemic hypertension: Therapy. In: Braunwald E, ed. *Heart Disease: A Textbook of Cardiovascular Medicine.* New York, NY: W.B. Saunders, 1984;922−51.

16 Multiple Risk Factor Intervention Trial Group. Multiple risk factor intervention trial: risk factors, changes and mortality results. *JAMA* 1982;248:1465−77.

17 Kaplan NM. Whom to treat: the dilemma of mild hypertension. *Am Heart J* 1981;101:867−70.

18 Sleight P. When and how far should we lower blood pressure? *Hypertension* 1983;5:(suppl III): III-14−16.

19 Taylor L, Foster MC, Beevers DG. Divergent views of hospital staff on detecting and managing hypertension. *Br Med J* 1979;1:715−16.

20 Editorial. Hypertension, risk, and left ventricular hypertrophy. *Lancet* 1984;i:941.

21 Sinaiko AR, Mirkin BL. CLinical pharmacology of antihypertensive drugs in children. *Pediatr Clin North Am* 1978; 25:137−57.

22 Oliver MF. Risks of correcting the risks of coronary disease and stroke with drugs. *N Engl J Med* 1982;306:297−8.

23 Berenson GS, Voors AW, Webber LS *et al*. A model for intervention of early essential hypertension in the 1980s. *Hypertension* 1983;5:41−53.

24 Report of the Second Task Force on Blood Pressure Control in Children. National Heart, Lung & Blood Institute. *Pediatrics* 1987;79:1−25.

25 Loggie JMH. An overview: which children with primary hypertension should be treated? In: Filer LJ, Lauer RM, eds. *Children's Blood Pressure. Report of the 88th Ross Conference on Pediatric Research.* Columbus, OH: Ross Laboratories, 1985;109−116.

19 Renal Parenchymatous Diseases Causing Hypertension

FRANK G. BOINEAU AND JOHN E. LEWY

Hypertension is a common feature of a variety of renal parenchymal diseases in children. It is a frequent problem when glomerular disease is present and in polycystic kidney disease. Hypertension occurs less often in obstructive uropathy and in chronic pyelonephritis with reflux. It is an unusual occurrence in children with primary interstitial disease until end-stage renal disease develops.

FREQUENCY OF HYPERTENSION IN RENAL DISEASE

Glomerular and small artery disease

Those glomerular and small artery diseases which are generally thought to be associated with a high prevalence of hypertension are shown in Table 19.1. A lower incidence of hypertension is found in the glomerular diseases listed in Table 19.2. When hypertension does occur in these diseases, it often does not develop until serious impairment of kidney function is present.

Chronic interstitial diseases

Table 19.3 illustrates the prevalence of hypertension in the more common of the chronic interstitial renal diseases found in children.

Prevalence of hypertension and status of renal function

In almost all types of progressive glomerular diseases, the incidence of hypertension increases in each group as renal function deteriorates. In a retrospective study by Vendemia and colleagues [1], 290 adult patients with renal parenchymal diseases were studied. The patients were divided into two major groups: 184 with glomerulonephritis and 106 with tubulointerstitial diseases. The patients in the first group were classified on clinical, histologic, and immunohistologic grounds as follows: 85 cases of immunoglobulin A (IgA) nephropathy, 40 cases of membranous glomerulopathy, 30 cases of membranoproliferative glomerulonephritis, and 29 cases of focal and segmental glomerulosclerosis. In the second group, there were 56 cases of polycystic kidney disease, 26 cases of chronic pyelonephritis, and 24 cases of analgesic nephropathy.

The patients were followed for a period ranging from 1 to 127 months. In all, 28% of those with glomerulonephritis and 60% of those with tubulo-interstitial disease interrupted medical control for more than 1 year and were removed from the study. The clinical course of the diseases were divided into four phases according to the level of renal function:

Phase I: "Normal renal function" was defined by a normal glomerular filtration rate (GFR) and a serum creatinine <1 mg/dl;

Table 19.1 Glomerular and small artery diseases associated with a high prevalence of hypertension

Acute postinfectious glomerulonephritis
Glomerulonephritis secondary to systemic vasculitides
Polyarteritis involving the kidney
Crescentic glomerulonephritis
Focal and segmental glomerulosclerosis
Cortical necrosis
Hemolytic–uremic syndrome

Table 19.2 Glomerular diseases associated with a moderate prevalence of hypertension

Membranous glomerulopathy
Membranoproliferative glomerulonephritis
Immunoglobulin nephropathy
Alport's syndrome

Table 19.3 Interstitial diseases associated with hypertension

Associated with low prevalence	Associated with high prevalence
Chronic pyelonephritis	Autosomal recessive polycystic kidney disease
Medullary cystic disease	Cyclosporine nephrotoxicity
	Allograft rejection

Phase II: "Mild renal failure" was defined by a GFR that was about 50% of normal and a serum creatinine between 1.1 and 3 mg/dl;

Phase III: "Severe renal failure" was defined by a GFR that was about 25% of normal and a serum creatinine between 3.1 and 7 mg/dl;

Phase IV: "End-stage renal failure" was characterized by GFR <10% of normal and a serum creatinine >7 mg/dl.

The results are shown in Figures 19.1 and 19.2.

The prevalence of hypertension in the different subgroups of glomerulonephritis is shown in Figure 19.1. In the late stages of renal failure, all the subgroups had a similar prevalence of hypertension of about 100%, whereas in the early phases the patients with focal and segmental glomerulosclerosis had a strikingly higher prevalence than those with the other three types of glomerulonephritis.

The prevalence of hypertension in the tubulointerstitial diseases is shown in Figure 19.2. The patients with pyelonephritis and those with analgesic nephropathy had a similar prevalence of hypertension in all four phases. The patients with poly-

cystic kidney disease showed the same prevalences throughout their course. There was a significant difference between polycystic kidney disease only in the intermediate phases.

The conclusions are that in various forms of progressive glomerular disease, hypertension occurs in virtually all patients as renal failure progresses. In chronic interstitial renal diseases which are common in children, hypertension occurs very frequently in those with polycystic renal disease and less often in those with chronic pyelonephritis. There are no pediatric studies similar to this study in adults; however, the conclusions of this study are probably similar to what would be found in a group of children and adolescents with chronic glomerular and tubulointerstitial diseases.

MECHANISMS LEADING TO HYPERTENSION IN RENAL DISEASE

The development of hypertension in progressive renal disease has been characterized by Brod and colleagues. [2]. The data are recorded in Table 19.4.

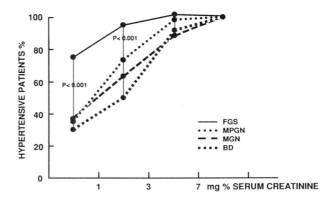

Fig. 19.1 The relationship between prevalence of hypertension and type of glomerular disease and plasma creatinine concentration. FGS = Focal glomerulosclerosis; MPGN = membranoproliferative glomerulonephritis; MGN = membranous glomerulonephropathy; BD = Berger's disease (immunoglobulin nephropathy). From [1], with permission.

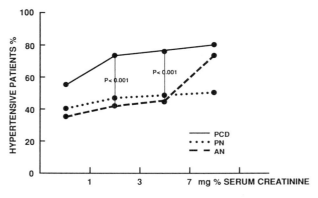

Fig. 19.2 The relationship between prevalence of hypertension and type of renal interstitial disease and plasma creatinine concentration. PCD = Polycystic kidney disease; PN = pyelonephritis; AN = analgesic nephropathy. From [1], with permission.

Table 19.4 Development of hypertension in patients with progressive renal disease. Adapted from [2]

| | | Normotensive renal patients ($n = 32$) | | | Hypertensive renal patients | | | |
| | | | | | Stage I–II ($n = 47$) | | | |
	Controls ($n = 17$)	Total	Normo-kinetic	Hyper-kinetic	Total	Normo-kinetic	Hyper-kinetic	Stage III ($n = 16$)
Blood pressure:systolic/ diastolic (mmHg)	128/76	132/81	133/82	130/79	170/105	170/105	170/104	190/114
Mean blood pressure (mmHg)	95	98	99	96	127	126	126	141
Cardiac index (l/min per m^2)	3.10	3.33	2.82	4.18	3.34	3.05	3.94	3.07
Blood volume (ml/m^2)	2833	3132	3002	3375	2931	3001	2802	3336
Total peripheral vascular resistance (dyn/s per cm^5)	1405	1398	1599	1063	1688	1772	1502	1980
Forearm vascular resistance (dyn/s per cm^5) $\times$ 10^{-5}	31.16	23.56	27.73	17.31	32.79	34.05	28.77	51.52
Forearm blood flow (ml/min per 100 ml)	4.01	3.87	3.64	4.24	3.47	3.52	3.14	4.03
Forearm venous distensibility (ml/100 ml per mmHg)	0.193	0.193	0.174	0.224	0.175	0.182	0.147	0.178

All values are means.

Ninety-seven patients with chronic renal parenchymal diseases and without anemia were studied. This group consisted of 32 normotensive (average blood pressure 132/81 mmHg) patients (age range 17–52 years), 49 patients (age range 19–55 years) with stage I or II hypertension (average blood pressure 170/105 mmHg), and 16 patients (age range 22–60 years) with stage III hypertension (average blood pressure 190/114 mmHg). The group consisted of patients with various types of glomerulonephritis and interstitial nephropathy including pyelonephritis, analgesic nephropathy, and polycystic renal disease. The age group included adolescents and adults. There were 17 healthy normotensive subjects studied as well.

On initial evaluation of all these patients the normotensive group with renal disease could be divided into two subgroups. There was a normokinetic group and a hyperkinetic group. The difference between these two subgroups was that the hyperkinetic group had a higher cardiac index, markedly increased circulating blood volume, lower total peripheral and forearm vascular resistance, hyperperfusion of the forearm, and increased venous distensibility within the forearm. All of these characteristics were significantly different ($p<0.03$) when

the hyperkinetic group was compared with the normokinetic group.

In the patients with renal disease and stage I–II hypertension (average blood pressure 170/105 mmHg) there were also two subgroups. One was normokinetic and the other was hyperkinetic. The main difference between the two was that the cardiac index was significantly greater in the hyperkinetic group compared with the normokinetic group. Total peripheral vascular resistance, blood volume, forearm blood flow, and forearm vascular resistance were similar in the two groups. In the patients with renal disease and with stage III hypertension (average blood pressure 190/114 mmHg), the cardiac index was the same as in the control group and no longer showed the elevation that was present in the patients with stage I and II hypertension. Total peripheral resistance was markedly elevated ($p<0.03$) in the patients with stage III hypertension when compared with healthy control subjects, normotensive patients with renal disease, and hypertensive patients with renal disease and stage I and II hypertension. The mean blood pressure in the normotensive patients with renal disease was 98 mmHg; in the patients with renal disease and stage I and II hypertension it was 127 mmHg, and in stage III hypertensive patients it was 141 mmHg. The difference between stage I—II and stage III was due entirely to a rise in total peripheral vascular resistance.

After 2—8 years, the patients were re-examined. Of the originally normotensive patients with renal disease, 29 were available for follow-up. There were 17 patients who were normokinetic on the original examination. Nine were still normotensive with a stable GFR and 8 had developed hypertension. Of the 8 who had developed hypertension, approximately half had a falling GFR. Of those who were originally hyperkinetic, 1 of 12 remained normotensive and 11 of 12 had developed hypertension. Most still had a stable GFR.

Of the patients who were hypertensive originally, 45 were available for follow-up evaluation. Thirty were normokinetic on original evaluation and 2 of these had their blood pressure return to normal. Twenty-eight of the 30 still had hypertension and approximately half had a falling GFR. There were 15 hyperkinetic patients in this group, one of whose blood pressure had returned to normal. Fourteen of the 15 remained hypertensive. Approximately one-third had a falling GFR. Thus 11 out of the 12 originally hyperkinetic normotensive patients with renal disease were now hypertensive, compared with only 8 out of 17 of the originally normokinetic normotensive patients with renal disease.

The authors' conclusions were that an inability of the diseased kidney to control plasma volume homeostasis leads to hypervolemia, which raises cardiac output in the patients with renal disease while they are still normotensive. As long as the arterioles adjust to the high output and the capacitance system to the high volume, blood pressure remains normal. When this adaptation of the peripheral circulation fails, blood pressure rises and the blood volume returns to normal. In this study peripheral plasma renin activity (PRA) did not correlate with any of the changes in blood volume, resistance, or cardiac index; only in the hypertensive patients with advanced renal disease and stage III hypertension did excessive renin production accompany the high blood pressure. Thus, until severe hypertension occurs, total peripheral resistance in hypertensive patients is variable but not usually elevated above that of healthy, control individuals. Likewise the cardiac index is generally elevated in the initial stage of hypertension with renal disease (stage I—II hypertension) and returns to the level of that of healthy control subjects when severe (stage III) hypertension occurs.

STRUCTURAL RENAL DISEASES THAT CAUSE HYPERTENSION
(see also Chapter 20)

Autosomal recessive polycystic kidney disease

Hypertension is usually present when autosomal recessive infantile polycystic renal disease is first recognized. In a study of 14 patients with this condition, Lieberman and colleagues [3] reported that 9 of 14 newborn babies and infants had recognized hypertension within the first 7 months of life. In all infants the hypertension was difficult to control and was an important contributing factor to their deaths. In 3 of the 5 infants who died, congestive heart failure developed during the course of their illness and hypertension probably contributed to its development.

In the 9 survivors, hypertension continued to be a problem in 6, who required antihypertensive medication. Progressive renal failure occurred in the 8 patients for whom data were available. It is of interest to note that hypertension was present early, and often before renal insufficiency developed. The cause of renal insufficiency in these infants [3] is unknown.

Autosomal dominant polycystic kidney disease

Generally referred to as adult polycystic kidney disease, autosomal dominant polycystic kidney disease usually presents after age 20 years. However, many cases have been recorded as presenting throughout the age range of pediatrics. Delaney and colleagues [4] reported a large series of 53 symptomatic patients with the disorder. Eight of these were recognized between the ages of 10 and 20 years. Hypertension was present in only 21% of the patients when the diagnosis was made. This is in marked contrast to the frequency with which hypertension occurs when the disease is first recognized in patients with autosomal recessive polycystic kidney disease. Other frequent manifestations of the autosomal dominant disease at onset of the illness include abdominal pain, urinary tract infection, gross hematuria and abdominal mass. As the disease progresses, the prevalence of hypertension increases to about two-thirds of all patients. Detailed studies of the mechanisms of hypertension in this disorder are lacking although some have reported that it is associated with an expanded plasma volume and low PRA [2,5,6].

In our own experience with 18 children with either autosomal dominant or autosomal recessive polycystic kidney disease, 6 children presented with the autosomal dominant type. They ranged in age from 1 day to 14 years. Hypertension occurred in only 1 patient whose medication has been able to be subsequently discontinued, with blood pressure remaining normal. Thus hypertension is not a common manifestation of autosomal dominant polycystic kidney disease when the disease presents in the pediatric age group. When it occurs it tends to be mild and is easily controlled with medications.

Evaluation of patients with suspected polycystic kidney disease

Polycystic kidney disease in children presents in a variety of ways. Autosomal recessive polycystic kidney disease often manifests itself by the presence of palpable bilateral flank masses. Due to their size, the kidneys can produce respiratory difficulty and even respiratory insufficiency [3]. The manifestations of autosomal dominant polycystic kidney disease are also quite variable. It may also present with bilateral flank masses so large as to cause respiratory insufficiency. The kidneys may be found to be either unilaterally or bilaterally enlarged by palpation on routine examination in infancy or childhood. The classic manifestations of abdominal pain, urinary tract infection, or gross hematuria do not characteristically occur in the pediatric age group.

With the advent of modern ultrasonography, the best initial evaluation of a child with suspected polycystic kidney disease is a careful abdominal ultrasound. This should include evaluation of the liver and kidneys in order to demonstrate whether there are definable cysts present in the renal and hepatic parenchyma. In autosomal recessive polycystic kidney disease, the cysts are usually quite small and one sees a pattern of increased echogenicity throughout both kidneys (which are massively enlarged). Cysts are not usually detected by ultrasound examination of the liver. Since hepatic fibrosis commonly occurs as the child grows older, evidence of that may be present on liver ultrasound examination. Ultrasound examination of the kidneys of both parents is extremely helpful in all cases of polycystic kidney disease in children. This is because the ultrasonic examination of the child may not be able to differentiate autosomal dominant from autosomal recessive polycystic kidney disease in early infancy. Disease may be found for the first time in the parent after the evaluation of the child with the suspected disorder.

In autosomal dominant polycystic kidney disease, the cysts are usually very large and present throughout the kidney which is also enlarged with an irregular surface if there are many cysts present. The cyst diameter ranges from several millimeters to several centimeters. In children the renal size is often only slightly increased and only a few cysts may be present. In the newborn infant the cysts may still be quite small and the kidney may have the ultrasonic appearance of the autosomal recessive type. Therefore it is mandatory that the parents as well as the siblings of the patient have an ultrasonic examination.

In difficult cases a liver biopsy may be helpful. In autosomal recessive polycystic kidney disease, there may be very small cysts present within the liver and in older children hepatic fibrosis may be present. In the autosomal dominant variety, cysts are usually present within the liver thus making the differentiation between the two types easier. Renal biopsy is rarely helpful since it is difficult to distinguish between the two types when the cysts are small [7, author's observations].

Intravenous pyelography with delayed films can be helpful in demonstrating the accumulation of contrast material within the cystic structures in the autosomal recessive type of polycystic kidney disease. The cysts are arranged in a radial fashion pointing toward the collecting system and have a sunburst appearance when films are taken about 12 h after injection of the contrast material. In the autosomal dominant variety, the calyceal system is usually splayed and distorted by the cysts which are near the collecting system. However the appearance is often normal when only a few cysts are present and therefore ultrasonography is a much more sensitive diagnostic tool for the early recognition of cysts in autosomal dominant polycystic kidney disease. Other imaging techniques, including computerized transaxial tomography, can be helpful in some cases but usually only complement the information found by ultrasonography and intravenous pyelography.

Medullary cystic disease

Medullary cystic disease is transmitted as an autosomal recessive disease in children and is associated with the presence of small renal cysts in the medullary region of the kidneys. There is usually progressive loss of kidney function as time goes on with renal failure occurring in most children in the second decade of life. Hypertension is uniformly absent in these children and indeed salt-wasting is common until end-stage renal disease occurs. Hypertension may then develop, presumably as a consequence of an expanded plasma volume with a secondary increase in cardiac output. In addition, anemia is usually present at that time and adds to the increased cardiac output [8].

Obstructive uropathy

Hypertension occurs infrequently in children with hydronephrosis. The exact frequency is unclear from the literature but probably depends upon whether obstructive uropathy is unilateral or bilateral. The frequency with which it occurs has been better characterized in children with a solitary hydronephrotic kidney [9]. In the report of Wehle and Walker [9], there were three causes of hydronephrosis: obstruction at the ureteropelvic junction, ureterovesical junction, or posterior urethral valves. The group with ureteropelvic junction obstruction had a mean creatinine clearance of 82 ml/min; the group with obstruction at the ureterovesical junction had a mean creatinine clearance of 73 ml/min, and the group with posterior urethral valves had a mean creatinine clearance of 63 ml/min. The children with obstruction at the ureterovesical junction had a creatinine clearance significantly reduced from normal ($p<0.01$). The groups with posterior urethral valve or ureteropelvic obstruction were too small for significant conclusions to be reached. Hypertension was defined as blood pressure greater than the 95th percentile on three different measurements. It was present in 14% of the children with ureteropelvic junction obstruction, 25% of the males but none of the females with ureterovesical junction obstruction, and 16% of the patients with posterior urethral valves. Thus in this series of 31 children, 5 or 16% either had hypertension at recognition of hydronephrosis or developed it during the course of their illness. Comparable figures in children with bilateral hydronephrotic kidneys or unilateral hydronephrotic kidneys with an opposite normal kidney are not available. The mechanisms of hypertension are unclear but sometimes activation of the renin−angiotensin−aldosterone system has been shown, with repair of the obstruction leading to normalization of blood pressure and PRA. For most cases the cause is unclear.

Evaluation and recognition of the cause of hypertension in these children is based upon imaging studies. Ultrasonography has proven especially valuable in demonstrating the dilated urinary tract.

In almost all instances of obstructive uropathy the dilated collecting system can be imaged by ultrasound [10]. Radioisotope scanning of the kidney can be especially helpful in determining whether the dilated collecting system found on ultrasound is indicative of obstruction or not. Dynamic renal scans using either ^{99m}Tc-diaminotetraethylpentacetic acid or ^{123}I-hippuran and intravenous administration of furosemide during the scan is a useful technique in differentiating whether a dilated urinary tract is obstructed or not [10]. Caution must be exercised in interpreting the response of a urinary system to furosemide if there is poor renal function or gross dilatation of the collecting system [10].

Hypoplastic kidneys

Bilateral hypoplasia of the kidneys is rarely associated with hypertension even when advanced renal insufficiency is present. Often children with this disorder lose excessive amounts of sodium from the kidney and as a consequence actually need oral salt supplementation to their diets [11].

Reflux nephropathy and pyelonephritis

In two studies of the relationship between reflux nephropathy and hypertension in children and adolescents, the frequency of hypertension varied from 10 to 20% [12,13]. All those who had hypertension also had renal scarring. In most, renal function was normal or near-normal, indicating that the appearance of hypertension in these patients is not necessarily related to the development of renal failure but rather to associated vascular lesions. In the paper by Wallace and associates [12] hypertension was present in 18% of the children with bilateral renal scars who had been operated on more than 10 years earlier for vesicoureteric reflux. Hypertension was observed in 11% of the cases with unilateral renal scarring. Of importance is the fact that although hypertension occurred only in patients with renal scarring, the extent of renal damage has no predictive value for the individual patient. Antireflux procedures do not usually result in improvement in hypertension if it is present before reflux is surgically corrected. Indeed, hypertension may develop after antireflux procedures are performed, even when the patient was normotensive at the time of the surgical procedure.

However, in a study by Gusmano and colleagues, 241 children with vesicoureteric reflux were reported. Hypertension developed in 5% (11 out of 241 patients) during the study. In all patients with hypertension the creatinine clearnace was reduced, ranging from 7 to 73 ml/min per 1.73 m^2 [14].

There has been some investigation into the mechanisms responsible for hypertension associated with reflux nephropathy and renal scarring. In a study by Dillon and Smellie [15], three separate groups of children with reflux nephropathy were studied to determine possible mechanisms responsible for hypertension. The data are summarized in Table 19.5. Group A consisted of 100 normotensive children, aged 2–15 years, who had radiologically demonstrable reflux nephropathy associated with previous vesicoureteric reflux. The peripheral PRA was measured in each; 8 of the 100 children had definitely elevated values that were above the normal range. The group as a whole had PRA values that did not decrease as expected with increasing age.

The second group (group B) consisted of 26 normotensive children with reflux nephropathy and scarring. Five of these children (19%) had a PRA value above the normal range for age. When compared with a similar age group of normal children, this group of normotensive children with reflux nephropathy had PRA values which were significantly higher ($p<0.05$). The PRA values in the normotensive children with reflux nephropathy did not follow the usual regression with age as the normal control group of children did.

A third group (group D) reported in this study consisted of 51 children with reflux nephropathy and scarring, and significant but nonmalignant hypertension. The PRA for the whole group was significantly elevated when compared to age-matched control patients (group C). In 36 of the 51 children PRA was markedly above the normal range and in 15 others the values were within the normal range but above the mean for the control group (group C). The PRA value of the group of hypertensive children (group D) was significantly increased ($p<0.001$) compared to that of the age-matched control subjects. Also, the peripheral PRA in this group of hypertensive patients was significantly increased ($p<0.005$) when compared to normotensive patients with reflux nephropathy and scarring (group B) [15].

In the same article, Dillon and Smellie [15] reported on 52 children with reflux nephropathy and hypertension, in whom bilateral renal vein renin measurements were performed. In 21 patients the reflux nephropathy and scarring was unilateral; in 24 it was bilateral but asymmetrical, and in 7 bilateral symmetrical scarring was present. In 33 patients, renal vein renin ratios were >1.5 and it is noteworthy that none of these had symmetrical renal disease. Thirteen patients with unilateral disease and 9 with bilateral asymmetrical disease underwent surgery. There were 20 nephrectomies, 1 nephrectomy together with a partial nephrectomy, and 1 partial nephrectomy. In 14 children the blood pressure returned to normal and in an additional 8 patients blood pressure control was significantly improved. Thus, renal vein renin ratios of >1.5 usually predicted surgical cure or improvement in the degree of hypertension. In 25 of the 52 patients studied, segmental renal vein samples were collected for measurement of PRA. In approximately half of these, the information proved useful, for it identified a segmental source of elevated renin production that was not detected by the main renal vein renin samples [16].

These measurements of PRA in peripheral blood, renal vein, and segmental renal vein blood strongly implicate renin in the hypertension seen in patients

Table 19.5 Plasma renin activity (PRA) in children with reflux nephropathy (RN). Adapted from [15]

	Normotensive with RN		Hypertensive with RN
	Group A	Group B	Group D
Number of patients	100	26	51
Number with elevated PRA	8	5	36
Group PRA	Did not fall with increasing age	Did not fall with increasing age	Increased ($p<0.001$) compared to normal children (group C*) and normotensive children with RN ($p<0.005$)

* Group C = age-matched control subjects.

with reflux nephropathy. Although not all of the PRA values in the hypertensive groups of patients were above the normal range for age, the values were probably inappropriately raised in relation to the blood pressure at that time.

Reflux nephropathy with scarring is usually easily recognized by intravenous pyelography. Cortical scars are present in the early nephrogram phase of the study. Subsequent films show blunting of the calyces in some but not all cases. However, scars may not be seen on intravenous pyelography even though they may be present. Added sensitivity can be obtained to demonstrate the presence of cortical scars by technetium ^{99m}Tc succimer dimercaptosuccinic acid (DMSA) scintigraphy [16]. Using DMSA imaging renal scars were present in 2 of 12 kidneys: these scars were missed by the intravenous pyelogram. Thus in approximately 10% of the kidneys with suspected reflux nephropathy, scars were not present on intravenous pyelograms but were found by DMSA scintigraphy.

Renal ultrasound is not as sensitive as intravenous pyelography in demonstrating cortical scars and the upper poles may be difficult to image [16]. Reflux can usually be demonstrated by voiding cystourethrography. Occasionally the reflux may have disappeared by the time the procedure is done but scarring is present on the intravenous pyelogram. It is assumed in older children that reflux in these cases has spontaneously disappeared but the residual effects remain.

Thus, in all children with hypertension, intravenous pyelography should be performed to determine if renal scars are present. In those children with hypertension in whom scars are not present but reflux nephropathy is suspected, a DMSA scan with technetium should be considered. Anatomic cortical perfusion defects may then be detected.

PRIMARY GLOMERULAR DISEASES THAT CAUSE HYPERTENSION

Acute nephritic syndrome

The acute nephritic syndrome is a clinical entity characterized, in its typical form, by the sudden development of edema, hypertension, gross hematuria, and diminished urine output. The best recognized etiology of the syndrome is acute post-streptococcal glomerulonephritis (APSGN). The frequency of hypertension in APSGN varies from 70 to 95% (Table 19.6) [17,18]. Powell and colleagues [19] studied 10 children aged 4–12 years with APSGN. All had an acute nephritic onset, an elevated anti-streptolysin-o (ASO) titer, and a reduction in the third component of complement. All patients except 1 were hypertensive on admission, with blood pressure ranging from 140/95 to 190/130 mmHg. During the period of oliguria, peripheral PRA was low in the hypertensive children, all of whom were edematous. There was a significant ($p<0.01$) degree of correlation between the percentage of weight loss after diuresis occurred and the PRA. There was also a highly significant correlation between the diastolic blood pressure on admission and subsequent weight loss ($r = 0.96$,

Table 19.6 Frequency of hypertension in glomerular diseases

Disease	Frequency of hypertension (%)	
	At onset	Follow-up
Acute nephritic syndrome	70–95	<5
Hemolytic–uremic syndrome	40–50	6–24*
Membranoproliferative glomerulonephritis	40	67†
Focal and segmental glomerulosclerosis	20	60
Diffuse mesangial hypercellularity	46	10
Crescentic glomerulonephritis	50	17†
Immunoglobulin nephropathy	6	6
Membranous nephropathy	6	NA
Systemic lupus erythematosus	28	NA
Henoch–Schönlein purpura	40	NA

* Chronic sequelae including hypertension.
† Excluding patients who developed end-stage renal disease.
NA = Data not available.

$p<0.001$). This direct relationship between the degree of salt and water overload and hypertension was noted in serial observations on each of the patients. Thus in this study by Powell and colleagues [19], the PRA was depressed compared with a control group of normal subjects. The degree of hypertension as noted by the diastolic blood pressure was directly related to excess body water accumulation and, by inference, expansion of the plasma volume.

These studies have been expanded and a more detailed functional evaluation of the renin—angiotensin—aldosterone system has been performed by Rodriguez-Iturbe and colleagues [18] in patients with the acute nephritic syndrome. Thirteen children with APSGN were studied. Their ages ranged from 4 to 14 years and the diagnosis of APSGN was based upon an elevated ASO titer, features of acute nephritic syndrome, and their subsequent course with complete resolution of disease. These patients were studied on two occasions. The first study (period A) was made during the acute nephritic syndrome within 48 h of admission to the hospital. The second study (period B) was made after the patients recovered from the acute nephritic syndrome, at which time the creatinine clearance and C3 complement had returned to normal and there was no edema, hypertension, or gross hematuria. Microscopic hematuria was still present. Period B studies were performed between 4 and 6 weeks after the initial admission. The patients had mild or moderate hypertension and none were treated with antihypertensive or diuretic drugs during period A or B.

During both periods of study, the patients were on a low-salt diet (10 mmol sodium per day). Compliance with the low-sodium diet was supervised during period A and for 3 days prior to studies in period B.

A control group of children was also studied. These children had normal kidney function and received one of three sodium intakes. The first group received sodium 10 mmol/day, group II received 150 mmol/day, and group III 300 mmol/day. In each case the urinary sodium excretion confirmed the prescribed sodium intake.

Plasma renin activity in period A of patients with APSGN was suppressed ($p<0.001$) compared with period B and it was comparable to the value in the sodium-loaded normal children receiving sodium 300 mmol/day. Plasma aldosterone followed the same pattern: there was suppression of the level in period A compared with period B, and the level in period A was similar to that in normal children receiving sodium 300 mmol/day. Urinary aldosterone excretion also followed the above patterns. During period B, PRA, plasma aldosterone, and urinary aldosterone values were similar to those of the normal children receiving a 10 mmol sodium diet. Significant correlations existed between PRA and plasma aldosterone ($p<0.001$) or urinary aldosterone ($p<0.001$) and were similar in control subjects. The severity of hypertension was correlated with fluid retention ($p<0.001$). Fluid retention was correlated with the suppression of PRA; 80% suppression of PRA was rapidly achieved with a 5—6% weight gain.

Thus in children with mild-to-moderate hypertension who have APSGN, the renin—angiotensin—aldosterone system appears to function physiologically and the degree of hypertension is strongly correlated with the degree of weight gain. This implies that there is a significant correlation between hypertension and expansion of plasma volume.

Management of hypertension in APSGN

There is considerable disagreement regarding levels of blood pressure in APSGN which require therapeutic intervention. Hypertension often resolves with bedrest alone. If the diastolic blood pressure is below 100 mmHg and decreases on bedrest, sodium restriction and continued bedrest are sufficient. If the blood pressure does not decline in 2—4 h or rises or symptoms of encephalopathy develop (headache, nausea, vomiting, seizures), treatment should be instituted promptly. Treatment of acute hypertensive emergencies is outlined in Chapter 31. Antihypertensive agents such as parenteral hydralazine and sublingual nifedipine are effective in treating hypertension associated with APSGN. Nitroprusside or diazoxide has been used successfully to treat severe acute hypertension. The cause of hypertension in APSGN is largely due to an expanded extracellular fluid volume. Diuretic administration can be important in promoting a diuresis and assisting in lowering the blood pressure: furosemide (2 mg/kg orally) is often effective. Improvement in encephalopathy has been seen in patients treated with intravenous furosemide even when only minimal or no changes in blood pressure have occurred. These observations imply that edema of the central nervous system plays an important role in hypertensive encephalopathy in APSGN [20].

Hemolytic—uremic syndrome

The hemolytic—uremic syndrome in children is characterized by petechiae, hepatosplenomegaly, jaundice, anemia, thrombocytopenia, and elevated serum creatinine. Hypertension occurs in 40—50% of children in the acute phase of the syndrome [21]. Powell and coworkers [19] measured PRA in 10 children with the hemolytic—uremic syndrome. They were aged 6 months to 8 years and all had typical features of the disorder. All had a prodrome of mild gastroenteritis in the week before admission, and presented with acute microangiopathic hemolytic anemia, thrombocytopenia, and acute renal failure. Five of the 10 were hypertensive with a diastolic blood pressure above 90 mmHg. In the other 5 children the diastolic blood pressure was never above 80 mmHg. Six were oliguric (<250 ml of urine/day) for 6—35 days and they were all treated with peritoneal dialysis. All of the hypertensive children had an elevated PRA compared to normotensive children without renal disease. In all children with hypertension, correction of the edema by either dialysis or fluid restriction did not return the blood pressure to normal. In 2 children the PRA was measured after blood pressure had returned to normal and antihypertensive drugs had been stopped. The PRA levels at that time were normal in both patients. Of the 5 children with diastolic blood pressure below 80 mmHg, PRA was normal in 4 but elevated in 1; however, that patient had been given an intravenous diuretic 12 h before the peripheral PRA was measured.

Kidney tissue was examined in 9 of the 10 children. In the 5 with hypertension, there was evidence of arterial luminal occlusion which was complete in 2 and partial in 3. Of the 5 children with diastolic blood pressure below 80 mmHg, 3 had evidence of partial arterial occlusion, 1 had no arterial luminal occlusion, and tissue was not obtained in the remaining child.

Thus, during the acute phase of the hemolytic—uremic syndrome when associated with hypertension, there is evidence of elevated PRA even without expanded total body water. In 4 of the 5 children with diastolic blood pressure below 80 mmHg PRA was normal. The renin—angiotensin—aldosterone system thus appears to be an important mechanism in the hypertension of this disease.

Long-term sequelae, including hypertension, proteinuria, decreased creatinine clearance, and cen-

tral nervous system abnormalities, continue in 6—24% of children who develop hemolytic—uremic syndrome [22].

In children with this condition who are hypertensive, drugs which reduce renin or its effector, angiotensin II, would be logical choices for its treatment.

Chronic glomerulonephritides

MESANGIOCAPILLARY (MEMBRANOPROLIFERATIVE) GLOMERULONEPHRITIS

Membranoproliferative glomerulonephritis (MPGN) is a chronic immune-mediated renal disease which over a protracted period of time may result in chronic renal failure. Hypertension is present in approximately 40% of cases when the disease is recognized [23]. The frequency of chronic hypertension is influenced favorably by the early use of alternate-day prednisone. In patients in whom alternate-day prednisone was initiated less than 1 year after clinical onset of MPGN, the frequency of hypertension did not change (average follow-up of 10.4 years). In those patients in whom alternate-day prednisone was initiated more than 1 year after the clinical onset of MPGN, the frequency of hypertension had increased to 75% after an average follow-up of 8.6 years. If those patients who developed end-stage renal disease were excluded from the calculations, those in whom alternate-day prednisone was started more than 1 year after clinical onset of MPGN developed hypertension—67% of the group with long-term follow-up [24]. Thus the frequency of hypertension is high at the onset of MPGN but does not increase when alternate-day prednisone is started early in the course of the disease.

FOCAL AND SEGMENTAL GLOMERULOSCLEROSIS

Focal and segmental glomerulosclerosis (FSGS) is not a single clinical entity but is a common end-event in numerous types of renal disease. Patients with FSGS may present with the nephrotic syndrome, hematuria and proteinuria, or proteinuria alone. This review of hypertension in FSGS will be restricted to children who have FSGS in association with the nephrotic syndrome. The frequency of hypertension in FSGS with nephrotic syndrome varies depending upon the size of the group reported and the referral pattern of the reporting center. In a large study by Ellis and colleagues [24], hypertension was initially present in 20% of children with FSGS and the nephrotic syndrome. With progression of the disease, the frequency of hypertension increased; in children with advanced renal insufficiency, the incidence of hypertension was 60%. With progression to end-stage renal disease, virtually all patients with FSGS developed hypertension.

In another study of idiopathic FSGS, Newman and colleagues [25] reported that 10% of children with FSGS initially had hypertension. On long-term follow-up, 60% of the same group had hypertension. The average length of follow-up was 7.6 years. All patients presented with normal renal function and all had the nephrotic syndrome at onset.

DIFFUSE MESANGIAL HYPERCELLULARITY

Children with idiopathic nephrotic syndrome found on biopsy to have diffuse mesangial hypercellularity had a poorer prognosis than those with minimal-change nephrotic syndrome [26]. In a combined study of the Southwest Pediatric Nephrology Study Group, 29 children with idiopathic nephrotic syndrome and diffuse mesangial hypercellularity were reported. At the onset of the nephrotic syndrome, hypertension was present in 46% of the children and impaired renal function in 24%. Follow-up evaluation on 26 of the children for a mean of 29 months revealed that only 2 patients (10%) still had hypertension. Thus hypertension in association with diffuse mesangial hypercellularity is often transient.

CRESCENTIC GLOMERULONEPHRITIS

Idiopathic crescentic glomerulonephritis is an uncommon clinical problem in children; however, it often progresses to end-stage renal disease. The clinical course and pathologic features were characterized in a study of 50 children in whom crescents were present in at least 50% of the glomeruli [27]. These 50 children had crescentic glomerulonephritis due to a variety of causes including immune complex disease, systemic lupus erythematosus, APSGN, IgA nephropathy, Henoch—Schönlein nephritis, vasculitis, antiglomerular basement membrane disease, and dense deposit disease. Hypertension was considered present if the diastolic pressure was above the 95th percentile for age. The overall frequency of

hypertension was 51% at clinical recognition of renal disease. In those patients with crescents present in 50—79% of the glomeruli, hypertension was present in 17%, while in those patients having crescents present in 80—100% of the glomeruli, hypertension was present in 73%. The mean systolic and diastolic blood pressure in the first group was 115/71 mmHg and in the second group 138/91 mmHg.

In this study, 49% of the patients (23 of 47) progressed to end-stage renal disease. Persistent elevation of blood pressure was noted in only 17% of the remaining 24 patients who did not progress to renal failure.

Thus crescentic glomerulonephritis often produces hypertension and renal insufficiency. In those patients who do not progress to end-stage disease and who have improvement in renal function, hypertension improves with time.

IMMUNOGLOBULIN NEPHROPATHY

The clinical presentation of children with IgA nephropathy has been described in two studies [28,29]. The Southwest Pediatric Nephrology Study Group [28] reported that 4 of 62 children (6%) had hypertension at the time of a diagnostic renal biopsy. Subsequently in 16 children followed for 5 or more years, 1 (6%) was hypertensive. Thus in this study hypertension was uncommon at the time of recognition of IgA nephropathy and did not develop on follow-up in most children.

In a study of IgA nephropathy in children and adults, Wyatt and associates [29] reported on 82 patients. Thirty-four were children or adolescents and presented at age 3—18 years. None in this age group presented with hypertension. With long-term follow-up (mean of 6 years) of 24 patients in the pediatric age group only 17% of those with a serum creatinine concentration at follow-up of 1.5 mg/dl or less had hypertension. Thus in children whose renal function did not markedly deteriorate with follow-up, hypertension did not usually develop. Thus as in the Southwest Pediatric Nephrology Study Group report [28], hypertension is not common at onset and does not usually develop on moderately long-term follow-up in IgA nephropathy.

MEMBRANOUS NEPHROPATHY

Membranous nephropathy is an uncommon renal disease in children. Habib and colleagues [30] reported on 50 children with this condition. Only 3 had an elevation in blood pressure at onset of the illness. The Southwest Pediatric Nephrology Study Group [31] reported on 11 children with membranous nephropathy in association with hepatitis B surface antigenemia. Of these 11 children, 3 (27%) had hypertension at the time of diagnosis. Thus hypertension is not common in children with membranous nephropathy in association with hepatitis B antigenemia.

VASCULITIC SYNDROMES

The three most common vasculitic syndromes in children include systemic lupus erythematosus, Henoch—Schönlein purpura, and polyarteritis nodosa. The first two are much more common than the last. In a report of glomerulonephritis in systemic lupus erythematosus in children, Garin and co-authors [32] reported that hypertension was present in 28% of 18 children with diffuse proliferative glomerulonephritis and 20% of 5 children with membranous nephropathy. During the course of therapy, which usually included prednisone, hypertension occurred more often.

In Henoch—Schönlein purpura, Meadow and colleagues [33] reported that 35 of 88 children had an acute nephritic syndrome with hypertension during the first 3 months after clinical onset. Thus up to 40% of children with this disorder developed hypertension. Long-term follow-up on the prognosis of Henoch—Schönlein nephritis in children was reported by Counahan and colleagues [34]. This study was a follow-up of all 88 children originally desribed by Meadow and colleagues [33]. The mean duration since illness of all patients was 10 years. Hypertension was a common problem in those who still had active renal disease. Hypertension was the sole finding in 5 of the 9 patients who were originally classified as having active renal disease and in these patients neither proteinuria nor hematuria was present. The authors recommend that children with Henoch—Schönlein nephritis be followed for at least 5 years after recognition of renal disease. Blood pressure must be carefully monitored even in those who have neither proteinuria nor hematuria.

Polyarteritis nodosa is an uncommon vasculitic syndrome in children. It is usually a rapidly progressive disorder which often results in death. Hypertension has been reported in 55% of adults who acquire polyarteritis nodosa and in a small

pediatric series, Ettenger and colleagues [35] reported that 4 of 9 children with polyarteritis nodosa had hypertension at the time of recognition of their illness. White and Schambelan [36] reported that in 2 adults with polyarteritis nodosa, both had markedly elevated PRA and urinary aldosterone excretion rates. Captopril, an angiotensin converting enzyme inhibitor, was effective in controlling the hypertension in both [36].

EVALUATION AND TREATMENT OF HYPERTENSION IN RENAL DISEASE

Because hypertension is a common problem in many different types of renal parenchymal disease, blood pressure should be carefully taken at each evaluation. The pressure should be recorded with the patient in a sitting position in a relaxed state with measurement of the first, fourth, and fifth Korotkoff sounds. Those children whose blood pressure is in the severe range of hypertension should have immediate treatment. Listed in Table 19.7 are the latest values for severe hypertension in children taken from the report of the Second Task Force on blood pressure control in children [37].

A summary of the drugs most often used to control severe hypertension in children is presented in Table 19.8 [37—39]. The guidelines for usage of various antihypertensive agents vary according to author and age of patient. In children who are obviously volume-overloaded, diuretic agents are aften useful in reducing the blood pressure. They have as a potential complication hypokalemia, which must be treated with either additional potassium in the diet or potassium chloride supplementation. Even if not used for initial therapy, diuretics are often added to

Table 19.7 Severe hypertension levels in children. Adapted from [37].

| Age group | Blood pressure (mmHg) | |
	Systolic	Diastolic
Newborn (8—30 days)	≥110	NA
Infant (<2 years)	≥118	≥82
Children (3—5 years)	≥124	≥84
Children (6—9 years)	≥130	≥86
Children (10—12 years)	≥134	≥90
Adolescents (13—15 years)	≥144	≥92
Adolescents (16—18 years)	≥150	≥98

NA = Not applicable.

Table 19.8 Oral drugs used to treat chronic renal hypertension in children. Modified from [33–39]

Drug	Initial oral dose (mg/kg per day)	Dose interval (h)	Maximum daily dose*	Peak action (h)	Duration of effect (h)	Most common side-effects
Vasodilators						
Hydralazine	1.0	4–6	200 mg/day	1–2	4–8	Tachycardia, fluid retention, headache
Minoxidil	0.1–0.2	12	20 mg/day	4	24–48	Fluid retention, tachycardia, hirsutism
Adrenergically active agents						
β-Adrenergic antagonists						
Propranolol	1–2	12	10 mg/kg per day	1–2	24	Insomnia, dizziness, depression, memory impairment, bradycardia, wheezing, reduced exercise tolerance
Atenolol	1	24	2 mg/kg per day	2–4	±24	Same as propranolol except wheezing rare
Metoprolol	1–2	12	5 mg/kg per day	2–4	24	Same as propranolol
Nadolol	40 mg (not/kg)	24	320 mg/day	3–4	24	Same as propranolol
Central α-adrenergic stimulators						
Methyldopa	5	12	40–60 mg/kg per day[†]		6–12	Depression, sedation, nightmares, fluid retention
Clonidine	0.005	12	0.03 mg/kg per day	2–4	6–12	Dry mouth, drowsiness, sedation, constipation, reactive hypertension with sudden cessation
α-adrenergic antagonists						
Prazosin	0.05–0.1	8	0.5 mg/kg per day	3	12	Syncope after first dose, fluid retention
Converting enzyme inhibitors						
Captopril						Reduced renal function, leukopenia, rash, headache, proteinuria, pruritis, cough, angioedema
<6 months	0.05	8	0.5 mg/kg per day	4	8–12	
>6 months	0.5	8	0.5 mg/kg per day	4	8–12	
Enalapril[‡]	2.5 mg/day	24	40 mg/day	3–4	8–12	Reduced renal function
Plasma volume-reducing drugs						
Chlorothiazide	10	12	250–500 mg/day	4	6–12	Plasma volume depletion, hypokalemia, hyponatremia, hyperuricemia
Furosemide	1–2	12–24	8 mg/kg per day	2	6–8	Plasma volume depletion, hypokalemia, hyponatremia, hyperuricemia
Spironolactone	1	8	200 mg/day	4	12–24	Hyperkalemia, gynecomastia
Calcium channel blocker						
Nifedipine	0.25	4–6	1 mg/kg per day	1	4–8	Dizziness, headache, flushing, nausea

* Maximum dose based on weight of 50 kg.
† Has cumulative effect. Dose increased at weekly intervals.
‡ To date used only in older adolescents.

other antihypertensive agents since plasma volume expansion will often result when vasodilators and adrenergically active agents are used. If GFR is reduced below approximately 60 ml/min per 1.73 m^2, the thiazide diuretics are usually ineffective and a loop diuretic agent such as furosemide must be used (see Table 19.8).

Adrenergically active agents are often used now as initial treatment for hypertension. They are effective antihypertensive drugs, especially the β-blocking agents. These include propranolol, atenolol, and nadolol, which have relatively few side-effects. In hypertension associated with renal parenchymal disease, cardiac output is often increased, and since the β-blocking agents reduce this they are particularly effective in lowering blood pressure. A recent addition to this group of drugs is labetalol. This is a combination β- and α-blocking agent that has been found to be useful in hypertension of various causes in adults. Thus far it has had relatively little use in pediatrics and therefore should be limited to older adolescents since the exact dosing for pediatric patients is not yet clear.

It is probably wisest initially to use a single antihypertensive agent, increasing its dosage at safe intervals until either the maximal dosage is achieved or side-effects occur from that drug. If minor side-effects occur the dose should be reduced; if serious side-effects occur then the medication must be stopped. Once a drug has been taken to its maximum useful dosage and blood pressure has not been reduced to a safe range then a second agent, usually in a different class, is added.

Vasodilators are often added after adrenergically active agents and diuretics have been tried in order to augment blood pressure reduction. Minoxidil is a particularly effective vasodilator but its well known side-effect, hirsutism, gives it limited usefulness in adolescents, especially females.

Angiotensin converting enzyme inhibitors may be particularly useful when excessive renin production is present or suspected. However they can result in a rising creatinine level and patients receiving them need to be monitored carefully. Captopril was the first to be introduced and has had favorable results in children with hypertension caused by excessive renin production or by a wide variety of renal parenchymal diseases. Another addition to this class of drugs is enalapril maleate. Enalapril has an advantage for it can be given once a day with a 24-h effect from the medication. It is currently best reserved for older adolescents since exact dosing in the pediatric age range is not yet available. It has had fewer reported side-effects than captopril in short-term studies. Because of reported leukopenia, the white blood count needs to be monitored weekly for the first month after starting captopril and then thereafter every 1–2 months for a year.

Calcium channel blocking agents are thought to reduce arteriolar tone by decreasing intracellular-free calcium. Although not extensively used in pediatrics, nifedipine is useful in treating acute hypertension. Nitrendipine and nicardipine which, like nifedipine, are dihydropyridine derivatives, have recently been released. They are similar to but longer-acting than nifedipine but have had limited pediatric use.

REFERENCES

1 Vendemia F, Fornasieri A, Velis O *et al*. Different prevalence rates of hypertension in various reno-parenchymal diseases. In: Blaufox MD, Bianchi C, eds. *Secondary Forms of Hypertension: Current Diagnosis and Management*. New York: Grune & Stratton, 1981.

2 Brod J, Bahlmann J, Cachovan M, Pretschner P. Development of hypertension in renal disease. *Clin Sci* 1983;64:141–52.

3 Lieberman E, Salinas-Madrigal L, Gwenn JL, Brennan LP, Fine RN, Landing BH. Infantile polycystic disease of the kidneys and liver. *Medicine* 1971;8:277–318.

4 Delaney VB, Adler S, Bruns FJ, Licinia M, Segel DP, Fraley DS. Autosomal dominant polycystic kidney disease: presentation, complications, and prognosis. *Am J Kidney Dis* 1985;5:104–11.

5 Leenen GH, Galla SJ, Redmond DP *et al*. Relationships of the renin–angiotensin–aldosterone system and sodium balance to blood pressure regulation in chronic renal failure of polycystic kidney disease. *Metabolism* 1975;24:589–603.

6 Nash DA. Hypertension in polycystic kidney disease without renal failure. *Arch Intern Med* 1977;137:1571–5.

7 Bernstein J. A classification of renal cysts. In: Gardner KD, ed. *Cystic Diseases of the Kidney*. New York: John Wiley, 1976.

8 Betts PR, Forrest-Hay I. Juvenile nephronophthisis. *Lancet* 1973;ii:475–8.

9 Wehle M, Walker RD. The child with solitary hydronephrotic kidney. *Urology* 1985;26:269–73.

10 Gordon I. Imaging the urinary tract. In: Holliday MA, Barrett TM, Vernier RL, eds. *Pediatric Nephrology*. 2nd edn. Baltimore: Williams & Wilkins, 1987.

11 Dillon MJ. Hypertension. In: Williams DI, Johnson JH, eds. *Pediatric Urology*. London: Butterworth Scientific. 1982.

12 Wallace DMA, Rothwell DL, Williams DI. The long-term follow-up of surgically treated vesico-ureteric reflux. *Br J Urol* 1978;50:479–84.

13 Smellie JM, Normand C. Reflux nephropathy in childhood. In: Hodson J, Kincaid-Smith P, eds. *Reflux Nephropathy*. New York: Masson Publishing, 1979.

14 Gusmano R, Perfumo F, Raspino M, Ginevri F, Verrina E,

Ciardi MR. Natural history of reflux nephropathy in children. *Contr Nephrol.* 1988;61:200−9.

15 Dillon MJ, Smellie JM. Peripheral plasma renin activity, hypertension and renal scarring in children. *Contr Nephrol* 1984;39:68−80.

16 Dillon MJ, Gordon I, Shah V. 99m-Tc-DMSA scanning and segmental renal vein renin estimations in children with renal scarring. *Contr Nephrol* 1984;39:20−7.

17 Lewy JE, Salinas-Madrigal L, Herdso PB *et al.* Clinico-pathologic correlations in acute poststreptococcal glomerulonephritis.*Medicine* 1971;50:433−501.

18 Rodriguez-Iturbe B, Baggio B, Colina-Chourio J *et al.* Studies on the renin−aldosterone system in the acute nephritic syndrome. *Kidney Int* 1981;19:445−53.

19 Powell HR, Rotenberg E, Williams AC, McCredie DA. Plasma renin activity in acute poststreptococcal glomerulonephritis and the hemolytic-uremic syndrome. *Arch Dis Child* 1974;49:802−7.

20 Repetto HA, Lewy JE, Braudo JL, Miteoff J. The renal functional response to furosemide in children with acute glomerulonephritis. *J Pediatr* 1972;80:660−6.

21 Campos A, Sibley R, Kim Y, Miller K, Michael AF. The hemolytic uremic syndrome. *Kidney* 1981;14:23−30.

22 Miller K, Kim Y. Hemolytic uremic syndrome. In: Holliday MA, Barratt TM, Vernier RL, eds. *Pediatric Nephrology.* 2nd edn. Baltimore: Williams & Wilkins, 1987.

23 McEnery PT, McAdams AJ, West CD. The effect of prednisone in a high-dose, alternate-day regimen on the natural history of idiopathic membranoproliferative glomerulonephritis. *Medicine* 1986;64:401−24.

24 Ellis D, Kapur S, Antonouych TT, Salcedo JR, Ynis EJ. Focal glomerulosclerosis in children: correlation of histology with prognosis. *J Pediatr* 1978;93:762−8.

25 Newman WJ, Fisher CC, McCoy RC *et al.* Focal glomerular sclerosis: contrasting clinical patterns in children and adults. *Medicine* 1976;55:67−87.

26 A report of the Southwest Pediatric Nephrology Study Group. Childhood nephrotic syndrome associated with diffuse mesangial hypercellularity. *Kidney Int* 1983;23:87−94.

27 A report of the Southwest Pediatric Nephrology Study Group. A clinico-pathologic study of crescentic glomerulonephritis in 50 children. *Kidney Int* 1985;27:450−8.

28 A report of the Southwest Pediatric Nephrology Study Group. A multi-center study of IgA nephropathy in children. *Kidney Int* 1982;22:643−52.

29 Wyatt RJ, Julian BA, Bhathern DB, Mitchell BL, Holland NH, Malluche HH. IgA nephropathy: presentation, clinical course, and prognosis in children and adults. *Am J Kidney Dis* 1984;4:192−200.

30 Habib R, Kleinknecht C, Gubler MC. Extramembranous glomerulonephritis in children: report of 50 cases. *J Pediatr* 1973;82:754−66.

31 A report of the Southwest Pediatric Nephrology Study Group. Hepatitis B surface antigenemia in North American children with membranous glomerulonephropathy. *J Pediatr* 1985;106:571−8.

32 Garin EH, Donnelly WH, Fennell RS, Richard GA. Nephritis in systemic lupus erythematosus in children. *J Pediatr* 1976;89:366−71.

33 Meadow SR, Glasgow EF, White RHR, Moncrieff MW, Cameron JS, Oqq CS. Schönlein−Henoch nephritis. *Q J Med* 1972;61:241−58.

34 Counahan R, Winterborn MH, White RHR *et al.* Prognosis of Henoch−Schönlein nephritis in children. *Br Med J* 1977; 2:11−14.

35 Ettenger RE, Nelson AM, Burke EC, Lie JT. Polyarteritis nodosa in childhood. *Arthritis Rheum* 1979;22:820−5.

36 White RH, Schambelan M. Hypertension, hyperreninemia and secondary hyperaldosteronism in systemic necrotizing vasculitis. *Ann Intern Med* 1980;92:199−201.

37 Report of the Second Task Force on Blood Pressure Control in Children−1987. *Pediatrics* 1987;79:1−25.

38 Portman RJ, Robson AM. Controversies in pediatric hypertension. In: Tune BM, Mendoza SA, eds. *Pediatric Nephrology.* New York: Churchill Livingstone, 1984.

39 Dillon MJ. Investigation and management of hypertension in children. *Pediatr Nephrol* 1987;1:59−68.

20 Focal and Diffuse Renal Parenchymal Lesions Associated with Hypertension: The Urologic Surgeon's Approach to Evaluation and Management

JOSE C. CORTEZ AND CURTIS A. SHELDON

Secondary and potentially curable forms of hypertension are more common in children than adults (Fig. 20.1). Renal parenchymal nonrenovascular disorders predominate, accounting for a majority of secondary causes. Despite this, a relative lack of investigation and paucity of long-term follow-up studies exist compared to the abundance of literature on the less common renovascular disorders. In this review we hope to increase the reader's awareness of these disorders, emphasizing their association with hypertension and their various surgical treatments. In addition, we will examine the experience and treatment of the child with bilateral versus unilateral renal parenchymal disease. The primary goals of treatment are: (a) normalization of blood pressure; and (b) maximal preservation of renal function.

Renal parenchymal disorders account for 73–78% of all causes of secondary childhood hypertension [2,3]. These figures vary depending on the age group, referral center, and referral bias (Figs 20.2 and 20.3) [5]. The likelihood that hypertension is due to secondary causes is age-related and occurs in 78% of 1–5-year-olds, 44% of 6–10-year-olds, and 32% of 10–15-year-olds [6]. In general, the younger the patient the higher the probability that hypertension is the result of potentially correctable disease. The various causes of renal parenchymal hypertension (RPHTN) are shown in Table 20.1. The most common disorders are reflux nephropathy, chronic pyelonephritis, and urinary obstruction.

Morbidity and mortality associated with RPHTN are determined by the nature of the underlying disease and the severity of the hypertension. For example, progression with renal damage has been seen in long-term follow-up studies of children with vesicoureteral reflux who have developed hypertension. Similarly, the development of hypertension in patients with renal scarring is a significant feature of those who developed end-stage renal disease. In studies of children with severe hypertension, mortality has been reported as high as 56% with an average duration of life (from diagnosis) of 14 months [7]. More recently with advances in antihypertensive therapy, surgical treatment, dialysis, and renal transplantation, the mortality has been reported at 17% [8].

Thus, the child with sustained hypertension should undergo careful and thorough evaluation for a correctable cause. Once identified, such a child requires antihypertensive medication or after careful patient selection, appropriate surgical treatment. These interventions may yield a successful result and potentially avoid morbid complications and mortality.

RENAL CONTROL OF BLOOD PRESSURE

Renal control of blood pressure is governed by two basic mechanisms involving the maintenance of

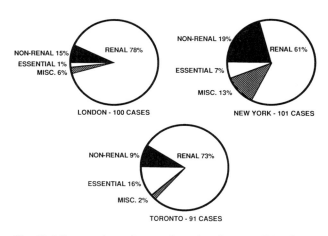

Fig. 20.1 Reports from three major referral centers [1] indicate that renal disease is the most common cause of persistent hypertension in hospitalized children. Misc. = Miscellaneous causes.

217

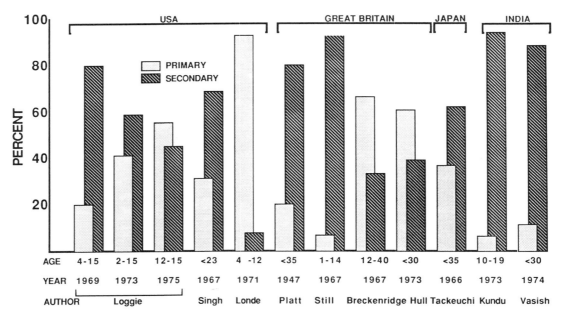

Fig. 20.2 The percentage of secondary and primary hypertension reported by different authors is influenced by age group, country of study, referral bias, referral patterns, and possibly patient selection [3,4].

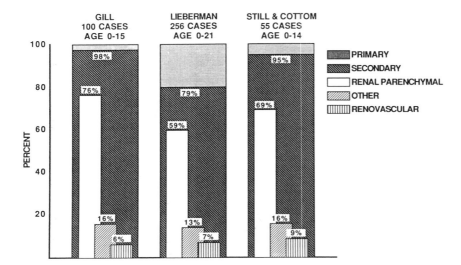

Fig. 20.3 Renal parenchymal disease accounts for the majority of causes of secondary hypertension in children [5].

extracellular fluid volume and the secretion of neuro-humoral substances. A basic understanding of these mechanisms is essential to a review of hypertension secondary to renal parenchymal disorders. Clinical and experimental evidence exists to suggest that these mechanisms may act singly or together in the patho-genesis of RPHTN.

Volume-dependent

Blood pressure is the product of cardiac output and

peripheral vascular resistance. Blood volume influ-ences blood pressure through its relation to the stroke volume and thus cardiac output. Figure 20.4 shows the renal mechanisms controlling body fluid and thus arterial pressure. Providing renal function is adequate, total body salt and water do not accumulate and blood pressure is maintained. In patients with poor renal function or reduced renal mass, hyper-tension may be volume-dependent and caused by accumulation of excess salt and water [9]. This occurs when intake exceeds the capacity of the kidney to

Table 20.1 The commonest causes of renal parenchymal hypertension.

Renal scarring
Reflux nephropathy
Chronic pyelonephritis

Hydronephrosis
Ureteral obstruction
Ureteropelvic junction obstruction

Hypoplasia/dysplasia
Segmental
Global
Occult renal tissue

Cystic diseases
Multicystic dysplastic kidney
Autosomal recessive (infantile) polycystic kidney
Autosomal dominant (adult) polycystic kidney
Solitary simple cyst

Tumors
Wilms' (nephroblastoma)
Juxtaglomerular cell
Mesoblastic nephroma

Trauma
Page kidney
Functionless post-traumatic segment

End-stage renal disease
Postrenal transplant

excrete the salt and water load. Likewise, patients with renal parenchymal disorders such as renal scarring (especially when extensive and bilateral) may have volume-dependent hypertension on the basis of decreased renal capacity to maintain salt and water balance. Hypertension has also been observed in the anephric human and animal secondary to accumulation of excess sodium and water. Clinically this is observed most commonly in the patient with end-stage renal disease.

Neurohumoral

The vasoactive substances produced by the kidney that influence blood pressure control are prostaglandins, the kinins, and renin. Renal parenchymal disorders may produce hypertension by alteration of the balance of these substances with local interruption of feedback interactions (see also Chapter 2).

Microscopic and histochemical studies have demonstrated adrenergic nerve terminals in direct contact with basement membranes of the glomerulus, juxtaglomerular apparatus, renal tubular epithelium and vasculature. Direct stimulation of these nerves results in an increase in arterial blood pressure that persists as long as the stimulus is present. Physiologic studies suggest that the renal sympathetic nervous system may play a specific role in blood pressure

Fig. 20.4 Arterial pressure is influenced by mechanisms that regulate sodium (Na⁺) and water (H₂O) balance. If renal function is adequate, total body sodium and water do not accumulate. Any excess load is excreted by the kidney. Renal parenchymal diseases that impair renal function may alter this delicate balance with a resultant decrease in the ability to excrete excess sodium and water. Subsequent accumulation of total body sodium and water increases the extracellular fluid (ECF) and blood volume compartments which ultimately affect autoregulatory mechanisms, total peripheral resistance, and cardiac output. This results in a volume-dependent increase in arterial blood pressure.

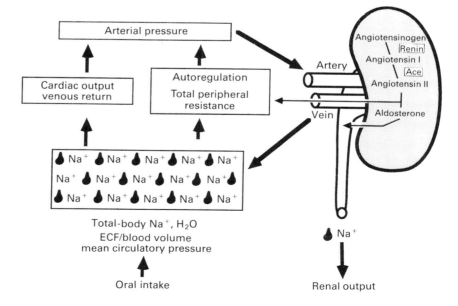

control by inhibiting renal sodium excretion. This may occur through several mechanisms, including: (a) redistribution or reduction of blood flow; (b) activation of the renin−angiotensin−aldosterone system; and (c) a direct effect on the tubule [10].

Prostaglandins

Both vasodilator and vasoconstrictor prostaglandins are produced by the kidney. The collecting tubules and interstitial cells produce those of the E series that have powerful local vasodilatory and natriuretic actions. The endothelial cells of the renal interlobular and afferent arterioles produce vasodilatory prostacyclins. Additionally, the cortical tubules and the glomeruli produce thromboxanes, which are powerful vasoconstrictors [10]. It has been suggested that renal parenchymal scarring may interrupt the corticomedullary hormonal balance resulting in a stimulus or disinhibition of the renin−angiotensin−aldosterone system [11].

Kinins

The role of renal kinins in control of blood pressure is unknown. Lysylbradykinin forms from kininogen (after activation by kallikrein) and is both vasodilatory and natriuretic. Its role in the pathogenesis of RPHTN is unproven [12].

Renin

The role of increased plasma renin activity (PRA) in the pathogenesis of RPHTN has been demonstrated clinically and experimentally. Hyperreninemia has been documented in children with different bilateral and unilateral renal disorders including renal scarring, urinary obstruction, and renal hypoplasia. The observation that removal of the renal unit secreting high renin results in blood pressure normalization suggests a causal relationship.

Mechanisms by which renal parenchymal disorders activate the renin−angiotensin−aldosterone system may be understood through models of experimentally induced hypertension. The Goldblatt [13] and Page [14] kidney models have been used to reproduce hypertension experimentally. These models may help us to understand the mechanisms by which renal parenchymal disorders affect control of blood pressure, water, and salt balance.

One-kidney Goldblatt model

The one-kidney Goldblatt hypertension model (Fig. 20.5) is produced by ipsilateral renal artery constriction and contralateral nephrectomy. Decreased renal perfusion results in an initial transient vasoconstrictor phase secondary to increased secretion of renin. Within 5−7 days the renal arterial pressure rises with a subsequent decrease in renin secretion. Blood pressure, however, continues to rise secondary to volume expansion. This volume expansion occurs in the absence of a contralateral compensatory renal unit and further suppresses renin secretion.

Two-kidney Goldblatt model

The two-kidney Goldblatt hypertension model (Fig. 20.5) is produced by constriction of the renal artery of one kidney in the presence of a normal functioning contralateral renal unit. Decreased renal perfusion of the constricted kidney activates baroceptor mechanisms with a resultant increase in the secretion of renin. This is followed by an increase in systemic blood pressure with increased perfusion of the contralateral kidney and contralateral suppression of renin secretion. Urinary sodium excretion is decreased in the constricted kidney secondary to a macula densa-mediated secretion of aldosterone resulting in increased tubular reabsorption of sodium. Increased contralateral renal sodium excretion results in a normovolemic state. Hypertension persists due to a continued increase in renin secretion from the kidney with a constricted artery. This model most closely resembles the development of hypertension in the patient with renal disease.

Page kidney

Renal parenchymal compression (Fig. 20.5) without renal artery stenosis may result in hypertension. This was demonstrated experimentally by Irvine H. Page in 1939 when he observed hypertension in animals after wrapping kidneys in a cellophane film [14]. He discovered that the cellophane wrap resulted in a perinephritis that formed a constricting perinephric fibrocollagenous hull. Increased PRA was observed in these animals and was postulated to be responsible for the development of hypertension by a mechanism similar to the Goldblatt model. Removal of the affected kidney or of the constricting hull resulted in

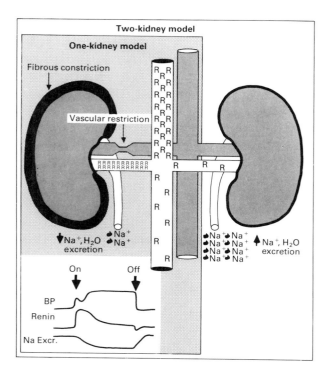

Fig. 20.5 One-kidney model Goldblatt hypertension results when vascular restriction (ON) of arterial blood flow to an ipsilateral kidney is present and contralateral nephrectomy is performed. Decreased perfusion is followed by an increase in the rate of renin (R) secretion with a subsequent acute increase in blood pressure. Sodium (Na^+) and water (H_2O) excretion from the compromised kidney drops accordingly. Over several days, as sodium and water accumulate from decreased excretion, blood pressure becomes less renin- and more volume-dependent. The increase in blood volume subsequently acts as an inhibitor of renin secretion. Blood pressure (BP), however, is maintained secondary to volume expansion. Removal of the vascular constriction (OFF) results in normalization of blood pressure from improved ability to handle excess sodium and water.

Two-kidney model Goldblatt hypertension is produced by ipsilateral vascular restriction (ON) without contralateral nephrectomy. Decreased perfusion is followed by increased renin secretion and decreased sodium and water excretion by the ipsilateral unit. Blood pressure rises secondary to increased renin secretion. The contralateral renal unit experiences an increase in renal perfusion pressure which results in contralateral suppression of renin secretion and contralateral tubular reabsorption of sodium. Thus, the perfused kidney excretes more sodium and water. The net effect is compensatory and results in a normal extracellular fluid volume.

Page kidney hypertension occurs when fibrous constriction of the renal parenchyma results in ischemia, in contrast to ischemia from vascular pedicle restriction. In patients with two kidneys, unilateral parenchymal fibrous constriction results in two-kidney Goldblatt hypertension. If fibrous parenchymal constriction occurs in a solitary kidney, one-kidney Goldblatt hypertension is produced.

normalization of blood pressures. Thus, Page demonstrated the development of hypertension secondary to ischemia caused by compression of the renal parenchyma. This effect has also been observed clinically by others in patients with fibrous encapsulation following renal trauma [15].

EVALUATION

Introduction

The evaluation of the child with hypertension requires an individualized approach based on clinical presentation, history, and physical examination (see Chapter 10) [16,17]. Because curable renal parenchymal disorders account for the majority of secondary causes, the clinician should inquire into any history of trauma, urinary tract infection, unexplained fevers, abdominal pain, flank pain, or gross hematuria. Likewise, palpation of an abdominal mass or auscultation of a bruit are important findings. The presence of any of these should support a prompt investigation identifying pathology that may have otherwise gone undetected. This investigation should then be directed at assessing renal parenchymal and collecting system anatomy, differential renal function, absence or presence of obstruction, and the physiologic significance of the lesion in causing hypertension. We will present only those investigations useful in evaluating and characterizing curable renal parenchymal disorders.

Renal ultrasound

In many cases, the history and physical examination yield few clues toward an etiology, making renal imaging an initial step in the evaluation. Renal imaging by ultrasound is a useful noninvasive tool in studying renal parenchymal and collecting system anatomy [18]. It is emphasized that this technique does not evaluate the physiologic significance of an abnormality. Rather, it helps direct further studies by suggesting an etiology based on size, shape, density (echogenicity), or anomaly. Ultrasound anatomic diagnoses and the renal abnormalities that may be associated with them are shown in Figure 20.6. It should be noted that the pathophysiologic process of renal scarring, reflux nephropathy, or chronic pyelonephritis may produce several ultrasound images and will require further differentiation by cystogram, and nuclear radioisotope scanning.

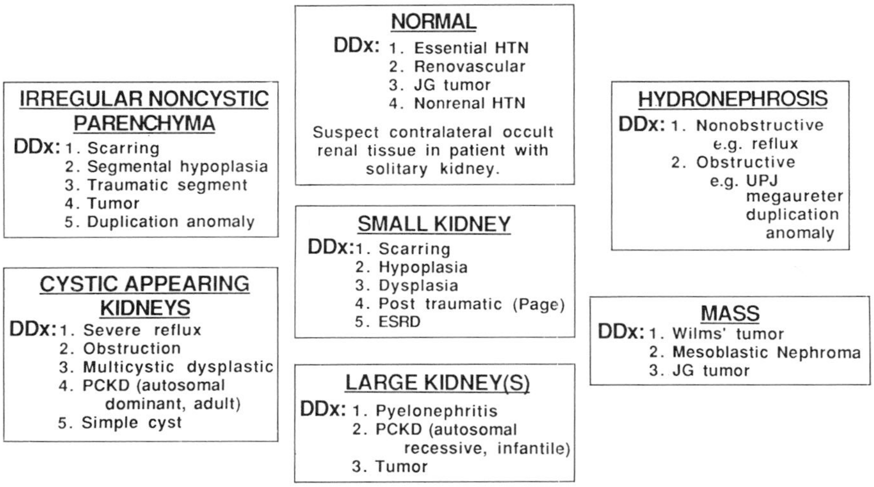

Fig. 20.6 Ultrasound imaging allows anatomic and structural examination that may help determine further studies in the hypertensive child. DDx = Differential diagnosis.

Be aware that a normal study may be seen in patients with the less common renovascular diseases and juxtaglomerular cell tumors. A solitary kidney in a hypertensive child should not be readily dismissed as normal since occult contralateral renal tissue hypersecreting renin has been described [19]. Patients with this problem may only be identified by invasive methods including angiography and renal vein and segmental vein renin sampling. Fortunately, these entities are uncommon and a normal study will (by anatomy only) exclude most of the curable renal parenchymal causes of hypertension.

Cystogram

Cystogram evaluation is indicated if there is a history of urinary tract infection or when ultrasound reveals findings that may represent any pathologic variant in the spectrum of vesicoureteric reflux as well as bladder or ureteral obstruction. This includes patients with irregular, cystic, small, large, or hydronephrotic kidneys (see Fig. 20.6).

Excretory urography

Although excretory urography has largely been replaced by ultrasound as a primary renal imaging modality, it is indicated when a parenchymal or collecting system abnormality requires further anatomic characterization and definition. This is especially important when planning surgical treatment of focal parenchymal (renal scars, simple cysts, segmental hypoplasia, etc.) and obstructive lesions (ureteropelvic junction obstruction, ureteral obstruction).

In situations where ultrasound is not available, the excretory urogram remains an acceptable primary imaging modality when not contraindicated by allergy, renal function, or cardiovascular instability. The solute osmotic load during an excretory urogram may constitute a risk in the child with severe hypertension, congestive heart failure, or respiratory distress.

Nuclear renography

Once a renal parenchymal process has been characterized anatomically, nuclear scanning is often necessary to assess the degree of function or obstruction.

Technetium 99 m dimercaptosuccinic acid (DMSA) is bound to albumin and localizes in functioning renal tubules. When localizing in the renal tubular mass, DMSA may identify areas of decreased or no function. This scan is useful in evaluating the parenchymal anatomy and function in patients with a history of trauma, scar, small kidney, large kidney, presumed solitary, ectopic, or cystic kidney [20].

Technetium 99 m diethylenetriaminepentaacetic acid (DTPA) is mostly filtered by the glomerulus without significant reabsorption or secretion. This characteristic makes it ideal for studying glomerular filtration rate, and radioisotope transit time (obstruction) through the collecting system allowing functional characterization of the anatomic abnormality. (Patients with hydronephrosis or duplication anomalies are best studied with this scan.) If obstruction is present, the rate of washout of DTPA is prolonged after a forced furosemide diuresis.

Summary

Renal ultrasound imaging is useful in the initial evaluation and anatomically excludes most causes of renal parenchymal hypertension. Further characterization of an abnormality then proceeds in a logical order excluding vesicoureteric reflux or obstruction when appropriate. Assessment of differential renal function is also an essential part of this exercise.

INVASIVE STUDIES

Angiography

The goal of angiography is to identify surgically treatable lesions and define their anatomy. Several clinical situations warrant further evaluation by angiography:
1 the child with severe persistent hypertension in the absence of other findings;
2 when a normal imaging evaluation is suspicious because of an elevated peripheral PRA;
3 when renovascular disease is suspected because of a bruit;
4 when tumor is suspected (abdominal mass);
5 when evaluating a presumed solitary kidney and searching for occult contralateral disease.

Angiography combined with renal vein renin sampling is useful in the investigation and management of childhood hypertension. At the Royal Hospital for Sick Children in Glasgow, Alroomi and associates [21] reported on studies in 42 children with persistent and severe hypertension. In 22 patients, renal vein renin sampling localized the source of renin by demonstrating its physiologic role in producing hypertension. Most of these patients underwent surgery and 80% were cured. Of significance, surgery was successful in all patients when these studies demonstrated unilateral disease with renin hypersecretion by that kidney (lateralization). Surgery was unsuccessful in the majority of patients with bilateral disease (40% cure rate).

Renal vein renin sampling and the concept of lateralization

In contrast to studies (ultrasound, excretory urog-

raphy, nuclear scanning, angiography) that help define the structural nature of a renal parenchymal abnormality, renin sampling helps establish a causal relationship by studying its physiologic significance. The mere presence of anatomic pathology does not prove that hypertension is secondary to it [22].

The diagnosis of renal parenchymal hypertension as a renin-dependent phenomenon is facilitated by the study of renin concentration from the inferior vena cava, main renal veins, and (when indicated) segmental veins. The diagnosis is dependent on three (lateralization) criteria [23] (Fig. 20.7) that describe the expected physiologic responses of the Goldblatt two-kidney, one-clip hypertension model:
1 renin hypersecretion from the suspect unit (V_1);
2 contralateral suppression of renin secretion from the normal unit (V_2);
3 decreased perfusion of the suspect unit as shown by an increased concentration of renal vein renin when compared to systemic (inferior vena cava) renin.

If a causal relationship exists between lesion and renin then removal of the lesion (providing disease is not present elsewhere) should result in normalization of blood pressure.

More recently, the yield of renal vein renin sampling has been improved by renin stimulation after converting enzyme inhibition [24]. Increased renin release from the suspect unit occurs when inhibition

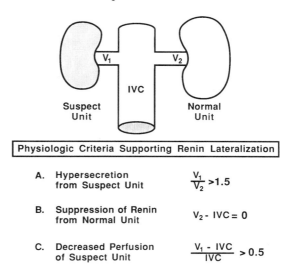

Physiologic Criteria Supporting Renin Lateralization	
A. Hypersecretion from Suspect Unit	$\frac{V_1}{V_2} > 1.5$
B. Suppression of Renin from Normal Unit	$V_2 - IVC = 0$
C. Decreased Perfusion of Suspect Unit	$\frac{V_1 - IVC}{IVC} > 0.5$

Fig. 20.7 Ipsilateral renin hypersecretion ($V_1:V_2$ ratio >1.5) and contralateral renin suppression [V_2 and inferior vena cava (IVC) renin approach equality] describe the concept of lateralizing renins. $V_1 - IVC/IVC > 0.5$ may occur when the suspect unit is poorly perfused or when suspect unit renal vein (V_1) renin is increased. $V_2 = $ Normal unit renal vein renin.

of angiotensin converting enzyme results in further decrease in perfusion of that unit. Converting enzyme inhibition thus enhances renin secretion and is useful when evaluating patients on β-blockers (renin secretion may be reduced) or whose renin sampling is inconclusive and if a renal lesion remains suspect.

Segmental renal vein renin sampling

Segmental renal vein renin sampling was first described by Schambelan and associates [25] in adult patients with segmental renovascular and parenchymal disease. They demonstrated that specific localization of these lesions was possible when main renal vein renin sampling was inconclusive. In addition, it has been shown that segmental sampling may also direct specific surgical treatment with successful results.

Segmental sampling is indicated in several circumstances:

1 when assessing the physiologic significance of a segmental or focal renal abnormality;

2 when previous imaging reveals no obvious renal abnormalities (as in the case of a small juxtaglomerular cell tumor);

3 when main renal vein renin sampling is inconclusive;

4 when planning a parenchymal sparing procedure.

Segmental renin samples are taken from upper, middle, and lower pole systems as well as main renal veins and inferior vena cava. Main renal vein renin interpretation is as described before (see Fig. 20.8). The renin values of the suspect segments are then evaluated by their ratios with renin values from the contralateral main vein or inferior vena cava [26]. Physiologic criteria of hypersecretion of renin from the suspect segment and the contralateral suppression of secretion apply as described previously (Fig. 20.8).

Parenchymal sparing surgery may be considered if segmental renal vein renin sampling reveals a focal source of renin. This has been described clinically in children where various lesions have been removed with resultant cure [26,27]. In many cases these segmental lesions would have otherwise been missed as main renal vein renin ratios were inconclusive (ratio <1.5) [28].

Summary

Main renal vein renin and segmental vein sampling are localization studies that are useful in assessing

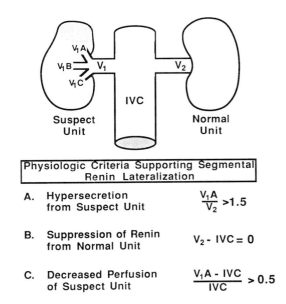

Fig. 20.8 Renin hypersecretion ratios may be calculated between the suspect segment (e.g. V_1A) and normal unit main vein (V_2) renin or inferior vena cava (IVC) renin. V_1A, B, and C are the suspect unit upper, middle, and lower pole regions respectively.

the presence and physiologic significance of lesions producing hypertension. It is stressed that the finding of increased renal vein renin suggests a causal relationship and in no way definitively predicts cure of hypertension [29].

REFLUX NEPHROPATHY

The most frequent cause of RPHTN in adolescent children is reflux nephropathy [7,8,30,31]. Renal scarring secondary to vesicoureteral reflux is a predominant feature and has been described in several clinical disorders under the various terms of chronic pyelonephritis, segmental hypoplasia, primary interstitial nephritis, Ask-Upmark kidney, and reflux nephropathy. Holland's review of 177 cases of hypertension with renal scarring and vesicoureteral reflux suggests that these disorders have similar clinical features and may represent a single disease process [31]. Although only 5 patients presented with coincident hypertension and urinary tract infection (UTI), a prior history of UTI was present in the majority of patients with chronic pyelonephritis, reflux nephropathy, or Ask-Upmark kidney. Likewise, the prevalence of vesicoureteral reflux was high in those patients studied (Fig 20.9).

The prevalence of hypertension with reflux neph-

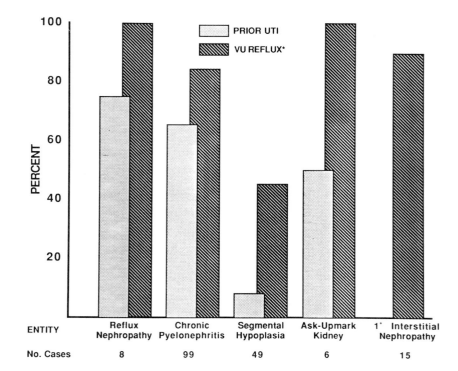

Fig. 20.9 Various diagnostic terms have been used to describe what may be a single disease process. Of 177 patients, 48% underwent voiding cystourethrography (VCUG). In most cases, the prevalence of vesicoureteral reflux and urinary tract infection was high. Prior history of urinary tract infection was not reported in those with primary (1°) interstitial nephritis.

ropathy is unknown. Calculations based on the prevalence of UTI and renal scarring estimate that as many as 50% of patients with renal scarring develop hypertension by age 30 [32]. The observed incidence of hypertension in patients with renal scarring ranges from 10 to 30% in different series [33−36]. Smellie suggests that hypertension associated with reflux nephropathy is age-related, with increased risk above age 15 [36]. Indeed, it has been observed that patients with this condition are at risk of developing delayed hypertension in adolescence and young adulthood [34].

Mechanism of hypertension in reflux nephropathy

It is suggested that hypertension with reflux nephropathy is secondary to activation of the renin−angiotensin−aldosterone system. Holland's review of 177 cases demonstrates an association between increased PRA and renal scarring, although many inconsistencies were noted with normal PRA occurring in many hypertensive patients [31]. Dillon's 1984 review of 51 patients with reflux nephropathy and hypertension revealed 36 patients with increased PRA [37]. A review of cases from Great Ormond Street Hospital (London) also found that the majority of patients with hypertension had an increased PRA. Of 15 patients with renal scarring, 9 had increased PRA

[30]. Further support for renin as a major factor in the hypertension associated with reflux nephropathy was seen in 6 children with reflux nephropathy who also had hypertensive encephalopathy. In these patients PRA was increased in 3 whose blood pressure was elevated at the time of PRA measurement and normal in 3 when the PRA was measured after blood pressure had normalized following institution of antihypertensive therapy [35,38]. Although the finding of normal PRA in some patients may suggest another mechanism for hypertension, Bailey [39] has demonstrated 2 patients with hypertension associated with reflux nephropathy and low PRA who had lateralizing renal vein renin studies (renal vein renin ratio greater than 1.5). This affirms the need for selective renal vein renin sampling in hypertensive patients despite normal peripheral PRA.

Elevated PRA has also been found in patients with reflux nephropathy but without hypertension. Savage and colleagues [30] reported that 8 of 100 normotensive children with reflux nephropathy had elevated PRA. Interestingly, after 5 years 2 of these 8 developed hypertension, suggesting that patients with reflux nephropathy and increased PRA are at higher risk for the development of hypertension [28]. Similarly, Smellie [36] and Dillon [37] reported 26 normotensive patients with reflux nephropathy, of whom 5 had elevated PRA.

Selective renal vein renin studies

The value of selective renal vein renin studies in the evaluation of hypertension associated with reflux nephropathy is controversial. Studies have shown that the PRA in the vein of a scarred kidney may be normal [30,40]. Bailey [41] has reported renal vein renin studies in both normotensive and hypertensive patients with reflux nephropathy. The renal vein renin ratio was greater than 1.5 in 3 normotensive and 2 hypertensive patients. The ratio was less than 1.0 in 1 normotensive and 3 hypertensive patients. These results may be explained by multiple factors, including technical sampling errors, or dilution of segmentally increased renin at the level of the main renal vein.

Support for selective renal vein renin sampling is demonstrated by Dillon and coworkers [42] who suggest that these studies do assist in identification of the renal unit producing increased renin. Selective renal vein renin studies in 52 hypertensive patients with reflux nephropathy revealed 33 with renal vein renin ratios greater than 1.5 with lateralization or localization that assisted in surgical treatment. Twenty-two of these patients had operative procedures: 20 had unilateral nephrectomy, 1 had a unilateral nephrectomy and contralateral partial nephrectomy, and 1 had a partial nephrectomy. There was a total of 14 cures and 8 patients with improved hypertension. Furthermore, in another series 50% of 44 patients with reflux nephropathy and hypertension required segmental renal vein renin studies in order to localize the source of hypertension. Additional large series provide supporting evidence that lateralizing renal vein renin studies may predict the success of surgical treatment [43,44].

In summary, strong evidence exists to suggest an association of increased renin secretion in patients with hypertension associated with reflux nephropathy. The findings of normal PRA or lack of lateralizing main renal vein renin in some patients may be secondary to multiple technical factors. Many of these patients may only be identified by segmental renal vein renin sampling. The opportunity to provide a surgical cure must not be overlooked.

Progression of patients with renal scarring to end-stage renal disease (ESRD)

Every patient with vesicoureteral reflux is at risk for renal injury. It is estimated that 12−30% of children

with ESRD have disease attributable to reflux nephropathy [45−47]. The number of children who progress from reflux nephropathy alone to ESRD is difficult to determine because end-stage pathology may represent other disorders that may or may not be associated with reflux. For example, small scarred hypoplastic kidneys may be seen in chronic pyelonephritis and global hypoplasia [48]. Arant [32] suggests that reflux nephropathy may be the single most common cause of chronic renal failure and ESRD in American children. He has reported experience at the Children's Medical Center in Dallas between 1980 and 1988 with 90 children and adolescents treated for ESRD. Of these, 19% had primary vesicoureteral reflux as the only identifiable cause of injury, with another 51% exhibiting urologic disorders associated with segmental renal atrophy that may have been secondary to previous vesicoureteral reflux.

While the prevalence of hypertension in patients with renal scarring is largely unknown, it has been observed that high blood pressure is a significant feature of those patients developing ESRD. Smellie's long-term study of children with vesicoureteral reflux published in 1979 showed progression of renal damage in those patients who developed hypertension [34]. Children with only reflux nephropathy may progress to ESRD and hypertension, despite having no further evidence of infection or renal scarring [48].

Delayed development of hypertension in patients with renal scarring

Patients with renal scarring secondary to reflux nephropathy continue to be at risk for development of hypertension despite successful antireflux surgery [38]. Wallace and co-authors [33] reported the development of hypertension in 18.5% of children with bilateral renal scarring and 11.3% of those with unilateral renal scars more than 10 years after antireflux surgery. Braren and associates [49] found 6 children who became hypertensive at a mean of 4 years following antireflux surgery (range 6 years). They represented 6 out of 35 or 17.1% of a series of children presenting with hypertension secondary to reflux nephropathy or obstructive uropathy over a 10-year period at Vanderbilt Children's Hospital. Hendren and associates [50] described a 14-year-old girl with marked atrophy of the left kidney who presented with hypertensive encephalopathy (blood pressure 280/125 mmHg). Seven years earlier she had undergone bilateral ureteral re-implantation for reflux. She underwent a left nephrectomy and at age 28 was normotensive on no antihypertensive medications.

Indeed, it has been observed in series of children with scarred kidneys, that hypertension remains a potential complication for many years. Taylor and associates [51] observed that age at presentation with hypertension in patients with scarred kidneys ranged between 4 and 16 years with most of the patients presenting between 8 and 12 years of age. Smellie [34] reported 83 children with reflux nephropathy, 11 of whom (13%) were hypertensive initially (6 with malignant hypertension), and 14 of whom (17%) developed hypertension over 4–20 years of follow-up. Thus, 30% of the 83 ultimately had courses complicated by hypertension.

HYDRONEPHROSIS

Hypertension associated with hydronephrosis has been well described in children and adults. Evidence exists to suggest that hypertension secondary to acute unilateral obstruction is most often renin-mediated [52]. Volume-dependent hypertension is common when obstruction is bilateral or chronic [53].

The observation of increased PRA with unilateral ureteral obstruction was first described clinically by Belman and co-authors in an adult female [54]. A hyperreninemic state with lateralization of renal vein renins to the affected side was followed by decreased PRA and normotension after successful corrective surgery (ureterolysis). Hyperreninemia has also been clinically described by others [55,56] in children with unilateral hydronephrosis. Experimental studies of peripheral PRA and blood pressure changes in dogs following acute unilateral ureteral occlusion demonstrate a transitory significant hypertensive and hyperreninemic state that persists for 4–6 weeks [52]. This suggests a correlation between unilateral obstruction and increased activity of the renin–angiotensin–aldosterone system with resultant hypertension.

Vaughan suggests that the "macula densa" theory best explains the mechanism of renin release in acute unilateral hydronephrosis. By this theory, acute unilateral ureteral obstruction results in decreased glomerular filtration rate and increased proximal reabsorption of sodium which results in decreased delivery of sodium to the macula densa with a resultant stimulus for renin release. In addition, Kawano and colleagues [55] have provided histologic evidence of hypergranularity and hypertrophy of the juxta-

glomerular cells in a 6-year-old male with massive ureteropelvic junction obstruction and hypertension, suggesting that renin release was involved in the etiology of the hypertension.

Hypertension associated with chronic (unilateral and bilateral) hydronephrosis is probably volume-dependent. In patients with this condition, PRA is not always elevated. Studies of 13 adult hypertensive patients with chronic hydronephrosis revealed that PRA was usually normal (78%) or low (15%) and that renal vein renin studies failed to show lateralization or contralateral suppression [53]. It is suggested that hydronephrotic atrophy results in tubular dysfunction and decreased renin secretion.

Several reports have demonstrated that increased PRA and lateralization of renal vein renin may predict the curability of hypertension following surgery for correction of obstruction. Weidman and associates' [57] series of 8 patients with unilateral hydronephrosis found 4 with renal vein renin ratios greater than 1.5 who were successfully treated by nephrectomy. Surgery was unsuccessful in 2 patients who had nonlateralizing renal vein renins (ratio less than or equal to 1.3).

Clinically, ureteropelvic junction obstruction associated with hypertension is frequently encountered in children and its presentation is varied. Symptoms may be absent [58], minimal [56] (anorexia and irritability), or severe, presenting with evidence of central nervous system involvement from malignant hypertension [59]. After diagnosing hypertension with obstructive uropathy, it is essential to direct treatment toward the normalization of blood pressure, correction of obstruction, and maximal preservation of renal function. In the past, the most commonly reported treatment has been nephrectomy [57]. However, reports of cure following surgical repair have shown that nephrectomy is not the only surgical option. Pyeloplasty results in relief from obstruction and preservation of renal mass. Several authors have reported success in achieving normotension with this procedure [49,50,56,58]. If surgical repair must be delayed because of medical reasons, it has been shown that a percutaneous nephrostomy is not only temporizing but may be predictive of the success of elective repair. Grossman and coworkers [59] reported a 28-month-old white male with malignant hypertension who presented with hemiparesis and facial nerve palsy from an intracerebral hemorrhage. Evaluation revealed a ureteropelvic junction obstruction. Placement of a nephrostomy tube confirmed the diagnosis and resulted in normotension off medication. Ultimately the patient underwent pyeloplasty which resulted in successful resolution of the obstruction and normotension after removal of the nephrostomy tube.

HYPOPLASIA/DYSPLASIA

Several forms of diffuse or segmental renal hypoplasia with or without dysplasia are recognized and have been associated with childhood hypertension. True congenital hypoplasia is rare and is identified by abnormal development of the renal lobules with a resultant decrease in the number of renal calyces. Dysplasia is generally absent. The more common acquired hypoplasia has been observed in patients with obstruction, reflux, or infection and is associated with different degrees of dysplasia [60].

The differentiation of these various forms is based on histologic rather than clinical findings. The radiographic diffusely small kidney may be hypoplastic, dysplastic, or atrophic. The segmental lesion may represent an acquired scar or a congenital abnormality. Confusion in diagnosis and etiology generally arises in the literature when renal scarring is interpreted as segmental hypoplasia [61].

Segmental hypoplasia

Segmental hypoplasia is a histopathologic entity first described by Ask–Upmark (1929) in patients with malignant hypertension. These patients had small kidneys with areas of normal histology separated by grooved areas of thinned aglomerular parenchyma that revealed thyroid-like tubules with small thick-walled arteries [62]. It is important to defer the diagnosis of segmental hypoplasia to histopathologic study. Cortical papillary segmental scarring is radiographically similar in appearance and has been incorrectly described under the term segmental hypoplasia. Likewise, the terms chronic atrophic pyelonephritis and reflux nephropathy have also been used to describe this radiographic picture. Thus, the controversy over the etiology of this disorder is confounded by confusing different entities with similar radiographic appearances.

Cortical papillary segmental scarring may not represent a single entity. Habib [63] demonstrated three main histologic patterns in segmental scars of coarsely scarred kidneys with dilated calyces and cortical thinning. The scars of segmental hypoplasia were characterized by thyroid-like tubules and tortuous obstructed vessels in the cortex. This appearance was most often associated with hypertension. The scars of chronic pyelonephritis were characterized by extensive inflammatory cell infiltrates. The third pattern was characterized by the presence of dysplastic structures and poorly developed overlying cortex suggesting a developmental anomaly. It is interesting to note that scars associated with dysplastic elements and inflammation were observed in patients with recurrent urinary infections associated with obstructive and nonobstructive urinary tract anomalies. This is consistent with findings of vesicoureteral reflux, pyelonephritis, or obstruction in patients with renal segmental hypoplasia.

Observations of segmental hypoplasia in patients with coexisting nonrenal congenital anomalies suggest a congenital origin in the etiology of Ask–Upmark kidney. Zezulka [64] (1986) reported 2 hypertensive patients with segmental hypoplasia and multiple anomalies, including congenital strabismus, keratoconus, clawed toes, pes cavus, bilateral first ribs, vertebral arch deficiencies, congenital hip dislocation, and supernumerary nipples. Factors that may be associated with acquired segmental hypoplasia (urinary tract infection, vesicoureteral reflux) were absent. Both patients underwent nephrectomy and the histology was consistent with Ask–Upmark kidney. These observations support the hypothesis that the Ask–Upmark kidney may be congenital in origin from an abnormality of organogenesis and development.

Goddard and associates [40] suggest that the renin–angiotensin–aldosterone system may play a role in the pathogenesis of hypertension in some forms of segmental hypoplasia. Histologic studies revealed increased juxtaglomerular cell counts in 5 of 15 patients suggesting hyperplasia of the juxtaglomerular apparatus. No juxtaglomerular apparatus cells were seen in the hypoplastic segments themselves, suggesting that increased renin secretion was from areas adjacent to the segments. In addition, measurements of PRA in 4 out of 6 patients were suggestive of inappropriate renin secretion and 1 child with terminal renal failure had an extremely high PRA. Hypertension was cured by nephrectomy.

Thus, evidence exists to suggest that segmental hypoplasia associated with hypertension may be the result of different processes with a similar radiographic presentation. It is likely that both congenital and acquired forms of this disorder exist. A congenital variant and its association with hypertension has been described by Ask−Upmark and others. The acquired forms may be better termed cortical papillary segmental scarring. Precise diagnosis should be made by histopathology with the term cortical papillary segmental scarring used to describe the radiographic features. It is suggested that segmental hypoplasia (Ask−Upmark kidney) is a congenital anomaly and that the forms associated with inflammation or dysplasia are acquired and the result of vesicoureteral reflux, obstruction, or infection.

Global hypoplasia

Global hypoplasia of the kidney has been associated with hypertension in children. Renal hypoplasia is secondary to subnormal growth and is distinct from cases that are termed Ask−Upmark kidney (segmental hypoplasia) or acquired atrophic kidney. The hypoplastic kidney lacks dysplastic elements such as primitive ducts, ductules, or cartilage. Tokunada and associates [65] described severe hyperreninemic hypertension in a 12-month-old male with a unilaterally hypoplastic kidney. There was no history of urinary tract infection. Evaluation revealed an elevated PRA with a normal left kidney and a poorly functioning right kidney as determined by DTPA scan and excretory urography. A nephrectomy was performed with subsequent normalization of blood pressure and a decrease in PRA. Pathologic evaluation revealed a small but normal-appearing pyelocalyceal system. The majority of glomeruli were sclerotic. Electron microscopy revealed immature epithelial cells in Bowman's capsule. The glomerular changes are implicated in the pathogenesis of hypertension in this entity.

Occult renal tissue

Hypertension in children with an apparently normal solitary kidney should undergo careful evaluation for occult contralateral nonfunctioning renal tissue. Fernbach and co-authors [19] reported a 9-year-old child where the diagnosis was made following selective renal vein renin studies. It was also suspected following cystoscopy in a 19-month-old female. The 9-year-old male was hypertensive on routine examination and PRA was measured and found to be increased. Intravenous urography and DTPA scan revealed a functioning solitary right kidney. Ultrasound failed to identify the left kidney. Evaluation

by arteriography and selective renal vein renin studies revealed an atrophic left kidney with lateralizing renins. A left nephrectomy was performed with cure of hypertension.

A 19-month-old hypertensive female with a solitary left kidney and left grade III vesicoureteral reflux was evaluated by cystoscopy prior to left ureteral reimplantation. Previous studies had failed to reveal the right kidney. The PRA was slightly elevated and selective renal vein renin studies were not done. At cystoscopy an unsuspected right ureteral orifice was discovered. The patient underwent a right flank exploration during which a small kidney was found. Right nephroureterectomy and left vesicoureteral reimplantation were performed with subsequent normalization of the blood pressure. It is important to note that in both cases renal ultrasound and DTPA radioisotope studies failed to show the presence of contralateral renal tissue. Elevated PRA and incidental discovery of a contralateral ureteral orifice were major clues indicating the need for further evaluation. In both cases the removed tissue consisted of a small kidney with hypoplastic and dysplastic elements. This report emphasizes the need for careful diagnostic evaluation of the hypertensive child with an apparently normal solitary kidney.

CYSTIC DISEASES OF THE KIDNEY
(see also Chapter 19)

Children with renal cystic disease may present with flank or abdominal masses, renal insufficiency, or hypertension. Many of these conditions are associated with a poor prognosis because of their propensity to progress to ESRD. Others follow a more benign course and produce symptoms by their local compressive effects. We will review the common genetic and nongenetic cystic diseases that have been associated with hypertension.

Multicystic dysplastic kidney disease

Multicystic dysplastic kidney disease, a nongenetic disease, is the most common renal cystic disease in children and a frequent cause of a unilateral abdominal mass in newborn babies and infants [66,67]. Complications of retained multicystic kidney include pain, infection, hypertension, and malignancy. Although the natural history of this disease is unknown and these complications appear to be uncommon, increased awareness of their occurrence may become more relevant as the trend toward nonoperative management increases the number of patients with retained multicystic kidneys. Hypertension has been observed in newborn infants, children, and adults with multicystic kidney disease but this is a rare problem [68—71].

Multicystic dysplastic kidney disease is usually unilateral and may present as a small-to-massively-enlarged nonfunctioning kidney. Bilateral disease has been reported and is incompatible with life. Morphologically, severe dysplasia with large or small cysts and primitive ducts is found. Accompanying ipsilateral ureteral or renal pelvic anomalies may be present including ureteral atresia and ureteropelvic junction obstruction. In some cases, the renal pelvis may be absent. Contralateral renal abnormalities are common and may occur in a third of the patients with this disease [71]. Obstructive lesions are the most common, especially ureteropelvic junction obstruction. Obstructive megaureter and ureteropelvic junction obstruction may occur in as many as 33% of patients [72]. If ipsilateral ureteral atresia is present, contralateral abnormalities appear to be more likely. The presence of contralateral lesions is important when evaluating the child with hypertension. Obstructive lesions and reflux nephropathy have by themselves been associated with hyperreninemic hypertension. When contralateral disease is present, cure of hypertension may not be possible.

Hypertension associated with multicystic kidney disease was first described by Javadpour and colleagues [68] in 1970 in an asymptomatic 6-year-old female. Their evaluation revealed a normal contralateral kidney and although an intravenous pyelogram and renal scan did not show the multicystic kidney, an aortogram and cystoscopy suggested the presence of an abnormal renal unit. The patient underwent exploration and nephrectomy with subsequent blood pressure normalization. Interestingly, the histopathologic evaluation revealed areas of hyperplasia of the juxtaglomerular apparatus, suggesting a renin-mediated mechanism for hypertension. Chen and coworkers [69] in 1985 reported severe hyperreninemic hypertension in a newborn infant with a multicystic dysplastic kidney and a normal contralateral kidney. Hypertension resolved after nephrectomy with a concomitant decrease in PRA to normal. No juxtaglomerular hyperplasia was noted in the kidney that was removed. Others have reported hypertension in patients with multicystic kidney disease without cure after nephrectomy [70,71]. In these

patients the absence of contralateral disease was not well documented and therefore remained a variable that may have predicted failure of therapy. Hypertension was also reported in a review of adults with multicystic dysplastic kidney disease [73]. Blood pressure apparently did not significantly change after nephrectomy; however, age and the possibility of essential hypertension may explain these failures.

Few long-term studies of patients with multicystic kidney disease exist. A review of 30 cases over 11 years at the Children's Hospital of Michigan in Detroit between 1975 and 1986 revealed only one 9-year-old with hypertension [70]. This patient had a normal PRA and the contralateral kidney was hypertrophied. It was felt that the hypertension was not related to increased renin secretion and at the time of the report, surgery had not been attempted. Interestingly, of 30 cases, 19 patients were followed conservatively (mean follow-up 33.5 months; range 2 to 101 months) and no morbidity or mortality from infection, hypertension, or tumor was noted.

The increased accuracy of noninvasive diagnosis has changed the management of multicystic kidney disease. Current controversy [66,74] exists as to the need for surgical treatment of the uncomplicated case. Complications such as pain, infection, hypertension, and malignancy are rare and when present are indications for surgical removal. The incidence of these complications is unknown and much of the emphasis for removal is based on historic and anecdotal experience and not on sound knowledge of the natural history of the disease. This dilemma will hopefully be resolved by careful study and follow-up of patients through the Multicystic Kidney Registry [75], Department of Pediatric Urology, University of Cincinnati at the Children's Hospital Medical Center. Through this, a better understanding of the risk factors that predispose certain patients to develop complications may help resolve the dilemma of choosing between surgical and conservative watchful management.

Autosomal recessive polycystic kidney disease

Autosomal recessive polycystic kidney disease (of infantile onset) is a congenital bilateral renal cystic disease that is expressed only in homozygotes. Cystic involvement of other organs and vascular aneurysms are not associated. Four clinical and morphologic forms have been characterized according to age of onset. Morphologically, the kidneys are large, spongy, with multiple diffuse small subcapsular cysts with medullary ductal ectasia. Presentation in the newborn period carries an ominous prognosis with death due to respiratory insufficiency secondary to the massively enlarged kidneys and pulmonary hypoplasia. Presentation in childhood carries a less ominous prognosis as progression to renal failure may be variable with some patients enjoying prolonged survival. Most children will develop systemic hypertension secondary to ESRD; this may require medical therapy [67,76].

Other cystic disease, such as medullary cystic disease–juvenile nephronophthisis complex — may also be associated with hypertension [67]. In these other genetically determined disorders, hypertension is usually present in the terminal phase of the disease secondary to progressive renal insufficiency.

Autosomal dominant polycystic kidney disease

Autosomal dominant polycystic kidney disease (of adult onset) usually becomes apparent in adulthood but may do so in early childhood. It is estimated that fewer than 10% of cases present in the first decade of life. Adults may present in their fourth or fifth decade with any of the recognized complications of this disorder such as pain, hematuria, infection, renal failure, or hypertension. Although a large proportion of adults (50%) may progress to ESRD it is difficult to predict which patients will do so [77]. The majority of symptomatic children, however, present in the terminal stages of their disease.

Glassberg and Filmer [67] reviewed the literature for all reported cases and found 29 cases of this disorder in infants younger than 6 months old. The 29 cases included 7 stillbirths, 2 abortions, and 20 livebirths. Of the liveborn infants, 13 died within 9 months of diagnosis (8 of these had acute renal failure associated with hypertension). Seven were alive (5 with good renal function, 2 with poor renal function).

Hypertension occurs in 50–75% of patients with autosomal dominant polycystic kidney disease and seems to present prior to deterioration in renal function. Initially it was thought to be secondary to the development of ESRD. However, its association in nonazotemic patients with autosomal dominant polycystic kidney disease suggests an alternate pathogenesis [78]. Hypertensive patients tend to have severe cystic involvement with larger kidneys as compared to normotensive patients [79]. Distor-

tion of the intrarenal architecture may produce local ischemia or tubular dysfunction resulting in hypertension.

Bell and associates [80] studied physiologic variables in hypertensive and normotensive patients with this disease who were nonazotemic (creatinine clearance greater than 70 ml/min), aged 20 to 50 years. The hypertensive group had increased cardiac preload and renal vascular resistance. The plasma volume and PRA were the same for both groups. However, the rise in PRA during angiotensin converting enzyme inhibition with captopril was significantly greater in the hypertensive group. This suggested that angiotensin converting enzyme blockade removed the negative inhibitory effect on renin release, resulting in a greater increase in PRA.

Conservative treatment has been advocated and centers around management of complications. Of these, the most lethal is progression of renal failure. Interestingly, it appears that treatment of hypertension and infection may delay the progression to ESRD [77]. Perhaps this occurs because functioning parenchyma is spared. Similarly, surgeons have attempted parenchymal-saving procedures to delay the lethal outcome. In 1911, Rovsing [81] suggested cyst puncture. More recently, Frang and colleagues [82] have demonstrated a decreased incidence of hypertension (from 33 to 3%) in patients aged 20–49 years who underwent excision of large cysts, puncture of small cysts, and removal of perihilar cysts. This observation has also been made by others who have performed cyst decompression to treat hypertension [83]. Presumably this results in decompression of functioning parenchyma with removal of forces that may cause atrophy, ischemia, or tubular dysfunction.

Solitary simple cysts

Simple renal cysts have been reported as a rare cause of hypertension. The pathogenesis appears to be related to activation of the renin–angiotensin–aldosterone system secondary to local ischemia. This is supported by laboratory observations of hyper-reninemia with lateralizing renal vein renins in 2 hypertensive adolescents. Blood pressure normalized after open decompression of the cysts [84,85].

RENAL PARENCHYMAL TUMORS

Hypertension has been observed in children with renal parenchymal tumors. These tumors include nephroblastoma (Wilms' tumor), hemangiopericytoma, and mesoblastic nephroma. The three mechanisms that may be etiologic in this form of hypertension are:

1 autonomous renin secretion;
2 ischemia from distortion or compression; and
3 arteriovenous shunting with decreased afferent arterial perfusion.

Nephroblastoma (Wilms' tumor)

In 1937, Pincoffs and Bradley [86] first described 4 children with hypertension and Wilms' tumor. In 2 they observed a significant fall in blood pressure after tumor removal followed by recurrence of hypertension with tumor regrowth. Until 1972 the incidence of hypertension in patients with Wilms' tumor was unknown. Sukarochana [87] reviewed 46 cases of Wilms' tumor seen at the Children's Hospital of Pittsburgh between 1955 and 1969. The incidence of hypertension was 63% and appeared to be related to increased renin production secondary to ischemia (one patient had a large arteriovenous fistula that may have contributed to hypertension by way of arteriovenous shunting). Nephrectomy normalized blood pressure in all cases, even if metastatic disease remained. This supports the hypothesis that compression or distortion of the renal or intrarenal vasculature with resultant ischemia leads to hypertension.

Autonomous renin secretion by a Wilms' tumor in a patient with severe hypertension has also been described. Ganguly [88] and associates reported high renin content in tumor extract when compared to adjacent parenchyma. Chemotherapy reduced the PRA and nephrectomy cured the hypertension. Hendren and associates [50] described the treatment of a 2-year-old male with hypertension and bilateral Wilms' tumors. Arteriography revealed bilateral renal vessel distortion. Intensive chemotherapy resulted in tumor shrinkage, diminished vessel distortion, and decreased blood pressure. Bilateral partial nephrectomies were performed to remove the tumors.

Juxtaglomerular cell tumors

Hemangiopericytomas are renin-secreting tumors that arise from the juxtaglomerular apparatus and usually present in young patients with severe hypertension. They are typically small and difficult to diagnose unless suspicion is high [89,90]. Robertson and associates [91] first described this syndrome in a severely hypertensive 16-year-old male with hypokalemia. Cure was achieved by nephrectomy.

Mesoblastic nephroma

Mesoblastomas may produce hypertension by their mass effect. Hendren and colleagues [50] described a newborn infant with hypertension and a large renal mass. Nephrectomy normalized the blood pressure.

RENAL TRAUMA

Hypertension secondary to renal trauma is an infrequent complication that confronts the surgeon and pediatrician [92–95]. Several reports suggest an incidence between 0.6 and 6% [96]. Recognition requires long-term follow-up as cases may present several years after the traumatic event [97], Increased awareness of delayed posttraumatic hypertension is necessary because of the trend for conservative nonoperative treatment of the majority of nonlife-threatening renal injuries [98–100]. It thus becomes more likely that the family physician or pediatrician will encounter such patients later and will need to stress regular measurement of blood pressure.

Hypertension in these patients may occur by several mechanisms including ischemia, infarction [97], or compression [15]. Page [14] first observed the effect of perinephric compression on blood pressure and renin production in an experimental model (Fig. 20.6). In his model, a fibrocollagenous inflammatory capsule produced changes in blood pressure. Clinical hypertension secondary to fibrous encapsulation of the kidney and compression of the parenchyma has also been described. Most cases are associated with normal PRA and are due to subcapsular hematomas secondary to trauma. Grim and associates [15] described hypertension in a 16-year-old male who had a history of blunt flank trauma 1 year earlier. Unilateral decreased vascular filling was found on aortography and there was lateralization of renal vein renins to the abnormal kidney. The patient's blood pressure was not controlled medically and he underwent open renal biopsy revealing a dense fibrous capsule over the posterior aspect of the kidney. A nephrectomy was performed with normalization of the blood pressure. Delayed hypertension has also been described in patients with a history of blunt renal trauma where a protracted period of normotension occurred prior to the development of severe hypertension [97].

Hypertension may also rarely occur from the functionless posttraumatic renal segment. Peterson [96] in 1986 reviewed 340 cases of renal trauma evaluated at Denver General Hospital between 1973 and 1983. Hypertension was discovered in only 3 (0.8%) at some point in their follow-up. Of these 3, hypertension in 1 patient was attributed to the presence of a functionless renal segment. (Thirteen patients in whom functionless renal parenchymal segments could be demonstrated were treated nonoperatively.) This patient, a child with blunt major trauma, developed hypertension. All patients remained asymptomatic and normotensive at 10-year follow-up.

Thus, a history of previous renal trauma is a risk factor for the development of hypertension that should alert the primary care physician. Such patients must be followed with serial blood pressure measurements. Hopefully increased knowledge of this delayed complication will not leave hypertension undetected, predisposing these children to increased morbidity and mortality.

MANAGEMENT APPROACH

Once a hypertensive child has been medically stabilized, and renal imaging reveals a parenchymal or collecting system abnormality, further management is based on:
1 response to medical treatment and general condition of the patient (see Figs 20.10 and 20.11);
2 pathology (e.g. tumor versus scar);
3 the presence of unilateral or bilateral disease;
4 the presence of focal or diffuse lesions;
5 renal function.

Patient selection and management have significantly evolved since Butler [101] in 1937 first demonstrated the reversal of hypertension following nephrectomy in a patient with a small pyelonephritic kidney. Subsequent reports of the result of nephrectomy in larger series of patients with unilateral renal parenchymal disease were rather disappointing with hypertension being cured or improved in 26–50% of patients. It is apparent that these results were affected by multiple factors such as age, presence of renal insufficiency, or presence of contralateral renal disease [102]. Reviews have demonstrated that careful patient selection in differentiation of unilateral from bilateral disease can result in increased success of surgical treatment.

Luke and associates [102] reviewed the results of nephrectomy in 34 patients with apparent unilateral parenchymal disease. This study demonstrated the difficulty in evaluating early reports of surgical treatment of hypertension secondary to renal parenchymal disease. The average age was 35 years. The total number of patients with hypertension cured plus those improved was 50%, with the remainder unimproved. Many of the patients had abnormal renal function; 3 had a nonfunctioning kidney with blood urea nitrogen >50 mg/dl. Their blood pressure was unaffected by nephrectomy. In addition, careful review revealed that 4 patients had an excretory urography or arteriograms showing evidence of contralateral disease. Three of these patients were not cured and 1 was improved on antihypertensive medication.

Treatment outcome is difficult to interpret in this group of patients affected by multiple variables; however, three conclusions can be drawn:
1 good results of surgery can be achieved in patients with true unilateral disease;
2 surgical success is more likely if renal function is normal;
3 success is more likely in younger patients.

Tumors and obstructive lesions

In patients with tumors, surgery is a diagnostic, staging, and therapeutic exercise that is dependent on renal function and the anatomic favorability for resection (see Figs 20.10 and 20.11). These patients are generally challenging as the goal of treatment is primarily to prolong life (curing the patient of the disease), therefore normalization of blood pressure (curing the hypertension) is a welcome additional benefit. The approach to these patients should follow the recommended evaluation and treatment protocols specific to that disease process.

Obstructive lesions are anatomic processes best treated by surgical reconstruction (parenchymal sparing) when feasible. This occurs when the obstruction is associated with an adequately functioning ipsilateral kidney and its repair is technically possible. For example, repair of a unilateral ureteropelvic junction obstruction will restore the normal anatomy, allow nonobstructive urine flow, rescue the jeopardized obstructed unit from further deterioration, and theoretically normalize blood pressure or allow for better control on medication. If hypertension remains poorly controlled, then removal may be necessary, especially if renin sampling suggests a causal physiologic relationship. Surgical removal of

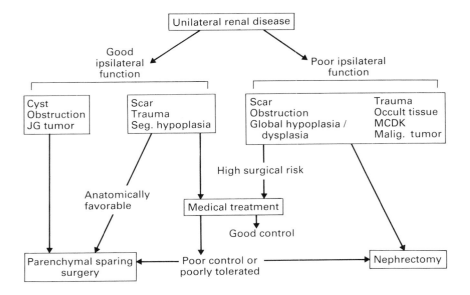

Fig. 20.10 Management of unilateral renal parenchymal hypertension is dependent on several factors. These include function of the diseased kidney, pathology and natural history of the disease process, anatomic favorability, surgical risk, and/or response to medical treatment. JG = Juxtaglomerular; Seg. = segmental; MCDK = multicystic dysplastic kidney; Malig. = malignant.

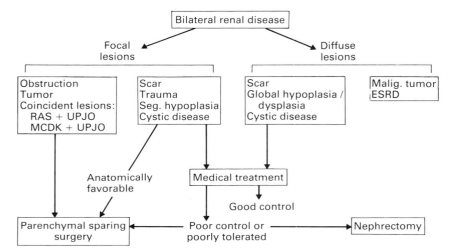

Fig. 20.11 Management of renal parenchymal hypertension in the patient with bilateral renal disease depends on whether the disease process is focal or diffuse. Other factors include the pathology and natural history of the disease, the anatomic favorability for resection, and/or response to medical treatment. RAS = Renal artery stenosis; UPJO = ureteropelvic junction obstruction; MCDK = multicystic dysplastic kidney; Seg. = segmental; MALIG. = malignant; ESRD = end-stage renal disease.

the obstructed unit is also indicated when poor function exists (less than 10% of total renal function) and the possible morbidity from reconstruction outweighs its potential benefits. These patients are better served by a simple nephrectomy (see Figs 20.10 and 20.11). In summary, tumors and obstructive lesions associated with hypertension are specifically surgical diseases. Their treatment has multiple potential benefits including normalization of or improvement in blood pressure control.

Unilateral versus bilateral disease

Management of nonobstructive and nonneoplastic disease is mostly dependent on the presence of unilat-

eral or bilateral lesions and the degree of renal function in the remaining parenchyma. Generally, unilateral disease in a normally functioning kidney has several treatment options (see Fig. 20.10). Surgery may not be necessary if control of blood pressure is adequate without exposing the patient to the side-effects of large doses of antihypertensive drugs. If hypertension persists, is poorly controlled, or is associated with poor ipsilateral function, then a surgical procedure tailored to remove part or all of the offending unit is indicated (Fig. 20.10).

These factors are appreciated when reviewing outcome of treatment in patients with renal scarring. Treatment success is related to the degree of renal scarring. Taylor and associates' [51] long-term follow-up of hypertension in 33 patients with scarred kidneys demonstrated that patients with unilateral scars and normal contralateral kidneys did best, despite surgical or nonoperative treatments. In this group of 20, 14 selected patients underwent operative treatment (12 nephrectomies, 2 partial nephrectomies) with none requiring antihypertensive drugs at follow-up of 2−11 years. Not surprisingly, all 4 patients with bilateral multiple renal scars required antihypertensive medication despite operative or medical forms of primary management. Three of these 4 patients (with severe uncontrolled hypertension and renal vein renin lateralization) continued to require antihypertensive medication despite excision of a nonfunctioning kidney. Patients with predominantly unilateral scarring and evidence of a single scar in the contralateral kidney had favorable results from surgery. Four patients in this group underwent nephrectomy because they had lateralizing renal vein renins (2 patients) and poorly controlled hypertension (2 patients). Three patients are off antihypertensive drugs and 1 is on reduced medication. Thus 21 (64%) of 33 patients with scarred kidneys were managed surgically with 17 of 21 (81%) cured and off antihypertensive medication. Fourteen of 17 patients had true unilateral disease. Three of 17 patients had a single scar in the remaining kidney. Of the remaining 4 who continued to require antihypertensive therapy, 3 had multiple bilateral scars. It is clear that the degree of renal scarring in the contralateral renal unit is important in predicting success from both operative and nonoperative therapies. In addition, a selected subset of patients with bilateral renal scarring may benefit from operative intervention.

Focal versus diffuse lesions

Careful differentiation of hypertensive patients with bilateral focal versus bilateral diffuse parenchymal disease may bring more patients into the realm of curability with precise surgical intervention (see Fig. 20.11). Hendren and associates [50] demonstrated that some patients with bilateral disease may have their hypertension corrected by surgery. One patient with bilateral vesicoureteral reflux and bilateral upper pole atrophy was cured of hypertension after bilateral upper pole partial nephrectomies and vesicoureteral re-implantation. This patient was normotensive after a 13-year follow-up. A second patient with hypertension, from a left nonfunctioning kidney associated with left vesicoureteral reflux occurring with a right

Table 20.2 A vast arsenal of techniques is available to the surgeon when planning the treatment of patients with renal parenchymal hypertension: Reconstructive and parenchymal-sparing techniques are preferred when possible.

Removal of renal unit[†]
Nephrectomy
    Unilateral
    Bilateral

Segmental nephrectomy
Unilateral
Bilateral

Relief of obstruction[‡]
Percutaneous nephrostomy
Pyeloplasty
Ureterocalicostomy
Ureteral reimplantation

*Ureteral Reimplantation***
Ureteral reimplantation
    Unilateral
    Bilateral

*Combination procedures for bilateral disease**
Nephrectomy
    With contralateral pyeloplasty
    With contralateral revascularization
    With contralateral reimplantation

*Segmental nephrectomy**
    Bilateral upper pole nephrectomy with bilateral ureteral
      reimplantation

Renal cysts
Excision
Decompression

---

* Procedures reported in literature as relieving hypertension
† Based on total and segmental ipsilateral renal function as estimated by dimercaptosuccinic acid radioisotope scan
‡ Success of reconstruction predicted by response to prior percutaneous nephrostomy
** Reimplantation alone unlikely to relieve hypertension

ureteropelvic junction obstruction, was normotensive 4 years after left nephrectomy and right pyeloplasty. A third patient with a left nonfunctioning kidney, left vesicoureteral reflux, and a right renal artery lesion was cured after left nephrectomy and right renal artery (autologous hypogastric arterial graft) reconstruction.

In contrast, 1 patient with bilateral diffuse parenchymal scarring from bilateral obstructed mega-ureters had successful re-implantation without improvement in blood pressure control. Hypertension was thought to be secondary to increased renin release (as determined by selective renal vein renins) from the upper pole of the scarred right kidney. This patient subsequently had a right nephrectomy because partial nephrectomy was not technically possible. The patient's hypertension was controlled with medication at 5-year follow-up. Thus, patients with bilateral focal parenchymal disease or coincident obstructive or renal vascular lesions may be approached surgically with a reasonable expectation of cure or improvement.

CONCLUSION

In summary, the differential diagnosis, mechanism, and treatment of renal parenchymal hypertension have been reviewed. The goals of all treatments are to normalize blood pressure while preserving renal mass. These goals may be achieved by careful patient selection and differentiation between unilateral (Fig. 20.10) and bilateral parenchymal disease (Fig. 20.11). Ideally, cases of true unilateral disease and bilateral anatomically favorable disease may be cured by precise surgical intervention (Table 20.2).

A subset of patients with diffuse disease may also be good surgical candidates. These include those with malignant tumors or ESRD. Finally, there exists a group of normotensive individuals who will require long-term blood pressure surveillance. These patients include those with reflux nephropathy, multicystic dysplastic kidney, simple solitary cysts, or a history of renal trauma. Increased awareness of the natural history of these disorders may reduce the subsequent morbidity and mortality from the development of hypertension.

REFERENCES

1 Rocchini AP. Childhood hypertension: etiology, diagnosis and treatment. *Ped Clin North Am* 1984;31:1259–73.
2 Loggie JMH. Systemic hypertension in children and adolescents. *Ped Clin North Am* 1971;18:1273–1310.
3 Londe S. Causes of hypertension in the young. *Ped Clin North Am* 1978;25:55–65.
4 Londe S, Bourgoignie JJ, Robson AM, Goldring D. Hypertension in apparently normal children. *J Ped* 1971;78:569–77.
5 De Swiet M. The epidemiology of hypertension in children. *Br Med Bull* 1986;42:172–5.
6 Lawson JD, Boerth R, Foster JG et al. Diagnosis and management of renovascular hypertension in children. *Arch Surg* 1977;112:1307–15.
7 Still JL, Cottom D. Severe hypertension in childhood. *Arch Dis Child* 1967;42:34–9.
8 Gill DG, Mendes da Costa B, Cameron JS et al. Analysis of 100 children with severe and persistent hypertension. *Arch Dis Child* 1976;51:951–6.
9 Guyton AC. Long term regulation of mean arterial pressure: the renal–body fluid pressure control system; long term functions of the renin angiotensin system; and mechanisms of hypertension. In: Guyton AC, ed. *Textbook of Medical Physiology.* Philadelphia: WB Saunders, 1981:259–73.
10 Kelleher SP, Schrier RW. The kidney in hypertension. In: Schrier RW, ed. *Renal and Electrolyte Disorders.* 3rd edn. Boston: Little, Brown, 1986:387–422.
11 Smith MC, Dunn MJ. Renovascular and renal parenchymal hypertension. In: Brenner BM, Rector FC, eds. *The Kidney.* 3rd edn. Philadelphia: WB Saunders, 1986:1221–51.
12 Ballermann BJ, Levenson DJ, Brenner BM. Renin, angiotensin, kinins, prostaglandins, and leukotrienes. In: Brenner BM, Rector FC, eds. *The Kidney.* 3rd edn. Philadelphia: WB Saunders, 1986:281–340.
13 Goldblatt H, Lynch J, Hanzal RF, Summerville WW. Studies on experimental hypertension: I. The production of persistent elevation of systolic blood pressure by means of renal ischemia. *J Exp Med* 1934;59:347–56.
14 Page IH. The production of persistent arterial hypertension by cellophane perinephritis. *JAMA* 1939;113:2046–8.
15 Grim CE, Mullins MF, Nilson JP, Ross G Jr. Unilateral "Page kidney" hypertension in man-studies of the renin–angiotensin–aldosterone system before and after nephrectomy. *JAMA* 1975;231:42–5.
16 Loggie JMH, New MI, Robson AM. Hypertension in the pediatric patient: a reappraisal. *J Ped* 1975;94:685–99.
17 Potter DE. The evaluation of the child with hypertension. Hypertension, fluid-electrolytes, and tubulopathies in pediatric nephrology. In: Strauss J, ed. *Proceedings of the Pediatric Nephrology Seminar VIII.* Boston: Martinus Nijhoff, 1982:123–32.
18 Dillon MJ. Clinical aspects of hypertension. In: Holliday MA, Barratt TM, Vernier RL, eds. *Pediatric Nephrology.* Baltimore: Williams & Wilkins, 1987:743–57.
19 Fernbach SK, Holland EA, Benuck I, Young S. Hypertension induced by occult renal tissue. *J Urol* 1987;138:842–4.
20 Menick MV, Uttley WS, Wild SR. The detection of pyelonephritic scarring in children by radioisotope imaging. *Br J Radiol* 1980;53:544–9.
21 Alroomi LG, Murphy AV, Nelson CS et al. Renal vein renin measurement and arteriography in the investigation and management of severe childhood hypertension. *Clin Chim Acta* 1985;150:103–9.
22 Stockigt JR, Noakes CA, Collins RD, Schambelan M. Renal-vein renin in various forms of renal hypertension. *Lancet* 1972;i:1194–8.
23 Sosa RE, Vaughan ED. Renovascular hypertension: background, pathophysiology, pathology and clinical evaluation. *AUA Update Series* 1989;8:138–43.
24 Thind GS. Role of renal venous renins in the diagnosis and management of renovascular hypertension. *J Urol* 1985;134:2–5.
25 Schambelan M, Glickman M, Stockigt JR, Biglieri EG. Selective renal-vein renin sampling in hypertensive patients with segmental renal lesions. *N Engl J Med* 1974;290:1153–7.

26 Lindstrom RR, Brosman SA, Paul JG et al. Segmental intrarenal catheterization in renin-mediated hypertension. J Urol 1977;118:10−12.

27 Parrott TS, Woodard JR, Trulock TS, Glenn JF. Segmental renal vein renins and partial nephrectomy for hypertension in children. J Urol 1984;131:736−9.

28 Javadpour N, Poppman JL, Scardino PT, Bartler FC. Segmental renal vein renin assay and segmental nephrectomy for correction of renal hypertension. J Urol 1976;115:580−2.

29 Vaughan ED. Editorial comment. J Urol 1984;131:739.

30 Savage JM, Dillon MJ, Shah V, Barrott TM, Williams DI. Renin and blood pressure in children with renal scarring and vesicoureteric reflux. Lancet 1978;ii:441−4.

31 Holland N. Reflux nephropathy and hypertension. In: Hodson CJ, Kincaid-Smith P, eds. Reflux Nephropathy. New York: Masson Publishing, 1979;251−62.

32 Arant BS. Reflux nephropathy. Kidney 1989;21:19−24.

33 Wallace MA, Rothwell DL, Williams DI. The long term follow up of surgically treated vesicoureteric reflux. Br J Urol 1978;50:479−84.

34 Smellie JM. Reflux nephropathy in childhood. In: Hodson CJ, Kincaid-Smith P, eds. Reflux Nephropathy. New York: Masson Publishing, 1979;242−50.

35 Holland N, Kotchen T, Bhathena D. Hypertension in children with chronic pyelonephritis. Kidney Int 1975;8:S243−51.

36 Smellie JM. Vesicoureteric reflux and renal scarring. Kidney Int 1975;8:65.

37 Dillon MJ. Peripheral plasma renin activity, hypertension and renal scarring in children. Contrib Nephrol 1984;39:68.

38 Stecker JF, Read BP, Poutasse EF. Pediatric hypertension as a delayed sequela of reflux-induced chronic pyelonephritis. J Urol 1977;118:644−6.

39 Bailey RR. Reflux nephropathy and hypertension. In: Hodson CJ, Kincaid-Smith P, eds. Reflux Nephropathy. New York: Masson Publishing, 1979;263−7.

40 Goddard C, Vallothon MB, Broyer M. Plasma renin activity in segmental hypoplasia of kidneys with hypertension. Nephron 1973;11:308−17.

41 Bailey RR. Renal vein renin concentration in the hypertension of unilateral reflux nephropathy. J Urol 1978;120−21.

42 Dillon MJ, Gordon I, Shah V. Tc(99m)-DMSA scanning and segmental renal vein renin estimations in children with renal scarring. In: Hodson CJ, Heptinstall RH, Winberg J, eds. Reflux Nephropathy Update. New York: Karger, 1984:28−35.

43 Vaughan ED, Buhler FR, Laragh JH et al. Hypertension and unilateral parenchymal renal disease. JAMA 1975;233:1177−83.

44 Delin K, Aurell M, Granerus G. Renin dependent hypertension in patients with unilateral kidney disease not caused by renal artery stenosis. Acta Med Scand 1977;201:345−51.

45 Bailey RR, Lynn KL. End stage reflux nephropathy. In: Hodson CJ, Heptinstall RH, Winberg J, eds. Reflux Nephropathy Update. New York: Karger, 1984:102−10.

46 Huland H, Busch R. Chronic pyelonephritis as a cause of end stage renal disease. J Urol 1982;127:642−3.

47 Baleshandeh K. Vesicoureteric reflux and end-stage renal disease. J Urol 1976;116:557.

48 Shortliffe LMD, Duckett JW. Renal scarring in children. AUA Update Series 1988;7:298−303.

49 Braren V, West JC, Boerth RC, Harmon CM. Management of children with hypertension from reflux or obstructive nephropathy. Urology 1988;32:228−34.

50 Hendren WH, Kim SH, Herrin JT, Crawford JD. Surgically correctable hypertension of renal origin in childhood. Am J Surg 1982;143:432−42.

51 Taylor RG, Azmy AF, Young DG. Long term follow up of surgical renal hypertension. J Ped Surg 1987;22:228−30.

52 Vaughan ED, Sweet RC, Gillenwater JY. Peripheral renin and blood pressure changes following complete unilateral ureteral occlusion. J Urol 1970;104:89−92.

53 Vaughan ED, Buhler FR, Laragh JH. Normal renin secretion in hypertensive patients with primarily unilateral chronic hydronephrosis. J Urol 1974;112:153−6.

54 Belman AB, Kropp KA, Simon NM. Renal-pressor hypertension secondary to unilateral hydronephrosis. N Engl J Med 1968;278:1133−6.

55 Kawano S, Yano S, Takahashi S, Nomura Y, Ogata J. A case of hypertension due to unilateral hydronephrosis in a child. Eur Urol 1986;12:357−9.

56 Carella JA, Silber I. Hyperreninemic hypertension in an infant secondary to pelviureteric obstruction treated successfully by surgery. J Ped 1976;88:987−9.

57 Weidman P, Beretta-Piccoli C, Hirsch D et al. Curable hypertension with unilateral hydronephrosis−studies on the role of circulating renin. Am Int Med 1977;87:437−40.

58 Nemoy NJ, Fichman MP, Sellers A. Unilateral ureteral obstruction. JAMA 1973;225:512−13.

59 Grossman IC, Cromie WJ, Wein AJ, Duckett JW. Renal hypertension secondary to ureteropelvic junction obstruction. Urology 1981;17:69−72.

60 Weiss MA, Mills SE. Atlas of Genitourinary Tract Disorders. Philadelphia: JB Lippincott, 1988:4.6−7.

61 Shindo S, Bernstein J, Arant BS. Evolution of renal segmental atrophy (Ask−Upmark kidney) in children with vesicoureteral reflux: radiographic and morphologic studies. J Ped 1983;102:847−54.

62 Ask−Upmark E. Uber juvenile maligne Nephrosklerose and ihr Vehaltris zu. Storungen in der nierenen Twicklung. Acta Pathol Microbiol Scand 1929;6:383.

63 Habib R. Pathology of renal segmental corticopapillary scarring in children with hypertension: the concept of segmental hypoplasia. In: Hodson CJ, Kincaid-Smith P, eds. Reflux Nephropathy. New York: Masson Publishing, 1979:220−39.

64 Zezulka AV. The association of hypertension, the Ask−Upmark kidney and other congenital abnormalities. J Urol 1986;135:1000−1.

65 Tokunada S, Takamura T, Asanai H et al. Severe hypertension in infant with unilateral hypoplastic kidney. Urology 1987;29:618−20.

66 Hartman GE, Smolik LM, Shochat SJ. The dilemma of the multicystic dysplastic kidney. Am J Dis Child 1986;140:925−8.

67 Glassberg KI, Filmer RB. Renal dysplasia, renal hypoplasia, and cystic disease of the kidney. In: Kelalis PP, King LR, Belman AB, eds. Clinical Pediatric Urology, 2nd edn. Philadelphia: WB Saunders, 1985:922−71.

68 Javadpour N, Chelouhy E, Moncada L, Rosenthal IM, Bush IM. Hypertension in a child with a multicystic kidney.

J Urol 1970;104:918—21.

69 Chen YH, Stapleton FB, Roy S III, Noe HN. Neonatal hypertension from a unilateral multicystic dysplastic kidney. *J Urol* 1985;133:664—5.

70 Vinocur L, Slovis TL, Perlmuttes AD, Watts FB Jr, Chang CH. Follow up studies of multicystic dysplastic kidneys. *Radiology* 1988;167:311—15.

71 Greene LF, Feinzaig W, Dahlin DC. Multicystic dysplasia of the kidney: with special reference to the contralateral kidney. *J Urol* 1971;105:482—7.

72 Peters CA, Mandell J. The multicystic dysplastic kidney. *AUA Update Series* 1989;8:50—5.

73 Ambrose SS, Gould RA, Trulock TS, Parrott TS. Unilateral multicystic renal disease in adults. *J Urol* 1982;128:366—9.

74 Stanisic TH. Review of the dilemma of the multicystic dysplastic kidney. *Am J Dis Child* 1986;140:865.

75 Wacksman J. Multicystic kidney registry in the management of multicystic kidneys. *Dial Ped Urol* 1987;10:4—6.

76 Bernstein J, Gardner KD Jr. Renal cystic disease and renal dysplasia. In: Walsh PC, Gittes RF, Perlmutter AD, Stamey TA, eds. *Campbell's Urology.* Philadelphia: WB Saunders, 1986:1760—803.

77 Herron KG, Grantham JJ. Autosomal dominant polycystic kidney disease. *AUA Update Series* 1988;8:250—4.

78 Nash DA. Hypertension in polycystic kidney disease without renal failure. *Arch Intern Med* 1977;137:1571.

79 Gabow PA, Heard E, Pretorius D *et al.* Relationship between renal structure and hypertension in autosomal dominant polycystic kidney disease. *Kidney Int* 1987;31:297.

80 Bell PE, Hossack KF, Gabow PA *et al.* Hypertension in autosomal dominant polycystic kidney disease. *Kidney Int* 1988;34:683—90.

81 Rovsing T. Treatment of multilocular renal cyst with multiple puncture. *Hospitalstid* 1911;4:105.

82 Frang D, Czvalinga I, Polzak L. A new approach to the treatment of polycystic kidney. *Int Urol Nephrol* 1988;20:13—21.

83 Yates-Bell JG. Rovsings operation for polycystic kidney. *Lancet* 1957;272:1.

84 Rose HJ, Pruitt AW. Hypertension, hyperreninemia and a solitary renal cyst in an adolescent. *Am J Med* 1976;61:579—82.

85 Babka JC, Cohen MS, Sode J. Solitary intrarenal cyst causing hypertension. *N Engl J Med* 1974;291:343—4.

86 Pincoffs MC, Bradley JE. The association of adenosarcoma of the kidney (Wilms' tumor) with arterial hypertension. *Trans Assoc Am Phys* 1937;52:320—5.

87 Sukarochana K. Wilms' tumor and hypertension. *J Ped Surg* 1972;7:573.

88 Gangurly A, Gribble J, Tune B, Kempson RL, Luetscher JA. Renin secreting Wilms' tumor with severe hypertension. *Ann Intern Med* 1973;79:835—7.

89 Eddy RL, Sanchez SA. Renin secreting renal neoplasm and hypertension with hypokalemia. *Ann Int Med* 1971;75:725—9.

90 Conn JW, Cohen EL, Lucas CP *et al.* Primary reninism. *Arch Intern Med* 1972;130:682—96.

91 Robertson DW, Klidjiana A, Harding LK, Walters G, Lee MR, Robb-Smith AHT. Hypertension due to a renin-secreting renal tumor. *Am Med* 1967;43:963—76.

92 Gonzales ET Jr, Guerriero WG. Genitourinary trauma in children. In: Kelalis P, King L, Belman A, eds. *Clinical Pediatric Urology.* 2nd edn. Philadelphia: WB Saunders, 1985:1125—56.

93 Peters PC, Sagalowslay AI. Genitourinary trauma. In: Walsh PC, Gittes RF, Perlmutter AD, Stamey TA, eds. *Campbell's Urology.* 5th edn. 1986:1192—247.

94 Kuzmarov IW, Morehouse DD, Gibson S. Blunt renal trauma in the pediatric population—a retrospective study. *J Urol* 1981;126:648—9.

95 Waterhouse K, Gross M. Trauma to the genitourinary tract—a 5 year experience with 251 cases. *J Urol* 1969;101:241—6.

96 Peterson NE. Fate of functionless post-traumatic renal segment. *Urology* 1986;27:237—42.

97 Mezoier A, Rainfoaz M, Lacombe M. Delayed hypertension after blunt renal trauma. *Am J Nephrol* 1988;8:108—11.

98 Mahmood AH, Pontes E, Pierce JM Jr. Surgical management of major renal trauma—a review of 102 cases treated by conservative surgery. *J Urol* 1977;118:7—9.

99 Mandour WA, Lai MK, Linke CA, Frank IN. Blunt renal trauma in the pediatric patient. *J Ped Surg* 1981;16:669—76.

100 Javadpour N, Guinan P, Bush IM. Renal trauma in children. *Surg Gynecol Obst* 1973;136:237—40.

101 Butler AM. Chronic pyelonephritis and arterial hypertension. *J Clin Invest* 1937;16:889—97.

102 Luke RG, Kennedy AC, Briggs JD, Struthers NW, Stirling WB. Results of nephrectomy in hypertension associated with unilateral renal disease. *Br Med J* 1968;3:764—8.

21 Hypertension in Children with Chronic Renal Insufficiency

NORMAN D. ROSENBLUM AND JULIE R. INGELFINGER

Hypertension is a common complication in the child with chronic renal insufficiency prior to and during dialysis and after renal transplantation. In this chapter we will discuss the pathophysiology, etiology, and management of hypertension in each of these settings.

PATHOPHYSIOLOGY OF HYPERTENSION IN RENAL INSUFFICIENCY

In renal insufficiency, the major factors leading to an increase in blood pressure are shown in Figure 21.1. Blood pressure is a function of cardiac output (CO) and total peripheral resistance (TPR). As glomerular filtration rate (GFR) and renal plasma flow (RPF) fall during the development of chronic renal failure, both CO and TPR increase.

The increase in CO is mediated by at least two factors: progressive anemia and an increase in extracellular fluid volume (ECFV). The importance of anemia as a determinant of increased CO has been shown by Kim and colleagues [2] who demonstrated that the difference in CO between normotensive and hypertensive patients disappeared when the anemia was corrected. The importance of an increased ECFV in producing hypertension is underlined by the ability to achieve normotension and a dry weight simultaneously with dialysis. Several studies have demonstrated that blood pressure varies directly with ECFV and with plasma or total body exchangeable sodium in patients with chronic renal failure [3]. An increase in ECFV is mediated by renal retention of sodium and water. This may result from a marked decrease in GFR. In this situation the total delivery of sodium and water to the renal tubules is diminished to such an extent that an overall retention of these substances results. Retention of sodium and water is also mediated by increases in the activity of angio-

tensin and aldosterone resulting from increased renin release which may be caused by several factors. For example, in certain types of renal failure ischemia of the afferent arteriole results in renin release.

An increase in TPR is often mediated by increases in circulating angiotensin. Elevated TPR may also be caused by decreased renal production of vasodepressor substances, such as prostaglandins which are hypotensive factors produced by the kidney medulla [4]. In addition, increases in TPR may be caused by changes in the activity of the autonomic nervous system, tissue edema causing vascular compression, and abnormalities of the vessel walls caused by perturbations in calcium and phosphorus metabolism.

There is, as yet, no agreement as to whether an elevation of CO or TPR or both together is most important in causing the hypertension of end-stage renal disease (ESRD) [2,3,5].

HYPERTENSION IN THE PATIENT WITH CHRONIC RENAL FAILURE PRIOR TO DIALYSIS

In contrast to the large number of studies of hypertension in patients receiving chronic dialysis, there are relatively few studies in hypertensive patients with chronic parenchymal renal disease prior to the initiation of dialysis. As noted above, the role of an increased ECFV has been well documented [2,5,6—8]. Studies of renin activity in these patients have revealed varying circulating levels [9]. Some of this variation is attributable to differences in the patients' volume status at the time of measurement. When plasma renin activity (PRA) is standardized for volume status, a better correlation exists between the blood pressure and PRA.

As seen clinically, children with chronic renal failure tend to fall into two distinct groups: those with glomerular disease, a majority of whom are hyperten-

239

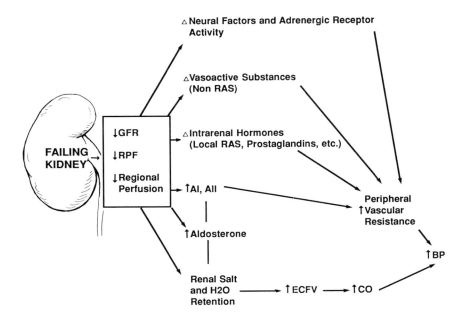

Fig. 21.1 In chronic renal insufficiency, decreases in glomerular filtration rate (GFR), renal plasma flow (RPF), and regional perfusion lead to changes (Δ) in neural factors, adrenergic receptor activity, intrarenal hormones, and nonrenin−angiotensin vasoactive substances. Increased angiotensin I (AI) and angiotensin II (AII) lead to a rise in peripheral vascular resistance and blood pressure. Increases in AI and AII also stimulate aldosterone production. This, as well as the decreased GFR and RPF, causes renal salt and water retention. The resultant increase in extracellular fluid volume (ECFV) leads to increased cardiac output (CO) and a rise in blood pressure. Anemia contributes to hypertension by increasing cardiac output. Adapted from [1].

sive, and those with renal dysplasia or hypoplasia in whom hypertension is less common. Of the children beginning dialysis at The Children's Hospital, Boston, 98% of those with glomerular disease have had predialysis hypertension as compared to only 23% of those with dysplasia or hypoplasia [10].

Treatment of hypertension in the patient with chronic renal failure prior to dialysis

Blood pressure must be lowered gradually in patients with chronic renal failure, since rapid lowering may lead to a loss of renal function in some. Irrespective of etiology, the majority of hypertensive patients have some element of volume expansion due to sodium retention and will benefit from diuretic therapy until there is a marked decrease in GFR. When the GFR is less than 10 ml/min, the renal responsiveness to diuretics is severely limited by the small amounts of sodium and water which are delivered to the renal tubules, the active site of the diuretic. Diuretics which interfere with renal potassium excretion should be avoided in patients with renal insufficiency, since potassium excretion in these patients is already limited. Thiazides are often not effective since they block a small proportion of the sodium handled by the tubule. A loop diuretic such as furosemide, ethacrynic acid, or bumetanide will provide a more effective natriuresis and diuresis.

Nondiuretic antihypertensive medication includ-

ing β-blocking agents and peripheral vasodilators may be efficacious. Both diuretics and antihypertensive drugs may have altered half-lives and elimination in patients with renal insufficiency. Dosages must be individualized and adjusted appropriately (Tables 21.1 and 21.2). Multiple antihypertensive agents may be required to control blood pressure adequately.

β-Blocking drugs are appealing in that they lower CO, a major determinant of blood pressure, and also interfere with renin release from the kidney. They should be used cautiously in patients who have decreased cardiac contractility and should be avoided in those with reactive airway disease. There are numerous β-blocking agents available, as shown in Table 21.2. At present, propranolol is the only one that is approved by the Food and Drug Administration for pediatric use in the USA. It has been reported to have a normal half-life in patients with renal failure. However, one report has documented massive retention of the metabolites of propranolol in uremia [12]. The clinical significance of this observation is not yet evident. β-Blocking agents that are excreted by the kidney, nadolol and atenolol, are given once per day. Converting enzyme inhibitors and calcium channel blocking drugs are being increasingly used in hypertensive patients with renal insufficiency. The limited information available suggests that both classes of agents hold promise for use in children with renal insufficiency [13,14].

Table 21.1 Diuretics in renal failure. Adapted from [11].

Drug	Oral absorption	Protein binding	Metabolism and elimination	Half-life (h) Normal	Half-life (h) Anephric	Dosage change with renal failure
Amiloride	Well absorbed	Not bound	Not metabolized; secreted into proximal tubule	6–9	?	Not effective and may induce hyperkalemia
Acetazolamide	Well absorbed	80% protein-bound; distributed in 30% of body weight	Not metabolized; 90% excreted in urine within 24 h	?	?	Not effective if GFR <30 ml/min
Bumetanide	Well absorbed	95% protein-bound	Rapid 80% urine excretion	$1–1\frac{1}{2}$	?	
Ethacrynic acid	Well absorbed	Unknown	Some hepatic metabolism; renal excretion of unchanged drug and metabolites	?	?	No change required; monitor hearing, renal function, and electrolytes
Furosemide	50% absorbed	90–95% absorbed	75% eliminated unchanged in urine	1	2–14	No change required; monitor renal function and electrolytes
Indapamide	Well absorbed	75% absorbed	70% renal, 20% gastrointestinal	14	?	Not effective if GFR <25 ml/min
Metolazone	?	?	?	?	?	May produce diuresis when GFR <20 ml/min
Mercurials	Poor	Unknown	Primarily renal elimination	2–3	22–48	Avoid repeated dose if GFR <25 ml/min because of nephrotoxic potential
Spironolactone	Well absorbed	90% protein-bound	Extensive hepatic metabolism; renal excretion of active and inactive metabolites	37	?	Not effective and may induce hyperkalemia if GFR <25 ml/min
Thiazides	50–70% absorbed	75% protein-bound	75% excreted in urine	12	Increased	Not effective if GFR <25 ml/min
Triamterene	50% absorbed	50% protein-bound	Extensive hepatic metabolism; renal excretion of small amounts of unchanged drug and metabolites	2	?	Not effective and may induce hyperkalemia if GFR <30 ml/min

GFR = Glomerular filtration rate.

Table 21.2 Antihypertensive drugs in renal failure

Drug	Metabolism/elimination	Half-life (h) Normal	Half-life (h) Anephric	Dosage change in renal failure	Effect of dialysis
Vasodilators					
Diazoxide	Excretion of unchanged drug and metabolites by kidney	20–36	↑	Slight ↓	Dialyzable
Hydralazine	Hepatic acetylation; renal excretion of metabolites	3	16	None ?	No data
Minoxidil	Mainly hepatic; renal excretion of 10% unchanged drug	1–4	1–4	None	No data
Nitroprusside	Renal excretion of thiocyanate	?	?	↓	Dialyzable; also thiocyanate dialyzable
Prazosin	Mainly hepatic; <5% excreted renally	9	?	Slight ↓	?
Terazosin	40% renal, 60% gastrointestinal	12	?	None ?	?
β-Blocking agents					
Propranolol	Mainly hepatic; renal excretion of metabolites	2–3	3–5	None	Not well dialyzable
Metoprolol	Mainly hepatic; renal excretion of metabolites	3–4	?	None	Not well dialyzable
Nadolol	Renal excretion	14–24	>24	GFR: 31–50 q. 24–36h 10–30 q. 24–48h <10 q. 40–60h	Dialyzable
Atenolol	Renal excretion; largely unchanged	6–9	>24	GFR: 15–35 half-dose <15 q.o.d.	Dialyzable
Timolol	Renal (20%)	3–4	↑	Slight ↓	Not well dialyzable
Pindolol	Primarily hepatic; also renal (40% unchanged)	3–4	Slight ↓	None	?
Labetalol	Hepatic metabolism	6–8	6–8	None	Dialyzable
Acebutolol	Hepatic metabolism; renal excretion of major metabolite	8–13	2–3× ↑	↓	Dialyzable
Esmolol	Hepatic metabolism	9 min	?	?	?
Adrenergically active agents					
Methyldopa	Renal excretion of 60% of unchanged drug plus metabolites	2–4	>4	Slight ↓	Dialyzable
Clonidine	60% renal excretion of metabolites	10–14	?	None	Not dialyzable
Guanabenz	Similar to clonidine	6	?	None	Not dialyzable
Guanfacine	Drug and metabolites excreted by kidney	13–17	?	?	Not dialyzable

Table 21.2 (*Continued*)

Drug	Metabolism/elimination	Half-life (h)		Dosage change in renal failure	Effect of dialysis
		Normal	Anephric		
Calcium channel blocking agents					
Nifedipine	80% of drug and its metabolites excreted via kidneys	2	?	↓	No data
Verapamil	Extensive hepatic metabolism; metabolites excreted in urine	4.5−12	?	Not known	Probably little
Diltiazem	Extensive hepatic metabolism	3.5	?	Not known	No data
Angiotensin converting enzyme inhibitors					
Captopril	Renal (40−50% unchanged)	1−3	↑	GFR: 15−30 slight ↓ → 5−15 half-dose → <5 quarter dose	Dialyzable
Enalapril	Renal	11	↑	As with captopril	Dialyzable
Lisinopril	Renal	12	↑	GFR: <20 half usual dose	Dialyzable
Miscellaneous					
Guanethidine	Renal excretion of unchanged drug (50%) and metabolites	120	?	None	No data
Reserpine	<1% in urine	50−100	?	None	Not dialyzable

GFR = Glomerular filtration rate (ml/min per 1.73 m^2).

HYPERTENSION IN PATIENTS ON DIALYSIS

The majority of patients who are hypertensive when starting dialysis will become normotensive upon attaining a dry weight [15] since their hypertension is mainly volume-dependent. Dry weight is not merely the absence of edema; it is that state at which further reduction of body water and sodium content results in hypotension. In the patient who is well ultrafiltered, accumulation of salt and water in the interdialytic period frequently results in hypertension which is then normalized by removal of fluid with the next dialysis. The severity of this form of hypertension in the majority of patients is related to their understanding of and compliance with dietary sodium and fluid restriction. As well, the ability to achieve full removal of accumulated volume with each dialysis is essential. Additional fluid removal can be achieved by using a dialyzer with a higher ultrafiltration coefficient and by increasing the transmembrane pressure.

The occasional patient in whom ultrafiltration fails to control the elevation in blood pressure should be evaluated for renin-dependent and other forms of hypertension. Early reports claimed that renin-mediated hypertension could be detected in ESRD patients by determining peripheral PRA. Subsequent observations have shown that such a clear separation of these patients is not possible by such means [16,17]. Diagnostic testing with inhibitors of the renin−angiotensin axis has been suggested as a means to predict renin−angiotensin-mediated hypertension and the potential response to native nephrectomy. Saralasin, a competitive angiotensin antagonist, which is no longer available, has been used for this purpose. Lifschitz and colleagues [18] studied 15 patients on hemodialysis with hypertension. Seven of 15 had a significant fall in systolic and diastolic blood pressure when treated with saralasin. Of these 7 responders, 5 underwent native nephrectomy and had a marked decrease in blood pressure. Of the 8 nonresponders, 2 had bilateral nephrectomy and both had persistent hypertension. Other inhibitors of the renin–angiotensin axis are available and have been used in a similar fashion. While angiotensin converting enzyme inhibitors such as captopril and enalapril [19] have not been studied in the pediatric age group, Vaughn and coworkers [20] have reported 2 adult patients with hypertension resistant to dialysis whose blood pressure was lowered with captopril. In patients with persistent renin-dependent hypertension, treatment with propranolol has been associated with lower mean arterial pressures and peripheral PRA in dialysed patients [21].

Bilateral native nephrectomy or transplant nephrectomy in the patient with a failed transplant should be considered in those individuals in whom no specific cause of hypertension has been found and/or in whom the hypertension is not controllable with antihypertensive drugs. The decision to perform nephrectomy should be weighed against the negative aspects of the anephric state, namely, loss of erythropoietin, loss of $1,25(OH)_2D_3$ production, and loss of urine output. It should also be based, as much as possible, on positive data implicating the kidney or kidneys to be removed as the source of the hypertension. In pediatric practice, present methods are limited but procedures such as challenge with angiotensin coverting enzyme inhibitors seem promising.

Patients receiving continuous ambulatory peritoneal dialysis (CAPD) have been reported to have better blood pressure control than those on hemodialysis [22,23]. This is probably due to continuous ultrafiltration on CAPD. A review of patients on hemodialysis and CAPD at The Children's Hospital, Boston, revealed that the fraction of patients with hypertension in each group was the same when the patients were well dialyzed [24].

Drug therapy of hypertension in the patient on dialysis

Hypertension in patients on dialysis is most often treated with β-blocking agents and converting enzyme inhibitors (Table 21.2). Propranolol has been used extensively and has been shown to be effective. While there are no published data regarding the use of other β-blocking agents in pediatric patients on dialysis, longer-acting preparations with cardiac selectivity such as atenolol may lead to improved patient compliance. In patients thought to have renin-mediated hypertension, the converting enzyme inhibitors captopril, enalapril, and lisinopril may be

useful. Their use is associated with few side-effects. However, their half-life is delayed in renal failure. Thus, low initial doses of converting enzyme inhibitors should be prescribed to avoid hypotension. Other types of antihypertensive medications have been used with success. The vasodilators hydralazine and prazosin are effective. Short-acting agents such as hydralazine should be withheld several hours before dialysis treatment to avoid hypotension during the dialysis. Methyldopa has been used effectively. It is dialyzable; thus, its dosage may require adjustment. Clonidine is well tolerated in the dialyzed patient and does not cause hemodynamic instability. Its use should be reserved for compliant patients since sudden withdrawal of the drug may cause rebound hypertension. Recently, calcium channel blocking agents have been found to be effective for treating dialysis-related hypertension. There is little experience with them in children and their role in patients on dialysis is still to be defined.

HYPERTENSION AFTER RENAL TRANSPLANTATION

Hypertension is an extremely common complication of renal transplantation in children. Its causes are many and are often related to the time elapsed since transplant. In the early posttransplant period, hypertension is almost universal and is secondary to a variety of factors including volume overload, poor perfusion of the transplant kidney, release of pressor substances by the transplant kidney, acute rejection, high-dose corticosteroid therapy, stenosis of the renal artery, and hypercalcemia. Late or sustained hypertension occurs less commonly and is most often due to chronic rejection, renal artery stenosis, urinary tract obstruction, intermittent high-dose steroid therapy, or recurrence of nephritis. These factors are discussed below.

Volume overload

Volume expansion and hypertension due to the infusion of large amounts of colloid and crystalloid fluids occurs in the first few days posttransplant. A high central filling pressure is desirable to ensure adequate function of the transplanted kidney. Large volumes of fluid may be required to achieve and maintain the desired central venous pressure. In small children who are the recipients of adult-sized kidneys this is particularly true. In our experience at The

Children's Hospital, Boston, all of these children have been hypertensive posttransplant. Hypertension due to volume expansion is transient, lasting 7–10 days, and is always responsive to diuretics in those with a well functioning graft. In those whose urine output is compromised, ultrafiltration with dialysis may be needed in the initial period.

Graft hypoperfusion

Hypoperfusion of an adult-sized kidney placed in a child would seem to be a plausible factor responsible for hypertension either because of the increased blood volume required to perfuse the graft or via the release of renin by a relatively underperfused graft. Existing data discount the theory that increasing renal mass leads to the development of hypertension. Using DLA-matched beagles it has been shown that pup recipients of adult kidneys do not develop hypertension [25]. Studies of cardiac output pre- and posttransplantation carried out at The Children's Hospital, Boston, showed that there was no significant increase in CO, nor did CO increase with increasing posttransplant blood pressure (unpublished data). Thus, at present, the importance of graft hypoperfusion as a determinant of hypertension remains to be elucidated.

Acute rejection

Hypertension is a well established sign of acute rejection [26]. Gunnels and co-authors [27], in their report of a patient with bilateral native nephrectomy and a renal transplant, documented hypertension with elevation of PRA and urinary aldosterone excretion in the face of a reduced creatinine clearance and a diagnosis of acute rejection 14 days posttransplant. After intensive immunosuppression using high-dose steroids, the creatinine clearance and hypertension improved, and the peripheral venous PRA and urinary aldosterone excretion returned to normal levels. The consistent demonstration of such findings is often difficult in the patient with acute rejection since the associated decrease in GFR will induce salt and water retention which may blunt the renin response. This is similar to Goldblatt's single-kidney hypertension model in which renin release is initially stimulated by decreased renal blood flow. Subsequent aldosterone-mediated salt and water retention, in turn, blunts the stimulus for renin release [28].

STEROID-RELATED HYPERTENSION

Hypertension may be related to the use of steroids. Several studies have correlated posttransplant steroid dosage with blood pressure. Popovtzer and associates [29] found a direct relationship between steroid dose and blood pressure in patients with well functioning transplants. Jacquot and colleagues reported a decrease in mean arterial pressure with time after transplant concomitant with a decrease in the use of steroids [30]. Hypertension has also been shown to resolve after conversion from daily to alternate-day steroids [31]. On the other hand, Rao and co-authors [32] and Bachy and colleagues [33] failed to confirm this relationship in their studies. It remains unclear whether the reported associations between decreased steroid dosage and lowered blood pressure are due to the steroid dosage itself or whether improved allograft function reflected by the ability to taper steroids is the main determinant of blood pressure in these patients. Finally, acute rises in blood pressure occur after high-dose steroid administration for rejection, despite the fact that the blood pressure may have been well controlled before the initiation of steroid therapy.

Cyclosporine A-related hypertension

Hypertension is a common occurrence in renal allograft recipients treated with cyclosporine A. The exact role of cyclosporine A in causing hypertension in this setting is difficult to determine due to the concomitant presence of pretransplant hypertension and allograft dysfunction caused by numerous factors. However, several studies comparing patients with renal transplants treated with cyclosporine A with those treated with other immunosuppressive regimens have indicated that significantly more severe hypertension develops during cyclosporine A therapy. In addition, elevated blood pressure has been consistently reported in patients with cardiac allografts [34], rheumatoid arthritis [35], myasthenia gravis [36], and uveitis [37] treated with cyclosporine A. While the mechanism of cyclosporine A-induced hypertension is incompletely understood, several interesting observations have been made. Several studies of patients with renal allografts [38] and bone marrow transplant recipients [39] have shown that PRA is not elevated. The GFR is often decreased [34,40], which may result in salt and water retention. Experimental studies in the rat have documented decreased GFR, RPF, and sodium excretion and increased renal vascular resistance and renal nerve activity after the administration of cyclosporine A [41]. Total peripheral resistance has been shown to be increased in cardiac transplant patients treated with cyclosporine A [42]. It has also been shown to stimulate the vascular release of vasoconstrictive prostaglandins and to inhibit the vascular release of vasodilatory prostaglandins *in vitro* [43,44]. Thus, cyclosporine A-induced hypertension may be secondary to decreased GFR and decreased excretion of sodium and water, and increased renal vascular resistance which may, in turn, provoke the release of vasoconstrictor hormones other than renin. Cyclosporine A also has direct effects on the systemic vasculature, causing an alteration in the normal secretion of vasodilatory and vasoconstrictive factors.

TRANSPLANT RENAL ARTERY STENOSIS

Renal artery stenosis occurs in approximately 5% of transplant recipients. It has several etiologies. The renal artery may be traumatized during the harvesting or the implantation of the graft. An extended period of warm ischemic time may cause injury to the artery. Humoral rejection may lead to renal artery stenosis, possibly related to the vascular deposition of immunoglobulin, complement, and fibrin [45]. Stenosis may develop along the suture line, particularly if a continuous suture is employed instead of interrupted sutures. Atheromatous plaque may be transplanted with the donor renal artery. Adhesions which form around the anastomotic site may cause late stenosis from extrinsic compression.

Renal artery stenosis has variable modes of presentation. It may present as gradually worsening sustained hypertension which is difficult to control even with multiple antihypertensive medications. On the other hand, a rapid, sudden increase in blood pressure may occur [46]. Finally, hypertension may appear at the same time as a rapidly rising creatinine, mimicking an acute rejection episode [47]. Since acute rejection is the most common diagnosis in the setting of hypertension and loss of function in a renal transplant, the possible existence of renal artery stenosis may be overlooked.

Radiologic evaluation of a patient for renal artery stenosis includes renal arteriography as the "gold standard." Digital subtraction angiography after di-

rect injection of the renal artery requires the use of a smaller amount of contrast material and visualizes the renal arteries as well as conventional arteriography [48,49]. Digital subtraction angiography with venous injection of contrast material usually visualizes the renal artery adequately but is not an adequate technique for evaluating renal artery branches [49]. As well, the degree of renal artery stenosis may be underestimated using this procedure [50]. Finally, duplex ultrasound scanning employing ultrasonographic visualization of the renal artery and Doppler flow measurements is now being examined as a noninvasive means of diagnosing renal artery stenosis [51,52].

In addition to these radiologic techniques, studies in adults suggest that diagnostic testing with captopril in renal allograft recipients with adequate renal function (creatinine clearance <2 mg/dl in the adult) and hypertension is an excellent predictor of significant renal artery stenosis. These patients with renal artery stenosis develop decreased effective RPF and reversible renal failure after treatment with captopril. However, renal insufficiency also develops in patients with chronic allograft rejection or sodium depletion who are treated with captopril [53]. Thus, the results of such testing are difficult to interpret in patients with early chronic rejection and hypertension. Finally, it is well established that the measurement of PRA is not a useful indicator of transplant renal artery stenosis. Plasma renin levels vary according to whether the patient has a single or multiple kidneys and whether diuretics are being used [54]. As well, in patients with a single kidney, normal PRA does not accurately predict the response of blood pressure to a renal revascularization procedure [55].

Therapy of renal artery stenosis should be directed toward its correction if at all possible. The techniques currently available include transluminal angioplasty and surgical revascularization [56]. While there are no published large series using transluminal angioplasty in children, adult series strongly suggest that it is safer and at least as efficacious as surgery for the initial treatment of transplant renal artery stenosis [57,58]. Medical management is reserved for those patients in whom repair is not possible or has been unsuccessful. In selecting a therapeutic agent for such patients, it should be noted that captopril may cause reversible renal insufficiency in the setting of a single transplanted kidney with renal artery stenosis [59].

MULTIPLE KIDNEYS AND POST RENAL TRANSPLANT HYPERTENSION

Just as native kidneys may be a source of hypertension in the patient with ESRD, the patient with a renal transplant may also be hypertensive due to the presence of nonfunctioning native kidneys. Numerous reports document a higher incidence of hypertension in patients with multiple kidneys posttransplant as compared to patients who have had prior nephrectomies of their native kidneys [55,60]. The native, diseased, nonfunctioning kidneys are thought to be responsible for a renin-mediated hypertensive state. Conflicting data on this subject are discussed below.

Several investigators have studied the value of renal vein renin ratios in predicting the blood pressure response to native nephrectomies. Castaneda and colleagues [61] found that these measurements were not predictive. Similar results were found by Curtis and coworkers [62] and Rao and co-authors [32]. In the study by Curtis and coworkers [62], 9 of 10 patients had a lower requirement for antihypertensive medicine after native nephrectomies. In contrast to the above findings, Linas and colleagues [63] studied 12 hypertensive transplant patients, one-half of whom had multiple kidneys. They showed increased renal vein renin levels coming from the native kidneys. They also demonstrated that saralasin infusion led to a significant decrease in systolic and diastolic blood pressures and a significant increase in venous PRA in patients with multiple kidneys. No data regarding outcome after native nephrectomies were reported.

The conclusion by Linas and colleagues [63] that "three-kidney" hypertensive transplant recipients have more renin-dependent hypertension than "single-kidney" hypertensive patients has been recently challenged. Curtis and co-authors [64] measured PRA in hypertensive adults with a single kidney and with three kidneys following transplantation. No differences in PRA were observed between these groups during a sodium-restricted period and during a period of normal sodium intake. In sum, there does appear to be an antihypertensive effect of native nephrectomy in some hypertensive patients with transplants who have good renal function, who do not have recurrent nephritis, and who are not on high doses of steroids. The response to this procedure may not be predicted by renal vein renin measurements. More studies using converting enzyme inhibitors are necessary to clarify their utility in predictive testing.

HYPERCALCEMIA AND POSTTRANSPLANT HYPERTENSION

Calcium homeostasis contributes to the regulation of blood pressure via changes in peripheral vascular resistance, cardiac output, or both [65,66]. Following transplant, serum calcium may be elevated due to hyperparathyroidism, vitamin D intoxication, or calcium infusion. Treatment of the hypercalcemia will lower the blood pressure.

Other causes

Children with previous glomerulonephritis are more likely to develop posttransplant hypertension [67], especially if the original renal disease recurs in the graft [24].

Renal transplant patients who develop acute pyelonephritis or transplant hydronephrosis have also been reported to develop hypertension at the same time [24].

CARDINAL FEATURES OF POSTTRANSPLANT HYPERTENSION

1 In the immediate posttransplant period most children develop hypertension.
2 Patients with stable renal function have less hypertension than those with chronic rejection. As a corollary, recipients of cadaveric kidneys who generally experience more rejection than recipients of kidneys from living related donors also experience more severe hypertension.
3 The most common etiologies of posttransplant hypertension are rejection and medication-related hypertension due to steroids and cyclosporine A.
4 Patients with prior glomerulonephritides are at greater risk for developing hypertension.

EVALUATION OF PATIENTS WITH POSTTRANSPLANT HYPERTENSION

An algorithm for the investigation of patients in the immediate postoperative period is shown in Figure 21.2. Perioperative fluid balance should be carefully documented, as should all vasoactive drugs that have

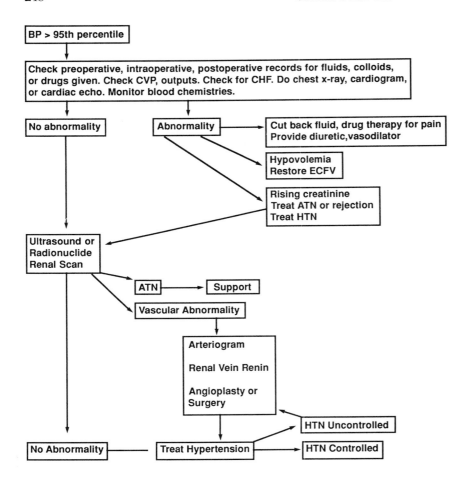

Fig. 21.2 Evaluation of postoperative, posttransplant hypertension. CVP = Central venous pressure; CHF = congestive heart failure; ATN = acute tubular necrosis; PRA = plasma renin activity; ECFV = extracellular fluid volume; HTN = hypertension. Adapted from [1].

been given. If the patient is euvolemic and does not have heart failure, then a renal ultrasound and a radionuclide renal scan should be performed. These may demonstrate acute tubular necrosis or a vascular abnormality. Patients with the latter should have the problem defined with a renal angiogram because surgery is often necessary. Acute tubular necrosis requires careful supportive care. Patients who are hypervolemic should be treated with fluid restriction and a diuretic. A vasodilator may be necessary to lower blood pressure but should be used carefully so as not to lower the blood pressure over-vigorously. However, should this occur, the hypovolemic patient will respond to restoration of the ECFV. Patients with a rising creatinine level require careful investigation of their fluid status and, often, a renal ultrasound and radionuclide scan.

Late or sustained hypertension may be investigated in a staged fashion, as presented in Figure 21.3. Abnormalities relating to urinary tract obstruction, ECFV, medications, and rejection should be looked for immediately. If found, appropriate treatment

should be instituted. Mild or moderate hypertension can be treated without further investigation unless the hypertension is refractory to treatment. In cases of severe hypertension, strong consideration should be given to looking for a vascular lesion by means of digital subtraction angiography, Doppler flow studies, or arteriography. If multiple kidneys are present, renal vein renin measurements may be made at the time of arteriography. The results of these studies may help to define further therapy.

TREATMENT OF HYPERTENSION IN THE TRANSPLANT PATIENT

Persistent hypertension should be treated with medication in addition to a trial of dietary sodium restriction. When renal function is normal, special consideration need not be given to drug metabolism. With renal insufficiency, some drugs require alteration of the dose and dosing interval and others, such as the diuretics, may not be of use. Steroid-related hypertension may be treated with diuretics

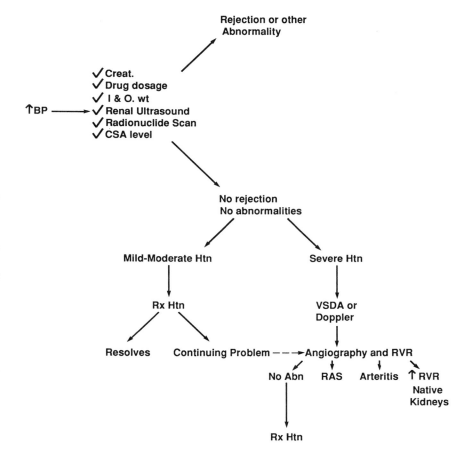

Fig. 21.3 Management of hypertension after the immediate postoperative period. BP = Blood pressure; I&O = intake and output; VDSA = venous digital subtraction angiography; RVR = renal vein renin; Abn = abnormality; RAS = renal artery stenosis; Rx = treat; HTN = hypertension. Severe hypertension warrants full investigation. Doppler flow or VDSA studies may obviate the need for arteriography in severe hypertension. While preliminary investigations may reveal rejection or another abnormality, search for a renal vascular abnormality should be considered if the hypertension does not respond to therapy and is severe in nature. Adapted from [1].

since it is partially volume-related. Vasodilators and β-blocking agents may be added. Renin-mediated hypertension is best treated with β-blockade and/or converting enzyme inhibition. As noted, the latter may cause azotemia in the solitary transplant kidney if there is renal artery stenosis.

ACKNOWLEDGMENTS

We thank Mrs Rosalie Curran and Ms Susan Purkis for their skillful secretarial assistance. This work was supported by grants NHLBI:HL 06913−02 and the Milton Fund (JR Ingelfinger).

REFERENCES

1 Ingelfinger JR. Hypertension in children with end-stage renal disease. In: Fine RN, Gruskin AB, eds. *End-Stage Renal Disease in Children*. Philadelphia: WB Saunders, 1984:340.

2 Kim KW, Onesti G, Schwartz AB, Chinitz JL, Swartz C. Hemodynamics of hypertension in chronic end-stage renal disease. *Circulation* 1972;46:456−64.

3 Kim KW, Onesti G, Swartz CD. Hemodynamics of hypertension in uremia. *Kidney Int* 1975;8:S155−62.

4 Muirhead EE, Brown GB, German GS *et al*. The renal medulla as an antihypertensive organ. *J Lab Clin Med* 1970;76:641−51.

5 Brod J, Fence V, Ulrych M. General and regional hemodynamics in hypertension in chronic renal disease. *Clin Nephrol* 1975;4:175−82.

6 Tarazi RL, Dustan HP, Frohlich ED, Gifford BW Jr, Hoffman GC. Plasma volume and chronic hypertension. Relationship to arterial pressure levels in different hypertensive diseases. *Arch Intern Med* 1970;125:835−41.

7 Davies DL, Bevvers G, Briggs JD *et al*. Abnormal relation between exchangeable sodium and the renin−angiotensin system in malignant hypertension and in hypertension with chronic renal failure. *Lancet* 1973;i:683−6.

8 Beretta-Piccoli C, Weidman P, DeChatel R, Reubi F. Hypertension associated with early end-stage kidney disease. *Am J Med* 1976;61:739−47.

9 Brass H, Ochs HG, Armbuster H, Heintz R. Plasma renin activity (PRA) and aldosterone (PA) in patients with chronic glomerulonephritis (GN) and hypertension. *Clin Nephrol* 1976;5:57−60.

10 Ingelfinger JR, Grupe WE, Levey RH. Posttransplant hypertension in the absence of rejection or recurrent disease. *Clin Nephrol* 1981;15:236−40.

11 Anderson RJ, Gamberstoglio JE, Schrier RW. Fate of drugs

in renal failure. In: Brenner BM, Rector FC Jr, eds. *The Kidney*. 2nd edn. Philadelphia: WB Saunders, 1981:2694.

12 Stone WJ, Walle T. Massive propranolol metabolite retention during maintenance hemodialysis. *Clin Pharmacol Ther* 1980;28:449–55.

13 Mirkin BL, Newman TJ. Efficacy and safety of captopril in the treatment of severe childhood hypertension: report of the International Collaborative Study Group. *Pediatrics* 1985;75:1091–100.

14 Scharer K, Rauh W, Ulmer HE. The management of hypertension in children with chronic renal failure. In: Giovanelli G, New MI, Gorini S, eds. *Hypertension in Children and Adolescents*. New York: Raven Press, 1981.

15 Vertes V, Cangiano JL, Berman LB. Gould A. Hypertension in end-stage renal disease. *N Engl J Med* 1969;280:978–81.

16 Weidman P, Maxwell MH, Lupu AN, Levin AJ, Massry SG. Plasma renin activity and blood pressure in terminal renal failure. *N Engl J Med* 1971;285:757–62.

17 Weidman P, Maxwell PH. The renin–angiotensin–aldosterone system in terminal renal failure. *Kidney Int* 1975;8(suppl):S219–34.

18 Lifshitz MD, Kirschenbaum MA, Rosenblatt SG, Gibney R. Effect of saralasin in hypertensive patients on chronic hemodialysis. *Ann Intern Med* 1978;88:23–7.

19 Fouad FM, Tarazi RC, Bravo EL, Textor SC. Hemodynamic and antihypertensive effects of the new oral angiotensin-converting enzyme inhibitor MK-421 (enalapril). *Hypertension* 1984;6:167–74.

20 Vaughn ED, Carey RM, Ayers CR, Peach MJ. Hemodialysis-resistant hypertension: control with an orally active inhibitor of angiotensin-converting enzyme. *J Clin Endocrinol Metab* 1979;48:869–71.

21 Lindner A, Douglas SW, Adamson JW. Propranolol effects in long-term hemodialysis patients with renin-dependent hypertension. *Ann Intern Med* 1978;88:457–62.

22 Salusky IB, Lucullo L, Nelson P, Fine RN. Continuous ambulatory peritoneal dialysis in children. 1982;29:1005–11.

23 Oreopoulos DG, Khanna R, Williams P, Vas SI. Continuous ambulatory peritoneal dialysis – 1981. *Nephron* 1982;39:293–303.

24 Ingelfinger JR. Hypertension in end-stage renal disease and renal transplantation. In: Ingelfinger JR, ed. *Pediatric Hypertension*. Philadelphia: WB Saunders, 1982.

25 Caldicott WJH, Ingelfinger JR. The influence of increased renal mass on cardiovascular function in immature dogs. *Ped Res* 1981;15:935–9.

26 Bennett WM, McDonald WJ, Lawson RK. Post-transplant hypertension: studies of cortical blood flow and the renal pressor system. *Kidney Int* 1984;6:99–108.

27 Gunnels JC Jr, Stickel DL, Robinson RR. Episodic hypertension associated with positive renin assays after renal transplantation. *N Engl J Med* 1966;274:543–7.

28 Helmer OM, Judson WE. The presence of vasoconstrictor and vasopressor activity in renal vein plasma of patients with arterial hypertension. *Hypertension* 1969;8:38.

29 Popovitzer MM, Pinnaggera W, Katz FH *et al*. Variation in arterial blood pressure after kidney transplantation. *Circulation* 1973;47:1297–305.

30 Jacquot C, Idatte JM, Bedrossian J, Weiss Y, Safar M, Bariety J. Longterm blood pressure changes in renal homotransplantation. *Arch Intern Med* 1978;138:233–6.

31 Curtis JJ, Galla JH, Kotchen TA, Lucas B, McRoberts JW, Luke RG. Prevalence of hypertension in a renal transplant population on alternate day steroid therapy. *Clin Nephrol* 1976;5:123–7.

32 Rao TKS, Gupta SK, Butt KMH, Kountz SL, Friedman EA. Relationship of renal transplantation to hypertension in end-stage renal failure. *Arch Intern Med* 1978;138:1236–41.

33 Bachy C, Alexander CPJ, van Ypersele de Strihon C. Hypertension after renal transplantation. *Br Med J* 1976;ii:1287–9.

34 Myers BD, Ross J, Newton L *et al*. Cyclosporine-associated chronic nephropathy. *N Engl J Med* 1984;311:699–705.

35 Berg KJ, Forre O, Bjerkhoel F *et al*. Side-effects of cyclosporine A treatment in patients with rheumatoid arthritis. *Kidney Int* 1986;29:1180–7.

36 Tindall RSA, Rollins JA, Phillips JT *et al*. Preliminary results of a double-blind, randomized, placebo-controlled trial of cyclosporine in myasthenia gravis. *N Engl J Med* 1987;316:719–24.

37 Palestine AG, Austin III HA, Balow JE *et al*. Renal histopathologic alterations in patients treated with cyclosporine for uveitis. *N Engl J Med* 1986;314:1293–8.

38 Bantle JP, Nath KA, Sutherland DER *et al*. Effect of cyclosporine on the renin–angiotensin–aldosterone system and potassium excretion in renal transplant recipients. *Arch Intern Med* 1985;145:505–8.

39 Textor SC, Forman SJ, Borer WZ *et al*. Sequential blood pressure, hormonal and renal changes during cyclosporine administration in bone marrow transplant recipients with normal renal function. *Clin Res* 1986;34:487.

40 Hamilton DV, Carmichael DJS, Evans DB, Calne RY. Hypertension in renal transplant recipients on cyclosporine A and corticosteroids and azathioprine. *Transplantation* 1982;37:597–600.

41 Moss NG, Powell SL, Falk RJ. Intravenous cyclosporin activates afferent and efferent renal nerves and causes sodium retention in innervated kidneys in rats. *Proc Natl Acad Sci USA* 1985;82:8222–6.

42 Greenberg ML, Uretsky BF, Reddy PS *et al*. Long-term hemodynamic follow-up of cardiac transplant patients treated with cyclosporine and prednisone. *Circulation* 1985;71:487–94.

43 Fan TP, Cox JH, Chishol PM. Mechanism of action of cyclosporine in preventing cardiac allograft rejection II. Graft tissue levels of prostacyclin and thromboxane. *Transplantation* 1987;43:343–5.

44 Perico N, Benigni A, Zoja C *et al*. Functional significance of exaggerated renal thromboxane A_2 synthesis induced by cyclosporine A. *Am J Physiol* 1987;251:F581–7.

45 Collins GM, Johansen K, Bookstein J *et al*. Transplant renal artery stenosis occurring in both recipients from a single donor. *Arch Surg* 1978;113:767–9.

46 Schramek A, Better OS, Adler O *et al*. Hypertensive crisis, erythrocytosis, and uraemia due to renal artery stenosis of kidney transplants. *Lancet* 1975;i:70–1.

47 Simmons RL, Tallent MB, Kjellstrand CM *et al*. Renal allograft rejection simulated by arterial stenosis. *Surgery* 1970;68:800–4.

48 Osborne RW, Goldstone J, Hillman BJ *et al*. Digital video subtraction angiography: screening technique for renovascular hypertension. *Surgery* 1981;90:932–9.

49 Working Group on Renovascular Hypertension. Detection,

evaluation and treatment of renovascular hypertension. *Arch Intern Med* 1987;147:820−9.

50 Wilms GE, Baert AL, Staessen JA, Amery AK. Renal artery stenosis: evaluation with intravenous digital subtraction angiography. *Radiology* 1986;160:713−15.

51 Greene ER, Venters MD, Avasthi PS, Conn RL, Jahnke RW. Non-invasive characterization of renal artery blood flow. *Kidney Int* 1981;20:523−9.

52 Taylor DC, Kettler MD, Moneta GL *et al.* Duplex ultrasound scanning in the diagnosis of renal artery stenosis: a prospective evaluation. *J Vasc Surg* 1988;7:363−9.

53 Curtis JJ, Luke RG, Welchel JD *et al.* Captopril and renal insufficiency. *N Engl J Med* 1984;309:667.

54 Kornerup HJ, Pedersen EB, Fjeldborg O. Kidney transplant artery stenosis. *Proc Eur Dial Transplant Assoc* 1977;34:377−85.

55 Grunfeld JP, Kelinkvech TD, Moreau JF *et al.* Permanent hypertension after renal homotransplantation in man. *Clin Sci Mol Med* 1975;48:391−403.

56 Barth KH, Brosilow SW, Kaufman SL. Percutaneous transluminal angioplasty of homograft renal artery stenosis in a 10 year old girl. *Pediatrics* 1981;67:675−7.

57 Lohr JW, MacDougall ML, Chonko AM *et al.* Percutaneous transluminal angioplasty in transplant renal artery stenosis: experience and review of the literature. *Am J Kidney Dis* 1986;7:363−7.

58 Greenstein SM, Verstandig A, McLean GK *et al.* Percutaneous transluminal angioplasty. *Transplantation* 1987;43:29−32.

59 Curtis JJ, Luke RG, Whelchel JD, Diethelm AG, Jones P, Dustan HP. Inhibition of angiotensin-converting enzyme in renal transplant recipients with hypertension. *N Engl J Med* 1983;308:377−81.

60 Cohen SL. Hypertension in renal transplant recipients: role of bilateral nephrectomy. *Br Med J* 1973;3:78−81.

61 Castaneda MA, Garvin PJ, Codd JE, Carney K. Selective post-transplantation bilateral native nephrectomy. *Arch Surg* 1983;118:1193−6.

62 Curtis JJ, Lucas BA, Kotchen TA, Luke RG. Surgical therapy for persistent hypertension after renal transplantation. *Transplantation* 1981;31:125−8.

63 Linas SL, Miller PD, McDonald KM *et al.* Role of the renin−angiotensin system in post-transplantation hypertension in patients with multiple kidneys. *N Engl J Med* 1978;298:1440−4.

64 Curtis JJ, Luke RG, Jones P, Diethelm AG, Whelchel JD. Hypertension after successful renal transplantation. *Am J Med* 1985;79:193−200.

65 Weidmann P, Massry SG, Coburn JW *et al.* Blood pressure effects of acute hypercalcemia: studies in patients with chronic renal failure. *Ann Intern Med* 1972;77:741−5.

66 Earll JM, Kurtzman NA, Moser RH. Hypercalcemia and hypertension. *Ann Intern Med* 1966;64:378−81.

67 Ingelfinger JR, Lazarus JM, Levey RH, Lowrie EG, Topor M, Grupe WE. Hypertension in pediatric renal transplant patients. *Ped Res* 1975;9:376−80.

22 Renovascular Hypertension in the Pediatric Age Group

WILLIAM J. FRY AND STEPHEN R. DANIELS

Renovascular disease is a potentially curable secondary form of hypertension. Most renovascular hypertension is due to a partial obstruction of the main renal artery. Obstruction may occur as a result of processes in the arterial lumen (thrombosis), the wall of the artery (fibromuscular dysplasia), or external forces compressing the artery (tumors). Renovascular hypertension can also result from involvement of only a branch renal artery.

In studies of adult patients with elevated blood pressure, the prevalence of renovascular hypertension ranges from less than 1% to approximately 20% depending on the selection criteria for inclusion [1]. The prevalence of renovascular hypertension in childhood is unknown. In the Muscatine study, Rames and colleagues measured blood pressure in 6622 predominantly white school children [2]. Approximately 13% had blood pressure greater than the 95th percentile at the first measurement, but less than 1% were found to have persistent blood pressure elevation. Of the 41 subjects with persistent hypertension, 2 (5%) were found to have renal artery stenosis. Daniels and associates found that 26 (3%) of 853 patients evaluated for elevated blood pressure at the Children's Hospital Medical Center, Cincinnati, Ohio had hypertension secondary to intrinsic renal artery stenosis [3]. Renovascular disease and coarctation of the aorta are the two most common causes of blood pressure elevation in children that are potentially remediable with surgery [4].

RENAL ARTERY

The normal renal artery is composed of three layers: the intima, the media, and the adventitia. All three may be involved in producing stenosis which leads to renovascular hypertension. The intima consists of an inner layer of endothelial cells supported by a basement membrane and a thin layer of subendothelial connective tissue.

The media is characterized by smooth muscle cells which are circumferentially distributed. Fibers of collagen and elastin are interspersed with the smooth muscle cells. The smooth muscle cell is capable of synthesizing elastin, collagen, actin, myosin, and mucopolysaccharide components of the extracellular ground substance [5]. When the artery is injured, the smooth muscle cells may migrate into the intima and develop phagocytic or fibroblastic characteristics [6]. At the inner and outer borders of the media are the internal and external elastic lamellae.

The adventitia is a matrix of loose connective tissue which contains macrophages, nerves, and vasa vasorum. The fibers of connective tissue are aligned in parallel and are tangential to the arterial lumen. These fibers are anchored to connective tissue fibers in the media.

PATHOLOGY OF THE RENAL ARTERY

There are a number of fibrous and fibromuscular lesions which can affect the renal arteries in children. Harrison and McCormack have developed a scheme of pathologic classification for these lesions based on the layer of involvement [7]. Their method of classification is outlined in Table 22.1. This system is useful for the pathologist; however, it has not as yet provided insight into the etiologic mechanisms involved in these problems.

In children, intimal fibroplasia, fibromuscular dysplasia, and vascular neurofibromatosis are the most common causes of renal arterial disease causing hypertension [8]. Intimal fibroplasia is a circumferential, often eccentric, accumulation of loose fibrous tissue-containing cells. Inflammation and lipid accumulation are not present. The vascular lesions of congenital rubella consist of intimal fibromuscular hyperplasia and may result in stenosis of the renal arteries [9].

Fibromuscular dysplasia produces a segmental nar-

Table 22.1 Pathologic classification of fibrous and fibromuscular lesions of the renal artery

Intima
Intimal fibroplasia

Media
(Focal, multifocal, or tubular stenoses, fibromuscular dysplasia with or without aneurysms)
    Medial fibroplasia
    Perimedial fibroplasia
    Medial hyperplasia
    Medial dissection

Adventitia
Periarterial fibroplasia

rowing of the renal artery which may or may not be associated with aneurysm formation. It can involve the main renal artery, segmental branches, or both. The sequential areas of thickening and thinning of the arterial wall produce the "string-of-beads" appearance described by angiographers [10]. The "string-of-beads" configuration is often seen in adult patients with fibromuscular dysplasia, but is less commonly seen in children. The thickened areas consist of a collagenous fibrous matrix. In the thin-walled regions the smooth muscle cells are absent and there is a deficiency of the elastic lamellae [8].

PATHOPHYSIOLOGY

The work of Goldblatt in the 1930's demonstrated that renal artery stenosis and renal ischemia could result in elevated blood pressure [11]. Since then, the pathophysiology of this process has been studied extensively in both human patients and animal models.

The primary response to renal artery stenosis and the resultant renal ischemia is the increased release of renin which occurs when pulse pressure is diminished in the afferent renal arterioles. This results in an elevation of blood pressure due to vasoconstriction which is mediated by increased circulating concentrations of renin and angiotensin. The process can be blocked by administration of an angiotensin converting enzyme inhibitor which reduces blood pressure to normal levels [11].

The secondary response to long-standing renal ischemia is the stimulation of aldosterone secretion which results in sodium retention and volume expansion. This rise in aldosterone is thought to be due

to chronic elevation of angiotensin concentrations. Angiotensin may have additional secondary effects in the central nervous system on the control of thirst and vascular tone [12,13].

The response to renal ischemia may differ depending on whether both kidneys are present and which kidney has stenotic lesions. If there is only one kidney, hyperreninemia may not be present in response to renal artery stenosis. In this situation, the mechanism of hypertension may be similar to that in anephric patients in whom volume excess rather than vasoconstriction is the predominant problem [13]. With chronic stenosis of a single renal artery when both kidneys are present, the hypertension may cause extensive nephrosclerosis of the contralateral kidney. In this situation, correction of the stenosis may not cure the elevated blood pressure, as the vascular changes in the contralateral kidney may be partially responsible for the hypertension [14].

ETIOLOGY (see also Chapters 23 and 32)

There are a number of causes of renovascular hypertension which have been described in children. These are outlined in Table 22.2. Intrinsic lesions are more common than extrinsic lesions in pediatric patients.

Fibromuscular dysplasia

Fibromuscular dysplasia is the most common cause of renovascular hypertension in most of the reported series. Boys and girls seem to be equally affected, and the lesion appears to be more common in whites than blacks [3,10,15−18]. The lesion was first described by Leadbetter and Burkland in 1938 [19]. It can occur in children of all ages, including infants [20].

Adventitial periarterial fibroplasia is a lesion of the outer media and external elastic membrane that is more common in teenage girls [21]. This lesion is often accompanied by signs of chronic inflammation within the connective tissue surrounding the renal artery.

Neurofibromatosis (von Recklinghausen's disease)

Vascular neurofibromatosis is the second most common cause of renovascular hypertension in most previously published reports [10,15,22]. However, there may be a problem with the identification of this lesion. In a review of pathologic specimens from children with renal artery stenosis, Blackburn found

Table 22.2 Causes of renovascular hypertension in children

Intrinsic
Intimal fibroplasia
   Congenital rubella
Medial fibromuscular dysplasia
Neurofibromatosis
Arteritis
   Takayasu arteritis
   Kawasaki disease
   Radiation
Thrombus
   Umbilical arterial catheterization
Trauma
   Blunt abdominal trauma
   Surgical trauma
Williams syndrome
Aneurysm
Embolism
Atherosclerosis
   Familial dyslipoproteinemia
Postrenal transplant stenosis

Extrinsic
Tumor
   Pheochromocytoma
   Wilms' tumor
   Neuroblastoma—ganglioneuroma
   Lymphoma
Congenital fibrous band
Retroperitoneal fibrosis
Perirenal hematoma

that many of the lesions that had previously been labeled as fibromuscular dysplasia were actually vascular neurofibromatosis on closer, more careful re-inspection [8]. The vascular lesions of neurofibromatosis can be separated into five classes:
1 pure intimal lesions;
2 advanced intimal lesions with medial changes;
3 nodular aneurysmal lesions with loss of medial elements;
4 periarterial nodular lesions; and
5 epithelioid lesions with cellular proliferation.

The arterial lesions of vascular neurofibromatosis are diagnostic [8]. However, the pathologic differences between vascular neurofibromatosis and fibromuscular dysplasia can be subtle, making it difficult to differentiate between the two without careful scrutiny. In patients with renal artery stenosis due to vascular neurofibromatosis, the other classic clinical features, such as café-au-lait spots, may be absent. Determination of the true relative prevalence of vascular neurofibromatosis and fibromuscular dysplasia awaits further study.

Arteritis

Daniels and colleagues reported that arteritis was the second most common cause of renovascular hypertension after fibromuscular dysplasia in their series [3]. Although the etiology of arteritis is usually unknown, two syndromes in which arteritis may involve the renal arteries in children have been recognized. With Takayasu arteritis, nonspecific symptoms of fever, malaise, arthralgia, and myalgia may last for several weeks. Patients may also develop skin lesions, such as erythema multiforme, and cardiopulmonary problems, such as pericarditis and pleuritis. The arteritis may involve large arteries, such as the aorta, as well as smaller arteries, including the renal arteries. Hypertension is usually a result of renal ischemia due to renal artery involvement. The diagnosis of Takayasu arteritis is established by clinical, radiographic, and pathologic examination. This disease appears to have a heavy predilection for young women [23] and onset is usually in the teenage years.

Kawasaki disease is a systemic inflammatory illness of unknown etiology. The sequelae of Kawasaki disease include arteritis with aneurysm formation. The most common site for aneurysms is the coronary arteries, but systemic arteries, including the renal arteries, may also be involved. Inoue and coworkers described systemic artery involvement in a series of 662 patients with Kawasaki disease [24]. Twenty-two patients had aneurysms in systemic arteries and 6 of the 22 had aneurysms of the renal arteries. However, none had developed renovascular hypertension. Hypertension has been reported in children with polyarteritis nodosa and renal artery involvement [25]. In fact, it has been suggested that Kawasaki disease and polyarteritis nodosa are manifestations of the same disease process [26].

Arteritis may also be caused by radiation for treatment of cancer. This may lead to subsequent renovascular hypertension [3,27].

Thrombosis

A relatively recently described cause of renovascular hypertension in infants is due to advances in neonatal intensive care. Infants have been found to develop elevated blood pressure from thrombosis of the renal artery following catheterization of the umbilical artery [28]. This is now probably the most common cause of severe hypertension in newborn infants

[29]. The prevalence of hypertension in infants who have undergone umbilical artery catheterization is reported as 3% [30]. Thrombi form on the catheter and then extend or embolize to the renal artery. Lou and co-authors have suggested the relationships of arterial hypertension to cerebral hemorrhage in the premature infant [31]. In some infants, cerebral hemorrhage may result from renovascular hypertension secondary to indwelling umbilical artery catheters. The relative risk of low versus high placement of umbilical artery catheters for causing renal artery thrombosis remains to be determined (see also Chapter 29).

Williams syndrome

Patients with Williams syndrome (idiopathic hypercalcemia of infancy) may develop systemic hypertension [32−34]. The cause of this elevation in blood pressure has often been attributed to renal failure secondary to hypercalcemia and nephrocalcinosis [32] or has remained unexplained [33,34]. The association of Williams syndrome with a wide variety of vascular anomalies, including hypoplasia and stenosis of both pulmonary and systemic arteries, has also been reported [33−35]. Daniels and coworkers have reported that hypertension in children with Williams syndrome may be related to peripheral vascular changes, including coarctation of the aorta and renal artery stenosis [36]. In their series, 3 of 5 patients with Williams syndrome, hypertension, and vascular anomalies had stenosis of the renal arteries. Two of those 3 patients also had associated long-segment narrowing of the aorta. The etiology of the vascular abnormalities in this syndrome remains unexplained. However, it has been suggested that the lesions can be progressive [37].

Atherosclerosis

Atherosclerotic disease is the most common cause of renovascular hypertension in adults. The lesions mainly affect the proximal third of the main renal artery and are seen mostly in men aged 40−70 years. This lesion is less common in blacks than whites [38] and is not present with increased frequency in individuals with diabetes, despite their propensity for vascular disease [39].

Arteriosclerotic lesions of the renal arteries are not common in children. When present, the lesion is similar to that seen in adults. Arteriosclerotic lesions are almost always associated with familial forms of hypercholesterolemia in which circulating levels of total cholesterol and low density lipoprotein-cholesterol are very high [40]. However, premature atherosclerosis also occurs with homocystinuria and may result in stenoses of peripheral vessels, including the renal arteries [41].

Extrinsic lesions

External compression of the renal artery may also produce hypertension. This situation has been reported to occur in patients with renal parenchymal tumors such as Wilms' tumor [42], and other abdominal tumors such as ganglioneuromas and neuroblastomas [43], with pheochromocytomas [44], and lymphomas [43]. It can also occur with problems other than tumors, including granulomatous disease [43], congenital fibrous bands [45], perirenal or subcapsular hematoma [46], and retroperitoneal fibrosis [47].

When renal artery compression is caused by a catecholamine-secreting tumor such as a neuroblastoma or a pheochromocytoma, it may be difficult to distinguish whether the blood pressure elevation is due to renal artery narrowing, catecholamine excess, or both. Making this distinction may have therapeutic implications as the mechanism of hypertension in these two entities is different and may require different management strategies.

CLINICAL PRESENTATION

The clinical presentation of children with renovascular hypertension is variable. Most commonly, the child is asymptomatic and is identified only by blood pressure measurement at a routine visit or at the time of a surgical procedure. Watson and co-authors found 9 of 17 patients to be asymptomatic at presentation [48] and Daniels and colleagues reported that 22 of 27 patients were asymptomatic [3].

When present, symptoms can range from mild to severe. Watson and co-authors described headaches, epistaxis, and anorexia in their patients [48], while Daniels and colleagues found 3 patients with hypertensive encephalopathy (1 of whom also had a cerebrovascular accident) and 2 with congestive heart failure [3]. The patients with encephalopathy or congestive heart failure were not significantly younger, nor did they have significantly higher blood pressure than the patients without presenting complications

[3]. Growth failure may also be observed at the time of presentation. Watson and co-authors reported 3 of 17 patients with failure to thrive [48]. Daniels and colleagues found that 37% of their patients with renovascular hypertension had height and/or weight below the 10th percentile for age and sex [3]. It is interesting to note that 50% of the patients with fibromuscular dysplasia in their series had growth failure. The reason for this is not well understood. Some of the other conditions associated with renal artery stenosis, such as Williams syndrome, may have growth failure as part of the syndrome.

The physical examination may provide clues to the presence of a renovascular lesion as a cause of hypertension. Patients should be examined for the features of disease entities such as neurofibromatosis and Williams syndrome, which may be associated with renal artery stenosis. The presence of an abdominal bruit, particularly if it is diastolic and lateral to the midline, may suggest a renal artery lesion. However, the occurrence of false-positive and false-negative abdominal bruits is well documented; this limits the clinical utility of this finding [49].

When the diagnosis of renovascular hypertension is under consideration, it is also useful to evaluate the patient for signs and symptoms of catecholamine excess which may occur when neurosecretory tumors impinge on a renal artery. These signs and symptoms include sweating, tremors, flushing, palpitations, tachycardia, and paroxysmal hypertension. If these are present along with evidence of renal artery stenosis, as previously noted, drug therapy may have to be chosen to address two different pathophysiologic mechanisms. The evaluation and treatment of hypertension associated with neurosecretory tumors is discussed in Chapter 25.

It is clear that not all children with elevated blood pressure need to be evaluated for renovascular hypertension. However, because it is often a silent entity, a high index of suspicion is required to identify children with renal artery stenosis. Several clinical characteristics can be helpful to make the decision to proceed with an evaluation which may include invasive testing, such as renal artery angiography. Children with severe hypertension who are very young and do not have a striking family history of hypertension should be considered for evaluation. Other indications for the suspicion of renovascular hypertension include the onset of hypertension after renal trauma, severe hypertension that is difficult to manage, evidence of deteriorating renal

function, and the presence of the clinical features of a disease that is associated with renal artery stenosis.

MEDICAL THERAPY

The goal of therapy for renovascular hypertension is to preserve viable renal tissue. This aim holds true for bilateral as well as unilateral renal artery disease, but may be difficult to accomplish when both kidneys are affected. Renovascular hypertension is potentially curable. This usually is accomplished with either a surgical procedure or transluminal balloon angioplasty.

Medical therapy for the reduction of blood pressure is indicated in the preoperative period. Preoperative blood pressure control is usually effective with the combination of a β-adrenergic blocking agent, a diuretic, and a vasodilator. An angiotensin converting enzyme inhibitor may be used in the situation where bilateral renal artery stenosis or a solitary kidney with renal artery stenosis has been excluded. However, when one of these conditions is present, the use of an angiotensin converting enzyme inhibitor may result in renal failure [50].

Medical therapy is also indicated for patients in whom surgery is not possible or is inadvisable either because of the location of the lesion or the size of the child. Daniels and co-authors reported 10 of 27 patients who received medical treatment alone. Four of them became normotensive without surgical intervention. Three had arteritis which subsequently resolved, and 1 had a renal artery stretch injury and thrombosis after blunt abdominal trauma [3]. Malin and associates have shown that newborn infants with renovascular hypertension as a result of thrombotic complications of umbilical artery catheterization can be successfully treated with aggressive medical management [51].

Pediatric patients with suspected renovascular hypertension should be referred to a tertiary care facility where there is experience in evaluating and treating this condition. Preoperative management may be difficult and requires the use of multiple antihypertensive agents. Ultimately, the definitive therapy for renovascular hypertension must be individualized depending on the etiology, location, and severity of the lesion, as well as the age of the child. Some renal artery lesions, particularly those associated with the arteritides, may resolve spontaneously and should be managed conservatively. Others require surgical intervention or transluminal balloon angioplasty.

SURGICAL THERAPY

The surgical management of children with renovascular occlusive disease presents a great challenge to the vascular surgeon. With the advent of improvements in cardiac care, anesthesia, and new surgical techniques, surgical therapy has become more frequent and there is increased ability for a safe and complete cure [22].

DIAGNOSTIC STUDIES

Physical examination

The surgical therapy will be based primarily on the total evaluation of the patient. There is no substitute for a careful assessment including a physical examination to determine the extent of the cardiac abnormality present, to include or exclude thoracic or abdominal aortic coarctation, and finally to determine if an abdominal mass is associated with the kidney. Unlike epigastric bruits, the discovery of a bruit in the costovertebral angle associated with hypertension is diagnostic of renovascular disease in over 80% of patients. Some children with severe hypertension are irritable and hyperactive. It may therefore be time-consuming and difficult to assess their physical findings completely. As there is a high association between neurofibromatosis and vascular anomalies in the abdominal aorta and renal arteries, the discovery of café-au-lait spots may be very helpful. In the presence of hypertension, café-au-lait spots indicate that further diagnostic studies should be pursued.

PLASMA RENIN ACTIVITY

Treatment of the hypertensive patient with antihypertensive drugs often may interfere with the accuracy of determinations of plasma renin activity (PRA). However the need to control the patient's blood pressure should be most important. Many drugs will elevate or suppress PRA, making renin levels in systemic blood and renal vein renin determinations inconclusive. The risk of stopping a medication that is effectively controlling the blood pressure may be tantamount to disaster and is not recommended for routine PRA determination. The advent of angio-tensin converting enzyme inhibitors has increased the accuracy of renin determinations and has made them a useful diagnostic modality. Fry and coworkers collected systemic blood for PRA before and after administration of an angiotensin converting enzyme inhibitor [52]. The same is true in the collection of blood for renal vein renin determinations. They have found an elevated renin production under these circumstances and in almost 100% of cases with an associated anatomic narrowing of the renal artery [53].

Sampling of blood for the determination of renal vein renin activity after angiotensin converting enzyme inhibitor stimulation requires samples from both renal veins and from the inferior vena cava above and below the renal veins. Ratios between the affected side and the normal side should be at least 1.5:1. This is to allow for the accepted margin of error for renin determinations. Renal systemic renin indices are defined as individual renal vein renin activity minus systemic renin activity, with the remainder divided by systemic renin activity. The renal systemic renin index in the affected kidney should be much larger than that of the normal side. Hyperreninemia originating from the kidney with a renovascular lesion should suppress the renin output from the contralateral "normal" kidney to unity. If the "normal" side is not suppressed, a total cure is unlikely. This probably signifies hypertensive damage to the "normal" kidney [54].

OTHER DIAGNOSTIC MODALITIES

The clinical response of the blood pressure to angiotensin converting enzyme inhibitors is helpful; however, it is not as diagnostically accurate as the determination of PRA. Intravenous pyelography has proven to be diagnostic of renal artery stenosis in only 30% of children examined [22]. Despite this lack of accuracy it is a good idea to utilize the intravenous pyelogram to rule out any congenital or acquired abnormality of the urinary tract that may cause or contribute to hypertension and alter the surgical approach.

The use of radioisotope renograms before and after the administration of the converting enzyme inhibitor captopril has demonstrated an increased accuracy in the diagnosis of occlusive renovascular disease [52]. However the use of captopril may cause impaired function in the face of renal artery occlusive disease. This may be due to the disruption of the autoregulation of glomerular filtration rate. Glomerular filtration rate becomes dependent on angiotensin II under conditions of low perfusion pressure. This may account for the change in renal function and is a reason not to use captopril in the treatment of renovascular hypertension. Serial urinalysis should be done after the institution of captopril therapy. Protein in the urine is indicative of glomerular filtration rate impairment. This should be a strong reason not to use captopril for a long period of time. A finding on the renogram after captopril administration is the virtual elimination of the radioisotope curve. This is seen in patients with a critical stenosis of the renal artery. The marked vasodilation in the renal parenchyma secondary to the action of captopril suddenly creates a greater outflow than the inflow restriction can accommodate. This finding is not only diagnostic of severe occlusive disease, but also is an absolute contraindication to the use of angiotensin converting enzyme inhibitors therapeutically [54]. It is in this setting that renal artery thrombosis occurs because of low flow, sludging, and clot formation. While the ability of renal scans to detect renovascular lesions is enhanced by the use of an angiotensin converting enzyme inhibitor, the accuracy of this test in the clinical setting is yet to be determined.

The refinement of ultrasonography and its combination with Doppler has opened up a new vista in noninvasive evaluation of renal blood flow [55]. The simultaneous visualization of the renal artery and determination of its flow characteristics has proven useful in the determination of renal artery occlusive disease. Flow characteristics in the aorta compared to the mid and distal renal artery have proven valuable in the determination of occlusive renal artery disease. With the use of ultrasound, the Doppler probe may be placed over the cortex of the kidney and wave form analysis will help to indicate the degree of blood flow in the kidney itself. When the two determinations are combined, Stanley and colleagues have found this technique to be exceedingly accurate, approaching a 90% agreement with arteriography [56] (Figs 22.1 and 22.2). In addition, it has been helpful in determining those patients who would have difficulty if they were treated with angiotensin converting enzyme inhibitors.

The routine determinations of blood flow in the renal artery and renal parenchyma are carried out and then a calculated dose (0.3 mg/kg) of captopril is given. The noninvasive studies are repeated 1 h after the drug has been given. Marked reductions in blood flow in the renal parenchyma are seen in those

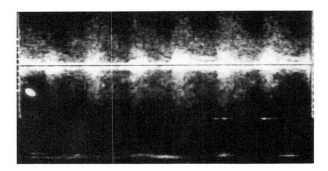

Fig. 22.1 Duplex scan through renal artery at the area of stenosis. Note the marked spectral broadening.

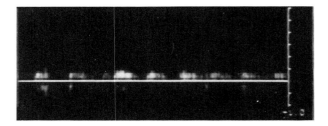

Fig. 22.2 Parenchymal flow in kidney. Note marked dampening of wave form with spectral broadening.

patients who have exceedingly tight stenosis of the renal artery and/or who will develop glomerulitis on extended therapy with angiotensin converting enzyme inhibitors (Figs 22.3 and 22.4). The number of patients who fall into the above categories represent only a small percentage who will have adverse reactions to angiotensin converting enzyme inhibitor therapy; they are nevertheless easily determined by this simple, straightforward examination. Since it does not necessitate the use of radioisotopes and is not invasive, it is very useful in children. As more experience is gained throughout the country and its accuracy is determined, it may become the diagnostic test of choice.

CARDIAC COMPLICATIONS OF RENOVASCULAR HYPERTENSION

Hypertensive cardiac damage in children poses a difficult problem in patient management. In Fry's experience this has been particularly true in children under the age of 5 years. It probably represents a failure of recognition of hypertension for extended

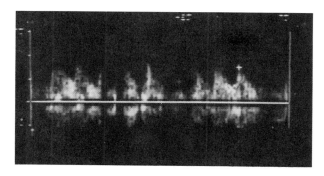

Fig. 22.3 Renal parenchymal wave form prior to captopril administration.

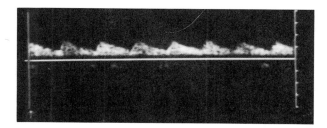

Fig. 22.4 Renal parenchymal wave form reduced after captopril administration. Note marked dampening of flow. Patient had a very tight renal artery stenosis and would have been a candidate for renal artery thrombosis if captopril therapy had been continued.

periods of time which results in an increase in left ventricular mass. The first presentation of long-standing hypertension may be with congestive heart failure. While it is at times exceedingly difficult to control blood pressure in children with renovascular hypertension, it is of great importance to optimize cardiac function prior to any operative intervention. In patients with cardiac damage due to hypertension it is important to utilize perioperative and intra-operative monitoring with the Swan–Ganz catheter. This allows the surgeon and the anesthesiologist carefully to evaluate cardiac output during a period of stress. Peterson and colleagues have shown in their laboratory, as have others, that a vasodilator, such as sodium nitroprusside, given alone, may cause severe ischemia at the apex of the heart [57]. It is therefore important that this drug should not be used unless the patient is receiving concomitant small doses of nitroglycerin which prevents the coronary steal often associated with nitroprusside. In the patient with cardiac damage, the root of the heart tends preferentially to receive coronary blood flow and rela-

tively small amounts are distributed to the apex of the heart. This becomes even more pronounced with the use of a drug such as sodium nitroprusside.

With each bout of left ventricular failure portions of the myocardium may become fibrotic. To avoid this unnecessary complication in the perioperative period, positive inotropic therapy should be used liberally.

SURGICAL INTERVENTIONS

The operative therapy for renal artery stenosis has traditionally been a bypass graft from the aorta to the renal artery distal to the area of stenosis. Since these vessels are small, the conduit of choice is autologous tissue and the internal iliac is the autologous artery of choice [56]. The chance for aneurysmal dilation is minimal and long-term follow-up studies have demonstrated the growth of this vessel with the growth of the child.

Approximately 50% of the time the internal iliac artery is not a viable conduit. This is because it is extensively involved with fibrodysplastic disease. Under these circumstances, it should not be used as a bypass graft. The distal saphenous vein can be used instead. Extreme care is taken in harvesting a segment of this vessel at the ankle. It is then immediately cooled, utilizing a buffered salt solution with heparin and papaverine added. It has been demonstrated that the use of papaverine greatly reduces the loss of endothelium within the vein graft. Fry has had little trouble with aneurysmal dilation under these conditons, and feels that when the internal iliac artery is not available, the distal saphenous vein is suitable as a bypass graft to the renal artery [22].

Great care must be taken in the anastomoses between the aorta and the graft and between the graft and the renal artery. Fry uses 8.0 and 9.0 suture material, utilizing magnification for these anastomoses. He also uses interrupted sutures, rather than a running suture, when nonabsorbable material is used. The advent of new absorbable sutures may negate the use of interrupted sutures and allow for the usual Carrel stitch to be used. It is important to note that intimal hyperplasia can occur at suture-lines between autologous tissues; therefore, it is important that these anastomoses should be spatulated so that their circumference is approximately three times greater than that of the circumference of the distal vessel.

Traditionally, the infrarenal aorta has been a very

suitable site for the takeoff of a bypass graft. This continues to be true in the majority of children. If coarctation of the abdominal aorta coexists, one may consider the hepatic artery as the takeoff point for a right renal bypass and the splenic artery as a takeoff for a left renal bypass. The splenic artery can be sacrificed just beyond its takeoff from the celiac axis without sacrificing the spleen. Splenic blood flow is preserved after ligation of the splenic artery as the spleen derives its blood flow from the short gastric vessels. The gastroduodenal artery is another artery which is appealing as a bypass to the right renal artery as no graft material is needed.

In children with Takayasu disease, the aorta may be so involved in the inflammatory process that it is not a suitable area for takeoff of a graft. Under such circumstances, the iliac arteries are usually spared and may be an acceptable point for a graft to originate. On occasion, the supraceliac aorta can be used as an originating area for a renal artery bypass. This can be done through the abdomen and requires little in the way of dissection. It allows for the takeoff of the graft above a coarctation or other abnormalities and has been a very suitable conduit [58].

Several authors advocate the routine auto-transplantation of the kidney in children with renovascular occlusive disease [57]. The kidney is removed and perfused. The renal artery is then repaired and the kidney is autotransplanted either back into its original site by suturing the graft to the aorta and re-anastomosing the renal vein, or it can be placed in the iliac fossa much like a routine renal transplant. If great care is taken, the ureter does not need to be divided and it will function well in either position. It may be necessary on occasion to divide the ureter in order to do multiple anastomoses in the parenchyma of the kidney *ex vivo*.

It is rarely necessary to do an *ex vivo* repair in children's renal arteries; however on those occasions when multiple branches are involved, it is a very good method that will allow for very careful, meticulous revascularization with preservation of renal function. The ischemic time in a child's kidney should not be longer than 30 to a maximum of 40 min. When the surgeon believes that it will take longer than this to revascularize the kidney adequately, it should be removed from the patient. Perfusion and cooling of the kidney should be done in order to preserve renal function.

In patients with orificial stenosis of a renal artery, it is appealing simply to re-implant the renal artery into the aorta. This can be done; however, there is always a degree of tension on the renal artery under these circumstances. It is well known that the resulting injury can cause intimal hyperplasia and re-occlusion of the vessel. Re-implantation, therefore, should only be utilized on rare occasions when no other suitable method of revascularization is available.

Patch angioplasty is one last possibility in the surgical approach to renal artery occlusive disease. We have no experience with this technique as we have felt that we should make every attempt to get beyond significant disease with a bypass graft in order to insure the best long-term results.

RENAL ARTERY STENOSIS ASSOCIATED WITH ABDOMINAL AORTIC COARCTATION

Abdominal coarctation is commonly associated with bilateral renal artery stenosis. In Fry's experience 70% of these patients have associated von Recklinghausen's disease.

The ideal operative approach would be to correct completely all of the congenital vascular abnormalities associated with this condition. This is not always feasible in children with severe hypertensive cardiac damage. The accompanying illustrations are of a 7-month-old child with an abdominal coarctation and bilateral renal artery stenosis (Figs 22.5 and 22.6). He had had four bouts of cardiac failure before a definitive diagnosis was made and represented a rather poor surgical risk. Because he did not tolerate his operative procedure well, the right renal artery was revascularized in one operation and the left renal artery at a second operation. The correction of the coarctation was left for a later time in order to allow for reduction in left ventricular hypertrophy. In this case, the hepatic artery and the splenic artery were used as they originated from a normal portion of the aorta. It is well recognized, however, that fibro-dysplastic disease may occur in the celiac axis at a later time and that this may require further operative intervention. This, then, was an expedient procedure in this patient to allow cardiac compensation and later repair of the coarctation.

Two methods of repair of abdominal coarctation are now popular. One is a large bypass graft from a normal thoracic aorta to a normal distal infrarenal aorta. Essentially, this bypasses the lesion. However, it does require a large graft and poses some difficulty

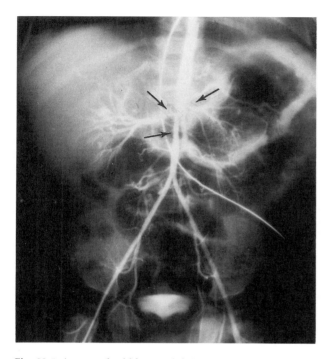

Fig. 22.5 A 7-month-old boy with bilateral renal artery stenosis (arrows) and coarctation originating below the celiac axis.

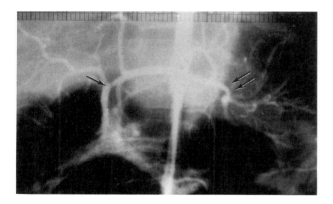

Fig. 22.6 Postoperative arteriogram showing patent right hepatorenal bypass (one arrow) and splenorenal bypass (two arrows).

for a takeoff of an aortorenal bypass. While there have been questions regarding the growth spurt of the child and whether a large bypass graft can accommodate this spurt, there have been no reported difficulties. The aorta becomes relatively fixed in the areas of the anastomoses and growth occurs above and below the insertion of the graft allowing for elongation of the trunk.

The most anatomical repair of abdominal coarc-tation is patch angioplasty of the aorta. The aorta is approached by mobilizing the left colon, the spleen, pancreas, and stomach, and reflecting them to the right. After the left crus is sectioned, this exposure allows visualization of the aorta from D9 or D10 down to the bifurcation. The left kidney is reflected to the right, as well, allowing a long segment of aorta to be exposed. The aorta can be clamped at the hiatus and the various branches occluded. A longitudinal arteriotomy is made with a gusset patch of dacron utilized to increase the size of the lumen. In the very young child, one must estimate the size of the adult aorta and fashion the size of the gusset patch to achieve this diameter. Obviously, this poses an early problem in that a relative aneurysm may be created. Great care must be taken, however, to make the patch large enough to accommodate ultimate growth or there will be a resultant stenosis of the aorta. Despite making a relative aneurysm in small children, there is not usually any difficulty with this technique since children readily grow to the size of the patch angioplasty.

This operation allows for aortorenal bypass either from the area of the gusset patch or other areas of the aorta. As it is completely anatomical, there is no problem with competitive flow and resultant throm-bosis in the area of the coarctation. Between the vascular surgery clinics at the University of Texas Southwestern Medical Center and the University of Michigan, 10 such patients have been treated with aortic patch angioplasty. Nine have done exceedingly well with no recurrent problems. One teenage patient at the University of Michigan developed an aneurysm. This was apparently due to congenital weakness in the media of the narrowed aorta. With an increased flow, she developed aneurysmal di-lation. This was successfully managed by Dr James Stanley who did a thoracic-abdominal aneurys-mectomy with an excellent result [56].

The need for careful evaluation and intensive peri-operative care of children with renovascular occlusive disease cannot be over-emphasized. To date, the only mortality in a series combined between the University of Michigan and the University of Texas Southwestern Medical Center has been 1 patient who died due to intractable congestive heart failure re-sulting from hypertension. The long-term results of operations in children for hypertension have been excellent with a 96% cured or improved rate. The chance for a complete cure of these children has been consistently above the 80% range.

REFERENCES

1 Kaplan NM. *Clinical Hypertension*. 4th edn. Baltimore: Williams & Wilkins, 1986:317−44.

2 Rames LK, Clarke WR, Connor WE, Reiter MA, Lauer RM. Normal blood pressures and the evaluation of sustained blood pressure elevation in childhood: the Muscatine study. *Pediatrics* 1978;61:245−53.

3 Daniels SR, Loggie JMH, McEnery PT, Towbin RB. Clinical spectrum of intrinsic renovascular hypertension in children. *Pediatrics* 1987;80:698−704.

4 Londe S. Causes of hypertension in the young. *Ped Clin North Am* 1978;25:55−65.

5 Jarmolych J, Daoud AS, Landau J, Fritz KE, McElvene E. Aortic media explants: cell proliferation and production of mucopolysaccharides, collagen and elastic tissue. *Exp Mol Pathol* 1960;9:171−88.

6 Poole JCF, Cromwell SB, Benditt EP. Behavior of smooth muscle cells and formation of extracellular structures in the reaction of arterial walls to injury. *Am J Pathol* 1971;62:391−404.

7 Harrison EG, McCormack LJ. Pathologic classification of renal arterial disease in renovascular hypertension. *Mayo Clin Proc* 1971;46:161−7.

8 Blackburn WR. Vascular pathology in hypertensive children. In: Loggie JMH, Horan MJ, Gruskin AB, Hohn AR, Dunbar JB, Havlik RJ, eds. *NHLBI Workshop on Juvenile Hypertension*. New York: Biomedical Information, 1984:335−64.

9 Esterly JR, Oppenheimer EH. Vascular lesions in infants with congenital rubella. *Circulation* 1967;36:544−54.

10 Stanley P, Gyepes MT, Olson DF *et al.* Renovascular hypertension in children and adolescents. *Radiology* 1978;129:123−31.

11 Barger AC. The Goldblatt memorial lecture, part 1: experimental renovascular hypertension. *Hypertension* 1979;1:447−55.

12 Buggy J, Fisher AE. Water and sodium intake: evidence for a dual central role for angiotensin. *Nature* 1974;250:733−5.

13 Davis JO. The pathogenesis of chronic renovascular hypertension. *Circ Res* 1972;40:439−44.

14 Thal AP, Grage TB, Vernier RL. Function of the contralateral kidney in renal hypertension due to renal artery stenosis. *Circulation* 1963;27:36−43.

15 Fry WJ, Ernst CB, Stanley JC *et al.* Renovascular hypertension in the pediatric patient. *Arch Surg* 1973;107:692−8.

16 Novick AC, Straffon RA, Stewart BH *et al.* Surgical treatment of renovascular hypertension in the pediatric patient. *J Urol* 1978;119:794−9.

17 Lawson JD, Boerth R, Foster JH *et al.* Diagnosis and management of renovascular hypertension in children. *Arch Surg* 1977;112:1307−16.

18 Stoney RJ, Cooke PA, String ST. Surgical treatment of renovascular hypertension in children. *J Ped Surg* 1975;10:631−9.

19 Leadbetter WF, Burkland CE. Hypertension in unilateral renal disease. *J Urol* 1938;39:611−26.

20 Makker SP, Lubahn JD. Clinical features of renovascular hypertension in infancy: report of a 9 month old infant. *Pediatrics* 1975;56:108−10.

21 McCormack LJ, Dustan HP, Meaney TF. Selected pathology of the renal artery. *Semin Roentgenol* 1967;2:126−38.

22 Stanley JC, Fry WJ. Pediatric renal artery occlusive disease and renovascular hypertension. *Arch Surg* 1981;116:669−76.

23 McKusick V. A form of vascular disease relatively frequent in the Orient. *Am Heart J* 1962;63:57−64.

24 Inoue O, Akagi T, Ichinose E, Kato H. Systemic artery involvements in Kawasaki disease. *Circulation* 1988;78:II-440.

25 McClain LG, Bookstein JJ, Kelsch RC. Polyarteritis nodosa diagnosed by renal arteriography. *J Ped* 1972;80:1032−5.

26 Landing BH, Larson EJ. Are infantile periarteritis nodosa with coronary artery involvement and fatal mucocutaneous lymph node syndrome the same? Comparison of 20 patients from North America with patients from Hawaii and Japan. *Pediatrics* 1977;59:651−62.

27 Gerlock AJ, Goncharenki VA, Ekelund L. Radiation-induced stenosis of the renal artery causing hypertension: case report. *J Urol* 1977;118:1064−5.

28 Plumer LB, Kaplan GW, Mendoza SA. Hypertension in infants−a complication of umbilical arterial catheterization. *J Ped* 1976;89:802−5.

29 Adelman RD. Neonatal hypertension. *Ped Clin North Am* 1978;23:99−110.

30 Adelman RD. The epidemiology of neonatal hypertension. In: Giovanelli G, New MI, Garini S, eds. *Hypertension in Children and Adolescents*. New York: Raven Press, 1981:21.

31 Lou HC, Lassen NA, Friis-Hansen B. Is arterial hypertension crucial for the development of cerebral hemorrhage in premature infants? *Lancet* 1979;i:1215−17.

32 Black JA, Butler NR, Schlesinger BE. Aortic stenosis and hypercalcemia. *Lancet* 1965;ii:546.

33 Schmidt RE, Gilbert EF, Amend TC, Chamberlain CR, Lucas RV. Generalized arterial fibromuscular dysplasia and myocardial infarction in familial supravalvar aortic stenosis syndrome. *J Ped* 1969;74:576−84.

34 Wiltse HE, Goldbloom RB, Antia AU, Ottesen OE, Rowe RD, Cooke RE. Infantile hypercalcemia syndrome in twins. *N Engl J Med* 1966;275:1157−60.

35 Ottesen OE, Autia AU, Rowe RD. Peripheral vascular anomalies associated with the supravalvar aortic stenosis syndrome. *Radiology* 1966;86:430−5.

36 Daniels SR, Loggie JMH, Schwartz DC, Strife JL, Kaplan S. Systemic hypertension secondary to peripheral vascular anomalies in patients with Williams syndrome. *J Ped* 1985;106:249−51.

37 Ino T, Nishimoto K, Iwahara M *et al.* Progressive vascular lesions in Williams syndrome. *J Ped* 1985;107:826.

38 Foster JH, Oates JA, Rhamy RK *et al.* Detection and treatment of patients with renovascular hypertension. *Surgery* 1966;60:240−52.

39 Munichoodappa C, D'Elia JA, Libertine JA, Gleason RE, Christlieb AR. Renal artery stenosis in hypertensive diabetics. *J Urol* 1979;121:555−8.

40 Oppenheimer EH, Esterly JR. Cardiac lesions in hypertensive infants and children. *Arch Pathol* 1967;84:318−25.

41 Boers GHJ, Smals AGH, Trijbels FJM *et al.* Heterozygosity for homocystinuria in premature peripheral and cerebral occlusive arterial disease. *N Engl J Med* 1985;313:709−15.

42 Sukarochana K, Tolentino W, Kieswether WB. Wilms' tumor and hypertension. *J Ped Surg* 1972;7:573−8.

43 Vermeulen F, Stos F, Delegher L *et al.* Surgical correction of renovascular hypertension in children. *J Cardiovasc Surg*

1975;16:21−34.

44 Naidich TP, Sprayregan S, Goldman AG, Spiegelman SS. Renal artery alterations associated with pheochromocytoma. *Angiology* 1972;23:488−99.

45 Silver D, Clements JB. Renovascular hypertension from renal artery compression by congenital bands. *Ann Surg* 1976;183:161−5.

46 Spark RF, Berg S. Renal trauma and hypertension. *Arch Intern Med* 1976;136:1097−100.

47 Castle CH. Iatrogenic renal hypertension: two unusual complications of surgery for familial pheochromocytoma. *JAMA* 1973;225:1085−8.

48 Watson AR, Balfe JW, Hardy BE. Renovascular hypertension in childhood: a changing perspective in management. *J Ped* 1985;106:366−72.

49 Korobkin M, Perloff DL, Palubinskas AJ. Renal arteriography in the evaluation of unexplained hypertension in children and adolescents. *J Ped* 1976;88:388−93.

50 Hricik DE, Browning PT, Kopelman R *et al*. Captopril induced functional renal insufficiency in patients with bilateral renal artery stenosis or renal artery stenosis in a solitary kidney. *N Engl J Med* 1983;308:373−6.

51 Malin SW, Baumgart S, Rosenberg HK *et al*. Nonsurgical management of obstructive aortic thrombosis complicated by renovascular hypertension in a neonate. *J Ped* 1985;106:630−4.

52 Geyskes GG, Oei HY, Puylaert CB, Dorhout Mess EJ. Renovascular hypertension identified by captopril-induced changes in the renogram. *Hypertension* 1987;9:451−8.

53 Stanley JC, Ernst CB, Fry WJ (eds). *Renovascular Hypertension*. Philadelphia: WB Saunders, 1984:157−60.

54 Fommei E, Bellina R, Bertelli P, Gazzetti P *et al*. Interactive functional imaging of renal scintigraphy after captopril in the detection of global and segmental hypoperfusion. *Contrib Nephrol* 1987;56:111−16.

55 Eidt JF, Fry RE, Clagett GP *et al*. Postoperative follow-up of renal artery reconstruction with duplex ultrasound. *J Vasc Surg* 1988;8:667−73.

56 Stanley JC, Ernst CB, Fry WJ (eds) *Renovascular Hypertension*. Philadelphia: WB Saunders, 1984;20−45,146−77, 277−326.

57 Peterson A, Brant D, Kirsh MM. Nitroglycerin infusion during infrarenal aortic cross-clamping in dogs: an experimental study. *Surgery* 1978;84:216−23.

58 Fry RE, Fry WJ. Supracoeliac aorto-renal bypass using saphenous vein for renal vascular hypertension. *Surg Gynecol Obstet* 1989;168:180−2.

23 Radiographic Evaluation and Intervention in the Child with Hypertension Related to Renal Disease

WILLIAM S. BALL JR

INTRODUCTION

The radiologist has always played an important role in the search for potentially curable causes of hypertension in children, including those arising from alterations in renal blood flow, which lead to excessive production of renin and angiotensin from the kidney. The excretory urogram (EU) was for years the "gold standard" of imaging the genitourinary system, but has now been replaced by more accurate diagnostic cross-sectional imaging including ultrasound, computerized tomography (CT), and magnetic resonance imaging (MRI). These newer modalities have significantly improved our ability to diagnose noninvasively many renal disorders that cause hypertension, including renal dysplasia or hypoplasia, chronic hydronephrosis, chronic pyelonephritis, glomerulonephritis, and tumors such as neuroblastoma and pheochromocytoma. Despite our recognition of essential hypertension in the pediatric age group, one of the most common secondary causes of hypertension remains primary renal artery fibromuscular disease. Even with the many advances in cross-sectional imaging, angiography continues to be our most valuable tool in the diagnosis and evaluation of renovascular disease in children.

The greatest change in the radiologist's role has been the transition from purely a diagnostician to that of also a therapeutic interventionalist. The development of small-vessel balloon dilatation catheters and safer, more effective, embolic delivery systems now provides the interventionalist with the tools to become directly involved in the management of children with renovascular hypertension. This new role requires the radiologist to be familiar not only with current cross-sectional imaging and interventional techniques, but with the changing concepts of hypertension in the pediatric population as well. It also requires a close association between the radio-logist and the clinical hypertension specialist managing the patient. This chapter primarily deals with the current integration of cross-sectional imaging and diagnostic angiography in the diagnosis of renal causes of hypertension in children. In addition, the latter part of this chapter will deal with the indications, patient selection, technical considerations, and results of renovascular interventional procedures as a means of managing hypertension.

RADIOGRAPHIC IMAGING

For years, the excretory urogram (EU) represented the "gold standard" of imaging the genitourinary tract. From the EU, it was possible to detect asymmetry in renal size, delay in excretion of contrast, or a dense persistent nephrogram indicating the presence of unilateral or bilateral renovascular disease (Fig. 23.1). Attempts to enhance the sensitivity of the EU included rapid-sequence filming soon after the injection of contrast, and this was known as the rapid-sequence urogram (RSU). Using the RSU, Stanley and colleagues reported a 65% sensitivity in diagnosing unilateral renovascular disease in children [1], with other authors reporting an accuracy, ranging from 24 to 54% [2,3]. The reliability of the RSU decreases further for bilateral renovascular disease [1]. Long-term studies in adults indicate that the sensitivity of the RSU is no greater than the standard pyelogram for detecting vascular disease [4]. The limitations of the pyelogram continue to be its inability to detect both early stenotic involvement of the main renal artery and segmental occlusions. It continues, however, to suffice as an adequate screening test for renal parenchymal disease or tumors when cross-sectional imaging is not readily available.

In most centers, ultrasound or CT has replaced the EU for evaluating the genitourinary tract in children. Ultrasound provides excellent anatomic detail of the

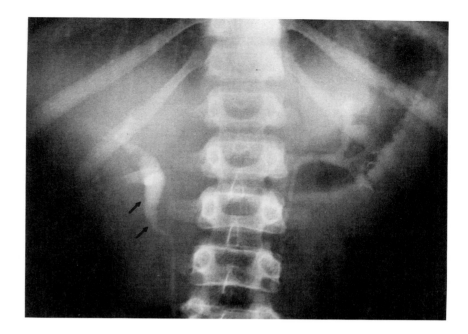

Fig. 23.1 A persistently dense right nephropyelogram and notching of the renal pelvis (arrows) due to extensive pelvocalyceal collateral blood flow are indirect evidence of a high-grade stenosis of the main renal artery.

kidneys in multiple projections without the use of ionizing radiation. Morphologic abnormalities which may secondarily cause excessive stimulation of the renin—angiotensin system, such as hydronephrosis, renal dysplasia, and chronic inflammatory disease, are easily detected on ultrasound [5,6] (Fig. 23.2). Despite its many advantages, ultrasound is incapable of anatomically visualizing renal vessels with suf-ficient resolution. Doppler ultrasound, with or without color, can enhance the ability of ultrasound to detect alterations in blood flow in both native and transplanted kidneys [7,8], but still lacks the resolution of angiography. Computerized tomography is also an effective diagnostic modality for renal parenchymal abnormalities, but is limited in the detection of renovascular disease despite the use of contrast

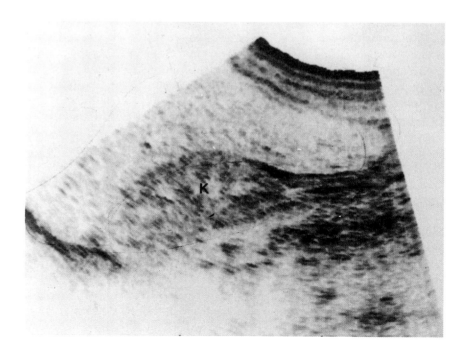

Fig. 23.2 Chronic pyelonephritis. On ultrasound, the right kidney (K) appears small and densely echogenic secondary to chronic scarring and inflammation.

enhancement. Rapid sequential axial images through the kidney during and following the bolus injection of intravenous contrast may improve the recognition of asymmetric renal blood flow, but lack the ability to image directly the vascular abnormality causing the alteration. More recently, magnetic resonance has also begun to play a role in imaging the kidneys (Fig. 23.3), but unlike CT, MRI has the additional potential to visualize renal vessels noninvasively by flow-related angiography. Perhaps in the future, magnetic resonance angiography may eventually replace the more invasive conventional angiogram in the diagnosis of renal artery stenosis.

All children with documented persistent hypertension should be screened with ultrasound in order to exclude renal parenchymal disease or tumor. Even with a negative screening examination, angiography is performed as the next step in the evaluation of suspected renovascular disease, especially in those patients with persistent moderate or severe hypertension who are very young at the time of diagnosis, or have hypertension associated with syndromes such as neurofibromatosis and Williams syndrome.

DIAGNOSTIC ANGIOGRAPHY

Over the past 10 years, diagnostic angiography has undergone considerable change in the form of patient selection, technique, improved safety, and the means by which data are recorded. Whereas in the past angiography was often performed routinely in all children with hypertension, the recognition of juvenile essential hypertension, improved laboratory studies, and advances in therapy have limited the use of angiography to those patients in whom there is a high index of suspicion for renovascular disease. Computerized collection and storage of angiographic data have also had a significant impact on renal angiography, by adding the new dimension of data postprocessing in order to improve information [9,10].

Digital venous subtraction angiography (DVSA), digital subtraction angiography (DSA), and standard conventional cut-film are all angiographic methods used to visualize and record images of the renal blood vessels following contrast injection. The process of DVSA combines the use of a central venous injection with computer-enhanced imaging over the region of interest. This technique is designed to eliminate arterial cannulation, and thus avoid the complications of direct arteriography in small chil-

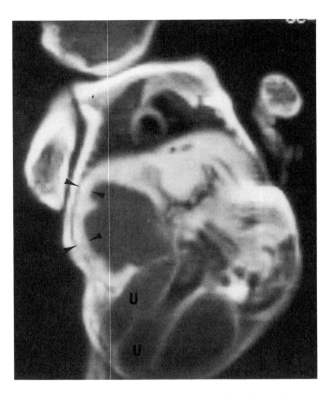

Fig. 23.3 Marked loss of renal cortex (arrowheads), and dilatation of the right collecting system and ureter (u), indicating distal obstruction, are well demonstrated on this coronal magnetic resonance image.

dren. With DVSA, contrast is injected through a centrally placed venous catheter located either within the superior vena cava or in the right atrium, advanced from a brachial or femoral venous approach. Shortly after injecting 1 ml per kg of full strength contrast over a 2-s interval, delayed enhanced images are collected, centering over the abdominal aorta and kidneys (Fig. 23.4). The angiogram produced represents a difference-image, formed by subtracting an unenhanced image obtained before the arrival of contrast from an enhanced image collected at the peak arrival of the contrast bolus within the region of interest.

The role of DVSA and its sensitivity in detecting renovascular disease have been met with mixed reviews [11–13]. Its shortcomings include image degradation due to motion misregistration artifact, the problem of overlapping vessels, and insufficient resolution necessary to visualize segmental and intrarenal arterial disease. Since segmental fibromuscular disease is not uncommon [14], its detection may go unnoticed using DVSA [12]. The careful screening

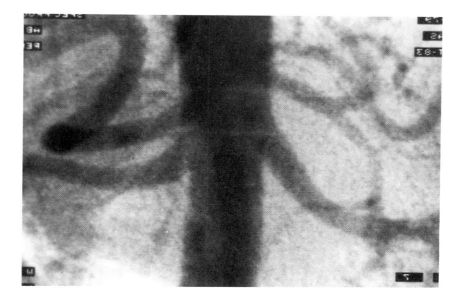

Fig. 23.4 There is excellent visualization of the abdominal aorta and main renal arteries (A) following a bolus injection of contrast within the right atrium and computerized enhanced imaging over the mid abdominal aorta.

and selection of patients for angiography, the need for multiple projections, and the high incidence of segmental disease require the selection of techniques (e.g. DSA, standard cut-film) that afford the highest resolution with the least chance for misdiagnosis.

Both DSA and conventional cut-film angiography require arterial cannulation. Improvements in catheter technology (e.g. smaller catheters) have led to increased safety with arterial cannulation even in the youngest and smallest of patients. In young uncooperative patients, direct arteriography is performed under general anesthesia using a standard Seldinger technique of femoral puncture. Each examination is begun with an abdominal aortogram in the anteroposterior projection, which is followed by oblique selective renal arteriography. For the abdominal aortogram in any age group, 1 ml of contrast per kg body weight is injected over a 2-s interval through either a pigtail or multiside-hole straight catheter centered just above the origin of the renal arteries. For selective arteriography, the amount of contrast injected depends on the size of the patient or renal artery, and ranges from 2 ml in infants under 10 kg to 9 ml in children over 50 kg. The injection is made through a directional catheter, and is administered as a rapid bolus over a 1–1.5-s period. For either abdominal aortography or selective renal arteriography with DSA, a 50% dilution of contrast is used, but at the same injection rate. Occasionally, the origins of the renal arteries are best visualized using a 15° obliquity with an aortic injection at the level of the renal ostia. Visualization of the segmental and intrarenal arteries requires selective injections, often in multiple projections, in order to improve resolution and avoid obscuring information due to overlapping vessels. Spasm encountered following selective renal arterial cannulation and injection should not be confused with focal fibromuscular disease. A repeat injection at a lower volume and pressure or a central injection into the abdominal aorta may help separate spasm from a true fibromuscular stenosis (Fig. 23.5). Complications of selective arteriography include intimal dissection and thrombosis secondary to excessive catheter manipulation, or from the "jet-effect" produced by a high-pressure injection [15] (Fig. 23.6). Excessive manipulation of the artery and unnecessary injections should be avoided, especially in the face of significant vascular disease in the contralateral kidney.

Selective renal arteriography is recorded using either conventional cut-film or computer digital storage. The advantages of computer-assisted angiography include reduction in contrast volume, lower injection pressure, the ability to use smaller catheters (thereby minimizing catheter-related complications), subtraction of unwanted background information, and postprocessing of images to enhance information (Fig. 23.7). Current computer subtraction systems with 512×512 or 1024×1024 pixel matrices have considerably improved digital resolution over earlier production units, but still lack the resolution of cut-film angiography. In most cases, it is wise to perform conventional angiography in at least one projection in order to take advantage of the excellent small-

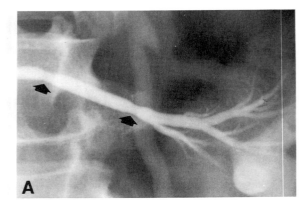

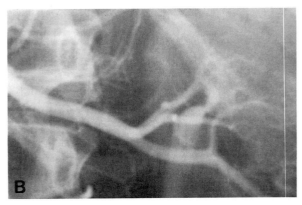

Fig. 23.5 Arterial spasm simulating fibromuscular disease. (A) Two areas of fibromuscular stenosis were suspected (arrows) following a selective renal arterial injection. (B) Both lesions subsequently proved to be spasm by their disappearance after a repeat injection into the central abdominal aorta.

vessel resolution and relative lack of susceptibility to motion artifact.

RENOVASCULAR DISEASE

The abdominal aorta in association with renovascular disease (see also Chapter 22)

Besides affecting the renal arteries, the abdominal aorta is frequently involved in neurofibromatosis [16], middle aortic syndrome [17], diffuse arteritis [18], and Williams syndrome [19], but often remains normal in the presence of juvenile idiopathic fibromuscular disease. Narrowing of the abdominal aorta, or coarctation, may be focal or diffuse, infrarenal or suprarenal. Smooth-walled abdominal coarctation of the infrarenal aorta can be found in association with both neurofibromatosis [16] (Fig. 23.8) and Williams syndrome [19]. In middle aortic syndrome [17], the

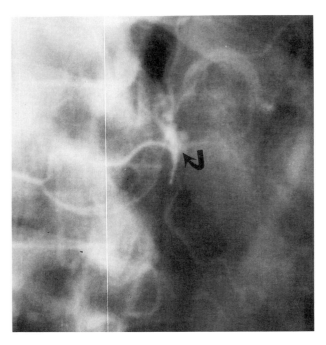

Fig. 23.6 Excessive catheter manipulation and high injection pressures resulted in this intimal dissection and extravasation of contrast (arrow) during a selective renal arteriogram. There was no compromise in renal arterial flow as a result, and bleeding ceased spontaneously after a short period of time.

coarctation is typically in the mid abdominal aorta at the level of the renal arteries (Fig. 23.9). A diffuse arteritis can produce focal or long-segment narrowing involving any portion of the abdominal aorta [18] (Fig. 23.10). Rarely, an acquired coarctation can result from radiation therapy [20], where the narrowing is limited to the radiation field-port utilized for treatment of renal or paraspinous tumors. Radiation induced coarctation can also produce renal artery stenosis and/or clinical hypertension [20]. In both middle aortic syndrome and in diffuse arteritis, the walls of the aorta are often irregular, whereas in postirradiation aortitis the coarctation usually appears late, at which time the walls are smooth. Proximal stenosis of the celiac and superior mesenteric arteries may likewise be encountered in idiopathic fibromuscular disease, diffuse arteritis, or neurofibromatosis.

Idiopathic fibromuscular disease (see also Chapter 22)

The most frequent cause of renovascular hypertension in the pediatric population remains fibromus-

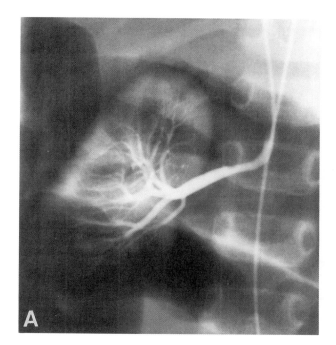

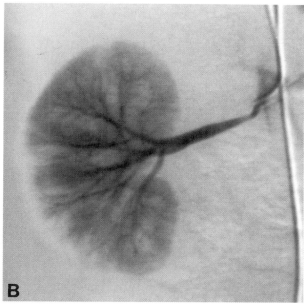

Fig. 23.7 (A) Poor visualization of the intrarenal vasculature on cut-film angiography is often a result of overlapping shadows. (B) Background information is eliminated by digital subtraction angiography with only a slight degradation in resolution.

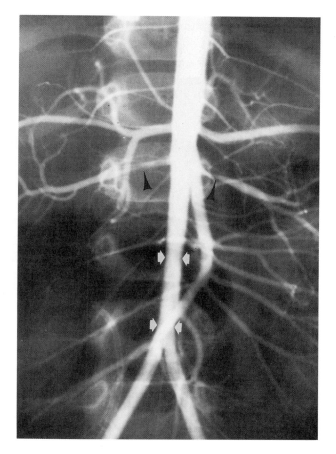

Fig. 23.8 Neurofibromatosis. There is mild diffuse hypoplasia of the infrarenal abdominal aorta from L2 to the bifurcation (arrows). Bilateral proximal tubular renal artery stenoses are also present; these are typical of the fibromuscular disease of neurofibromatosis (arrowheads).

cular disease (FMD) [21]. Most references to this disorder in children fail to distinguish between the idiopathic form and that found in association with neurofibromatosis, tuberous sclerosis, or Williams syndrome. Juvenile idiopathic fibromuscular disease (JIFD) most commonly affects the medial or muscular layer of the artery [22], whereas in neurofibromatosis and Williams syndrome, proliferation of the intimal layer predominates [23]. Despite attempts to categorize the pathology of arterial involvement [24], considerable overlap exists between the radiographic appearance of both the idiopathic and syndromic forms of FMD. Unilateral stenoses are reported as being more common [24]; however, Lawson and co-authors recorded bilateral involvement in 44% of children studied [22]. The right renal artery is also said to be more frequently involved in adults [24], but there is little evidence in children that the right is involved more often than the left [25]. Our own experience supports a slight predilection for unilateral rightsided disease; however, bilateral stenoses are common enough to warrant careful investigation of both sides when performing angiography.

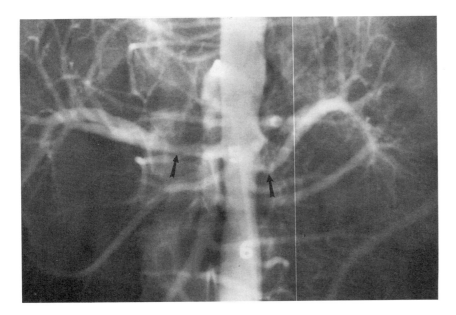

Fig. 23.9 Middle aortic syndrome. The mid abdominal aorta demonstrates a mild coarctation proximal and distal to the renal artery ostia. Proximal stenoses of both renal arteries (arrows) are also present.

Idiopathic FMD in adults typically produces a stenosis in the mid or distal main renal artery [26], often with disease extending into the ventral and dorsal segmental branches. In JIFD, the distribution of involvement is similar to that found in adults (Fig. 23.11), whereas ostial and proximal stenoses are more characteristic of the syndromic form of FMD [26]. Not infrequently with JIFD, the stenotic lesion may be isolated to the segmental branches (Fig. 23.12). On occasion, the focal stenosis may involve the proximal renal artery, but rarely is there ostial narrowing (Fig. 23.13). The "string-of-beads" appearance, so often reported in adults with medial or muscular fibroplasia [27], is uncommon in children (Fig. 23.14), where lesions are more often focal, multifocal, or tubular in appearance (Fig. 23.15).

The degree of poststenotic dilatation depends upon the severity of the stenosis (Fig. 23.16). Poststenotic dilatation appears as a smooth-walled ectasia of the artery distal to the stenosis, which helps differentiate this entity from the eccentric and saccular appearance of an aneurysm. Poststenotic dilatation and multiple aneurysms of the main renal artery or segmental branches can occur in combination [28]. As with poststenotic dilatation, the aneurysms are usually located distal to the stenotic segment, and typically measure 1–3 cm in diameter [28] (Fig. 23.17). Giant aneurysms may be found in association with fibromuscular disease in older patients, but are uncommon in the pediatric population [29].

Little is known about the natural history of FMD.

In a series of 55 patients of indeterminate age reported by Sheps and coworkers, one-third demonstrated progression of disease with time [30]. Rarely, spontaneous regression or a "waxing-and-waning" course may occur [31,32] (Fig. 23.18). A slow progression to a higher-grade stenosis or complete occlusion of the renal artery may produce little change clinically due to the recruitment of collateral circulation over time. With complete occlusion of the renal artery, the kidney comes to rely solely on collateral circulation from adrenal, capsular, lumbar, or ureteric branches (Fig. 23.19). When a high-grade stenosis involves a segmental branch, collateral circulation may be primarily intrarenal [33] (Fig. 23.20).

Fibromuscular disease in syndromes

Neurofibromatosis, Williams syndrome, and rarely tuberous sclerosis may manifest clinically with hypertension of renovascular origin. In the adult with neurofibromatosis, pheochromocytomas account for most cases of hypertension [34], whereas in patients less than 18 years of age with von Recklinghausen's disease, hypertension is more closely related to FMD of the renal arteries [35]. As mentioned previously, the abdominal aorta is not uncommonly involved in neurofibromatosis. Bilateral involvement is more common in this disorder than in JIFD (Fig. 23.21), and there is a greater predilection for the stenosis to include the ostium as well as the proximal segment of the main renal artery (Fig. 23.22). Focal stenotic

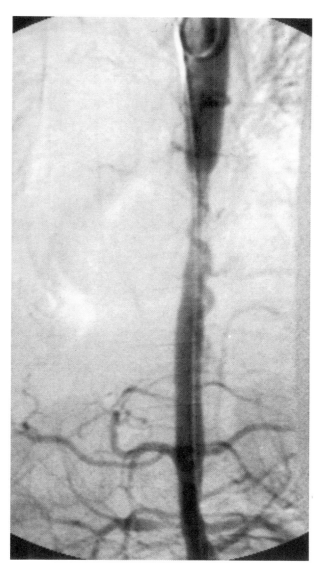

Fig. 23.10 Diffuse arteritis. A severe irregular coarctation of the aorta resulted from a diffuse progressive arteritis of unknown etiology.

lesions often appear smooth and tubular, reflecting a greater degree of intimal proliferation and hyperplasia [23]. Less commonly, the entire main renal artery may appear diffusely hypoplastic, and aneurysms may develop distal to the stenotic lesions. On occasion, the pattern of renal artery stenosis in a patient with known neurofibromatosis may overlap with the radiographic appearance of other forms of FMD, making their separation difficult by angiography alone.

Daniels and co-authors [19] reported the association of renal artery stenosis and hypertension in 3 of 5 patients presenting with Williams syndrome. Little is known about the patterns of fibromuscular renal artery disease leading to stenosis in this disorder. Unlike in neurofibromatosis, aortic supravalvar coarctation and peripheral pulmonary stenoses are common in Williams syndrome [36]. Despite the apparent differences, the radiographic pattern of renal arterial disease may be similar to that found in neurofibromatosis, limiting their differentiation angiographically.

HYPERTENSION ASSOCIATED WITH RENAL PARENCHYMAL DISEASE
(see also Chapters 19 and 20)

Rarely, severe hypertension may result from either diffuse chronic pyelonephritis [37] or from segmental renal scarring or hypoplasia [38,39]. The appearance of chronic pyelonephritis on EU and cross-sectional imaging is that of a small lobulated kidney with marked diffuse renal cortical loss (Fig. 23.2) and adjacent calyceal dilatation. The term Ask−Upmark kidney is used to designate a particular form of renal segmental dysplasia not uncommonly presenting with hypertension [39,40]. This unusual form of dysplasia is most often unilateral, and rarely bilateral [40]. Although there is controversy over whether the Ask−Upmark kidney is congenital or acquired, the most likely etiology is from segmental scarring due to chronic reflux nephropathy [41]. The kidney is small and displays a deep transverse circumferential groove on the cortical surface of either the mid or upper pole. The adjacent calyx is usually dilated.

Angiography is rarely indicated for the diagnosis of chronic pyelonephritis or segmental hypoplasia, but may be required to exclude FMD if severe or unstable hypertension is present. The angiographic differentiation of chronic pyelonephritis from severe FMD is usually not difficult. With chronic inflammation, the main renal artery is normal or diffusely small in caliber from decreased flow to the scarred kidney. Often the segmental and interlobar arteries are normal; however, the more peripheral arcuate and interlobular arteries are frequently lost or distorted due to cortical scarring (Fig. 23.23). In severe cases, significant intrarenal collateral circulation develops, but extrarenal collateral circulation may be lacking due to preservation of flow in the main renal artery. In segmental hypoplasia, the main renal artery and its ostium may be minimally decreased in caliber, but lacks the focal changes of fibromuscular

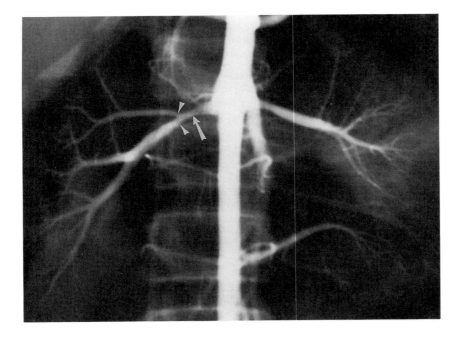

Fig. 23.11 Bilateral juvenile idiopathic fibromuscular disease. Stenotic fibromuscular narrowing of the mid and distal right main renal artery (arrow) extends to involve the proximal segmental branches as well (arrowheads). Despite the extensive mid to distal involvement, there is sparing of the ostium and proximal main renal artery.

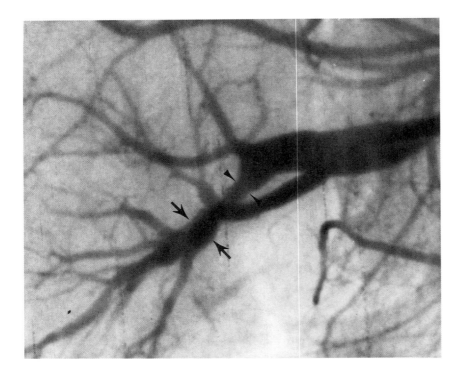

Fig. 23.12 Segmental juvenile idiopathic fibromuscular disease. A severe stenosis involves the proximal ventral segmental artery (arrowheads) producing moderate poststenotic dilatation (arrows). The main renal artery including the ostium was normal.

disease. The intrarenal vessels are normal in the uninvolved portions of the kidney, whereas the vasculature leading to the hypoplastic band is narrowed, crowded together, and displays pruning of the interlobular arteries due to medial hypertrophy and occasionally intimal proliferation [41].

Congenital hypoplasia of the kidney is rarely associated with hypertension in children [42]. In this condition, the kidney is diffusely small with a smooth contour. There is little or no calyceal distortion, although the number of calyces may be deficient. The kidney is often in a more medial location along the

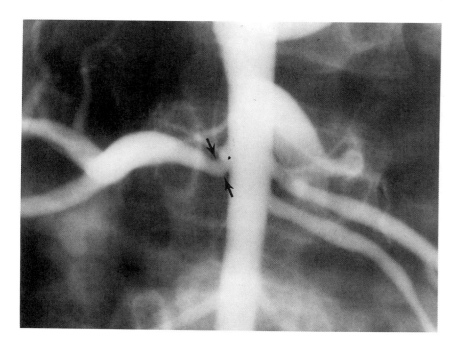

Fig. 23.13 Less commonly seen is proximal involvement of the main renal artery (arrow) in idiopathic juvenile fibromuscular dysplasia. Note the sparing of the ostium (asterisk) despite the proximal location of the stenosis.

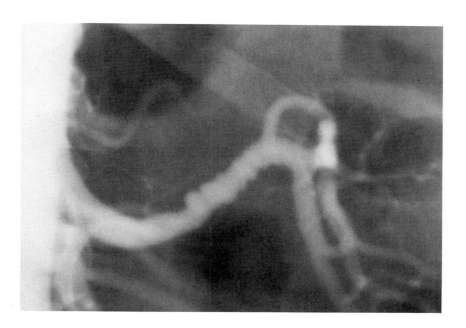

Fig. 23.14 A typical "string-of-beads" appearance indicates the presence of fibromuscular dysplasia throughout the mid and distal main renal artery. This pattern is only rarely seen in children.

spine due to its shorter main renal artery [42]. The recognition of a "miniature" yet architecturally preserved kidney on EU or cross-sectional imaging indicates this diagnosis, and often precludes the necessity for angiography. Angiography is only warranted if the diagnosis is in doubt, or to exclude FMD in the presence of severe or poorly controlled hypertension. The angiographic features include a small, smooth-walled main renal artery and ostium which measures

approximately 20% of normal size and lacks the focal changes associated with FMD [42]. Although the intrarenal arteries are diffusely small, their appearances lack the distortion seen in chronic pyelonephritis.

Severe hydronephrosis secondary to obstruction rarely produces hypertension by activation of the renin–angiotensin system [43]. Moreover, the hypertension may or may not resolve following relief of the

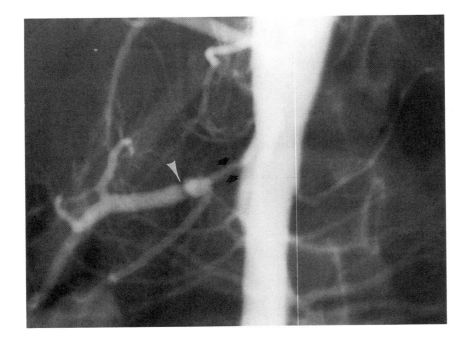

Fig. 23.15 The long tubular stenosis in the proximal main renal artery is more indicative of intimal proliferation, and contrasts with the more focal segment (arrowheads) in the mid artery from medial hyperplasia.

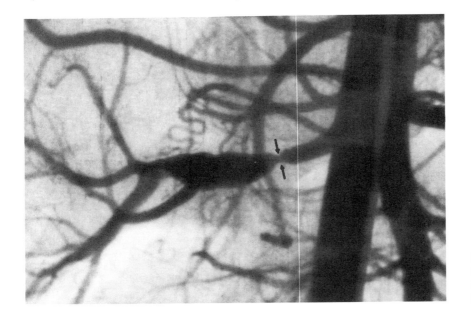

Fig. 23.16 Moderate poststenotic dilatation characterized by fusiform ectasia of the artery lies distal to a focal fibromuscular stenosis (arrows).

obstruction. Hydronephrosis is best diagnosed on the delayed images of an EU or by cross-sectional imaging, where often the cause and the level of the obstruction can be identified. Angiography is not indicated in a patient with hydronephrosis when excessive renin production ceases following elimination of the obstruction.

Angiographically, hydronephrosis is easily differentiated from FMD by a normal main renal artery and thinning, stretching, and displacement of intrarenal vessels around massively enlarged calyces (Fig. 23.24). Tortuosity and pruning of intrarenal vessels may be encountered if there has been co-existent chronic inflammation.

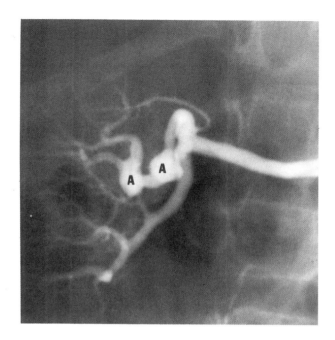

Fig. 23.17 Aneurysms (A) are often associated with fibromuscular disease, and are differentiated from poststenotic dilatation by their saccular appearance and eccentric location.

RENAL TRANSPLANTATION

Angiography continues to play an important but limited role in the management of patients with persistent hypertension following renal transplantation [44,45]. Hypertension immediately after transplantation may result from excessive renin production from the native kidneys, acute rejection, or secondary to thrombosis of the graft. In the acute phase, cross-sectional imaging and radionuclide studies are sufficient for evaluation, without angiography. Angiography may be of benefit in the established transplant, however, when there is persistent or a new onset of hypertension secondary to acquired renal artery stenoses or chronic rejection [46–49]. In most cases, chronic rejection can be identified using sonography (Fig. 23.25), isotope renography, and percutaneous biopsy. In the absence of proof of rejection, angiography may become necessary to

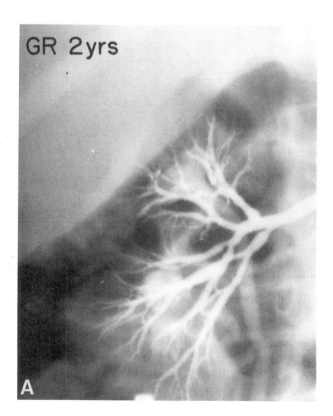

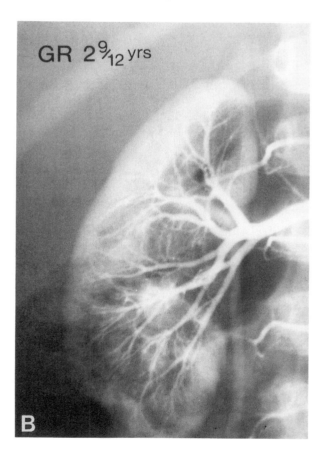

Fig. 23.18 (A) Multiple segmental and subsegmental fibromuscular stenoses were identified angiographically in this 2-year-old hypertensive child. (B) After 9 months, spontaneous regression of the lesion was accompanied by spontaneous clinical improvement in the hypertension.

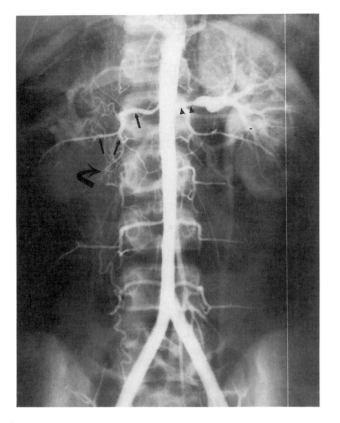

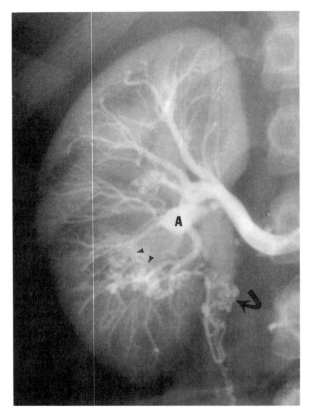

Fig. 23.19 A complete fibromuscular occlusion of the right renal artery has led to extensive collateral circulation derived from lumbar arteries (arrows) and a rich pelviureteric plexus (curved arrow). A long-segment proximal stenosis of the left renal artery (arrowheads) is also present.

Fig. 23.20 An aneurysm (A) and multiple intrarenal segmental arterial occlusions are identified in the mid and lower pole of the right kidney. Collateral circulation is derived from the periureteric plexus (curved arrow), and from intrarenal collaterals (arrowheads).

exclude arterial lesions which may further limit the life of the graft.

Stenoses of the transplanted renal artery may occur at the anastomosis secondary to scarring, suture granulation, or cross-clamping at the time of transplantation [50] (Fig. 23.26). A stenosis distal to the anastomosis may be due to ischemia of the graft, cross-clamping or, rarely, chronic rejection [51]. Significant abnormalities of the intrarenal vasculature, including narrowing, focal occlusion, pruning, and irregularity of vessels, should indicate chronic rejection rather than decreased flow due to an arterial stenosis [46] (Fig. 23.27). In the absence of obvious arterial disease involving the graft, venous sampling for measurement of plasma renin activity (PRA) from both the native kidneys and from the transplant is often necessary to locate the cause of persistently elevated peripheral PRA. Prior to the performance of

angiography, the radiographer should be fully aware of the type of anastomosis and its location. For diagnostic evaluation, arterial access can be either from the contralateral or ipsilateral femoral artery. Stenoses occurring directly at the anastomosis of a renal artery with the iliac vessel may be difficult to identify, and often a central iliac injection in multiple obliquities is required to eliminate overlapping vessels. A subselective injection is then performed to evaluate the intrarenal vasculature, but excessive manipulation of the graft should be avoided to minimize complications which might result in arterial thrombosis.

PERCUTANEOUS TRANSLUMINAL ANGIOPLASTY

Percutaneous transluminal angioplasty (PTA) has been used extensively in the treatment of atheroscle-

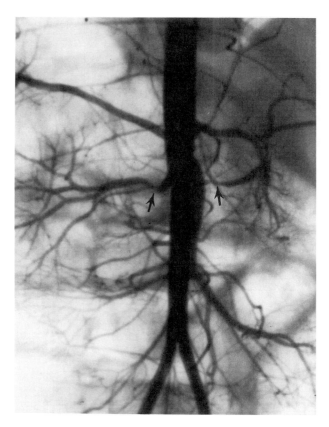

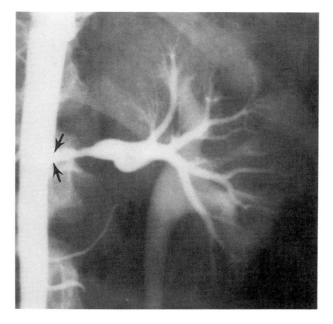

Fig. 23.22 Neurofibromatosis. A long-segment proximal renal arterial stenosis is often accompanied by ostial narrowing (arrows).

Fig. 23.21 Neurofibromatosis. There is extensive fibromuscular disease causing narrowing of proximal renal arteries (arrows). The tubular long-segment stenosis of the proximal left renal artery is typical of the intimal hyperplasia in this disorder.

rotic renal arterial occlusion [52,53], but is now gaining similar popularity for the dilatation of stenoses secondary to FMD [54,55]. The procedure is now considered both a safe and effective means of treating stenosis of the renal artery due to either primary FMD (Fig. 23.28) or following surgical re-implantation in children.

Technique

Renal angioplasty was not widely accepted in children until the development of new small-diameter, low-profile balloons. Balloons originally designed for coronary and peripheral small-vessel angioplasty are available in sizes from 2 to 5 mm in diameter (Fig. 23.29). The smaller balloons are mounted on 3.7−5 French gauge catheters, which can be safely introduced into the femoral artery of even the young child. Balloons made of more resilient materials offer

the possibility of increasing the success of dilating arteries with previously resistant FMD found in association with neurofibromatosis and Williams syndrome.

The technique of renal angioplasty in children is similar to that which is described in adults [57,58]. Prior to the angioplasty, selective arteriography is performed to identify the location of the lesions and the severity of the stenosis. Diagnostic angiography is often performed in combination with sampling of renal venous blood for measurement of PRA. Rarely should angioplasty be performed at the same time as the diagnostic angiogram. In usual circumstances, PTA is delayed until the levels of PRA are available. This is done in order to determine accurately the site of excess renin production, and to identify which side is most affected when there is bilateral involvement. Angioplasty is usually performed in children under general anesthesia because of the length of the procedure and to insure patient cooperation.

Sos and colleagues [59] demonstrated the value of selecting a balloon catheter which slightly overstretches the stenotic segment. From a standard cut-film angiogram, a balloon size is selected equal to the diameter of the prestenotic renal arterial segment. By not correcting for magnification, a balloon size is

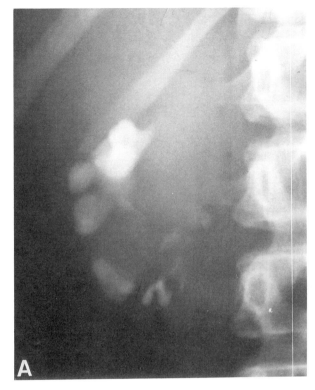

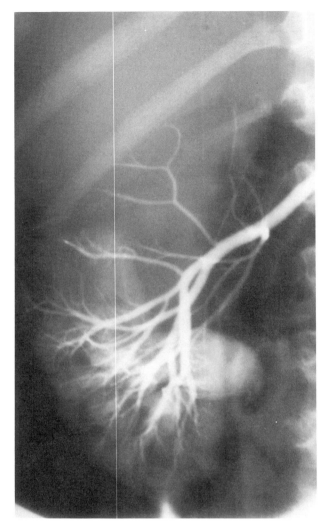

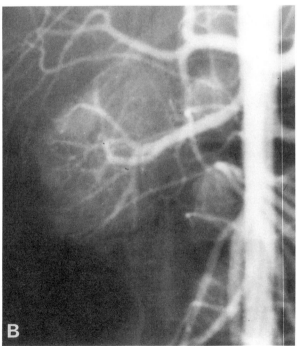

Fig. 23.24 Marked hydronephrosis involves the upper pole moiety of this duplicated right kidney. At arteriography, the normal vasculature of the lower pole moiety contrasts with the hydronephrotic stretching, narrowing, and displacement of the upper pole vessels around dilated calyces.

Fig. 23.23 Chronic pyelonephritis. (A) Chronic inflammation has led to marked renal cortical loss and adjacent calyceal dilatation. (B) At arteriography, the main renal artery is normal; however, there is severe pruning and distortion of intrarenal vessels secondary to scarring.

thus chosen which will slightly overstretch the stenotic lesion. When both main renal artery and segmental stenoses are present, the proximal lesions are dilated first in order to improve flow distally. If there is bilateral involvement, the most difficult side, or the side with the highest value of PRA, is dilated first. In general, a more conservative approach of dilating only one side at a time is taken in children to minimize the risk of rendering the patient anephric in the event of bilateral thrombosis. The contralateral side is then dilated in 4–6 weeks, depending

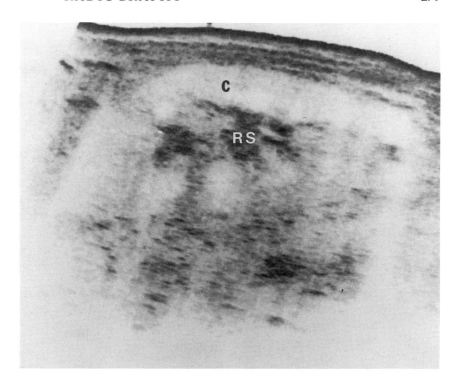

Fig. 23.25 Sonography revealed a swollen and enlarged transplant kidney, a hypoechoic cortex (c), and a hyperechoic central renal sinus (RS) complex compatible with chronic rejection.

upon the response of the hypertension to the first procedure.

The stenotic segment is initially traversed with a directional angiographic catheter and a flexible-tipped steerable wire guide. Once the catheter and wire guide are distal to the stenosis, a pressure gradient can be determined across the lesion during gradual withdrawal of the catheter, leaving the wire guide in place. One should not attempt to measure pressure gradients across a very tight stenosis or a distal segmental lesion in order to avoid excessive catheter manipulation which may lead to spasm and thrombosis. With the wire guide left distal to the stenosis, the catheter is then withdrawn and replaced by the appropriate dilating balloon. In order to avoid thrombotic complications during balloon dilatation, the child is fully heparinized with 100 U per kg body weight prior to insufflation of the balloon. Three attempts at dilatation are performed for a period of 20−30 s each, or until the balloon no longer deforms. If difficulty is encountered in crossing the stenotic lesion, a smaller lower-profile balloon is selected for the initial dilatation, followed serially by larger-diameter balloons. Advancement of a balloon across a tight stenosis is further facilitated by using a stiffer wire guide such as the Rosen wire (Cook, Bloomington, IN) or a Cope-mandril (Cook, Bloomington, IN); however, extreme care must be taken to prevent inadvertent advancement of the wire during dilatation which may lead to distal complications.

Following successful dilatation of a stenosis in the main renal artery, smaller-diameter balloons can be passed distally to dilate any segmental lesions. If considerable spasm is encountered in the initial dilatation of a proximal stenosis, the distal lesions are left for a second procedure. Infusion of heparinized saline through the tip of the dilating catheter during inflation of the balloon may help prevent distal thrombosis, especially when dilating segmental lesions. Finally, repeat angiography is performed to evaluate the success of the procedure, and to search for the presence or absence of extravasation, spasm, or thrombosis complicating the dilatation. Intravenous heparinization is maintained for 36 h after dilatation, and the child is discharged on aspirin (64 mg) every other day for a minimum of 6 weeks.

Results of angioplasty

Balloon dilatation of renal arteries involved with FMD in adults has produced excellent immediate and

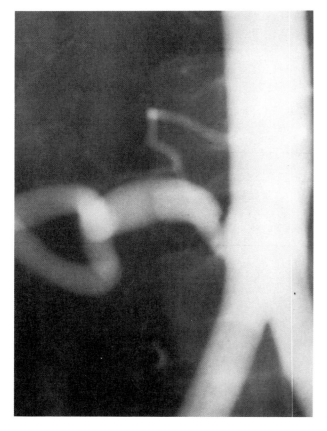

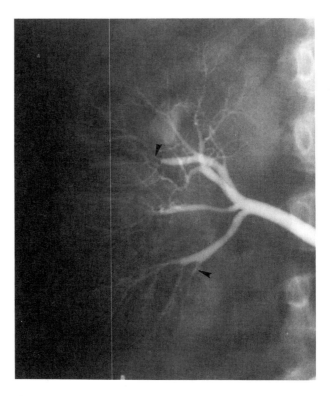

Fig. 23.27 An angiogram of a right pelvic transplant reveals marked pruning (arrowheads), distal segmental occlusion, and irregularity of the intrarenal vessels consistent with chronic rejection.

Fig. 23.26 A stenosis has developed at the proximal anastomosis of a transplanted renal artery to the lower abdominal aorta. Such stenoses are likely due to suture granulation or cross-clamping at the time of surgery.

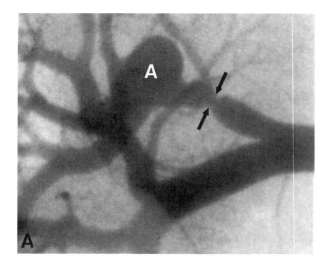

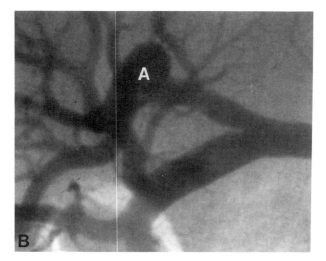

Fig. 23.28 (A) A segmental fibromuscular stenosis (arrows) is accompanied by a distal aneurysm (A) in this 7-year-old male with hypertension. (B) Following balloon dilatation, the stenotic lesion has resolved, coinciding with a clinical return to a normotensive state. From [56], with permission.

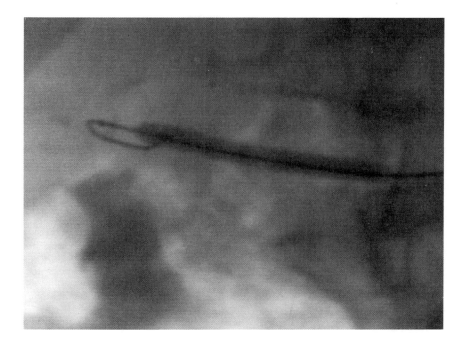

Fig. 23.29 Low-profile coronary and peripheral small-vessel angioplasty balloons ranging in size from 2 to 5 mm in diameter are ideal for dilating distal renal artery stenoses. From [56], with permission.

long-term results [60,61]. In a report on 31 patients who underwent dilatation for FMD, Tegtmeyer demonstrated angiographic improvement in all cases, with only a single case of restenosis at 1-year follow-up [60]. Thirty-two per cent of his patients became normotensive following dilatation, and an additional 68% were judged "improved" with their blood pressures more easily controlled with less medication. Other reports have described similar initial results, with a long-term patency rate up to 3 years of 83–100% [61–63]. There are fewer published series on PTA in children due to the lower incidence of FMD in the pediatric population [64,65]. The first successful renal artery angioplasty in a child was reported by McCook and co-authors in 1980 [66]. Since then, Stanley and colleagues have reported on the successful use of PTA in 5 children with JIFD; this has led to a greater acceptance of the procedure in the pediatric population [64]. All 5 children became normotensive, with only a single case of recurrent hypertension secondary to restenosis. Mali and co-workers felt the success of angioplasty could be predicted depending upon whether there was a short stenosis in the mid or distal renal artery, a short stenosis at or near the origin, or a long stenosis near the origin [67]. In their series of 12 children and adolescents, a more acceptable result was achieved with short stenotic lesions, whereas origin and long-segment stenoses, often associated with neuro-

fibromatosis, were refractory to dilatation [67]. Percutaneous transluminal angioplasty is most successful in dilating JIFD; the initial and long-term results are similar to those reported in adults. The application of balloon angioplasty in children with neurofibromatosis and perhaps Williams syndrome has been less rewarding [67,68]. The lack of uniform success with dilatation in FMD occurring in these syndromes may be due to the greater intimal proliferation, longer segments of involvement, and the frequency of ostial narrowing. The high atmospheric balloon should improve the results of dilating intimal FMD with predominantly circumferential involvement, but ostial hypoplasia is unlikely ever to respond to balloon angioplasty.

Renal artery stenosis in the transplanted kidney is also amenable to balloon dilatation [69,70] (Fig. 23.30) using similar techniques for dilating FMD in native kidneys. Prior knowledge of the type of anastomosis and its location is important before determining whether the ipsilateral or contralateral iliac artery will be cannulated for angioplasty. Both proximal and distal stenoses involving the transplanted artery can be easily dilated with a balloon technique. Excessive manipulation of the renal arteries should be avoided, since often coexistent mild rejection may increase the risk of arterial spasm.

Operative re-implantation of a stenotic renal artery may be complicated in time by restenosis at the

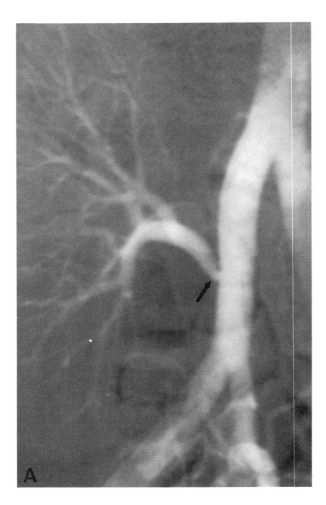

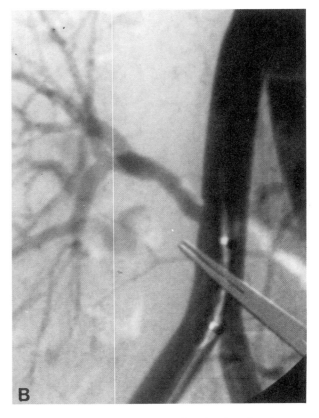

Fig. 23.30 (A) A proximal stricture has developed at the anastomosis of the transplanted artery with the common iliac artery (arrow). (B) The vessel appeared widely patent following successful balloon dilatation, and coincided with clinical improvement in the hypertension.

surgical anastomosis. The approach and technique for dilating graft stenoses are similar to those previously described in native and transplanted renal arteries (Fig. 23.31). Ectasia of a venous bypass graft should not be confused with poststenotic dilatation distal to an anastomotic stricture.

Arterial spasm constitutes the most significant risk of balloon angioplasty. The resultant decrease in blood flow may lead to spontaneous thrombosis of the renal artery. Pretreatment of patients with vasodilators is of only minimal benefit in reducing the risk. If spasm is encountered during the performance of balloon angioplasty, it may be relieved by the intra-arterial infusion of nitroglycerin at a rate of 0.25–1 μg/kg per min. Although alterations in systemic blood pressure are unusual at this dosage, patients must be constantly monitored for hypotension during the infusion. Thrombotic complications are minimized by heparinizing the patient prior to

balloon dilatation. However, despite adequate heparinization, spontaneous thrombosis may still result from intimal injury. In the event of thrombosis, a direct infusion of urokinase can be effective in lysing the clot. The dosage of urokinase has not been established in children; however, dosages of 500–2000 U/min are well tolerated. This infusion is continued directly into the clot for a period of 30–120 min, and continued as long as there is evidence of clot lysis and improvement in flow. Failure to lyse the clot may necessitate surgical embolectomy.

Rupture of the renal artery from excessive force of dilatation at the stenotic site is a rare complication of balloon angioplasty that has not, to our knowledge, been reported in children. In the event of an arterial rupture where there is extravasation of contrast, the balloon can be re-inflated at the leak to minimize hemorrhage. With the artery occluded by the balloon, a distal infusion of heparinized saline may help

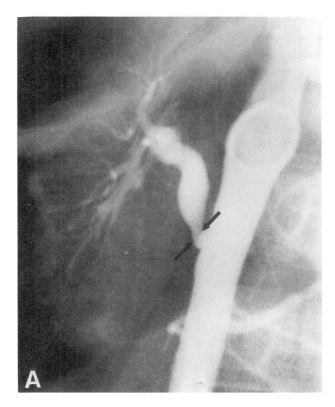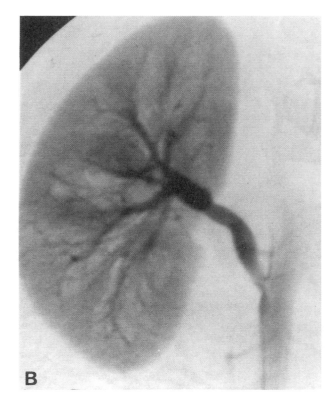

Fig. 23.31 (A) Autologous re-implantation of the renal artery to the abdominal aorta is complicated by a proximal stenosis at the anastomosis (arrows). There is only moderate angiographic improvement following balloon dilatation, but it was accompanied by significant clinical improvement in this child's hypertension.

prevent thrombosis of the kidney until a surgical correction can be achieved.

RENAL EMBOLIZATION

Ablation of the kidney through a transcatheter approach has been advocated in adults for the control of hyperproteinuria in nephrotic syndrome [71] and for the management of malignant hypertension [72,73]. There is less experience with similar techniques of embolization in children. In general, every attempt should be made to preserve any residual renal function in order to avoid the long-term risks of dialysis and renal transplantation in the young patient. None the less, ablation may be of benefit in controlling hypertension when a segmental artery stenosis cannot be successfully dilated or treated surgically [74], when malignant hypertension accompanies a small nonfunctioning or virtually nonfunctioning kidney,

or when there is excessive renin production from native kidneys following renal transplantation [75].

Technical aspects

A variety of agents including gelfoam sponge, polyvinyl alcohol, absolute alcohol (ethanol), and stainless steel minicoils can be used in children to ablate the renal artery. Gelfoam affords excellent biocompatibility, but is gradually resorbed over several weeks leading to recanalization of the artery. It can, however, be used in combination with other agents such as ethanol to provide a permanent occlusion of the renal artery. Polyvinyl alcohol is used most often for the permanent occlusion of both small and medium-size renal arteries, and comes either as particles or as a sponge which can be cut and shaped into plugs. Although absolute alcohol in its liquid form can be easily administered through a catheter for permanent occlusion, complications can result from its inadvertent reflux into distal aortic branches or collateral vessels [76]. The proper delivery of absolute alcohol requires the use of an occlusion balloon or wedging of the catheter into the target artery to prevent unwanted reflux.

Stainless steel minicoils provide a very safe and effective means of occluding larger renal vessels. The coils come in a variety of helix diameters ranging from 2 to 8 mm, and are excellent for occluding the main renal artery following distal embolization with gelfoam, polyvinyl alcohol, or absolute alcohol. Thrombosis around the coil fixates the device *in situ*, thereby preventing any risk of its migration into the aorta.

Particulate embolic agents (gelfoam, polyvinyl alcohol) and liquid agents (absolute alcohol) are easily embolized through catheter sizes as small as 3 French, but when possible a 5 French catheter is selected in order to minimize the risk of inadvertent plugging of the lumen by the agent. There are currently available stainless steel or platinum coils which will pass through catheters as small as 3 French gauge.

Embolization of segmental branches of the kidney is best achieved through a coaxial catheter system in which a 3 French catheter is passed through a 5 French sheath placed in the main renal artery (Fig. 23.32). This system allows for ease of distal maneuverability, and provides the means to quickly replace the inner catheter in the event of plugging by the embolic agent. Following each embolization an angiogram is performed to determine the progression of thrombosis, and to identify early reflux which may make further embolization unsafe.

Care is taken to maintain sterility during the embolization to prevent contamination which might lead to abscess formation within the infarcted kidney. In order to minimize the risk of infection, cefazolin sodium (500 mg) or a similar broad-spectrum antibiotic may be added to the embolic solution and begun systemically just prior to the procedure and continued for 5–7 days postembolization.

Mild transient leukocytosis, low-grade fever, and flank pain are expected side-effects of complete renal ablation. Persistent leukocytosis or fever greater than 101°F can indicate a complicating infection within the infarcted kidney. Serial cross-sectional imaging may be necessary to rule out the development of an abscess. Flank pain usually peaks between 3 and 5 days after embolization, and gradually subsides over the next 2 weeks. Narcotic analgesia is often needed within the first 72–96 h following the procedure, but is rarely necessary beyond this time period.

Results

Medical renal ablation in FMD should only be considered in children who are poor operative risks, or who have lesions which cannot be treated surgically.

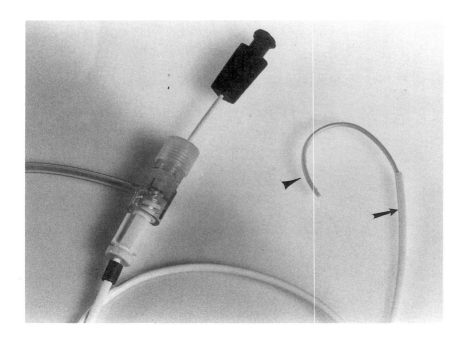

Fig. 23.32 A coaxial catheter system may aid in embolization of the renal vasculature, and consists of a 5 or 6 French guiding sheath (arrow), through which a 2 or 3 French embolization catheter (arrowhead) is passed into the distal renal vasculature for superselective ablation. From [56], with permission.

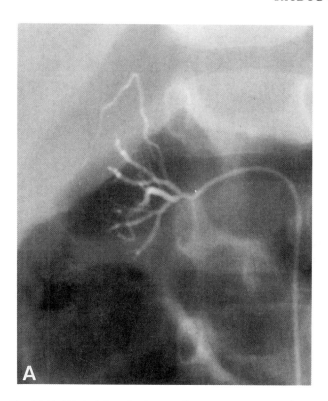 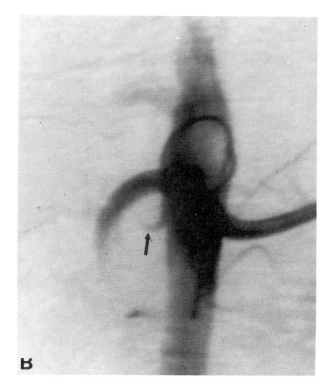

Fig. 23.33 (A) A right selective renal arteriogram was performed in this 4-year-old male presenting with malignant hypertension, and revealed a small shrunken end-stage kidney with marked pruning of the renal vasculature. (B) A significant improvement in the hypertension was achieved by complete ablation (arrow) of the right kidney with absolute alcohol. From [56], with permission.

Reuter and coworkers described the successful use of controlled renal infarction of a segment of the kidney distal to a nonoperable segmental renal artery stenosis which was not amenable to balloon dilatation in a 15-year-old male [77]. Warren and associates [78] reported similar success in treating a 5-year-old girl with hypertension by ablating the right upper pole of the kidney distal to a segmental stenosis. Rarely, uncontrollable or malignant hypertension secondary to a nonfunctioning unilateral end-stage renal moiety can be treated successfully by complete ablation of the remaining tissue (Fig. 23.33). Prior to any ablation, radionuclear split renal function studies should be performed to insure that the contralateral side is functioning normally, and that the ipsilateral involved kidney does not contribute significantly to the renal reserve. When time permits, sampling of renal venous blood for measurement of PRA should be performed prior to embolization to insure that the contralateral side is not contributing significantly to excess renin production. In a similar fashion, controlled renal infarction can be used to prevent end-stage native kidneys from producing persistent hypertension after renal transplantation. In such cases, embolization should be undertaken with extreme caution during periods of maximum immunosuppression of the patient from the pharmacologic treatment of rejection. During these periods of immunosuppression, the risk of infection within the infarcted kidney may be increased. If possible, elective medical ablation should be performed during intervening periods of maximum immunocompetency. When such a situation cannot be avoided, surgical nephrectomy is likely safer and a more direct means of assuring complete removal of the offending organ.

REFERENCES

1 Stanley P, Gypes MT, Olson DL, Gates GF. Renovascular hypertension in children and adolescents. *Radiology* 1978;129:123−31.

2 Stanley JC, Fry WJ. Surgical treatment of renovascular hypertension *Arch Surg* 1977;112:1291−7.

3 Korobkin M, Perloff DL, Palubinskas AJ. Renal arterio-

graphy in the evaluation of unexplained hypertension in children and adolescents. *J Pediatr* 1976;88:388−93.

4 Thornbury JR, Stanley JC, Fryback DG. Hypertensive urogram: a non-discriminatory test for renovascular hypertension. *AJR* 1982;138:43−9.

5 Slovis TL. Pediatric renal anomalies and infections. In: Babcock DS, ed. *Neonatal and Pediatric Ultrasonography*. New York, NY: Churchill-Livingstone, 1989:157−85.

6 Leonidas JC, McCauley RGK, Klauber GC *et al.* Sonography as a substitute for excretory urography in children with urinary tract infection. *AJR* 1985;144:815−19.

7 Nichols BT, Rittgers GE, Norris CS, Barnes RW. Non-invasive detection of renal artery stenosis. *Bruit* 1984;8:26−9.

8 Taylor KJW, Morse SS, Rigsby CM *et al.* Vascular complications in renal allografts: detection with duplex Doppler US. *Radiology* 1987;162:31−8.

9 Gones AS, Pais SO, Barbaric L. Digital subtraction angiography in the evaluation of hypertension. *AJR* 1983;140:779−83.

10 Clark RA, Alexander ES. Digital subtraction angiography of the renal arteries—prospective comparison with conventional arteriography. *Invest Radiol* 1983;18:6−10.

11 Tonkin IL, Stapleton FB, Roy S III. Digital subtraction angiography in the evaluation of renal vascular hypertension in children. *Pediatrics* 1988;81:150−8.

12 Busch HP, Strass LG, Hoevels J, Georgi M. Fibromuscular dysplasia, a pitfall in intravenous digital subtraction angiography. *Eur J Radiol* 1984;4:42−3.

13 Buonocore E, Meaney TF, Borkowski GP *et al.* Digital subtraction angiography of the abdominal aorta and renal arteries. *Radiology* 1981;139:281−6.

14 Stringer DA, deBruyn R, Dillon MJ, Gordon I. Comparison of aortography, renal vein renin sampling, radionuclide scans, ultrasound and the IVU in the investigation of childhood renovascular hypertension. *Br J Radiol* 1984;57:11−12.

15 Olbert F, Denck H, Wicke L. Komplikationen bei Katheterangiographien. Ursachen und deren Behandlung. *Wien Med Wochenschr* 1973;123:293.

16 Syme J. Neurofibromatosis as a cause of renovascular hypertension. *Australas Radiol* 1980;24:62−6.

17 Scott HW, Dean RH, Boerth R *et al.* Coarctation of the abdominal aorta: pathophysiologic and therapeutic considerations. *Ann Surg* 1979;189:746−57.

18 Gotsman MS, Beck W, Schrire V. Selected angiography in arteritis of the aorta and its major branches. *Radiology* 1967;88:232−48.

19 Daniels SR, Loggie JMH, Schwartz DC, Strife JL, Kaplan S. Systemic hypertension secondary to peripheral vascular anomalies in patients with Williams syndrome. *J Pediatr* 1985;106:249−51.

20 Colquhoun J. Hypoplasia of the abdominal aorta following therapeutic irradiation in infancy. *Radiology* 1966;86:454−6.

21 Daniels SR, Loggie JMH, McEnery PT, Towbin RB. Clinical spectrum of intrinsic renovascular hypertension in children. *Pediatrics* 1987;80:698−704.

22 Lawson JD, Boerth R, Foster JG *et al.* Diagnosis and management of renovascular hypertension in children. *Arch Surg* 1977;112:1307−16.

23 Salyer WR, Salyer DC. Vascular lesions of neurofibromatosis. *Angiology* 1974;25:510−19.

24 Bookstein JJ, Abrams HL, Buenger RE *et al.* Radiologic aspects of renovascular hypertension: III. Appraisal of arteriography. *JAMA* 1972;221:368−74.

25 Makker ST, Moorthy B. Fibromuscular dysplasia of renal arteries: an important cause of renovascular hypertension in children. *J Pediatr* 1979;95:940−5.

26 Fry WJ, Ernst CB, Stanley JC, Brink B. Renovascular hypertension in the pediatric patient. *Arch Surg* 1973;107:692−8.

27 Harrison EG Jr, Hunt JC, Bernatz PE. Morphology of fibromuscular dysplasia of the renal artery in renovascular hypertension. *Am J Med* 1967;43:97−112.

28 Eliot J, Andre M, Meutse B *et al.* Dysplasie, fibreuse des arteres renales avec aneurysmes sacciformes. *Radiol Electrol* 1973;55:245−6.

29 Castaneda-Zuniga W, Zollikofer C, Valdez-Davila O, Nath PH, Amplatz K. Giant aneurysms of the renal arteries: an unusual manifestation of fibromuscular dysplasia. *Radiology* 1979;133:327−30.

30 Sheps SG, Kincaid OW, Hunt JC. Serial renal function and angiographic observations in idiopathic fibrous and fibromuscular stenosis of the renal arteries. *Am J Cardiol* 1972;30:55−60.

31 Siegler RL, Miller FJ, Mineau E, Moatamed F. Spontaneous reversal of hypertension caused by fibromuscular dysplasia. *J Pediatr* 1982;100:83−5.

32 Goncharenko V, Gerlsek AJ Jr, Shaff MI, Hollifield JW. Progression of renal artery fibromuscular disease in 42 patients as seen on angiography. *Radiology* 1981;139:41−5.

33 Kirks DR, Fitz CR, Korobkin M. Intrarenal collateral circulation in the pediatric patient. *Pediatr Radiol* 1977;5:154−9.

34 Tilford DL, Kelsch RC. Renal artery stenosis in childhood neurofibromatosis. *Am J Dis Child* 1973;126:665−8.

35 Holt JF. Neurofibromatosis in children. *AJR* 1978; 130:615−39.

36 Ottesen OE, Autia AU, Rowe RD. Peripheral vascular anomalies associated with the supravalvar aortic stenosis syndrome. *Radiology* 1966;86:430−5.

37 Holland NH, Kotchen T, Bhathena D. Hypertension in children with chronic pyelonephritis. *Kidney Int* 1975; 52(suppl):43−51.

38 Habib R, Kourtecuisse V, Ehrensperger J *et al.* Hypoplasie segmentaire du rein avec hypertension arterielle chez l'enfant. *Ann Pediatr (Paris)* 1965;12:262−79.

39 Meares EM Jr, Gross DM. Hypertension owing to unilateral renal hypoplasia. *J Urol* 1972;108:197−200.

40 Himmelsarb E. The Ask-Upmark kidney. *Am J Dis Child* 1975;129:1440−4.

41 Arant BS Jr, Sotelo-Avila C, Bernstein J. Segmental "hypoplasia" of the kidney (Ask-Upmark). *J Pediatr* 1979;95:931−9.

42 Cha EM, Kandzari S, Khoury GH. Congenital renal hypoplasia angiographic study. *Radiology* 1972;114:710−14.

43 Belman AB, Kropp KA, Simon NM. Renal-pressor hypertension secondary to unilateral hydronephrosis. *N Engl J Med* 1968;278:1133−6.

44 Brasch WF, Walters W, Hammer HJ. Hypertension and surgical kidney. *JAMA* 1940;115:1837−41.

45 Lacombe M. Arterial stenosis complicating renal allotransplantation in man: a study of 38 cases. *Ann Surg* 1975;181:283−8.

46 Bachy C, Van Ypersele C, Strihou D, Alexandre GP, Troch R.

Hypertension after renal transplantation. *Dialysis Transplant Nephrol* 1976;12:461−70.

47 Lindfors O, Laasonen L, Fyhrquist F, Cock B, Lindstrom B. Renal arterial stenosis in hypertensive renal transplant recipients. *J Urol* 1977;118:240−3.

48 Staple TW, Chiang DTC. Arteriography following renal transplantation. *Am J Roentgenol Rad Ther Nucl Med.* 1967;101:669−80.

49 Tilney NL, Rocha A, Strom TV. Renal arterial stenosis in transplant patients. *Ann Surg* 1975;199:454−60.

50 Gerlock AJ, McDonell RC, Smith WC *et al*. Renal transplant artery stenosis: percutaneous transluminal angioplasty. *AJR* 1983;140:325−31.

51 Kaude JV, Hawkins IF. Angiography of renal transplants. *Radiol Clin North Am* 1976;14:295−308.

52 Tegtmeyer CJ, Kellum CD, Ayers CR. Percutaneous transluminal angioplasty of the renal artery: results and long term follow-up. *Radiology* 1984;153:77−84.

53 Martin LG, Price RB, Casarella WJ *et al*. Percutaneous angioplasty in clinical management of renovascular hypertension: initial and long term results. *Radiology* 1985;155:629−33.

54 Stanley P, Senac MO Jr, Bakody P *et al*. Percutaneous transluminal dilatation for renal artery stenosis in a 22-month-old hypertensive girl. *AJR* 1983;140:983−4.

55 Barth KH, Brusilow SW, Kaufman SL, Ferry FT. Percutaneous transluminal angioplasty of homographed renal artery stenosis in a 10 year old girl. *Pediatrics* 1981;67:675−7.

56 Towbin RB, Ball WS Jr. Pediatric interventional radiology. *Radiol Clin North Am* 1988;26:419−40.

57 Tegtmeyer CJ, Dyer R, Teates CD *et al*. Percutaneous transluminal dilatation of the renal artery; techniques and results. *Diag Radiol* 1980;135:589−99.

58 Sos TA, Saddekni S, Sniderman KW *et al*. Renal artery angioplasty: techniques and early results. *Urol Radiol* 1982;3:223−31.

59 Sos TA, Pickering DG, Sniderman KW *et al*. Percutaneous transluminal renal angioplasty in renovascular hypertension due to atheroma or fibromuscular dysplasia. *N Engl J Med* 1983;309:274−9.

60 Tegtmeyer CJ, Elson J, Glass TA *et al*. Percutaneous transluminal angioplasty: the treatment of choice for renovascular hypertension due to fibromuscular dysplasia. *Radiology* 1982;143:631−7.

61 Martin EC, Mattern RF, Bare L *et al*. Renal angioplasty for hypertension: predictive factors for long term success. *AJR* 1981;137:921−4.

62 Mahler F, Probst P, Haertel M *et al*. Lasting improvement of renovascular hypertension by transluminal dilatation of atherosclerotic and non-atherosclerotic renal artery stenoses. *Circulation* 1982;65:611−17.

63 Colapinto RF, Stronell RD, Harries-Jones EP *et al*. Percu-

taneous transluminal dilatation of the renal artery: follow-up studies on renovascular hypertension. *AJR* 1982; 139:727−32.

64 Stanley P, Hieshina G, Mehringer M. Percutaneous transluminal angioplasty for pediatric renovascular hypertension. *Radiology* 1984;153:101−4.

65 Lund G, Sinaiko A, Castaneda-Zuniga WR *et al*. Percutaneous transluminal angioplasty for treatment of renal artery stenosis in children. *Eur J Radiol* 1984;4:254−7.

66 McCook TA, Mills SR, Kirks DR *et al*. Percutaneous transluminal renal artery angioplasty in a $3\frac{1}{2}$ year old hypertensive girl. *J Pediatr* 1980;97:958−60.

67 Mali WP, Puijlaert CB, Kouwenberg HJ *et al*. Percutaneous transluminal renal angioplasty in children and adolescents. *Radiology* 1987; 165:391−4.

68 Miller GA, Ford KK, Braun SD *et al*. Percutaneous transluminal angioplasty versus surgery for renovascular hypertension. *AJR* 1985;144:447−50.

69 Raynaud A, Bedrossian J, Remy P *et al*. Percutaneous transluminal angioplasty of renal transplant arterial stenoses. *AJR* 1986;146:853−7.

70 Whiteside CI, Cardella CJ, Yeung H *et al*. The role of percutaneous transluminal dilatation in the treatment of transplant renal artery stenosis. *Clin Nephrol* 1982;17:55−9.

71 Henrich WL, Goldman M, Dotter CT *et al*. Therapeutic renal arterial occlusion for elimination of proteinuria. *Arch Intern Med* 1976;136:840−2.

72 Eliscu EH, Haire HM, Tew FT, Newton LW. Control of malignant renovascular hypertension by percutaneous transluminal angioplasty and therapeutic renal embolization. *AJR* 1980;134:815−17.

73 Adler J, Einhorn R, McCarthy J *et al*. Gelfoam embolization of the kidneys for treatment of malignant hypertension. *Radiology* 1978;128:45−8.

74 LiPuma JP, Dresner I, Alfidi JR, Sun Yoon Y. Embolization of an occluded segmental renal artery via collateral circulation in a child. *AJR* 1981;136:603−4.

75 Fletcher EWL, Thompson JF, Chalmers DHK *et al*. Embolization of host kidneys for the control of hypertension after renal transplantation: radiology aspects. *Radiology* 1984; 57:279−84.

76 Cox G, Lee KR, Price HI *et al*. Colonic infarction following ethanol embolization of renal cell carcinoma. *Radiology* 1982;145:343−5.

77 Reuter SR, Pomeroy PR, Chuang VP, Kyung JC. Embolic control of hypertension caused by segmental renal artery stenosis. *AJR* 1976;172:389−92.

78 Warren WC, Warshaw BL, Hymes LC, Sones PJ Jr. Selective embolization of stenotic intrarenal artery for control of hypertension. *J Pediatr* 1982;101:743−5.

24 Coarctation of the Aorta

BARRY MARCUS AND ARNO R. HOHN

INTRODUCTION

As a result of modern diagnostic technology, coarctation of the aorta is today largely a disorder of infants and young children. In this age group it may account for about 20% of those who are found to be hypertensive [1,2]. On occasion, coarctation may have escaped detection until older childhood or adolescence. Those providing health care for the young must take their patients' blood pressure. If the pressure is high, palpation of pulses should be attempted in both upper and lower extremities and blood pressures from all four limbs must be obtained. Once a discrepancy is found, a two-dimensional echocardiogram with Doppler study can be used to confirm the diagnosis of coarctation in most cases.

EMBRYOLOGY AND ANATOMY OF COARCTATION

Consideration of embryologic theories of etiology offers insight to the hypertension found in coarctation of the aorta. Of the explanatory hypotheses proposed, faulty union of the aortic arches with the descending aorta is no longer accepted. While constriction of ductal tissue in the aorta has been found to cause aortic constriction after palliation for the hypoplastic left heart syndrome, this mechanism is also not generally felt fully to account for aortic coarctations [3]. Most hold that fetal hemodynamic forces mold the disorder [4]. It is thought that decreased antegrade aortic blood flow develops. This leads to a proportionate increase in pulmonary and then ductus arteriosus flow. A posterior aortic shelf forms and may deflect ductal flow proximally into the left subclavian artery and distally into the descending aorta. Ductal constriction may impact on this process after birth. Although sufficient fetal ascending aorta flow exists

to supply the first arch branches, there is reduced isthmic flow. Tubular hypoplasia of the isthmus results from this process. In extreme cases isthmic atresia occurs causing interrupted aortic arch. Anomalies, such as malalignment ventricular septal defects which divert blood from the aorta, promote the process described. However, defects like tetralogy of Fallot which increase ascending aortic flow are seldom associated with coarctation of the aorta.

Current anatomic classifications of aortic coarctation are based on the elaborated embryologic concepts. Thus, in infants and young children, coarctations are labeled as "periductal" in recognition of the fact that the aortic constriction may be at, above, or below the site of ductal entry (Fig. 24.1). In older individuals, where the site of coarctation is generally distal to the ligamentum arteriosum, the terminology of "adult coarctation" is in common usage (Fig. 24.2).

PATHOPHYSIOLOGY OF HYPERTENSION

Mechanical factors

Over the years it has become increasingly clear that the hypertension found in coarctation of the aorta is not simply the result of the anatomic aortic narrowing. Indeed mechanical factors as a cause of hypertension in coarctation have been discredited by such arguments as that infrarenal coarctation fails to produce hypertension and that proximally transplanted kidneys relieve hypertension in coarctation [6]. These arguments do not take into account the fact that renal depressor mechanisms can normalize blood pressure in infrarenal coarctation [7]. Nor do they recognize that the cervical kidney adds a low resistance circuit to the proximal circulation which could also lower blood pressure [6]. In experimentally in-

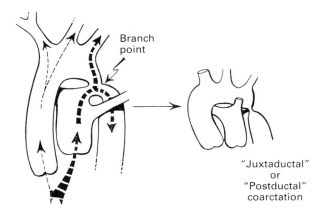

Fig. 24.1 (Left) Fetal blood flow pattern and (right) coarctation anatomic profiles generally presenting in the newborn baby and infant. From [5], with permission.

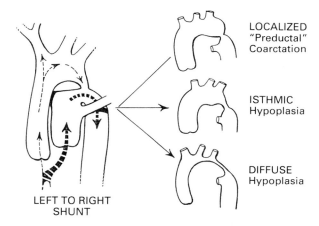

Fig. 24.2 (Left) Fetal blood flow pattern and (right) coarctation anatomic profile with closed ductus in the older child. From [5], with permission.

duced narrowing of the aorta, hypertension follows immediately and the embryologic considerations previously cited make it likely that a chain of events is initiated by the mechanical factor of aortic narrowing.

Renal mechanisms

Beginning with the studies of Goldblatt and colleagues of aortic constriction in 1939 [8] and the studies of cervical renal autotransplantation by Scott and Bahnson [6], renal factors in the hypertension of coarctation of the aorta have received considerable attention. Investigations of the renin–angiotensin system (RAS) have led many to conclude that it plays

an important role in the hypertension of coarctation. Findings such as a greater elevation of plasma renin activity (PRA) following exercise in patients with unoperated coarctations compared to subjects without coarctation, and excessive activity of the RAS determined by saralasin testing before and after operative repair of coarctation [7] give credibility to the notion of involvement of the RAS in coarctation. The inverse relationship of angiotensin II to volume has been experimentally shown to be true for acutely induced aortic constriction [9]. On the other hand, with chronic experimental coarctation the relationship is less clear. Mechanisms not involving angiotensin II and/or volume retention may exist. Renal sympathetic nerves have been felt to play a role in the hypertension of coarctation, for removal of these nerves in animals with experimental coarctation reduces their blood pressure excess by about one-half over levels found prior to creation of the coarctation [10].

Nonrenal neural mechanisms

Neural mechanisms like baroreceptor-mediated responses have been demonstrated to have a role in the hypertension of acute experimental aortic constriction. In chronic animal models of coarctation there is a resetting of the baroreceptors and few of the changes seen with the acute response can be found. Subtle changes in sympathetic nervous system activity do however exist as evidenced by alterations in vascular resistance and decreased levels of plasma norepinephrine [11].

Regional vascular factors

Reactivity of various regional vascular beds is thought to be altered in coarctation of the aorta and thus to contribute to the pathophysiology of hypertension. However conflicting information has been reported with respect to regional vascular factors such as degree and location of waterlogged arterial walls, i.e. excess vascular wall water content [11,12]. Therefore, further and more controlled studies are required to determine the significance of regional vascular factors in coarctation.

CLINICAL PATTERNS

In the evaluation of individuals for coarctation, consideration must be given to the fact that the clinical picture in the infant with coarctation is characteristically different from that seen in the older child. These two age groups will therefore be discussed separately [1,13−18].

Infantile coarctation complex

Among infants presenting with coarctation, associated cardiovascular anomalies are the rule with isolated coarctation occurring in only 10% of these babies [16]. The most commonly associated abnormalities include proximal aortic arch hypoplasia in three-fourths of the patients, and patent ductus arteriosus in two-thirds [1,13,14,16]. Bicuspid aortic valve is also frequent [1,13−16]. Coarctation can be but one feature of multiple left-sided lesions present in an individual patient including combinations of mitral valve, supramitral, and aortic valve abnormalities [1,13]. Ventricular septal defect in the muscular portion of the ventricular septum has been noted in more than 50% of infants with coarctation [13,14,16]. The left subclavian artery can be underdeveloped in association with its proximity to the coarctation site. Thus, coarctation in the infant generally presents as a complex; the coarctation is but one part of a combination of lesions. Its clinical presentation reflects the pathophysiologic interaction among the various associated lesions in a particular patient [14].

The coarctation complex of lesions causes the majority of infants with it to present generally with symptoms of congestive heart failure. Shortness of breath with feedings, excessive sweating, and poor weight gain are noted by history. On examination, the infant with symptomatic coarctation is often quite ill. Tachypnea and tachycardia are common. Depending on the associated defects, a variety of murmurs can be appreciated [14,15]. Hepatomegaly is often present. Cardiomegaly, present on chest X-ray, and right ventricular hypertrophy by electrocardiogram (ECG) are classic in the infant with symptomatic coarctation. The ECG findings reflect intrauterine blood flow patterns which enhance right ventricular stress in the presence of the coarctation complex. Upper extremity systolic hypertension with notably lower pressure in the lower extremities and full upper extremity pulses with reduced or absent lower extremity pulses may be found. However, a widely patent ductus arteriosus may allow for equalization of upper and lower extremity blood pressure and pulses.

Coarctation in childhood

Unlike the infant who presents with a symptomatic coarctation complex, the older child is generally asymptomatic [1,13,15,18]. In long-standing coarctation, a history of increased fatigability, leg weakness and, rarely, lower extremity claudication may be elicited. Congestive heart failure is rare. Coarctation that presents in the older child may be a clinically isolated lesion. However, in about two-thirds of these patients, there is a bicuspid aortic valve [17]. The proximal aorta is generally normal or dilated and, most often, the ductus has closed.

Physical examination is diagnostic with normal-to-increased upper extremity pulses and delayed, decreased, or absent femoral pulses. Upper extremity systolic hypertension associated with a pressure gradient between the upper and lower extremities is the rule. Lower extremity systolic blood pressure is significantly lower than the upper extremity pressure, but frank proximal hypertension may occasionally not be found owing to the presence of large collaterals around the coarctation. A nonspecific systolic murmur heard along the left mid or upper sternal border and at mid thoracic level posteriorly over the spine may emanate from turbulence across the coarctation site [1,13,15]. A systolic ejection murmur at the base of the heart can indicate a bicuspid aortic valve. Systolic or continuous murmurs in the back either reflect the coarctation directly or (especially if over the scapulae) represent collaterals. Liver size is typically normal.

The chest X-ray characteristically reveals a normal cardiac size. If the thoracic aorta is dilated proximally and distally to an indentation, coarctation may be suspected. In patients beyond 5 years of age, rib notching is increasingly noted with age. The ECG may be normal, or can manifest left ventricular hypertrophy in the older child with long-standing coarctation. An ECG variant with incomplete right bundle branch block is seen in about 10% of children with coarctation of the aorta [1,13].

DIAGNOSTIC CRITERIA

In virtually all older children and a majority of infants with coarctation, clinical criteria suffice for diagnosis [1,13−15,17,18]. These include
1 differential systolic blood pressure with upper

extremity pressure greater than that in the lower extremity;

2 femoral pulses delayed, decreased, or absent, relative to normal or full upper extremity pulses;

3 presence of collaterals on physical examination by murmur or palpation.

Chest X-ray can corroborate the diagnosis made by physical examination by revealing an hourglass configuration of the thoracic aorta and/or rib notching (i.e. collaterals). Two-dimensional echocardiography with Doppler is particularly effective in the infant not only for visualizing the coarctation (Fig. 24.3), but also for identifying associated defects [19,20]. In the older child, where echocardiographic imaging of the aortic arch is technically more difficult, magnetic resonance imaging and digital subtraction angiography have been shown to define the aortic arch anatomy well [21–23]. Cardiac catheterization is generally reserved for patients with particularly complex anatomy, those with a history of prior surgical repair, or to assess collaterals in those patients suspected of having coarctation with sparse collaterals, i.e. those with significant proximal hypertension [1,13,14].

THERAPY

Historically, the accepted treatment of coarctation

has been surgical [1,13–15]. There are, however, instances where medical therapy perioperatively is necessary. [24]. Balloon angioplasty of recoarctation in the cardiac catheterization laboratory has been utilized favorably in the treatment of residual or recurrent coarctation postoperatively, and is being investigated with regard to the treatment of native coarctation [25–29]. With these thoughts in mind, discussion of medical, surgical, and balloon catheter angioplasty treatment of coarctation follows.

Medical therapy

In infancy, coarctation often leads to congestive heart failure [14]. Medical therapy is often necessary to stabilize the infant prior to surgery, or to delay surgery until a more optimal time. In the young infant presenting with acute severe heart failure precipitated by closure of a previously patent ductus arteriosus, prostaglandin E_1 effects dramatic, often lifesaving, relief of the obstruction, allowing the patient to proceed to surgery or balloon angioplasty in a compensated, nonemergency state [24]. In infants with less severe, subacute congestive heart failure, standard anticongestive therapy is frequently utilized to optimize their condition, allow for growth, and if possible, allow for semi-elective timing of intervention within the first year of life. It should, how-

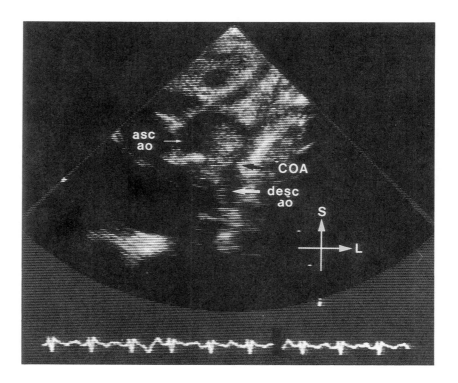

Fig. 24.3 Two-dimensional echocardiographic image of the aortic arch in a newborn infant with coarctation of the aorta. Suprasternal notch view demonstrates the ascending aorta (asc ao), site of coarctation obstruction (COA), and thoracic descending aorta (desc ao). L = Left; S = superior.

ever, be stressed that the definitive treatment of hypertension secondary to coarctation should be either surgical or by balloon angioplasty—*not* medical.

In the older child, the presence of upper extremity hypertension or a resting right arm—leg systolic blood pressure gradient of 30 mmHg or greater are indications for surgery or balloon angioplasty, provided that adequate collateral vessels are present around the coarctation site (see section on paraplegia, below). Left arm versus leg blood pressure measurements may not reveal or may underestimate the pressure gradient across the coarctation because the left subclavian artery—which supplies the left arm—may originate directly adjacent to or below the site of coarctation obstruction. The optimum age for intervention in the older child is 3—5 years [1,13]. Severe upper extremity hypertension warrants urgent surgical intervention or balloon angioplasty in view of the risks of cerebrovascular accident or myocardial overload ischemic injury. Temporizing with medical therapy is not indicated.

Surgical correction

Although surgery to repair coarctation has been performed for over 40 years, a number of operative issues remain controversial [1,13,14,30—37]. The timing of elective surgery is one such issue. The earlier in life the repair is done, the higher the risk of recurrent obstruction, but the lower the risk of residual postoperative hypertension. Conversely, later timing of elective surgery lowers the risk of residual obstruction but, if preoperative duration of upper extremity hypertension is prolonged, may increase the risk of residual hypertension [36,37]. Preoperative level of upper extremity (right arm) systolic blood pressure may be the best determinant of surgical timing [37]. Most authorities favor elective coarctation repair at 3—5 years of age. If marked hypertension or, rarely, heart failure occurs in the older child, earlier repair should be undertaken [1]. In symptomatic infants or newborn babies with the coarctation complex, the clinical status often dictates that early surgery must be performed. Such surgery is indicated on an urgent basis if measures to combat congestive heart failure are not successful in stabilizing the patient. In the newborn infant requiring stabilization with prostaglandin E_1 as described above [24], early operation is necessary.

The type of operation employed is also a contro-

versial issue at present [30,31,33]. Three operations are primarily utilized:

1 end-to-end anastomosis of the aorta after resection of the coarctation segment (Fig. 24.4);

2 synthetic patch aortoplasty involving placement of a patch (i.e. dacron) across an incised portion of the aorta to widen the aorta with concomitant removal of the coarctation ledge (Fig. 24.5); and

3 patch aortoplasty utilizing the left subclavian artery for the patch (Fig. 24.6).

In the last procedure, the left subclavian artery is ligated (as would be performed for a Blalock—Taussig shunt) and a flap of proximal subclavian tissue is turned down as a patch aortoplasty to widen the aorta at the level of the coarctation site. There is concomitant removal of the coarctation ledge.

In older children, either the end-to-end resection or the synthetic patch aortoplasty is utilized. It appears that the surgeon's preference is the major factor influencing the choice of operation, and that successful relief of coarctation can be accomplished with either technique. Currently, at our institution, end-to-end anastomosis is favored by our surgeons. The major concern regarding the end-to-end anastomosis is whether late aortic narrowing—particularly in the infant or small child—and subsequent hypertension can be avoided [31,36]. With synthetic patch aortoplasty, aortic aneurysm formation opposite patch placement may become a late problem [32]. In our experience, in infants the subclavian patch aortoplasty is presently the procedure of choice. It appears to offer the greatest relative likelihood of early success regarding relief of obstruction and allows for growth at the repair site using biologic tissue. This avoids using prosthetic patch material, although late restenosis or aortic aneurysm formation may occur [34,35]. Of the three operations mentioned above, relative risk with regard to the development of late postoperative hypertension is known only for the end-to-end anastomosis. The patch aortoplasties have not been followed for long enough time periods to provide a clear-cut comparative risk estimate for this problem.

Balloon angioplasty

Over the past several years, use of the balloon catheter in the cardiac catheterization laboratory to dilate the residual or recurrent coarctation site following unsuccessful surgical repair has found favor [25—27,29]. Balloon angioplasty is in many centers the procedure

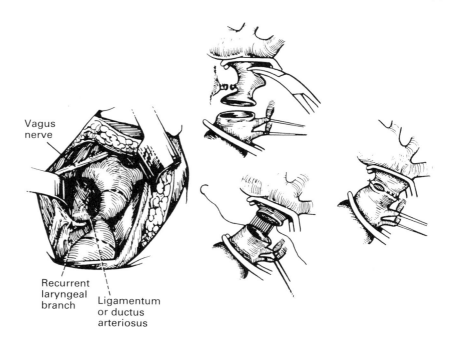

Fig. 24.4 Resection of coarctation with primary end-to-end anastomosis. From [5], with permission.

Vagus nerve

Recurrent laryngeal branch

Ligamentum or ductus arteriosus

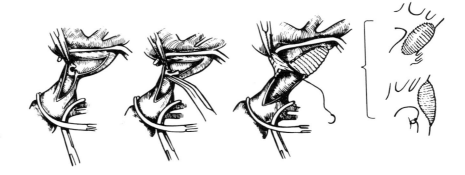

Fig. 24.5 Synthetic (dacron) patch aortoplasty. The coarctation obstruction is excised. The patch is then placed. From [5], with permission.

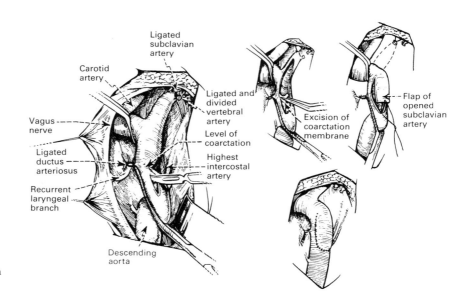

Fig. 24.6 Subclavian patch aortoplasty. The coarctation obstruction is excised. Subclavian artery tissue flap is then turned down and used as a patch. From [5], with permission.

Ligated subclavian artery

Carotid artery

Ligated and divided vertebral artery

Level of coarctation

Highest intercostal artery

Excision of coarctation membrane

Flap of opened subclavian artery

Vagus nerve

Ligated ductus arteriosus

Recurrent laryngeal branch

Descending aorta

of choice for residual or recurrent coarctation [25–27]. The surgical approach to these particular patients is notably difficult in part because the operative field is complicated by the presence of numerous adhesions, making access difficult. In addition, there is distorted operative anatomy so that results are frequently less satisfactory than when an unoperated or native coarctation is approached.

The balloon size is determined relative to neighboring proximal aortic arch. The balloon is inserted via retrograde aortic passage to the coarctation site over a soft guide wire. After inflation to full expansion with dilute saline the lumen of the coarctation segment is proportionately dilated. Preliminary results among patients with postoperative residual or recurrent coarctation suggest that the balloon catheter approach compares favorably with the surgical approach in short-term outcome [25–27,29]. Long-term follow-up is awaited to determine whether late aortic aneurysm formation or recurrence of obstruction occurs; either may temper the early optimistic results in these patients.

Reports assessing the role of balloon angioplasty in the treatment of native coarctation are increasingly favorable in terms of successful relief of gradient and satisfactory uncomplicated follow-up [25,28]. However, pending long-term follow-up regarding persistent relief of obstruction and occurrence rate of aortic aneurysm formation at the site of balloon angioplasty, it is not presently clear whether balloon angioplasty will ultimately be considered an alternative approach to surgery in the treatment of native coarctation.

Balloon angioplasty does not appear to be associated with paradoxical hypertension after the procedure—as often occurs after surgical repair (see below) [38,39]. This difference in hypertension occurrence is associated with relatively reduced sympathetic nervous system stimulation, catecholamine release, and PRA following balloon angioplasty compared with surgical intervention [38,39].

POSTOPERATIVE PROBLEMS

Postoperative (paradoxical) hypertension

Hypertension following corrective surgery for coarctation was initially reported by Sealy and colleagues in 1957 [40]; they coined the term "paradoxical hypertension." Approximately two-thirds of patients who undergo corrective surgery manifest paradoxical hypertension at some time during their postoperative course [7,36,40–49]. Three categories have been described:

1 early—within the first 12–24 hours following surgery;

2 late—onset 2–5 days postoperatively; and

3 persistent—hypertension that continues beyond 1 month after surgery to correct coarctation [40–43].

EARLY PARADOXICAL HYPERTENSION

Surgery for correction of coarctation of the aorta is associated with marked stimulation of the sympathetic nervous system in the immediate postoperative period. Several investigators have noted a dramatic elevation in the level of circulating plasma norepinephrine among patients recovering from surgery for coarctation repair as compared with patients who have undergone other types of surgical procedures [7,42–44,47]. This elevation is most notable within the first 24 h postoperatively and has been temporally associated with the occurrence of early paradoxical hypertension [42–44,47]. The precise reason why surgical repair of coarctation elicits this particularly marked sympathetic nervous system stimulation is unclear. One concept is that the abrupt postoperative fall in proximal aortic blood pressure provokes an intense baroreceptor-mediated response, with a resultant brisk sympathetic discharge [40,41,46]. A second hypothesis is that surgical manipulation of the thoracic aorta in the region of the aortic isthmus, possibly via stimulation of intra-aortic stretch receptors, elicits an intense release of catecholamines. Patients who undergo surgery for repair of thoracic aortic aneurysms also have a propensity for early postoperative hypertension [43,48].

In early paradoxical hypertension there is a moderate-to-severe elevation in systolic blood pressure [42–44,47]. In our experience, initial antihypertensive therapy involves propranolol, provided that cardiac function and the cardiac conduction system are intact (Table 24.1). Hydralazine may be used in addition if further blood pressure control is needed. At our institution, captopril has occasionally been used in this setting. For the rare occurrence of hypertensive crisis associated with central nervous system symptoms, or for particularly severe hypertension, we use diazoxide or nifedipine as initial therapy. We have occasionally used nitroprusside when severe hypertension required continuous therapy to maintain control. The course of early paradoxical hypertension includes a depressor response to β-blocker or

Table 24.1 Treatment of paradoxical postoperative hypertension (HBP) without residual anatomic obstruction*

Type of postoperative HBP	Mild–moderate HBP	Severe HBP
Early (≤1 week postop.)	Propranolol 0.05–0.1 mg/kg per dose i.v. q. 6 h p.r.n. or Hydralazine 0.15 mg/kg per dose i.v. q. 4–6 h p.r.n.	Propranolol + hydralazine If hypertensive crisis: Diazoxide 3–5 mg/kg per dose i.v. bolus q. 4 h p.r.n. (maximum dose 150 mg) or Nifedipine 0.22–0.5 mg/kg per dose sublingual q. 4 h p.r.n. ± Nitroprusside 0.5–4 µg/kg i.v. continuous infusion
Late (1–4 weeks postop.)	Propranolol (oral) 0.5–1 mg/kg per dose p.o. q.i.d. or Captopril 0.1 mg/kg per starting dose p.o. t.i.d. Dose range for newborn infants: 0.1–0.3 mg/kg per dose Dose range for older children: 0.1–2 mg/kg per dose	Propranolol (oral) + captopril
Persistent (≥4 weeks postop.)	Propranolol (oral) or Captopril	Propranolol (oral) + captopril

* If residual anatomic obstruction is present, then balloon dilation aortoplasty or surgery is considered.

vasodilator therapy initially and self-limited outcome in the majority of patients. If untreated, the patient is at risk for the postcoarctectomy syndrome (see below).

In 1985, Gidding and associates reported that the prophylactic use of propranolol—for 2 weeks before coarctation surgery and throughout the first postoperative week—was effective in the prevention of paradoxical hypertension in the first week after surgery [47]. Further experience is awaited to assess the impact of this regimen in this setting.

LATE PARADOXICAL HYPERTENSION

Hypertension occurring late—2–5 days postoperatively—is generally preceded by early paradoxical hypertension [41–43]. Investigation into the pathogenesis of late paradoxical hypertension has implicated the RAS [41–43]. Elevated PRA has been found in association with the rise in blood pressure in these patients [43]. Saralasin, a competitive antagonist of

angiotensin II at the vascular receptor level, has been shown to effect a reduction in blood pressure in late paradoxical hypertension [7]. However, saralasin is no longer available for clinical use but inhibitors of the enzyme that converts angiotensin I to angiotensin II are available—the angiotensin converting enzyme inhibitors.

The cause of heightened renin–angiotensin activity is not precisely understood but several possibilities have been proposed. The increased activity of the sympathetic nervous system noted in patients after coarctation repair leads to stimulation of the RAS [7,42–44]. The fall in proximal aortic blood pressure associated with repair of a coarctation may trigger heightened baroreceptor output including reflex stimulation of the renin–angiotensin axis via the sympathetic nervous system [7,42–44,46]. Another hypothesis is that there is reactive vasoconstriction of blood vessels, below the coarctation site, to the newly acquired pulsatile flow. This may lead to release of neural and/or hormonal mediators, effecting stimulation of the RAS [6]. Redistribution of renal blood flow within the kidney following repair of a coarctation may also affect the renin–angiotensin axis.

Unlike the early form, late paradoxical hypertension involves primarily an elevation of diastolic blood pressure and is generally less severe. Treatment involves use of β-blocker therapy or angiotensin converting enzyme inhibitors [7, 42, 43]. We recommend propranolol, provided cardiac function and the cardiac conduction system are intact, or captopril (Table 24.1). If parenteral therapy is required and cardiac function and conduction are intact, intravenous propranolol may be effective. The natural history of the late paradoxical hypertension is self-limited, resolving within 2 weeks in the majority of patients studied [40,41,43]. Patients with significant late paradoxical hypertension are at increased risk for the postcoarctectomy syndrome (see below) [50–53].

Postcoarctectomy syndrome

Sealy in 1953 described the occurrence of mesenteric arteritis following repair of coarctation and labeled this the postcoarctectomy syndrome [50]. It is characterized by abdominal symptoms on or about the third postoperative day [50–53]. Abdominal pain, tenderness, paralytic ileus, development of gastrointestinal signs, or symptoms of bowel necrosis, bleeding, or melena are noted and findings may progress to those of an acute abdomen. More than 90% of patients who develop this syndrome have associated marked early paradoxical hypertension. Abdominal surgery, required in a subset of these patients, has revealed a necrotizing mesenteric arteritis of small arterial vessels mainly involving the small bowel. Histologic examination of these vessels has revealed intimal changes and thromboses. It has been proposed that the postcoarctectomy syndrome results from injury to the small blood vessels distal to the coarctation site after corrective surgery. The vessels are thought to be injured by the newly acquired pulsatile flow in the presence of postoperative paradoxical hypertension [50–53].

With present awareness of the possibility of developing postcoarctectomy syndrome in association with untreated postoperative hypertension, this previously common problem is seldom seen. Prompt recognition and treatment of early paradoxical hypertension and avoidance of the premature introduction of feedings in the early postoperative period usually prevent the syndrome. However, when found, treatment includes bowel rest, intravenous nutrition, treatment of associated hypertension, and serial close observation for the development of gastrointestinal signs or symptoms requiring surgical intervention.

Paraplegia

This disastrous complication following repair of coarctation is fortunately quite rare [54]. The pathogenesis of the event is incompletely understood, but likely represents compromise of blood flow to the spinal cord during surgery [54]. Relative paucity of collateral flow and/or prolonged aortic cross-clamp time during repair, especially in the presence of elevated core temperature, are thought to be associated with increased risk [54]. Cases of paraplegia, however, have occurred in the absence of any of these factors. Intense investigation is underway to develop methods to monitor spinal cord and lower body perfusion and to detect spinal cord jeopardy intraoperatively. Variations in operative technique and choice of surgery are employed if spinal cord jeopardy is suspected. Unfortunately, no operative technique, including cardiac bypass methods, completely prevents the risk of paraplegia.

Persistent postoperative hypertension

Approximately 1 in 5 patients with late paradoxical hypertension will have persistent postoperative hypertension [18, 36, 55]. Persistent postoperative hypertension is that present for more than 1 month following surgery. Depending on the age at surgery, the specific anatomy, and the length of follow-up, between 15 and 33% of all patients undergoing coarctation repair will have persistent postoperative hypertension [18,31,36,55].

HYPERTENSION ASSOCIATED WITH RESIDUAL OR RECURRENT COARCTATION

In two-thirds of patients with persistent hypertension postoperatively, an anatomic explanation can be found [18,36]. Physical examination reveals the presence of residual gradient between upper and lower systolic blood pressure and/or disparity between upper and lower extremity pulses. If these differences are equivocal at rest, exercise testing has been shown to unmask the presence of postoperative aortic obstruction [45]. An upper extremity systolic blood pressure greater than 200 mmHg during or immediately following intense aerobic exercise is suspicious for residual obstruction and further evaluation should be considered [45]. If residual obstruction is confirmed by echocardiography, magnetic resonance imaging, digital subtraction angiography, and/or cardiac catheterization, then either balloon angioplasty or re-operation should be pursued. With regard to evaluation for recurrent or residual coarctation obstruction in the older child, aortic anatomic assessment by magnetic resonance imaging combined with physiologic Doppler echo flow profiling can frequently yield a diagnosis non-invasively [20−22].

PERSISTENT POSTOPERATIVE HYPERTENSION WITHOUT OBSTRUCTION

The hypertension in this group of patients can be systolic or diastolic and upper-to-lower extremity assessments of pulses and blood pressure are without disparity or gradient [36,46,55]. Several possible mechanisms have been proposed to explain this phenomenon: the first is increased proximal aortic impedance or abnormal vascular reactivity [46,55,56]. Utilizing histochemical analysis of specimens of aortic wall−coarctation site from experimental animals−the aortic wall has been found to be less distensible and to have increased impedance relative to aortic wall from control animals [46]. The proximal aortic wall in specimens of coarctation has also been found to have an abnormal vascular reactivity to catecholamines [46]. Increased forearm vascular reactivity to norepinephrine in patients with hypertension after repair of coarctation, compared to normotensive controls, has been reported [56]. In humans, differences in exercise-induced maximal muscle blood flow in the precoarctation versus distal vascular bed have been described in association with long-standing coarctation. This is consistent with reduced capacitance in the proximal vascular bed, possibly stemming from the effects of chronic systolic hypertension [46].

A second proposed mechanism for hypertension in this setting is an altered baroreceptor response. Investigations in children who have had surgical repair of their coarctation but who have persistent hypertension have demonstrated an altered baroreceptor set-point with reduced sensitivity [57,58]. The baroreceptor reflexes tend to maintain blood pressure at preoperative levels. Baroreceptor readaptation to normal blood pressure levels is delayed postoperatively or does not occur. Accompanying the heightened baroreceptor set-point is an increase in baseline sympathetic tone in these patients [57].

A third mechanism for hypertension may be an altered RAS response. An abnormally increased PRA in association with either salt restriction or diuresis has been demonstrated in patients with repaired coarctation who have persistent postoperative hypertension when compared to patients with hypertension and normal baseline RAS. Angiotensin receptor blockade with saralasin reduced blood pressure in the group with hypertension and repaired coarctation but did not reduce blood pressure in the control subjects. It is suspected that a lack of adjustment of the responsiveness of the renin−angiotensin axis to the normalized hemodynamics of renal blood flow following repair of coarctation is responsible [7,42,43]. The heightened baroreceptor reset described above, with its accompanying increased level of sympathetic tone, may also directly trigger an increased RAS response [7,42,43].

These three mechanisms may all be active and interactive−to varying degrees−in the individual patient with persistent postoperative hypertension not due to residual obstruction. In view of the above, we recommend β-blocker therapy or angiotensin converting enzyme inhibitors as antihypertensive treatment for this subgroup of patients (Table 24.1).

Many questions remain regarding this subgroup. It is not clear, for example, why certain patients with no residual aortic obstruction remain hypertensive while others do not. Some published literature suggests that the age at time of repair and the preoperative degree of hypertension are key variables [35,36], but can other factors be implicated? The optimal therapeutic regimen and natural history await further investigation.

ABDOMINAL COARCTATION

This rare condition should be considered in any patient who presents with the typical clinical picture of coarctation but in whom evaluation of the anatomy of the thoracic aorta proves negative for obstruction [48]. Presence of an abdominal bruit may be a very helpful diagnostic clue. The potential surgical anatomy of abdominal coarctation is more varied than in thoracic coarctation. Therefore, aortography is routinely required to define both the coarctation site and any involvement of neighboring vessels, including renal arteries. The surgical approach can then be tailored to the specific anatomy. Postoperative paradoxical hypertension may occur following repair of abdominal coarctation and should be watched for and managed as with thoracic coarctation.

PSEUDOCOARCTATION

The term pseudocoarctation refers to an unusually tortuous thoracic aorta without anatomic obstruction [59]. The aorta may be kinked but an obstructive coarctation shelf is not found. Collaterals do not develop. Pulses and blood pressures above and below the coarctation are normal and do not manifest the disparity and gradients seen with coarctation. Surgery is not indicated unless an aortic aneurysm develops. The propensity of an unusually tortuous aorta to aneurysm formation is reported in the literature [59]. Magnetic resonance imaging, in concert with echocardiography, are the noninvasive techniques of choice for evaluation in this condition [20−22]. If noninvasive physiologic evaluation with echo Doppler does not confirm the clinically assessed absence of upper-to-lower extremity systolic blood pressure gradient, then cardiac catheterization is necessary to rule out true coarctation.

SUMMARY

For those interested in hypertension, coarctation of the aorta offers intriguing problems to solve regarding mechanisms of hypertension at various stages of the disorder. From a clinical standpoint, coarctation of the aorta should be considered in any child or adolescent with hypertension, or in infants with early cardiac decompensation. In general the diagnosis can be made clinically with noninvasive laboratory confirmation; invasive assessment is usually reserved for unusual or complex situations. Management has classically involved surgical intervention resulting in removal or patch reconstruction of the obstructed portion of the aorta. The technique of balloon catheter angioplasty has been utilized in patients with recurrent or native coarctation, and initial results are encouraging, such that it is the procedure of choice in many centers for recurrent coarctation and may become an alternative to surgery for native coarctation. Further follow-up is ongoing regarding the long-term efficacy and complications of this technique for the treatment of coarctation.

From the study of paradoxical hypertension after operation, much pathophysiologic information has evolved. The pathophysiology of persistent postoperative hypertension without residual or recurrent obstruction may involve an interaction between the sympathetic limb of the autonomic nervous system and the RAS, resulting in a heightened blood pressure set-point. In patients with this problem blood pressure does not return to normal. Persistent abnormal proximal aortic impedance may also play an important role. In patients without overt residual or recurrent obstruction, treatment of persistent paradoxical hypertension involves β-blocker therapy or use of angiotensin converting enzyme inhibitors.

Although the record of coarctation surgery is extensive, many important questions remain incompletely answered with regard to the optimal operative and postoperative management of this fascinating condition.

REFERENCES

1 Keith JD. Coarctation of the aorta. In: Keith JD, Rowe RD, Vlad P, eds. *Heart Disease in Infancy and Childhood*. 3rd edn. New York: Macmillan, 1978;736−70.

2 Leuman EP. Blood pressure and hypertension in childhood and adolescence. *Ergeb Inn Med Kinderheilkd* 1979;43:109−83.

3 Lang P, Jonas RA, Norwood WI, Mayer JE, Casteneda AR. Palliation for aortic atresia−hypoplastic left heart syndrome: an update. *Circulation* 1985;72(suppl III):260.

4 Edwards JE, Christensen NA, Clagett OT, McDonald JR. Pathologic considerations in coarctation of the aorta. *Proc Mayo Clin* 1948;23:234.

5 Moulton AL. Coarctation of the aorta. In: Arciniegas E, ed. *Pediatric Cardiac Surgery*. Chicago: Year Book, 1985;95−107.

6 Scott HW, Bahnson HT. Evidence for a renal factor in the hypertension of experimental coarctation of the aorta. *Surgery* 1951;30:206−17.

7 Parker FB Jr, Farrell B, Streeten DHP, Blackman MS, Sondheimer HM, Anderson GH Jr. Hypertensive mechanisms in coarctation of the aorta. Further studies of the renin−angiotensin system. *J Thorac Cardiovasc Surg* 1980;80:568−73.

8 Goldblatt H, Kahn JR, Hanzel RF. Studies on experimental hypertension. The effect on blood pressure of constriction of the abdominal aorta above and below the site of origin of both main renal arteries. *J Exp Med* 1939;69:649−74.

9 Bagby SP, Bauer GM. Vascular reactivity to angiotensin II in canine neonatally induced coarctation hypertension. *Kidney Int* 1983;23:166.

10 Whitlow PL, Katholi RE. Neurohumoral activity and the role of renal nerves in canine coarctation of the aorta. *Am J Cardiol* 1982;49:888.

11 Bagby SP. Dissection of pathogenetic factors in coarctation hypertension. In: Loggie JMH *et al.*, eds. *NHLBI Workshop on Juvenile Hypertension*. New York: Biomedical Information,

1984;253−66.

12 Bell DR, Overbeck HW. Increased resistance and impaired maximal vasodilation in normotensive vascular beds of rats with coarctation. *Hypertension* 1979;1:80−5.

13 Gersony WM. Coarctation of the aorta. In: Adams FA, Emmanouilides GC, Riemenschneider TA, eds. *Moss' Heart Disease in Infants, Children, and Adolescents.* 4th edn. Baltimore: Williams & Wilkins, 1989;243−55.

14 Rowe RD, Freedom RM, Mehrizi A, Bloom KR, eds. Syndrome of coarctation of the aorta. In: *The Neonate With Congenital Heart Disease.* Philadelphia: WB Saunders, 1981;166−92.

15 Perloff JK, ed. Coarctation of the aorta. In: *The Clinical Recognition of Congenital Heart Disease.* 3rd edn. Philadelphia: WB Saunders, 1987;125−60.

16 Becker AE, Becker MJ, Edwards JE. Anomalies associated with coarctation of the aorta−particular reference to infancy. *Circulation* 1970;41:1067−75.

17 Glancy DL, Morrow AG, Simon AL, Roberts WC. Juxtaductal aortic coarctation−analysis of 84 patients studied hemodynamically, angiographically, and morphologically after age 1 year. *Am J Cardiol* 1983;51:537−51.

18 Liberthson RR, Pennington DG, Jacobs ML, Daggett EM. Coarctation of the aorta: review of 234 patients and clarification of management problems. *Am J Cardiol* 1979;43: 835−40.

19 Smallhorn JF, Huhta JC, Adams PA, Anderson RH, Wilkinson JL, Macartney FJ. Cross-sectional echocardiographic assessment of coarctation in the sick neonate and infant. *Br Heart J* 1983;50:349−61.

20 Marx GR, Allen HD. Accuracy and pitfalls of Doppler evaluation of the pressure gradient in aortic coarctation. *J Am Coll Cardiol* 1986;7:1379−85.

21 von Schulthess GK, Higashino SM, Higgins SS, Didier D, Fisher MR, Higgins CB. Coarctation of the aorta: MR imaging. *Radiology* 1986;158:469−74.

22 Boxer RA, LaCorte MA, Singh S *et al.* Nuclear magnetic resonance imaging in evaluation and follow-up of children treated for coarctation of the aorta. *J Am Coll Cardiol* 1986;7: 1095−8.

23 Moodie DS, Yiannikas J, Gill CC, Buonocore E, Pavlicek W. Intravenous digital subtraction angiography in the evaluation of congenital abnormalities of the aorta and aortic arch. *Am Heart J* 1982;104:628−34.

24 Heymann MA, Berman W Jr, Rudolph A, Whitman V. Dilatation of the ductus arteriosus by prostaglandin E_1 in aortic arch abnormalities. *Circulation* 1979;59:169−73.

25 Rao PS. Balloon valvuloplasty and angioplasty in infants and children. *J Pediatr* 1989;114:907−14.

26 Huhta JC. Angioplasty for recoarctation (editorial). *J Am Coll Cardiol* 1989;14:420−1.

27 Cooper SG, Sullivan ID, Wren C. Treatment of recoarctation: balloon dilation angioplasty. *J Am Coll Cardiol* 1989;14: 413−19.

28 Morrow WR, Vick GW, Nihill MR *et al.* Balloon dilation of unoperated coarctation of the aorta: short and intermediate-term results. *J Am Coll Cardiol* 1988;11:133−8.

29 Lock JE, Bass JL, Amplatz K, Fuhrman BP, Castaneda-Zuniga W. Balloon dilation angioplasty of aortic coarctation in infants and children. *Circulation* 1983;68:109−16.

30 Hesslein PS, McNamara DG, Morriss MJH, Hallman GL, Cooley DA. Comparison of resection versus patch aortoplasty for repair of coarctation in infants and children. *Circulation* 1981;64:164−8.

31 Smith RT Jr, Sade RM, Riopel DA, Taylor AB, Crawford FA Jr, Hohn AR. Stress testing for comparison of synthetic patch aortoplasty with resection and end to end anastomosis for repair of coarctation in childhood. *J Am Coll Cardiol* 1984;4:765−70.

32 Clarkson PM, Brandt PWT, Barratt-Boyes BG, Rutherford JD, Kerr AR, Neutze JM. Prosthetic repair of coarctation of the aorta with particular reference to Dacron onlay patch grafts and late aneurysm formation. *Am J Cardiol* 1985;56: 342−6.

33 Waldhausen JA, Nahrwold DL. Repair of coarctation of the aorta with a subclavian flap. *J Thorac Cardiovasc Surg* 1966; 51:532−3.

34 Beekman RH, Rocchini AR, Behrendt DM *et al.* Long-term outcome after repair of coarctation in infancy: subclavian angioplasty does not reduce the need for reoperation. *J Am Coll Cardiol* 1986;8:1406−11.

35 Martin M, Beekman RH, Rocchini AP, Crowley DC, Rosenthal A. Aortic aneurysms after subclavian repair of coarctation of the aorta. *Am J Cardiol* 1988;61:951−3.

36 Maron BJ, Humphries JO, Rowe RD, Mellits ED. Prognosis of surgically corrected coarctation of the aorta: a 20 year postoperative appraisal. *Circulation* 1973;47:119−26.

37 Daniels SR, James FW, Loggie JMH, Kaplan S. Correlates of resting and maximal exercise systolic blood pressure after repair of coarctation of the aorta: a multivariable analysis. *Am Heart J* 1987;113:349−53.

38 Choy M, Rocchini AP, Beekman RH *et al.* Paradoxical hypertension after repair of coarctation of the aorta in children: balloon angioplasty versus surgical repair. *Circulation* 1987; 75:1186−91.

39 Lewis AB, Takahashi M. Plasma catecholamine responses to balloon angioplasty in children with coarctation of the aorta. *Am J Cardiol* 1988;62:649−50.

40 Sealy WC, Harris JS, Young WG Jr, Callaway HA Jr. Paradoxical hypertension following resection of coarctation of aorta. *Surgery* 1957;42:135−47.

41 Sealy WC. Coarctation of the aorta and hypertension. *Ann Thorac Surg* 1967;3:15−28.

42 Rocchini AP, Rosenthal A, Barger AC, Castaneda AR, Nadas AS. Pathogenesis of paradoxical hypertension after coarctation resection. *Circulation* 1976;54:382−7.

43 Fox S, Pierce WS, Waldhausen JA. Pathogenesis of paradoxical hypertension after coarctation repair. *Ann Thorac Surg* 1980;29:135−41.

44 Benedict CR, Grahame-Smith DG, Fisher A. Changes in plasma catecholamines and dopamine β-hydroxylase after corrective surgery for coarctation of the aorta. *Circulation* 1978;57:598−602.

45 Freed MD, Rocchini AP, Rosenthal A, Nadas AS, Castaneda AR. Exercise-induced hypertension after surgical repair of coarctation of the aorta. *Am J Cardiol* 1979;43:253−8.

46 Sehested J, Baandrup U, Mikkelsen E. Different reactivity and structure of the prestenotic and poststenotic aorta in human coarctation: implications for baroreceptor function. *Circulation* 1982;65:1060−5.

47 Gidding SS, Rocchini AP, Beekman R *et al.* Therapeutic effect of propranolol on paradoxical hypertension after repair of coarctation of the aorta. *N Engl J Med* 1985;312:1224−8.

48 Scott HW Jr, Dean RH, Boerth R, Sawyers JL, Meacham P, Fisher RD. Coarctation of the abdominal aorta: pathophysiologic and therapeutic considerations. *Ann Surg* 1979;189:746−57.

49 Sealy WC. Paradoxical hypertension after repair of coarctation of the aorta: a review of its causes. *Ann Thorac Surg* 1990;50:323−9.

50 Sealy WC. Indications for surgical treatment of coarctation of the aorta. *Surg Gynecol Obstet* 1953;97:301.

51 Trummer MJ, Mannix EP Jr. Abdominal pain and necrotizing mesenteric arteritis following resection of coarctation of the aorta. *J Thorac Cardiovasc Surg* 1963;45:198−209.

52 Ho ECK, Moss AJ. The syndrome of "mesenteric arteritis" following repair of aortic coarctation. *Pediatrics* 1972;49:40−5.

53 Verska JJ, DeQuattro V, Wooley MM. Coarctation of the aorta. The abdominal pain syndrome and paradoxical hypertension. *J Thorac Cardiovasc Surg* 1969;58:746−53.

54 Brewer LA III, Fosburg RG, Mulder GA, Verska JJ. Spinal cord complications following surgery for coarctation of the aorta. *J Thorac Cardiovasc Surg* 1972;64:368−81.

55 Simsolo R, Grunfeld B, Gimenez M *et al.* Long-term systemic hypertension in children after successful repair of coarctation of the aorta. *Am Heart J* 1988;115:1268−73.

56 Gidding SS, Rocchini AP, Moorehead C, Schork MA, Rosenthal A. Increased forearm vascular reactivity in patients with hypertension after repair of coarctation. *Circulation* 1985;71:495−9.

57 Beekman RH, Katz BP, Moorehead-Steffens C, Rocchini AP. Altered baroreceptor function in children with systolic hypertension after coarctation repair. *Am J Cardiol* 1983;52:112−17.

58 Sehested J, Schultze G. Vasomotor wave and blood pressure response to erect posture after operation for aortic coarctation. *Br Heart J* 1982;48:357−63.

59 Dungan WT, Char F, Gerald BE, Campberg SG. Pseudocoarctation of the aorta in childhood. *Am J Dis Child* 1970;119:401−6.

25 Catecholamine-producing Tumors that Cause Hypertension: Diagnosis and Management

JENNIFER M. H. LOGGIE

Pheochromocytoma, neuroblastoma, ganglioneuroblastoma, and ganglioneuroma are all tumors of neuroectodermal origin that can cause hypertension secondary to the production of excess catecholamines. However most children with neuroblastomas do not have an increase in circulating norepinephrine and epinephrine. In one study, all patients with neuroblastoma had high plasma dopa whereas plasma catecholamines were not consistently increased [1]. The most common pattern of urinary catecholamines and their metabolites from children with neuroblastoma is one of excess dopamine, with disproportionately high levels of vanillylmandelic acid (VMA), and homovanillic acid (HVA). Norepinephrine and epinephrine levels are usually normal. When they are high, hypertension may be a clinical feature. In contrast, in patients with pheochromocytomas, norepinephrine and epinephrine usually occur in excess in the urine although their metabolites, VMA and metanephrines are also proportionately increased. Most patients with pheochromocytomas have a predominance of norepinephrine secretion and are thus hypertensive. If epinephrine is the predominant free amine, and norepinephrine production is not much increased, the patient may present with tachycardia and/or arrhythmias rather than hypertension. This is an unusual occurrence.

Pheochromocytomas arise from the chromaffin cells of the sympathoadrenal system. These cells occur in association with the celiac, mesenteric, renal, adrenal, hypogastric, testicular, and prevertebral sympathetic nerve plexuses. They are also found adjacent to other sympathetic nerves, e.g. those innervating the bladder. Ectopic sites also occur. Thus pheochromocytomas may arise anywhere where sympathetic tissue has occurred during development and they have been described in locations extending from the neck to the urinary bladder (Fig. 25.1). In adults the major sites for these tumors are the medulla of the adrenal gland, the paraganglia cells of the sympathetic nervous system, and the organ of Zuckerkandl at the aortic bifurcation. Multiple tumors occur in only 8% of cases; however, 70% of patients with familial pheochromocytomas have bilateral tumors that arise in the adrenal glands. In contrast, it has been reported that only 50% of children with pheochromocytomas had solitary, intraadrenal tumors; 24% had tumors in both adrenals and 32% had more than one tumor either within the adrenal glands or in extra-adrenal sites [3].

Neuroblastomas also arise from neural crest elements, including the thoracolumbar sympathetic ganglia and adrenal medulla. They do not arise in the brain or spinal cord. The most common primary site

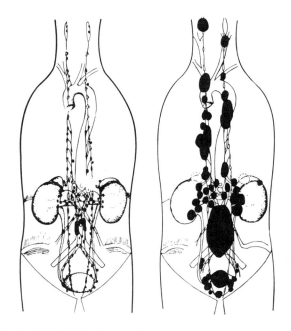

Fig. 25.1 (Left) Distribution of chromaffin tissue in the human newborn infant; (right) distribution of pheochromocytomas reported in the literature. From [2].

301

is in the adrenal gland and three-fourths of neuroblastomas are intra-abdominal with only one-fourth being intrathoracic. Of the intra-abdominal tumors, half have the adrenal gland as their primary site with the rest arising in the pararenal, paravertebral, and pelvic areas. Intrathoracic neuroblastomas are nearly all in the posterior mediastinum, usually in the upper third.

It is helpful when dealing with catecholamine-producing tumors to understand the basic biosynthesis and metabolism of these amines. This is shown in Figure 25.2. Tyrosine hydroxylase is the rate-limiting step in the biosynthetic process. The catecholamines are primarily inactivated by catechol-O-methyltransferase (COMT) and monoamine oxidase (MAO). The end-products of the metabolism of norepinephrine and epinephrine by COMT are normetanephrine and metanephrine respectively. Vanillylmandelic acid is formed through several steps after the inactivation of norepinephrine and epinephrine by MAO. Dopamine is also inactivated by the action of COMT and MAO. Homovanillic acid is the major metabolite formed through the activity of MAO on dopamine.

Norepinephrine, epinephrine, dopamine, VMA, metanephrines, and HVA can all be measured in urine. They are used to make the diagnosis of pheochromocytoma and neuroblastoma. However several other conditions that occasionally cause increased excretion of catecholamines, their metabolites, or both have been reported [4]. These include astrocytoma [5], retinoblastoma [6], autonomic hyperreflexia, toxemia of pregnancy or eclampsia with convulsions, hypertensive crisis associated with administration of MAO inhibitors, and carcinoid tumor [4].

NEUROBLASTOMA

Neuroblastoma is the third commonest tumor of childhood and the most common solid tumor. It affects 9 children per million annually in the USA and is very rare after the age of 14 years. Under 5 years of age the male : female ratio is 1.4. Rarely the tumor has been reported as a familial entity with autosomal dominant inheritance [7]. Intrathoracic neuroblastomas comprise 25% of all intrathoracic tumors in children.

It is of interest that there is a high incidence of occult neuroblastoma found in newborn infants who die from other causes [8]. It is presumed that most of

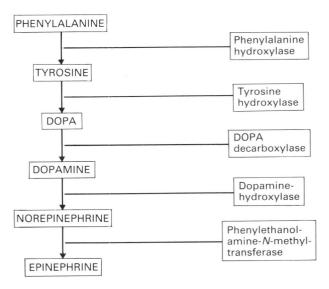

Fig. 25.2 Biosynthetic and metabolic pathway of catecholamines.

these tumors are suppressed by the immune system. Even when metastases are present in the newborn infant with a neuroblastoma there may be regression or maturation of tumor cells with survival.

Histologically neuroblastomas may be completely undifferentiated or may show gradations of maturation to ganglioneuroma. Some 25–50% show either local or diffuse calcification.

Clinical presentation

Children with neuroblastoma classically present with an abdominal mass which may be associated with fatigue and lassitude secondary to anemia. The mass may cross the midline and this may help to differentiate it from Wilms' tumor. Sometimes there is a history of nausea, vomiting, anorexia, abdominal pain or swelling, change in bowel habit, weight loss, and fever. If the tumor is intrathoracic in location it can cause pneumonia and respiratory difficulty. Tumors located in sympathetic ganglia along the cervical, thoracic, or lumbar spine may invade through the intervertebral foramina causing compression of the spinal cord and neurologic signs and symptoms.

Metastases usually involve the reticuloendothelial system and bone. In the latter location they may be either reactive or lytic and may cause pain. Metastases to the orbit may cause dislocation of the globe and if there is bone marrow involvement, pallor, ecchymoses, and infection may suggest leukemia.

Subcutaneous metastases may be generalized giving a scattered eruption of firm, nontender, blueish, mobile nodules—the so-called "blueberry muffin" appearance.

As noted earlier, hypertension is not a common finding in children with neuroblastoma. However it sometimes occurs in association with tachycardia and increased sweating; the tumor behaves much like a pheochromocytoma. It remains unclear why this happens but in our experience it can be seen with tumors of all gradations of maturity, including ganglioneuroma. One 15-year-old female presented to us with a history that prior to dental surgery she had a normal blood pressure. Approximately 15–20 min after anesthetic induction her blood pressure rose to 220/130–140 mmHg. She also developed sinus tachycardia with atrial bigeminy. At a later time when she was asymptomatic, she was found to have elevated plasma norepinephrine and abdominal computerized tomography (CT) showed a left adrenal mass measuring 2.5 × 2.5 cm on axial scans. After surgical removal this was found to be a ganglioneuroma. When last seen, 3 years after tumor removal, the girl had a normal blood pressure and had not had any further hypertensive episodes.

It may not be possible on clinical grounds to determine if catecholamine excess is the cause of hypertension in young children and infants with neuroblastomas. These tumors, when intra-abdominal, may produce caudal and anterior displacement of the kidney with lateral rotation of the upper pole. Extrinsic distortion of the calcyceal system may occur and, theoretically, there may also be distortion and/or stretching of the renal arteries. This could lead to a functional renal artery narrowing with overproduction of renin by a relatively ischemic kidney. Therefore it is very important to measure urinary catecholamine and metabolite excretion before selecting antihypertensive drugs since β-blocking agents may worsen the hypertension of catecholamine excess.

Wilms' tumor, the fourth most common cancer in childhood, also occurs in young children and may present as an abdominal mass with hypertension [9]. It can usually be differentiated from neuroblastoma on the basis of appropriate imaging studies. However it should be noted that neuroblastoma has been reported on occasion to be intrarenal both by imaging and at surgery [10]. With Wilms' tumor, urinary catecholamines and their metabolites are normal.

Treatment of hypertension

It has been said that treatment of hypertension in association with neuroblastoma is difficult, that there is poor correlation between levels of excretion products and hypertension, and that generally α-blockade is unnecessary [11]. This has not been the experience at the Children's Hospital Medical Center, Cincinnati, OH over the past 25 years. Children with neuroblastoma and hypertension have often had high urinary levels of *free* catecholamines rather than only their metabolites and dopamine, and they have responded well to α-blockade with phenoxybenzamine or, on occasion, prazosin. Tachycardia has been controlled with β-blocking agents after α-blockade has been established. Some children have also received α-methyl-1-tyrosine (Demser) and have had a salutary response. Clearly if there is no correlation between increased urinary free catecholamines and blood pressure, conventional antihypertensive drugs would be preferable to α-blockade. In these cases a renin–angiotensin–aldosterone mechanism may be responsible for the hypertension.

PHEOCHROMOCYTOMA

It has been estimated that about 0.1% of the adult population with persistent diastolic hypertension have pheochromocytomas. A higher incidence has been found at referral centers, probably because more complex patients are seen there. It must also be remembered when calculating the prevalence of pheochromocytoma that about 50% of adults with this tumor have paroxysmal rather than persistent hypertension [4].

The incidence of pheochromocytoma in children with hypertension is not clear. In one of the only extensive reviews of this condition in childhood, written in 1963, Stackpole and co-authors [3] noted that hypertension was sustained in 90% of children with this tumor. This may not be the case nowadays when blood pressure measurement is much more routine in children than it was then, so that patients with tumors may be found earlier than before.

We have evaluated over 1000 hypertensive children in the past 25 years and have had only 7 proven pheochromocytomas. Two other children with histories, clinical, and biochemical findings highly suggestive of pheochromocytoma have not had tumors localized by current imaging techniques. The rest of our small population of children with tumors producing an excess of catecholamines with associated hypertension have had neuroblastoma [7], ganglioneuroblastoma (1), or ganglioneuroma (1).

Pheochromocytoma may occur at any age during childhood and has been reported in the newborn period [12] as well as in the first year of life [13]. There is also one report of a premature infant girl with congenital pheochromocytomas in both adrenal glands [14]. In females, it has been reported that 62% with pheochromocytomas presented between 11 and 15 years of age, i.e. around menarche [3]. In males there is no such clustering by age and approximately two-thirds of all prepubertal children with the tumor are boys. After puberty, the incidence in females increases. In our small series of patients, 5 of the 7 with proven pheochromocytomas were males, as were the 2 patients with a highly suspicious clinical and biochemical presentation.

Pathologic conditions sometimes associated with pheochromocytomas

Familial pheochromocytoma occurring with tumors or hyperplasia of the thyroid and parathyroid glands has been designated as multiple endocrine neoplasia (MEN) type 2. The tumors do not necessarily present in the different glands at the same time. The co-existence of pheochromocytoma, medullary thyroid carcinoma, mucosal neuromas, thickened corneal nerves, alimentary tract ganglioneuromatosis, and, frequently, a marfanoid habitus is also familial and is designated MEN type 2b or 3. Thyroid carcinoma is found with both familial and sporadic pheochromocytomas and, when the two coexist, pheochromocytomas occur in both adrenal glands in 70% of patients. Hyperparathyroidism also occurs with both familial and sporadic pheochromocytoma, although much less commonly with the latter [4]. In the case of the familial entities, inheritance is as an autosomal dominant trait.

Excess elaboration of cortisol or adrenocorticotrophic hormone by a pheochromocytoma may lead to the coexistence of Cushing's syndrome. Sometimes hyperplasia of the adrenal cortex has been shown to coexist with pheochromocytoma and this may also result in evidence of cortisol excess. One case has been reported of a 16-month-old female with Cushing's syndrome and pheochromocytoma [15]. Her hirsutism was first noticed at 6 months of age.

In addition to secreting adrenocorticortrophic hormone and cortisol, it has been reported that pheochromocytomas may also secrete other hormones [16]. Viale and coworkers [17] have reported a case of an adrenal pheochromocytoma producing vasoactive intestinal polypeptides, somatostatin, and calcitonin. The patient with this tumor had the watery diarrhea syndrome (WDHH) which has also been reported with malignant pheochromocytoma [18]. By the end of 1986, 7 patients with the combination of WDHH and adrenal pheochromocytoma had been reported [18]. More often this syndrome occurs with pancreatic tumor or hyperplasia [19]. Recently a child with an adrenal ganglioneuroblastoma that produced gut hormones and presented as a pseudo-obstruction has been reported [20]. Acromegaly has also been reported to have been caused by a plurihormonal adrenal medullary tumor [21]. In addition the previously reported coexistence of acromegaly, pheochromocytoma, and hyperparathyroidism has been thought to represent a form of MEN [4].

It is well known that neurofibromatosis may be associated with pheochromocytoma [22]. In adults with this condition, the incidence of the tumor is said to be less than 1%. However, in children with neurofibromatosis, renal artery disease is said to be a commoner cause of hypertension than is pheochromocytoma [23]. Pheochromocytoma also occurs in association with von Hippel–Landau disease (cerebellar hemangioblastoma with retinal angioma), Sturge–Weber disease, and tuberous sclerosis.

Clinical presentation

Pheochromocytoma has been called the great mimic because of the protean nature of its manifestations. The symptoms are due either to the pharmacologic effects of excessive circulating levels of norepinephrine and epinephrine or to the complications of hypertension. The commonest symptom is headache. These vary in intensity, character, and location but they may be abrupt and severe with sudden rises in blood pressure, even when persistent hypertension is present.

At the onset, it must be mentioned that children with this tumor, like adults, may display marked emotional lability. Therefore one should always seek information regarding recent changes in behavior when evaluating hypertensive children and adolescents. One child with episodes of vertigo, drowsiness, and arm spasms was diagnosed as neurotic for 2 years before his death. At autopsy a left suprarenal tumor was found and it was noted that blood pressure had never been measured during one of his "attacks."

Of the 71 cases of pheochromocytoma reported by Hume in 1960 [24], 81% had headaches, sweating was prominent in 68%, nausea in 56%, and visual changes and weight loss in 44%. These symptoms — other than headache — were said to be commoner in children than adults. In addition 25% of children had polyuria and polydipsia and convulsions occurred in 23%. Reddish-blue mottling of the skin, a puffy red cyanotic appearance of the hands, and polyphagia may also occur. In addition some children have palpitations, pallor, abdominal pain, nervousness, weakness, and fatigue. One of our patients presented with severe throbbing headaches, polyphagia, weight loss, and palpitations. He had papilledema and was originally admitted on the neurosurgical service as having a possible brain tumor. Another boy presented with fever of unknown origin of about 6–8 weeks' duration and he was admitted for an immunologic evaluation on the hematology service where it was noted that he also had hypertension. On the other hand, a teenage male who was completely asymptomatic presented with a tumor that was visible through the anterior abdominal wall. After hospitalization he did, however, have acute, severe headaches when he lay prone or when his abdomen was palpated. He had a malignant pheochromocytoma with widespread skeletal metastases.

Many of the signs of pheochromocytoma are similar in both children and adults. They include sustained or paroxysmal hypertension, tachycardia, fever, pallor, and hyperhydrosis. Arrhythmias may also occur and hypertensive retinopathy may be present. Infrequently a palpable mass occurs in the abdomen, as in the boy described above.

It is important to recognize that the episodic symptoms of pheochromocytoma may occur as rarely as every few months or as often as many times in a single day. They may be transient in nature or last for hours or days. Typically, attacks become more frequent — though not necessarily more severe — with the passage of time. A number of things may elicit an attack and these are listed in Table 25.1.

Differential diagnosis

It is our experience that children with pheochromocytomas usually have symptoms and/or signs suggesting the diagnosis. However, because of its varied

Table 25.1 Factors that can precipitate symptoms and signs in patients with pheochromocytoma

Miscellaneous
Massage or steady pressure for 1–2 min in the area of a tumor
Compression of the tumor by body position
Postural changes (especially bending)
Increased intra-abdominal pressure from any cause, e.g. tight clothes
Anxiety or emotional stress
Trauma
Pain
Pressure on the carotid sinuses
Bladder distension
Intubation for anesthesia

Activities
Exercise
Hyperventilation
Valsalva maneuver
Micturition (especially with bladder pheochromocytoma)
Straining at stool
Smoking
Shaving
Gargling
Sneezing
Sexual intercourse
Childbirth
Ingestion of food or alcohol containing tyramine (e.g. cheese, beer, wine)

Drugs
Histamine
Glucagon
Epinephrine
Tyramine
Methacholine
Nicotine
Adrenocorticotrophic hormone (corticotropin)
Phenothiazines
Succinylcholine
General anesthesia

Diagnostic procedures
Angiography

presentation, the tumor must always be kept in mind when seeing any hypertensive child, or children and adolescents with headaches that sound as if they are of a vascular nature. It is not unusual for the blood pressure to rise quite high during a migraine headache and this may confuse the picture.

Children with hypertension from any cause may have features like those of pheochromocytoma such as tachycardia, anxiety, irritability, or even encephalopathy. The diagnosis must always be entertained and the tumor screened for if there are any suggestive signs or symptoms. In asymptomatic patients with sustained, moderate, or severe hypertension, screening should also be done, particularly if they have conditions known to coexist with pheochromocytoma.

It should be kept in mind that in children pheochromocytomas have been reported encircling the renal arteries or obstructing ureters so that one may be misled into believing that the etiology of the hypertension is renal or renovascular.

Acute, severe hypertension with sudden onset of headache is sometimes seen with a variety of drug ingestions. Usually these can be identified by screening the urine for toxic substances.

One should also bear in mind that adolescents or their parents who have access to vasopressor drugs may have pseudopheochromocytoma with factitious symptoms [4]. Other rare causes of paroxysmal hypertension include porphyria, clonidine withdrawal, and Guillain–Barré syndrome.

Pheochromocytomas are generally quite vascular tumors and hemorrhagic necrosis may occur. This complication can present as an acute abdomen with or without hypotension. Other tumors, predominantly epinephrine-secreting, can present with arrhythmias without hypertension and may be difficult to diagnose. Although a couple of our patients with pheochromocytomas have had glucosuria, it is our experience that diabetes mellitus does not usually present a differential diagnostic problem with pheochromocytoma in childhood.

Diagnostic evaluation

When a pheochromocytoma is suspected, urine should be collected to measure the 24-h excretion of norepinephrine, epinephrine, dopamine, VMA, and metanephrines. If only one of these free amines and their metabolites is used for screening, the measurement of total metanephrines gives the highest yield of positive results in adults with pheochromocytomas [25].

In patients having intermittent hypertension with episodic symptoms it may be necessary to do fractional collections of urine. This is because with paroxysmal symptoms of short duration, the amount of catecholamines excreted during the attack may not increase the 24-h totals into abnormal ranges. A fractional collection should cover the period of the attack and there should be a second collection made as a control during an asymptomatic period of the same duration.

When a pheochromocytoma is suspected and urinary catecholamines and their metabolites are consistently normal, it may be necessary to measure plasma catecholamines. Unfortunately few laboratories have data on the normal plasma levels of norepinephrine, epinephrine, and dopamine in children of various ages. However values in excess of the normal adult ranges are clearly also abnormal for children and adolescents. Plasma catecholamines may be high in the absence of increased urinary levels of free amines and they should be measured when urinary levels are normal or equivocal and clinical suspicion of pheochromocytoma is high.

In the past, intravenous phentolamine was used as a screening diagnostic test for patients with hypertension who were suspected of having pheochromocytoma. It is rarely used nowadays since safer and more accurate studies are available. Furthermore false-positive tests, with a marked drop in blood pressure, occurred particularly in patients receiving some antihypertensive drugs or barbiturates. Drugs that provoke a release of catecholamines by a pheochromocytoma include histamine, glucagon, and tyramine. Histamine is contraindicated in asthmatic patients and the tyramine test is unreliable [4].

Although provocative pharmacologic testing is rarely used nowadays, it can still be a useful maneuver in patients with normal or only mildly elevated blood pressure and paroxysmal symptoms suggestive of pheochromocytoma. Plasma and urinary catecholamines and their metabolites are measured in conjunction with the pharmacologic provocation. These tests and how to perform them are well described in a monograph about pheochromocytoma by Manger and Gifford [4].

The advent of CT increased the ability to localize pheochromocytomas preoperatively [26]. It was more productive and less hazardous than the performance of angiography. Tumors in 2 different children are demonstrated by CT in Figure 25.3. Additional imaging studies, such as magnetic resonance imaging (MRI), or scintigraphy with metaiodobenzylguanidine (MIBG) are now also available. However it should be noted that the injection of radiographic contrast media or glucagon during special imaging procedures may precipitate the release of catecholamines with hypertension and/or arrhythmias. Despite all of these new technologies it may still be difficult to localize pheochromocytomas, especially in children, in whom they are more often extra-adrenal and multiple than in adults. Nor is it clear

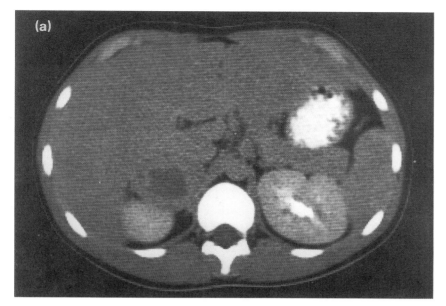

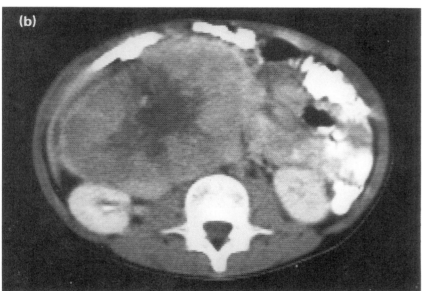

Fig. 25.3 (a) Computerized tomography scan showing a right suprarenal mass, measuring 5 × 4.5 × 6 cm. The mass displaces the right kidney inferiorly. The nonenhancing, low-density center represents necrosis or hemorrhage. A benign right adrenal pheochromocytoma was removed from this 15-year-old boy. (b) Computerized tomography scan showing a 15 × 8 cm mass that is anterior and inferior to the right kidney, displacing it posterolaterally. It also has a nonenhancing, low-density center. This was a malignant pheochromocytoma in a 13-year-old male who had multiple skeletal metastases.

whether MRI, CT, or MIBG scintigraphy is best for localizing pheochromocytomas in children since this has not been studied in any large series.

Quint and colleagues [27] have compared MRI, CT, and I-131 MIBG scintigraphy in localizing pheochromocytoma and paraganglioma in adults. Their study was biased by the fact that patients were selected on the basis of positive findings with scintigraphy and then directed to CT and MRI. None the less, some observations of value were made. The data suggested that MRI, CT, and scintigraphy were nearly equivalent in the evaluation of primary adrenal pheochromocytoma. MRI and scintigraphy were somewhat superior to CT in identifying primary extra-adrenal tumors. Screening for recurrent and metastatic disease was thought to be best with scintigraphy since the whole body can be scanned. For more precise anatomic definition MRI was better than CT when recurrent tumor was present.

An advantage of CT is that it is more widely available and can be performed rapidly. Its sensitivity in identifying primary adrenal pheochromocytomas is 92–100% [28,29]. Its disadvantages include its mediocre accuracy in identifying extra-adrenal tumors and the need to use intravenous contrast material. This can cause release of catecholamines with an abrupt rise in blood pressure in patients who are without adequate α-blockade. Also CT cannot reliably show the difference between an incidental adrenal cortical adenoma and a pheochromocytoma in a hypertensive patient. In addition, surgical clip artifacts pose a problem with CT when recurrent tumor is under investigation.

The advantages of MRI are that it appears capable of differentiating between an incidental adrenal adenoma, and a pheochromocytoma. In addition to tissue characterization, MRI is useful for studying anatomic areas that are problems with CT. Therefore tumors adjacent to the inferior vena cava, the urinary bladder, and the heart are shown better with MRI. In their series, Quint and associates [27] found sagittal and coronal MRI scans very helpful in identifying intrapericardial tumors. Disadvantages of MRI include the fact that it is expensive and time-consuming.

Scintigraphy, as mentioned earlier, has the advantage that whole-body scanning can be done. This is particularly important in the detection of extra-adrenal pheochromocytomas and metastatic disease. The sensitivity is approximately 90% and the specificity 95%. The use of I-123 MIBG, instead of I-131 MIBG, increases the sensitivity and provides better resolution. Disadvantages of scintigraphy include its limited availability and poor anatomic location of lesions. In addition the study takes up to 3 days to complete. I-131 MIBG scintigraphy has a false-negative rate of about 13%, largely because of inadequate tracer uptake within tumor [30]. It can, however, demonstrate adrenal medullary hyperplasia which occurs mainly in patients with MEN-2 syndromes.

Prior to the availability of new imaging techniques, central venous sampling for the measurement of plasma catecholamines could be useful for localizing pheochromocytomas. A step-up in values in a given location suggested the anatomic site of tumor [31]. The place of venous sampling in an era of improved imaging techniques is unclear but it may still be useful when these resources are limited. Its use is compared with that of CT and I-131 MIBG scintigraphy in 4 children by Turner and coworkers [32].

The diagnosis of malignant pheochromocytoma is usually made by the surgeon at the time of tumor removal. If for some reason malignancy is suspected preoperatively, metastases should be sought primarily in bone, lung, and liver. MIBG scintigraphy can be very helpful in delineating the extent of tumor spread; however, conventional bone and liver scans may have to be performed as well. If malignancy is diagnosed only intraoperatively, these studies should be done postoperatively.

The differentiation between a benign and malignant tumor is important prognostically. However it should be noted that patients with malignancy, and even widespread metastases, have lived for many years even though effective chemotherapy was not available. Manger and Gifford [4] commented that of 18 patients with malignant pheochromocytomas, 13 had curative resections attempted and 5 had palliative procedures. Twelve of the 18 patients died of the disease within 1 month to 17 years after the primary operation. The median survival time was 5.6 years but 3 patients lived 20 or more years after primary surgical treatment even though they had continued evidence of disease. Malignancy was more common with extra-adrenal tumors and patients with pulmonary metastases had a poorer prognosis than other patients.

In adults, pheochromocytoma is malignant in 10% of cases. In children the incidence is less clear. In our small series of children with pheochromocytoma only 1 of the 8 proven tumors was malignant. This adolescent had extensive skeletal metastases at the time of presentation and underwent two abdominal debulking procedures. After 5 years on α- and β-blocking agents as well as α-methyl-1-tyrosine for 3 years, he opted to discontinue all of his drugs. When last seen at a social visit, 7 years after diagnosis, his blood pressure was measured at 272/164 mmHg.

Whenever a pheochromocytoma is thought to be familial, the immediate relatives should be screened for evidence of pheochromocytoma, medullary thyroid carcinoma, and hyperparathyroidism. They should be seen periodically thereafter and any patient with MEN type 2 or 3 should receive genetic counseling.

Management

It is infrequent for patients with pheochromocytomas to present as urgent surgical problems. However if hypertension is severe or there are serious arrhythmias, urgent medical treatment may be indicated. This usually consists of the administration of α-blocking agents with or without β-blocking agents. The antihypertensive drugs used to treat other forms of hypertension are not usually helpful, with the exception of sodium nitroprusside and prazosin hydrochloride [4,33].

It continues to be debated whether patients with nonemergent pheochromocytomas should be routinely treated with α-blockade before surgical removal is attempted. In centers with teams very experienced in the management of these tumors, routine α-blockade is not considered mandatory [4]. In fact, it is argued that adequate blockade may mask the surgeon's ability to find by palpation additional tumors that have not been localized preoperatively by imaging techniques. In children, in whom tumors are often multiple or extra-adrenal, this may be particularly true. None the less, in centers where pheochromocytomas are seen infrequently, preoperative α-blockade is probably the better part of valour. Certainly anesthesia and surgery are usually less eventful when the cardiovascular system has been stabilized.

Medical management

As discussed, medical management of pheochromocytoma is indicated routinely before surgery under some circumstances. It is also indicated when there are serious complications of hypertension, or if the tumor has metastasized or is not entirely resectable. Even when malignant tumors cannot be completely removed, debulking may make medical management easier since lesser amounts of catecholamines may be produced.

In some patients, tachycardia may be marked either before or during α-blockade and it may be felt that a β-blocking agent is indicated. It must be remembered that β-blockade should not be induced without prior α-blockade. In the absence of α-blockade, a β-blocking drug such as propranolol will overcome any vasodilating effect of epinephrine and may lead to the aggravation of hypertension [4].

α-BLOCKADE

Phenoxybenzamine, phentolamine, and prazosin are all drugs that have been used in the treatment of hypertension secondary to catecholamine excess. They all have α-blocking properties; prazosin may be useful when it is felt that hypertension should be treated, but its etiology has not yet been confirmed by measurement of increased catecholamines. However we have not been impressed that it produces as smooth a blockade as phenoxybenzamine.

For over two decades, phenoxybenzamine has been used to control the hypertension associated with pheochromocytoma. It also will control the excess sweating seen in some patients with this tumor. Phenoxybenzamine combines irreversibly with postganglionic α-adrenergic receptors and has no effect on β-receptors. Its onset of action occurs several hours after oral administration and its effects are cumulative with daily dosing. The duration of action as an α-receptor blocking agent is 3−4 days after a single dose and its half-life is about 24 h. Only the oral form of the drug is available for clinical use in the USA. An intravenous form is investigational and has not been used extensively. However it is said that blockade after a single dose by this route is very persistent, lasting 3−4 days [34]. Since the onset of action is slow, the drug is not suitable for intra-operative management of pheochromocytoma. In addition, phentolamine and sodium nitroprusside, which are much quicker and shorter-acting, are both effective and readily available for intravenous administration.

Phenoxybenzamine has not been carefully studied in children. The initial pediatric dose recommended is 0.2 mg/kg up to a maximum of 10 mg in 24 h [35]. Dosage is increased gradually at 2−4 day intervals and a maintenance dose of 0.4−1.2 mg/kg per day in 2−4 divided doses is recommended. In adolescents, adult dosing guidelines are applicable with a starting dose of 10 mg twice a day, increased by 10 mg every other day. In fact, the total daily dose of phenoxybenzamine is one that achieves adequate blood pressure control without serious adverse effects. These include postural hypotension (which may be severe), reflex tachycardia, a stuffy nose, and gastrointestinal irritation. Other side-effects such as drowsiness and confusion are less common.

It should be mentioned that the action of drugs such as dopamine, ephedrine, epinephrine, metaraminol, methoxamine, and phenylephrine may all be altered in the presence of α-blockade with phenoxybenzamine [35]. If hypotension secondary to an overdose of drug occurs, the usual pressor agents are ineffective and epinephrine is contraindicated as it may cause further hypotension. The fall in blood pressure due to phenoxybenzamine-induced α-blockade is often responsive to the infusion of extra volume. Intravenous infusion of levarterenol bitartrate may also be useful but may sometimes not produce a rise in blood pressure. Manger and Gifford have reported that infusion of angiotensin caused its usual pressor effect in 1 patient given intravenous phenoxybenzamine who was unresponsive to intravenous norepinephrine [4].

Phentolamine, which produces α_1- and α_2-blockade and antagonizes the effects of both circulating epinephrine and norepinephrine, is no longer available for oral administration in the USA. It was said to be erratically absorbed, giving less smooth control of blood pressure than phenoxybenzamine. The intravenous form is still available and is sometimes used intraoperatively to control the pressor crises that may occur with pheochromocytoma. Parenteral administration may cause acute and prolonged hypotension, tachycardia, and cardiac arrhythmias. As with phenoxybenzamine, the effects of several sympathomimetic agents are altered in the presence of phentolamine.

Labetalol, which has a selective α_1-blocking effect, has one-sixth to one-tenth the potency of phentolamine, and its β-blocking effect is one-fourth to one-sixth that of propranolol. In humans, the ratios of α-to β-blockade have been estimated to be about 1:3 and 1:7 following oral and intravenous administration respectively [36]. The intravenous form of labetalol has been used successfully to lower blood pressure in patients with pheochromocytomas. However, it should be noted that a pressor response may occur instead of a depressor effect.

β-BLOCKADE

Tachycardia and arrhythmias may be a feature in patients with pheochromocytoma either before or after α-blockade. To counteract these problems, β-blockade is often undertaken. Since it was one of the first β-blocking agents available, propranolol has been used the most in this situation. Other than the advantage of extensive experience with its use, propranolol is also known not to block the uptake of I-131 MIBG, which is important when scintigraphy is proposed for diagnostic purposes.

The pharmacology of the β-blocking agents is described in Chapter 13. They should be avoided in patients with asthma, and have a variety of side-effects, including occasionally serious mental depression. It is important to reiterate that they should not be used until α-blockade is established since they may exacerbate hypertension, necessitating an increase in dose of the α-blocking agent. Adequate α- and β-blockade is present in patients with pheo-

chromocytomas when blood pressure and heart rate (or arrhythmias when present) are controlled. It is said that one of the advantages of phenoxybenzamine is that it reverses the hypovolemia that may accompany pheochromocytoma.

METYROSINE (α-METHYL-1-TYROSINE)

Metyrosine reduces catecholamine biosynthesis up to 75% by blocking tyrosine hydroxylase activity in converting tyrosine to dihydroxyphenylalanine (dopa). This is the initial and rate-limiting step in the production of catecholamines. Patients with pheochromocytoma who are receiving the drug have reduced blood pressure and decreased excretion of urinary catecholamines.

Metyrosine has been used successfully in the preoperative management of patients with pheochromocytoma, as well as in those with inoperable or malignant tumors or contraindications to surgery. We have also used it in the management of neuroblastoma with catecholamine excess. The initial adult dose is usually 250 mg four times daily with increases in increments of 250−500 mg daily until an effective dose has been reached. The maintenance dose is usually between 2 and 3 g/day in four divided doses by mouth. The pediatric dose has not been established but we have used an initial dose of 10−15 mg/kg per day in four divided doses. We have titrated upwards in 100−200 mg increments per day every few days until blood pressure has been controlled.

Metyrosine is well absorbed from the gut and has a half-life of about $3\frac{1}{2}$ h. Reduction in urinary catecholamines is usually seen in 2−3 days. After discontinuation, the levels return to those seen before treatment within 3−4 days and the blood pressure gradually increases to pretreatment levels within 2−3 days. Most of the drug is excreted unchanged by the kidneys [37].

Adverse effects include diarrhea, extrapyramidal effects, other central nervous system effects including mood changes, and crystalluria or urolithiasis. In order to minimize the risk of crystalluria a high fluid intake is recommended (in adults at least 2000 ml when on a 2 g/day dose).

Surgical management

Patients with pheochromocytomas may have a reduction of blood volume even when α-blockade is adequate. Therefore there are those who recom-

Table 25.2 Differential diagnosis of pheochromocytoma

Hyperthyroidism
Hyperdynamic β-adrenergic circulatory state
Vascular headaches (e.g. migraine)
Renal parenchymal or renal arterial disease with hypertension
Intracranial lesions (e.g. tumors)
Autonomic hyperreflexia
Familial dysautonomia
Neuroblastoma, ganglioneuroblastoma, ganglioneuroma

mend routine preoperative measurement of total blood volume, plasma volume, and red cell mass. Before surgery, whatever component is reduced may be replaced. Alternatively empiric volume replacement may be undertaken intraoperatively. The objective is to avoid the profound and prolonged drop in blood pressure that sometimes occurs after tumor removal. Intra- and postoperative infusion of pressor agents is rarely necessary if proper attention is given to adequate volume replacement, as gauged by an acceptable blood pressure level.

If bilateral adrenalectomy is contemplated either because of bilateral tumors or for some other reason, steroid replacement may have to be started just before anesthesia is induced and continued indefinitely thereafter.

Clearly, during surgery blood pressure, heart rate, and rhythm have to be carefully and appropriately monitored by the anesthetist. There also must be good venous access available for the infusion of volume expanders and drugs. Phentolamine may be given intravenously as either an infusion or a bolus to control high blood pressure. Alternatively, hypertension may be managed with intravenous sodium nitroprusside. In our experience, patients with pheochromocytomas have blood pressures that are very sensitive to control with this agent, which has the additional advantage of having a very transient effect when the infusion is stopped. Lidocaine and propranolol have both been used effectively to control intraoperative rhythm disturbances.

Intubation is a time when severe hypertensive crises may occur in patients who are not adequately α- and β-blocked or who have not been properly prepared with muscle relaxants and anesthesia. Other crises may occur during manipulation of tumors by the surgeon.

The case has been made that an anterior transabdominal approach is mandatory when operating for pheochromocytoma [4]. This is particularly true in children in whom these tumors are not infrequently extra-adrenal, bilateral, or multiple. The entire abdomen must be carefully explored. It has also been suggested that, in children in whom one adrenal gland has been removed because of tumor, the other should be biopsied even if it appears to be normal. This is because Stefanini and co-authors observed that a tumor in the contralateral adrenal gland was not palpable and the gland looked normal in 5% of patients [38].

Postoperatively, patients who have been α-blocked with phenoxybenzamine may continue to have drug effect for 2 or 3 days. This means that a normal or low blood pressure does not preclude the existence of a missed tumor. Low blood pressure should be managed with volume replacement: care must be taken that urine output is adequate and that fluid overload does not occur. If hypertension has been prolonged or severe, left ventricular function may be compromised. In addition, in some patients, catecholamine myocarditis may contribute to suboptimal cardiac function [39,40].

The occurrence of hypertension soon after surgical removal of a pheochromocytoma indicates one of the following three situations: the presence of pain; the presence of residual tumor either unrecognized at operation or with metastases, or the presence of inadvertent renal artery ligation. Appropriate diagnostic studies and therapy should differentiate between these causes.

In any patient with a pheochromocytoma, histamine-releasing drugs should be avoided, since they may precipitate the release of catecholamines. On the other hand, the use of phenothiazines as antiemetics may result in profound hypotension.

Postoperative follow-up

Since tumor recurrence has been reported in nearly 10% of patients who have had a pheochromocytoma removed [14], long-term follow-up is mandatory. Initially patients should be seen two or three times a year and then yearly for 5–10 years. If there is any suspicion of tumor recurrence, catecholamine measurements should be undertaken. Patients suspected of having familial pheochromocytomas should be followed for the rest of their lives. They should be evaluated periodically for evidence of medullary thyroid carcinoma and hypoparathyroidism, as well as pheochromocytoma.

As already noted, patients with inoperable or

metastatic pheochromocytomas may be managed in the long term with the α- and β-blocking drugs with or without metyrosine. While effective chemotherapy for malignant tumors is only now being reported [41,42], long-term survival was possible in the past if the complications of hypertension and serious arrhythmias could be prevented. It should be noted that I-131 MIBG is being used as both a diagnostic and a therapeutic agent in malignant pheochromocytoma.

Pheochromocytoma during pregnancy [43–45]

Pregnancy occurs in adolescent females for whom pediatricians may be the responsible caregivers. It is therefore important to note briefly that unrecognized pheochromocytoma is a life-threatening condition for the mother and her fetus. In 1971 Schenker and Chowers reviewed 86 cases of pheochromocytoma in pregnancy [43]. If the tumor had been undiagnosed, over half of the mothers and their fetuses died. If the diagnosis was made during pregnancy, the maternal mortality was 17.3% but the fetal mortality was only slightly decreased. Therefore, any teenager presenting with significant hypertension of unknown origin should be screened for pheochromocytoma with urine and/or plasma catecholamines.

REFERENCES

1 Goldstein DS, Stull R, Eisenhofer G et al. Plasma 3,4 dihydroxyphenylalanine (Dopa) and catecholamines in neuroblastoma or pheochromocytoma. *Ann Intern Med* 1986;105:887–8.

2 Page LB, Coupland RE. Pheochromocytoma. In: *Disease-a-Month*. Chicago: Year Book, 1968.

3 Stackpole RH, Melicow MM, Uson AC. Pheochromocytoma in children. Report of 9 cases and review of the first 100 published cases with follow-up studies. *J Pediatr* 1963;63:315–30.

4 Manger WM, Gifford RW Jr, eds. *Pheochromocytoma*. New York: Springer-Verlag, 1977.

5 Evans CH, Westfall V, Atuk NO. Astrocytoma mimicking the features of pheochromocytoma. *N Engl J Med* 1972;286:1387–9.

6 Kontras SB. Urinary excretion of 3-methoxy-4-hydroxymandelic acid in children with neuroblastoma. *Cancer* 1962;15:978–86.

7 Knudsen AG, Strong LC. Mutation and cancer: neuroblastoma and pheochromocytoma. *Am J Hum Genet* 1972;24:514–32.

8 Hayes FA, Smith EI. Neuroblastoma. In: Pizzo PA, Poplack DG, eds. *Principles and practice of Pediatric Oncology*. Philadelphia: JB Lippincott, 1989:607–22.

9 Loggie JMH. Evaluation and management of childhood

10 Rosenfield NS, Leonidas JC, Barwick KW. Aggressive neuroblastoma simulating Wilms' tumor. *Radiology* 1988;166:165–7.

11 Ingelfinger JR. *Pediatric Hypertension*. Philadelphia: WB Saunders, 1982:199.

12 Greenberg RE, Gardner LI. Pheochromocytoma in father and son. Report of the eight affected kindred. *J Clin Endocrinol* 1959;19:351–3.

13 Linde P. Unusual tumor (pheochromocytoma) in infant 5 months old. *Nord Med* 1924;12:897.

14 Gifford RW Jr, Kvale WF, Maher FT et al. Clinical features, diagnosis and treatment of pheochromocytoma: a review of 76 cases. *Mayo Clin Proc* 1964;39:281–302.

15 Neff FC, Tice G, Walker GA, Ockerblad N. Adrenal tumor in female infant. *J Clin Endocrinol* 1942;2:125.

16 Sano T, Saito H, Inaba H et al. Immunoreactive somatostatin and vasoactive intestinal polypeptide in adrenal pheochromocytoma. An immunochemical and ultrastructural study. *Cancer* 1983;52:282–9.

17 Viale G, Dell'orto O, Moro E et al. Vasoactive intestinal polypeptide, somatostatin and calcitonin-producing adrenal pheochromocytoma associated with the watery diarrhea (WDHH) syndrome—first case report with immunohistochemical findings. *Cancer* 1985;55:1099–106.

18 Nigawara K, Suzuki T, Hirotsugu T et al. A case of recurrent malignant pheochromocytoma complicated by watery diarrhea, hypokalemia, achlorhydria syndrome. *J Clin Endocrinol Metab* 1987;65(5):1053–6.

19 Morrison AB. Islet cell tumor and the diarrheogenic syndrome. In: Fitzgerald PJ, Morrison AB, eds. *The Pancreas*. Baltimore: Williams & Wilkins, 1985:185.

20 Malik M, Connors R, Schwarz KB, O'Dorisio TM. Hormone-producing ganglioneuroblastoma simulating intestinal pseudoobstruction. *J Pediatr* 1990;116:406–8.

21 Roth K, Wilson D, Eberwine J et al. Acromegaly and pheochromocytoma: a multiple endocrine syndrome caused by a plurihormonal adrenal medullary tumor. *J Clin Endocrinol Metab* 1986;63:1421–5.

22 Veyre B, St Pieree A, Laffet G et al. Association pheochromocytoma-neurofibromatosis. *Nouv Presse Med* 1975;4:2873–6.

23 Guthrie GP Jr. Adrenal disorders causing hypertension in children. In: Kotchen TA, Kotchen JM eds. *High Blood Pressure in the Young*. Littleton, MA: John Wright, 1983:209–26.

24 Hume DM. Pheochromocytoma in the adult and child. *Am J Surg* 1960;99:458–96.

25 Kaplan MN, Cramer NJ, Holland OB. Single voided urinary metanephrine assays in screening for pheochromocytoma. *Arch Intern Med* 1977;137:190–3.

26 Ganguly A, Henry DP, Yune HY et al. Diagnosis and localization of pheochromocytoma. *Am J Med* 1979;67:21–6.

27 Quint LE, Glazer GM, Francis IR et al. Pheochromocytoma and paraganglioma: comparison of MR imaging with CT and I-131 MIBG scintigraphy. *Radiology* 1987;165:89–93.

28 Welch TJ, Sheedy PF, van Heerden JA et al. Pheochromocytoma: value of computed tomography. *Radiology* 1983;148:501–3.

29 Francis IR, Glazer GM, Shapiro B et al. Complementary roles of CT and ^{131}I-MIBG scintigraphy in diagnosing pheochro-

hypertension. *Surg Clin North Am* 1985;65:1623–49.

mocytoma. *Am J Radiol* 1983;141:719−25.

30 Shapiro B, Copp JE, Sisson JC *et al*. Iodine-131 metaiodobenzylguanidine for the locating of suspected pheochromocytoma: experience in 400 cases. *J Nucl Med* 1985;26:576−85.

31 Pekkarinen A, Scheinin TM, Nänto V. Localization of pheochromocytoma by vena caval catheterization and determination of plasma catecholamines. *Ann Chir Gynaecol Fenn* 1967;56:419−23.

32 Turner MC, de Quattro V, Falk R *et al*. Childhood familial pheochromocytoma. Conflicting results of localization techniques. *Hypertension* 1986;8:851−8.

33 Wallace JM, Gill DP. Prazosin in the diagnosis and treatment of pheochromocytoma. *JAMA* 1978;240:2752−3.

34 Nickerson M, Collier B. Drugs inhibiting adrenergic nerves and structures innervated by them. In: Goodman LS, Gilman A, eds. *The Pharmacologic Basis of Therapeutics*. 5th edn. New York: Macmillan, 1975;533−64.

35 Phenoxybenzamine (systemic). In: *Drug Information for the Health Care Professional*. Rockville: United States Pharmacopeial Convention, 1990:2230−1.

36 Beta-adrenergic blocking agents (systemic). In: *Drug Information for the Health Care Professional*. Rockville: United States Pharmacopeial Convention, 1990:620−41.

37 Metyrosine (systemic). In: *Drug Information for the Health Care Professional*. Rockville: United States Pharmacopeial

38 Stefanini P, Baglioni A, Fiorani P. Le pheochromocytome. *Lyon Chir* 1969;65:195.

39 Schaffer MS, Zuberbuhler P, Wilson G *et al*. Catecholamine cardiomyopathy: an unusual presentation of pheochromocytoma in children. *J Pediatr* 1981;99:276−9.

40 Imperato-McGinley J, Gautier T, Ehlers K *et al*. Reversibility of catecholamine-induced dilated cardiomyopathy in a child with a pheochromocytoma. *N Engl J Med* 1987;316:793−7.

41 Siddiqui MZ, Von Eyben FE, Spanos G. High voltage irradiation and combination chemotherapy for malignant pheochromocytoma. *Cancer* 1988;7:275−8.

42 Averbuch SD, Steakley CS, Young RC *et al*. Malignant pheochromocytoma: effective treatment with a combination of cyclosporin, vincristine and dacarbazine. *Ann Intern Med* 1988;109:267−73.

43 Schenker JG, Chowers I. Pheochromocytoma and pregnancy. *Obstet Gynecol Surg* 1971;26:739−47.

44 Burgess GE. Alpha blockade and surgical intervention of pheochromocytoma in pregnancy. *Obstet Gynecol* 1979;53:266−70.

45 Lyons CW, Colmorgen GHC. Medical management of pheochromocytoma in pregnancy. *Obstet Gynecol* 1988;72:450−1.

Convention, 1990:1891−2.

26 Miscellaneous Causes of Hypertension in Children

RUSSELL W. CHESNEY AND AARON L. FRIEDMAN

INTRODUCTION

Reviews of the characteristics of hypertension in children list as causes a number of etiologic factors that defy conventional pathophysiologic classification [1]. This chapter is intended as a source of information regarding the incidence, clinical features, pathophysiology, and treatment of some of these unusual causes of hypertension. In writing it, we have struggled with the total lack of recent information concerning the features of hypertension in many of these disorders and with the fact that many of the articles were written in an era before the role of catecholamines, prostaglandins, salt intake, the renin−angiotensin−aldosterone system, and vascular volume status was understood or could be accurately determined. We can appreciate why many reviewers have left these conditions merely listed in a table of secondary causes of hypertension and have not delved deeper into the mystery of the associated hypertension. Finally, we intend to indicate where we are speculating about the pathogenesis or therapy of a given cause of hypertension.

POLIOMYELITIS

Hypertension occurs secondary to poliomyelitis (Heine−Medin's disease) in two situations: during the acute phase of the disorder [2,3] and long after the acute phase has ceased, when the disorder is quiescent [4]. Hypertension during the acute phase occurs in anywhere from 7 to 60% of children and young adults with a much higher incidence of abnormally elevated blood pressure recordings being found in patients with more severe disease, involving paralysis of more limbs [2,3,5,6]. Hypertension is more frequent in males in a 2:1 ratio [3] and is far more commonly detected in fatal cases (more than 50%) and in children with bulbar paralysis (more than 33%) [7].

Although many of the publications from the 1940s and 50s do not indicate the method by which blood pressure was determined, in most instances a value of 145/95 mmHg was chosen as a cut-off point. Moreover, in many instances the blood pressure values recorded were much greater and malignant hypertension has been reported in association with bulbar encephalomyelitis [8]. In patients with respiratory difficulties, higher blood pressure readings are often recorded and retinal arteriolar changes, such as nicking and flame hemorrhages, are not uncommon [9]. In a report of a series of children with poliomyelitis from Delhi [5], 122 of 182 patients with severe disease demonstrated elevated blood pressures. Thus, this condition may be an important cause of hypertension among unimmunized children living in urban and rural areas of the underdeveloped world [10,11].

Although hypertension in the acute phase of poliomyelitis is generally self-limited, it may persist for months [2,3]. Indeed, it has been recognized for more than 45 years that hypertension can be detected many years after the original attack [4,11]. Most patients with chronic hypertension have involvement of two or more limbs and in patients with involvement of all four limbs as well as the trunk muscles, the incidence of hypertension in one series was 74% [11]. Not only are mean blood pressure values significantly higher in subjects 10−15 years after an attack of poliomyelitis, but blood pressure is also elevated in other paralytic disorders [12]. The incidence of chronic hypertension in poliomyelitis is approximately 15−25%, clearly higher than in control populations [4,11−14]. What is uncertain from these large series reporting chronic hypertension is whether the elevation in blood pressure has persisted from the original attack. Patients with more mild disease have blood pressure values exceeding 145/95 mmHg at an incidence of 5.7%, but with more severe involvement, elevated blood pressure levels are found in 22% of the subjects [14]. A strong association between the chronic use of respirators and bulbar involvement with elevated blood pressure values has also been shown, whereas family history of hypertension, the presence of renal calculi, pyuria, proteinuria, and hypertension in the acute phase of the disease are not more common among hypertensive subjects [13]. Hypertension also appears to involve both the systolic and diastolic phase of blood pressure [11,12].

The pathogenesis of hypertension during the acute phase of an attack of poliomyelitis is unclear. The ascribed mechanisms for hypertension were suggested in the era when epidemics of poliomyelitis occurred. These mechanisms did not consider autonomic nervous system dysfunction or changes in cardiovascular reflexes brought about by the changes in posture that attend an attack of poliomyelitis. Approximately a quarter of a century ago, it was shown that renal vasoexcitatory materials were found in the circulation of patients with both poliomyelitis and the Guillain–Barré syndrome (GBS) [15]. Prevailing hypotheses in the 1950s argued over the possibility of a neurogenic or a hypoxic origin of hypertension during the acute attack [5]; however, it is clear that an elevation in blood pressure often preceded a measured decline in respiratory vital capacity in patients with bulbospinal disease [3]. Some authorities postulated that hypertension was part of a central nervous system alarm reaction to hypoxia, the fear of paralysis, and/or ischemia of the vasomotor center [5,7]. It is clearly established that the vasomotor center will respond to cerebral ischemia by excitation which will increase peripheral vasoconstriction, peripheral resistance, and cardiac output [16]. Autopsy studies in hypertensive patients with bulbar involvement showed that autonomic nuclei in the hypothalamus and medullary reticular substance are involved with inflammatory changes in fatal acute attacks [3].

Although data are nonexistent, it is also tempting to speculate that hyperactivity of the sympathetic nervous system and the increased activity of the renin–angiotensin system found in GBS are germane to the acute-phase hypertension of poliomyelitis. Furthermore, postural changes and hypercalcemia, which may contribute to hypertension following fractures (see below), may also be important etiologic factors.

Late-phase hypertension may be related to autonomic hyperactivity [3], but it is clearly more common in patients with multiple-limb paralysis and atrophy.

This atrophy of skeletal muscles may result in a reduction in the number of blood vessels ("vessel drop-out") with a loss of capacitance vessels [12,13]. With any increase in cardiac output, blood pressure will rise since no channels are free to open and reduce the pressure in the system.

Virtually nothing has been written concerning the treatment of either acute- or late-phase hypertension in poliomyelitis. In the absence of established guidelines for therapy, it would seem prudent to individualize therapy. One could potentially use agents that would overcome autonomic hyperactivity such as β-blocking agents or captopril in the acute phase, and employ vasodilators and β-blocking agents in treating late-phase disease, but the use of these agents has not been validated.

GUILLAIN–BARRÉ SYNDROME

Hypertension in GBS is similar to poliomyelitis-related blood pressure changes in that its incidence is higher in more severe disease. During the height of paralysis, patients often have hypertension in association with tachycardia, which resolves as muscle function improves [17–21]. Hypertension in GBS is an acute-phase event and late-phase hypertension is not evident if recovery is complete.

Many, perhaps most, patients with GBS-associated hypertension have evidence of autonomic dysfunction. At the height of paralysis in these patients it is possible to demonstrate an elevation in the plasma levels of norepinephrine (+253%) and cortisol (+205%) and in urinary vanillylmandelic acid levels (+253%) [18]. It is uncertain whether increased cortisol reflects autonomic dysfunction.

Patients without hypertension and tachycardia do not have abnormal levels of these compounds. Further, at the time of recovery, the levels of cortisol, vanillylmandelic acid, and norepinephrine fall to the normal range.

This dysautonomia in GBS may well arise because of baroreceptor deafferentation which leads to resting tachycardia and hypertension [22]. Studies in normal subjects have indicated that lidocaine blockade of the glossopharyngeal and vagus nerves in the neck will deafferentate both arterial and cardiopulmonary baroreceptors. Muscle nerve sympathetic activity then appears to increase since it is normally under a state of strong baroreceptor inhibition [22]. Microelectrode recordings of muscle nerve sympathetic activity in patients with GBS indicate increased activity, not found in normal individuals or post recovery [18]. These findings have given rise to the hypothesis that increased muscle nerve sympathetic activity is related to a decrease in inhibition of the central vasomotor centers caused by abnormalities in the afferent limbs of the arterial and intrathoracic baroreflexes. Since many factors influence plasma vanillylmandelic acid and norepinephrine concentrations and since the measurement of muscle nerve sympathetic activity is difficult, some caution must be exercised in accepting the hypothesis [17]. However, this mechanism would account for the findings of hypertension and tachycardia in GBS patients. Further, it is possible that in poliomyelitis a similar mechanism is involved, although no direct evidence of the loss of baroreceptor function has been shown in the hypertension associated with this disease.

A further pathophysiologic mechanism for the hypertension in GBS involves activation of the renin−angiotension system [23,24]. Stapleton and colleagues [22] have described a child with GBS and hypertension who had normal levels of urinary catecholamines, but increased activity of the renin−angiotensin system. The finding of raised plasma renin activity (PRA) indicates that renin release is possibly stimulated by increased sympathetic tone [25]. In a single case, the finding of hypertension, a high hematocrit in association with increased activity of the sympathetic nervous system, and high PRA actually appeared when the man had only leg weakness [24]. Subsequently, he developed the full-blown picture of GBS.

Given increased activity of the sympathetic nervous and renin−angiotensin systems, it is appropriate to treat these patients with a β-blocking agent such as propranolol [23] or metoprolol. Even though captopril has been used successfully in many patients with increased activity of the renin−angiotensin system, this agent should be used with caution in patients with the GBS. Indeed, several patients receiving captopril therapy have been reported as developing a possible drug-induced Guillain−Barré neuropathy [26,27].

The prognosis for hypertension in GBS is excellent since all hormonal abnormalities return to normal with recovery [18,19,23,24].

TURNER'S SYNDROME

Turner's syndrome or XO gonadal dysgenesis is associated with hypertension in approximately 20−25% of patients with this condition [28,29]. No single cause of hypertension has been identified in this chromosomal disorder and both anatomic and endocrine causes of blood pressure elevation have been identified [1,29].

The cardiovascular anomalies of Turner's syndrome are complex and often directly account for hypertension [28]. Among the described lesions are coarctation of the aorta, renal artery stenosis, kinking or pseudocoarctation of the aorta, and renal artery branch stenosis [1,28−31]. The mechanisms and diagnostic evaluation or hypertension found in association with renal artery stenosis and coarctation of the aorta have been discussed in Chapters 23 and 24. It is very important to completely rule out these anatomic causes in all cases of hypertension in conjunction with Turner's syndrome. New techniques, including echocardiography, digital subtraction angiography, and noninvasive nuclear scans, simplify the process of evaluation. None the less, more than 90% of patients with Turner's syndrome will not have an anatomic lesion readily identifiable.

The use of estrogenic or androgenic steroids to induce puberty and to improve growth rates during adolescence can be associated with the development of hypertension [32−34]. While all women receiving estrogens should have their blood pressure monitored, it is obviously important that girls with Turner's syndrome should be carefully followed. The monitoring of blood pressure is particularly important because of the recent appreciation that girls with Turner's syndrome have a high incidence of bicuspid aortic valves [35,36], which in turn can be associated with dissecting aortic aneurysms [31,36,37]. Bicuspid aortic valves are also associated with dilatation of the aortic root and are probably the most common cardiac finding in Turner's syndrome [35].

Potential renal causes of hypertension include the occurrence of horseshoe kidneys, the presence of a single kidney, and renal malrotation [28,29,38]. The incidence of horseshoe kidneys may be as high as 50%. However, an association between this anomaly and hypertension is questionable. Chronic glomerulonephritis has also been rarely found in association with Turner's syndrome; a renal biopsy in 2 cases showed membranoproliferative glomerulonephritis [39,40].

Although Hashimoto's chronic lymphocytic thyroiditis has been reported with increased frequency in Turner's syndrome [28], patients have also been described who present with Graves disease or hyperthyroidism, which can lead to systolic hypertension [41].

Despite the observation, made in 1966, that hypertension is common [42] and that as many as 30% of adult patients with Turner's syndrome are hypertensive [28], a systematic detailed examination of the renin—angiotensin—aldosterone system has not yet been made. In one series of more than 200 patients with this syndrome, such risk factors as family history, karyotype, renal disease, hormone therapy, and cardiovascular changes other than coarctation did not appear to be more prevalent in hypertensive patients than in those with normal blood pressure values [28]. Obesity was a risk factor for hypertension in this series.

The therapy of hypertension in this disorder is empiric. After radiologic and ultrasonographic evaluation of the aorta, the heart, and the kidneys to rule out surgically remediable lesions, it would seem logical to use weight reduction and other non-pharmacologic approaches in managing milder degrees of hypertension. A β-blocking agent in appropriate doses should probably be the first drug tried, since, at least theoretically, these agents may be useful in preventing dissection of the aortic root lesions as well as in lowering blood pressure. Vasodilators and converting enzyme inhibitors could potentially be contraindicated if aortic root dilitation or renal artery stenosis is shown to exist since they could potentially reduce renal blood flow and lead to azotemia. It should also be appreciated that no controlled drug trials of the treatment of hypertension in Turner's syndrome have been reported.

GENITOURINARY SURGERY

Hypertension in patients with urologic disorders is well described. One aspect of this general category of hypertension is elevations in blood pressure with genitourinary surgery. Berens and colleagues described 16 patients who developed hypertension at the completion of or within 2—3 days of urologic surgery [42]. Patients ranged in age from 1 to 11.5 years and their hypertension persisted for 1—13 days. In all but 1 of the instances reported, the patients had hypertension, and in all but 3 the patients had surgery on and/or catheterization of a ureter. The authors compared the group undergoing genitourinary surgery with a group of patients who underwent surgery not involving the urinary tract.

They found that patients with genitourinary surgery manifested their postoperative hypertension for a much longer period of time. Belman and Lewy described 6 patients with severe hydronephrosis and mild renal insufficiency (serum creatinine 1—3 mg/dl) who underwent permanent cutaneous urinary diversions [43]. These 6 patients developed an increase in their blood pressure as compared to preoperative values in the immediate postoperative period. The authors state that all patients had a return to their normal preoperative blood pressure values within 6 weeks. Fonkalsrud and Smith reported that 9 of 50 patients undergoing ileal conduit urinary diversion developed hypertension [44].

The cause of this form of hypertension has not been clearly delineated. Authors have speculated that the renin—angiotensin—aldosterone system is involved in the transient hypertension that occurs with urinary tract surgery [45]. Belman and Lewy [43] demonstrated elevated peripheral PRA in 6 children during hypertensive phases following urinary diversion. All patients in this study had hydronephrosis—often unilateral—as their underlying disease. Hyperreninemic hypertension occurred following the urinary diversion, and the authors suggested that the procedure resulted in sustained renin release [44,46—48]. In the report by Berens and colleagues, unoperated hydronephrosis was the predominant presurgical diagnosis [42]. Although the authors did not measure PRA, they believed that the renin—angiotensin—aldosterone system led to hypertension directly or indirectly through enhanced sympathetic tone. Numerous reports have documented hypertension with hydronephrosis, especially unilateral disease [47,49,50] in both adults [47—51] and children [43—46,52]. Hyperreninemia has been considered the major pathophysiologic mechanism. However, hydronephrosis and hypertension without hyperreninemia have also been reported [53,54].

Hypertension associated with urinary tract surgery is not limited to patients with hydronephrosis. Hicks and co-authors reported 8 children with vesicoureteral reflux and hypertension [54]. Gabriel and Heslop reported hypertension with ureteric ligation [55], and hypertension during transurethral surgery has also been documented. The hypertension during transurethral surgery was associated with the absorption of large volumes of irrigating solution and represents another mechanism by which hypertension can develop with urologic surgery [56]. Finally, in patients with cervical and thoracic cord lesions uro-

logic procedures may result in severe hypertension
[57]. This hypertension is the result of autonomic
hyperreflexia, which represents the exaggerated, un-
inhibited spinal cord reflex to the presence of urinary
tract distension or urinary tract manipulation.

HYPERTENSION WITH ORTHOPEDIC PROCEDURES

Hypertension has been found in children who have
undergone orthopedic surgery. Early reports documented elevated blood pressure following leg-
lengthening procedures [58–61]. Yosipovitch and
Palti [60] were able to demonstrate in animal studies
that the rise in blood pressure following leg lengthening was mediated through a reflex response to
tension developed in the sciatic nerve. Harandi and
Zahu reported hypertension following repair of a
flexion contracture of the knee [61]. They suggested
that the hypertension was caused by stretching of the
sympathetic network surrounding blood vessels.

Orthopedic immobilization has also been shown
to result in hypertension. In a report by Turner and
associates, children with orthopedic immobilization
had a fourfold higher incidence of hypertension
compared to other hospitalized children [62]. They
characterized the hypertension in immobilized children as mild, transient, not associated with other
symptoms, and having no consistent etiology. They
speculated on a number of causes for immobilization-
associated hypertension. These included sympathetic
stimulation, as proposed by Harandi and Zahu, and
hypercalcemia secondary to immobilization. Elevated
serum ionized calcium, which can be present after
immobilization, has been shown to increase vascular
tone.

Regardless of the cause, mobilization often resulted
in a normalization of blood pressure. In some
patients, despite continued casting, blood pressure
returned to normal when the children were able to
ambulate.

Further observations regarding hypertension and
orthopedic procedures were provided by Linshaw
and colleagues [63]. They reported 5 children who
developed hypertension associated with traction
for fractures. In 3 of the 5 cases, lower extremity traction was used, and in 2 cases traction was used on
the upper extremity. These authors measured PRA
and found it elevated in 1 patient. They suggested,
however, that in patients who are immobilized and
in whom bedrest may lead to sodium and water

Table 26.1 Miscellaneous causes of hypertension in children not involving renal parenchyma

Poliomyelitis
Guillain–Barré syndrome
Turner's syndrome
Genitourinary surgery
Fractures
Drugs
Glucocorticoids
Phencyclidine (PCP or angel dust)
Burns
Leg traction and other orthopedic procedures
Cyclic vomiting with dehydration

Table 26.2 Causes of hypertension in Guillain–Barré syndrome

Increased catecholamine release
Increased renin–angiotensin system activity
Increased cortisol secretion
Arterial and thoracic baroreceptor deafferentation

Table 26.3 Reported causes of hypertension in Turner's syndrome

Coarctation of the aorta
Renal artery stenosis
Renal malrotation (?)
Horseshoe kidney (?)
Chronic glomerulonephritis
Thyrotoxicosis
Estrogen replacement
Androgens to promote growth (?)
Obesity

retention, even normal PRA may be "inappropriate"
for the patients' expanded extracellular volume.

BURN HYPERTENSION

Transient hypertension may complicate the clinical
course of children with extensive burns, particularly
in those suffering from deep third-degree burns
[64–69]. The exact incidence of burn hypertension is
difficult to determine from the rather sparse clinical
literature on this subject but is said to vary between
10.4 and 89.7% of patients [68]. Several pathogenic
mechanisms have been postulated and may be at
play either alone or in combination. Volume depletion with subsequent elevation of PRA and enhanced production of angiotensin II has been noted

[65]. Fluid administration, as a part of burn resuscitation, and the use of topical compounds containing sodium chloride which is absorbed have also been postulated to cause hypertension [66]. It should also be noted that the presence of hypertension correlates with elevated PRA, plasma aldosterone values, cortisol concentrations, and cardiac index [1].

It has also been found in a study of 8 hypertensive and 7 normotensive children with the same extent of burn that hypervolemia and elevated total peripheral resistance were hallmarks of the hypertensive children [67]. Hypertensive and normotensive children did not differ in terms of PRA, catecholamines, aldosterone, or electrolyte values. However, the authors of this study speculated that the initial neuro-endocrine response to burns included activation of the renin—angiotensin system.

Therefore, several mechanisms appear to underlie the hypertension associated with burns in children. The therapy varies according to the etiology of the hypertension and again should be individualized. Finally, it should be appreciated that burn-healing leads to resolution of hypertension. However, while the child is undergoing burn care, he or she may develop hypertensive encephalopathy and seizures [69]; thus, this complication can greatly influence the management of the burned patient.

HYPERTENSION AND DRUGS

Hypertension is associated with a large variety of pharmaceutical agents. The number of drugs leading to hypertension is beyond the scope of this review. We will focus on certain agents with which hypertension is common or of particular significance.

Glucocorticoids

Hypertension is a common occurrence with glucocorticoid excess. Approximately 20% of patients receiving pharmacologic doses of glucocorticoids develop hypertension, whereas 80% of patients with endogenous glucocorticoid excess (Cushing's syndrome) develop elevated blood pressure [70–73]. The incidence of cardiovascular complications in patients with Cushing's syndrome may be as high as 40% [74,75].

The mechanisms by which glucocorticoids cause hypertension are by no means firmly established. At least five have been postulated [76]. These include:

1 *Changes in sodium transport.* Glucocorticoids increase renal Na^+-K^+-ATPase activity which favors increased sodium reabsorption by the kidney [77]. However, it is unclear if this finding is indeed important in the pathophysiology of glucocorticoid-induced hypertension.

2 *Effect on vascular smooth muscle.* Some authors have shown an enhancement of the pressor response to epinephrine following pretreatment with cortisol or other glucocorticoids [78–80]. Others have shown no effect of glucocorticoids on vascular responsivity [81].

3 *Hemodynamic.* Glucocorticoids are thought to shift interstitial volume to the plasma volume compartment. The response of the vasculature to this increase in plasma volume is to increase total peripheral resistance and thereby maintain an elevated blood pressure. This hypothesis remains unproven and data regarding plasma volume and extracellular volume with glucocorticoids show little, if any, change in the volume compartments [82,83].

4 *Hormonal changes.* Speculation has focused on the role of the renin—angiotensin system as a factor in glucocorticoid-mediated hypertension. Because many glucocorticoids have little if any mineralocorticoid activity, the postulate presumes a rise in renin activity leading to an increased circulation of angiotensin and secondarily circulating aldosterone. Glucocorticoids have been shown by some investigators to elevate plasma renin substrate and activity [84]. Others have not documented a change in PRA [85]. Further, captopril does not prevent glucocorticoid-induced hypertension [86]. Preliminary work has suggested involvement of the sympathetic nervous system with glucocorticoid-induced hypertension [87]. Other studies have suggested prostaglandin-mediated effects of glucocorticoid leading to reduced vasodilator activity [88,89]. The last two postulates will require further study.

5 *Direct action.* Whitworth [76,90] has suggested that the hypertensive action of glucocorticoids is a separate (from any glucocorticoid or mineralocorticoid activity) action. She has suggested that the hypertensinogenic receptor is in the central nervous system. As with the other proposed mechanisms, more study is clearly needed to strengthen this hypothesis. In most instances withdrawal of the glucocorticoid or reducing the dose reverses the hypertension. Many antihypertensive drugs are effective. A glucocorticoid antagonist has been studied in Cushing's syndrome and has been shown to ameliorate hypertension as well as other features of Cushing's syndrome [91].

Cocaine, phencyclidine, and sympathomimetic agents

Use of a number of illicit drugs is associated with the development of hypertension. Two drugs known to have hypertension as an important aspect of their toxicity are cocaine and phencyclidine (PCP).

Cocaine (benzoylmethylecgonine) has received a great deal of attention because of its addictive nature, easy accessibility, and the deaths of young athletes from overdoses. Its local anesthetic effect is probably due to its ability to block the initiation and conduction of nerve impulses by altering sodium ion permeability during depolarization [92]. Systemically, cocaine blocks the re-uptake of neurotransmitters (norepinephrine and dopamine) at presynaptic sites leading to excess neurotransmitter. In this way activation of the sympathetic nervous system leads to vasoconstriction, hypertension, and tachycardia. Further, the postsynaptic sites are sensitized to the effects of catecholamines such as epinephrine and norepinephrine [93]. Deaths have been associated with cocaine: cardiovascular events (myocardial infarction, arrhythmia, hypertension) are the most common [94].

Phencyclidine made its "street" appearance in the late 1960s as "angel dust." Its mechanism of action is unclear: purported ones are stimulation of opiate receptors: stimulation of α-adrenergic receptors, and inhibition of cholinesterase activity. Mild toxicity is associated with mainly central nervous system symptoms but with higher doses hypertension and tachycardia are frequently present (approximately 50%) and circulatory collapse due to acute myocardial depression is seen with very high doses [95].

The sympathomimetic agents are widely used in medicine. Amphetamines are used to treat hyperactivity and are abused as agents to overcome fatigue or for diet control and weight reduction. Pseudoephedrine, ephedrine, and phenylpropanolamine are used as decongestants, and oxymetazoline, xylometazoline etc. are used in topical decongestant sprays. Isoproterenol, metaproterenol, terbutaline, etc. are used as bronchodilators. All these agents have the potential to cause hypertension, especially when used frequently and in high doses [96].

ACKNOWLEDGMENT

This study was supported in part by National Institutes of Health grants AM31682 and AM37223.

REFERENCES

1 Ingelfinger JR. *Pediatric Hypertension*. Philadelphia: WB Saunders, 1982:159.
2 McDowell FH, Plum F. Arterial hypertension associated with acute anterior poliomyelitis. *N Engl J Med* 1951;245: 241−5.
3 Vickers HD. Anterior poliomyelitis, relation to hypertension in young adults. *NY State J Med* 1940;40:55.
4 Coryllos E. Etiology and occurrence of arterial hypertension in poliomyelitis: a review of the literature. *Arch Pediatr* 1983;70:122−34.
5 Sehgal H, Olseroi M. A clinical study of severe form of acute poliomyelitis in children. *Indian Pediatr* 1977; 14:47−53.
6 Kemp E. Arterial hypertension in poliomyelitis. *Acta Med Scand* 1951;157:109−18.
7 Ohry A, Ezra D, Brooks ME. Malignant hypertension after encephalopoliomyelitis. *Harenfvah* 1981;101:360−1.
8 Neubauer H, Mainzer K. Hypertensive arteriolopathy in poliomyelitis. *Klin Augenheilk* 1963;142:708−12.
9 Sancheti KH, Sahasiabudhe BG, Bahingare RK. Clinical profile of 3005 polio children in a rural population. *Indian J Pediatr* 1979;46:237−44.
10 Zimanyi J, Prohaszka M, Szondy M, Ormai S. Arterial hypertension after poliomyelitis. *Acta Med Scand* 1959;164:497−505.
11 Welner A, Yosipovitch ZH, Groen JJ. Elevated blood pressure in children and adolescents with residual paralysis and deformities from poliomyelitis and other crippling disorders. *J Chronic Dis* 1966;19:1157−64.
12 Ostfeld AM. Sustained hypertension after poliomyelitis. *Arch Intern Med* 1961;107:551−7.
13 Kohn LA. The incidence of hypertension long after poliomyelitis. *J Chronic Dis* 1967;20:269−73.
14 Shorr E, Swerfoch BW. Hepato-renal vasotropic factors in blood during chronic essential hypertension in man. *Trans Assoc Am Phys* 1961;61:350−60.
15 Greyton AC. *Textbook of Medical Physiology*. Philadelphia: WB Saunders, 1981:206−87.
16 Johnson RH. Autonomic dysfunction in clinical disorders with particular references to catecholamine release. *J Auton Nerv Syst* 1983;7:219−32.
17 Ahmad J, Kham AS, Siddiqui MA. Estimation of plasma and urinary catecholamines in Guillain−Barré syndrome. *Jpn J Med* 1985;24:24−9.
18 Fagius J, Wallin BG. Microneurographic evidence of excessive sympathetic outflow in the Guillain−Barré syndrome. *Brain* 1983;106:589−600.
19 Radhadrishnau K, Chopra JS, Khattri HN. Cardiovascular dysautonomia in Guillain−Barré syndrome. *J Assoc Phys India* 1982;30:493−4.
20 Sainani GS, Deshpaude DV. Dysautonomia and Guillain−Barré syndrome. *J Assoc Phys India* 1982;30:491−2.
21 Fagius J, Wallin BG, Sundliof G, Nerhed C, Englesson S. Sympathetic outflow in man after anesthesia of the glossopharyngeal and vagus nerves. *Brain* 1985;108:423−38.
22 Stapleton FB, Skoglund RR, Duggett RB. Hypertension associated with the Guillain−Barré syndrome. *Pediatrics* 1978;62:588−90.

23 Richards AM, Nicholls MG, Beard ME, Parkin PJ, Espinei EA. Severe hypertension and raised hematocrit: unusual presentation of Guillain–Barré syndrome. *Postgrad Med J* 1985;61:53–5.

24 Laufer J, Passwell J, Keren G, Brandt N, Cohen BE. Raised plasma renin activity in the hypertension of the Guillain–Barré syndrome. *Br Med J* 1981;282:1272–3.

25 Atkinson AB, Brown JJ, Lever AF, Robertson JI. Combined treatment of severe intractable hypertension with captopril and diuretic. *Lancet* 1980;ii:105–8.

26 Atkinson AM, Brown JJ, Lever AF et al. Neurologic dysfunction in two patients receiving captopril and cimetidine. *Lancet* 1980;ii:36–7.

27 Loggie J. Systemic hypertension. In: Moss AJ, Adams FH, Emmanoulidies GC, eds. *Heart Disease in Infants, Children and Adolescents*. 3rd edn. Philadelphia: WB Saunders, 1983;692–707.

28 Hall JG, Sybert VP, Williamson RA, Risher NL, Reed SD. Turner's syndrome. *West J Med* 1982;137:32–49.

29 Nivelon JL, Mabille JP, Turc C et al. Turner's syndrome with generalized arterial hypertension, pseudocoarctation of the aorta (kinking) and a ring-form X chromosome. *Pediatrics* 1970;33:383–92.

30 Lie JT. Aortic dissection in Turner's syndrome. *Am Heart J* 1982;103:1077–80.

31 Levine LS. Treatment of Turner's syndrome with estrogen. *Pediatrics* 1978;62:1178–83.

32 Dewhurst CJ, De Koos EB, Haines RM. Replacement hormone therapy in gonadal dysgenesis. *Br J Obstet Gynaecol* 1975;82:412–16.

33 Root AW. Use of oxandrolone in Turner's syndrome. *J Pediatr* 1980;96:166–9.

34 Miller MJ, Geffner ME, Lippe BM et al. Echocardiography reveals a high incidence of bicuspid aortic valve in Turner's syndrome. *J Pediatr* 1983;102:47–50.

35 Slater DN. Turner's syndrome associated with bicuspid aortic stenosis and dissecting aortic aneurysm. *Postgrad Med J* 1982;58:436–8.

36 Strader WJ III, Wachtel HL, Lundberg GD Jr. Hypertension and aortic rupture in gonadal dysgenesis. *J Pediatr* 1971;79:473–5.

37 Litvak AS. The association of significant renal anomalies with Turner's syndrome. *J Urol* 1978;120:671–2.

38 Goodyer PR. Turner's syndrome, 46X, del (X) (pII), persistent complement activation and membranoproliferative glomerulonephritis. *Am J Nephrol* 1982;2:272–5.

39 Glasier CM. A 6-year-old girl with Turner's syndrome and proteinuria (clinical conference). *Urol Radiol* 1981;3:189–90.

40 Kawai K. A case of Turner's syndrome with hyperthyroidism. *Endocrinol Japan* 1978;25:631–4.

41 Haddad HM, Wilkius L. Congenital anomalies associated with gonadal aplasia: review of 55 cases. *Pediatrics* 1959;23:885–902.

42 Berens SC, Lunde LM, Goodwin WE. Transitory hypertension following urologic surgery in children. *Pediatrics* 1966;58:194–200.

43 Belman AB, Lewy PR. Acute transient renin-mediated hypertension in children following urinary diversion. *Urology* 1984;3:693–6.

44 Fonkalsrud EW, Smith JP. Permanent urinary diversion in infancy and childhood. *J Urol* 1965;94:132–8.

45 Munof AJ, Baralt JFP, Melendez MT. Arterial hypertension in infants with hydronephrosis: report of 6 cases. *Am J Dis Child* 1977;131:38–43.

46 Riehle RA Jr, Vaughan ED Jr. Renin participation in hypertension associated with unilateral hydronephrosis. *J Urol* 1981;126:243–6.

47 Garrett J, Polse SL, Morrow JW. Ureteral obstruction and hypertension. *Am J Med* 1970;49:271–7.

48 Weidmann C, Beretta-Piccoli C, Hirsch D, Reubi FC, Massry SG. Curable hypertension with unilateral hydronephrosis. *Ann Intern Med* 1977;87:437–40.

49 Schwartz DT. Unilateral upper urinary tract obstruction and arterial hypertension. *NY State J Med* 1969;69:668–71.

50 Wise HM. Hypertension resulting from hydronephrosis. *JAMA* 1975;231:491–2.

51 Carella JA, Silber I. Hyperreninemic hypertension in an infant secondary to pelviureteral obstruction treated successfully by surgery. *J Pediatr* 1976;88:987–9.

52 Vaughan ED Jr, Buhler FR, Laragh JH. Normal renin secretion in hypertensive patients with primary unilateral chronic hydronephrosis. *J Urol* 1974;112:153–6.

53 Palmer JM, Zwerman FG, Assaykeen TA. Renal hypertension due to hydronephrosis with normal plasma renin activity. *N Engl J Med* 1970;283:1032–3.

54 Hicks CC, Woodard JR, Walton KN, Filandi GP. Hypertension as a complication of vesicoureteral reflux in children. *Urology* 1976;7:587–93.

55 Gabriel R, Heslop RW. Reversible hypertension and hypertension and hyperreninemia after accidental ureteric ligation. *Br Med J* 1977;2:999–1000.

56 Neder RM, O'Higgins JW, Aldrete JA. Autonomic hyperreflexia in urologic surgery. *JAMA* 1970;213:867–9.

57 Mark LC, Marx F, Arkins RE et al. (Anesthesia Study Committee of New York State Society of Anesthesiologists): Clinical Anesthesia Conference. Hypertension during transurethral surgery. *NY State J Med* 1966;66:979–80.

58 Wilk LH, Bagley CE. Hypertension, another complication of the leg lengthening procedure. *J Bone Joint Surg* 1963; 45A:1263–5.

59 Axer A, Elkon A, Eliahu HE. Hypertension as a complication of limb lengthening. *J Bone Joint Surg* 1974;45A:520–3.

60 Yosipovitch ZH, Palti Y. Alterations in blood pressure during leg lengthening. *J Bone Joint Surg* 1967;49A:1352–9.

61 Harandi BA, Zahu A. Severe hypertension following correction of flexion contracture of the knee. *J Bone Joint Surg* 1974;56A:1733–8.

62 Turner MC, Ruley EJ, Buckley KM, Strife CF. Blood pressure elevation in children with orthopedic immobilization. *J Pediatr* 1979;95:989–92.

63 Linshaw MA, Stapleton FE, Gruskin AB, Baluarte HJ, Harbin GL. Traction related hypertension in children. *J Pediatr* 1979;95:994–6.

64 Lieberman E. Clinical assessment of the hypertensive patient. In: Kochen TA, Kotchner JM, eds. *Clinical Approaches to High Blood Pressure in the Young*. Boston: John Wright/PSG 1983:244–6.

65 Dillon MA. Clinical aspects of hypertension. In: Holliday MA, Barratt TM, Vernier RL, eds. *Pediatric Nephrology*. 2nd edn. Baltimore: Williams & Wilkins, 1987:743–57.

66 Brizio M, Moltini L, Moller A, Coutler LC. Incidence of post-burn hypertension crisis in patients admitted to two burn centers and a community hospital in the United States. *Scan J Plast Rescontr Surg* 1970;13:21−8.

67 Popp MB, Friedberg DL, MacMillan BG. Clinical characteristics of hypertension in burned children. *Am Surg* 1980;191:473−8.

68 Popp MB, Silberstein EB, Srivastava LS. A pathophysiologic study of the hypertension associated with burn injury in children. *Ann Surg* 1981;193:817−24.

69 Douglas BS, Broadfoot MJ. Hypertension in burnt children. *Aust NZ J Surg* 1972;42:194−6.

70 Savage O, Copeman WSC, Chapman L, Wells MV, Treadwell BLJ. Pituitary and adrenal hormones in rheumatoid arthritis. *Lancet* 1962;i:232−4.

71 Treadwell BLJ, Sever ED, Savage O, Copeman WSC. Side effects of long term treatment with corticosteroids and corticotrophin. *Lancet* 1964;i:1121−3.

72 Greminger P, Tenschert W, Vetter W, Luscher T, Vetter H. Hypertension in Cushing's syndrome. In: Mantero F, Biglieri EG, eds. *Endocrinology of Hypertension*. London: Academic Press, 1982:103−10.

73 Soffer L, Lannacore A, Gabrilove J. Cushing's syndrome. *Am J Med* 1961;30:129−34.

74 Welbourn RB, Montgomery DAD, Kennedy TL. The natural history of treated Cushing's syndrome. *Br J Surg* 1971; 58:1−16.

75 Ross EJ, Lynch DC. Cushing's syndrome − killing disease: discriminatory value of signs and symptoms aiding early diagnosis. *Lancet* 1982;ii:646−9.

76 Whitworth JA. Mechanisms of glucocorticoid-induced hypertension. *Kidney Int* 1987;31:1213−24.

77 Charney AN, Silva P, Besarab A, Epstein FH. Separate effects of aldosterone, DOCA and methylprednisolone on renal Na$^+$-K$^+$-ATPase. *Am J Physiol* 1974;227−345.

78 Handa M, Kondo K, Suzuki H, Saruta T. Dexamethasone hypertension in rats: role of prostaglandins and pressor sensitivity to norepinephrine. *Hypertension* 1984;6:236−41.

79 Lecomte J, Grevisse J, Beaumarriage M. Potentiation per l'hydrocortisone des effets moteurs del l'adrenaline. *Arch Int Pharmacodyn* 1959;119:133−7.

80 Anderson WP, Harris DT. Blood pressure responses to prolonged infusions of adrenaline and noradrenaline in conscious dogs. *Clin Exp Hypertens* 1983;6:1469−84.

81 Kohlman-Ribeiro A, Marson-Saragoca M, Ramos OL. Methylprednisolone induced hypertension: role for the autonomic and renin−angiotensin systems. *Hypertension* 1981;3(suppl II):107−11.

82 Conway FJ, Hatton R. The effect of β-adrenergic blockade on the development of deoxycorticosterone acetate in the dog. *Br J Pharmacol* 1977;60:289−90.

83 Conway FJ, Hatton R. Development of deoxycorticosterone acetate hypertension in the dog. *Circ Res* 1977; 43(suppl 1):82−6.

84 Drakoff LR, Selvadurai R, Sutter E. Effect of methylprednisolone upon arterial pressure and the renin angiotensin system in the rat. *Am J Physiol* 1975;228:613−17.

85 Okuno T, Suzuki H, Saruta T. Dexamethasone hypertension in rats. *Clin Exp Hypertens* 1981;3:1075−86.

86 Elijovich R, Drakoff LR. Mechanism of the response of captopril in glucocorticoid hypertension. *Clin Exp Hypertens* 1982;4:1795−814.

87 Waeber B, Gavras H, Bresnahan MR, Gravras I, Brunner HR. Role of vasoconstrictor systems in experimental glucocorticoid hypertension in rats. *Clin Sci* 1983;65:255−61.

88 Hong S, Levine L. Inhibition of arachadonic acid release from cells as the biochemical action of anti-inflammatory corticosteroids. *Proc Natl Acad Sci USA* 1976;73:1730−4.

89 Rascher W, Dietz R, Schomig A *et al.* Modulation of sympathetic vascular tone by prostaglandins in corticosterone-induced hypertension in rats. *Clin Sci* 1979;57:235s−7s.

90 Scoggins BA, Butkus A, Coghlan JP *et al.* The role of "mineralocorticoids," "glucocorticoids" and "hypertensioninogenic" steroids in ACTH-induced hypertension. In: Kaufman W, Wambach G, Helber A, Meurer KA, eds. *Mineralocorticoids and Hypertension* Berlin: Springer-Verlag, 1983:113−27.

91 Nieman L, Chrousos GP, Kellner C *et al.* Successful treatment of Cushing's syndrome with the glucocorticoid antagonist RU486 (abstract). In: *Endocrinology: Proceedings of the 7th International Congress of Endocrinology, Quebec City, 1−7 July 1984*. The Hague: Excerpta Medica.

92 Cregler LL, Mark H. Medical complications of cocaine abuse. *N Engl J Med* 1986;315:1495−1500.

93 Ritchie JM, Greene NM: Local anesthesics. In: Gilman AG, Goodman LS, Rall TW, Murad F, eds. *The Pharmacological Basic of Therapeutics*. 7th edn. New York: Macmillan, 1985:309−10.

94 Fischman MW, Schuster CR, Resnekov L *et al.* Cardiovascular and subjective effects of intravenous cocaine administration in humans. *Arch Gen Psychiatry* 1976;33:983−9.

95 McCaron MM, Schulze BW, Thompson GA *et al.* Acute phencyclidine intoxication. Clinical patterns, complications and treatment. *Ann Emerg Med* 1981;10:290−7.

96 Arena JM, Drew RH. *Poisoning*. 5th edn. Springfield, IL: Charles Thomas 1985:631−5.

27 Blood Pressure in Young Athletes

JAMES L. CHRISTIANSEN AND WILLIAM B. STRONG

It has been estimated that 17 million young people in the USA participate in organized sports, with 7 million involved in interscholastic competition at the secondary school level [1]. It is also estimated that 2–5% of the adolescent population have elevated arterial blood pressure [2]. This would suggest that between 140 000 and 350 000 young athletes have elevated blood pressure. The magnitude of this problem warrants consideration. The injudicious labeling of a young athlete as having high blood pressure may have immediate detrimental effects in terms of poor self-image, not to mention the long-term ramifications on further athletic training, employment potential, and insurance premiums [3].

Prudent recommendations concerning eligibility of such athletes for competition and participation are necessary. Unfortunately, the practicing physician is faced with a paucity of information on this topic, with few articles specifically addressing the problem in a comprehensive fashion [3–5]. Therefore, the objectives of this chapter will be to:
1 review the physiologic parameters of the cardiovascular response and adaptation to dynamic and static exercise;
2 evaluate the role of exercise in blood pressure control;
3 describe the special features of hypertension in athletes;
4 evaluate the risk of blood pressure elevation for sudden death or disease progression during sports participation;
5 review current therapy of hypertension in the context of athletic performance, and
6 provide rational guidelines for the management of athletes with blood pressure elevation.

CARDIOVASCULAR RESPONSE TO STATIC AND DYNAMIC EXERCISE

Dynamic exercise (often referred to as aerobic) involves change in muscle length and joint movement, with rhythmic contractions of large muscle groups [6]. Running, swimming, and bicycling are primarily dynamic forms of exercise. Static (isometric) exercise involves development of a relatively large force with use of a smaller muscle mass, with little or no change in muscle length or joint movement. This would occur in the contraction of skeletal muscles against fixed objects [6]. Weight lifting, wrestling, and field events such as the shot-put and hammer-throw have a major static component, as does line blocking in football. The hemodynamic response to each form of exercise is distinctive.

Dynamic exercise evokes a marked increase in heart rate, cardiac output, and oxygen consumption ($\dot{V}o_2$). Normally, systolic blood pressure increases with the intensity of the work load, diastolic blood pressure remains unchanged, and mean blood pressure rises [6,7]. Systemic vascular resistance (SVR), a calculated number (SVR = MAP/CI, where MAP = mean arterial pressure, and CI = cardiac index), invariably decreases since the magnitude of increase in cardiac output generally exceeds that of the pressure change. Furthermore, the extent to which the heart rate and systolic blood pressure increase during dynamic exercise may depend on the muscle groups being used. For example, at a given level of $\dot{V}o_2$, performance of arm work effects a greater blood pressure, lower cardiac output, and greater change in peripheral resistance than the performance of leg work [8].

Static exercise, as tested during isometric hand grip or free weight lifting with intra-arterial blood pressure monitoring, produces a smaller increase in cardiac output and $\dot{V}o_2$ with a marked rise in mean arterial pressure. Systemic vascular resistance remains within normal limits or increases since cardiac output and mean arterial blood pressure tend to rise proportionally [9,10]. The observed increase in diastolic blood pressure is thought to be due to an increase in cardiac output, but may also be due to reflex effects originating in the active muscles [11]. These responses are elicited by contraction of even a small muscle mass, resulting in a progressive increase in blood pressure as the contraction is sustained. An important factor in determining the blood pressure response to static exercise is percentage of maximum contraction exerted by a given muscle group; the mass of muscle involved is less important [11]. In comparison, when the same subject performs static or dynamic exercise which evokes similar increases in $\dot{V}o_2$, an increase in mean arterial pressure occurs only with the static effort [7]. In one study, intra-arterial blood pressure monitoring during weight lifting by means of the single arm curl and double leg press documented average peak blood pressures of 255/190 and 320/250 mmHg respectively [10]. This degree of blood pressure elevation was thought to be due to a contribution of the mechanical compression effect of contracting muscles, the pressor reflex of static contraction, and the superimposition of an elevated intrathoracic pressure (during maximal lifts) caused by the Valsalva maneuver.

Thus, dynamic exercise may be thought of as primarily producing a volume load, and static exercise as producing a pressure load on the left ventricle [12]. In hypertensive patients, the hemodynamic response to dynamic exercise parallels that of normotensive individuals, but the peak level of arterial pressure is higher [13]. A similar pattern is observed with static exercise. In reality, few physical activities can be described as purely dynamic or static, especially when consideration is given to factors such as the position played on a team and training regimens used prior to and throughout the competitive season. Nevertheless, in formulating guidelines as to recommendations for competitive athletes with hypertension, the 16th Bethesda Conference on cardiovascular abnormalities in the athlete attempted to classify sports in terms of dynamic and static demands [12]. Table 27.1 presents that classification.

MORPHOLOGIC AND FUNCTIONAL CARDIAC ADAPTATIONS TO CHRONIC EXERCISE

Hearts of athletes engaged in predominantly static exercise show distinct differences in cardiac morphology when compared to those of athletes involved in predominantly dynamic exercise. Both static and dynamic exercise change several factors that are important in determining myocardial oxygen demand [14,15]. These are heart rate, wall tension, and con-

tractile state of the ventricle. Wall tension is affected by pressure development and ventricular volume. In dynamic exercise, there is a large increase in heart rate and an increase in stroke volume. This is achieved by both an increase in end-diastolic volume (Frank–Starling mechanism) and a decrease in end-systolic volume (increased contractile state). Static exercise evokes a smaller increase in heart rate and little change in the end-diastolic and end-systolic volumes of the left ventricle. However, arterial pressure and contractile state of the ventricle are increased.

The morphologic sequelae of these changes were first described in cross-sectional studies comparing athletes to sedentary control subjects. An echocardiographic comparison of a group of long-distance runners and swimmers (dynamic exercise athletes) with a group of wrestlers and shot-putters (static exercise athletes) demonstrated an increase in left ventricular mass common to both groups, with only the dynamic athletes exhibiting an increase in left ventricular internal dimension [16]. In contrast, only the static athletes showed significant increases in the thickness of the septum and posterior left ventricular wall. Thus, the heart of the athlete engaged in endurance sports exemplifies that of a chronic volume overload characterized by hypertrophy associated with chamber enlargement, while the heart of the athlete involved in static exercise typifies that of a chronic pressure overload with chamber volume similar to normal but with increased wall thickness [6]. The conclusion that these adaptations result from intense exercise training, rather than as a result of genetic predisposition or because of an enhanced cardiac growth response to training, cannot be established by cross-sectional studies.

Longitudinal studies offer several advantages over cross-sectional studies in assessing the cardiac adaptations to chronic exercise training [6]. First, in the use of randomly selected subjects, it may be assumed that a genetic predisposition for a training effect is not present and findings can be readily extrapolated to the general population. Second, because a subject serves as his or her own control, variations within experimental groups are minimized as a major source of error in comparing sedentary and trained groups. Nevertheless, in comparing longitudinal studies with cross-sectional studies between athletes and nonathletes, Schaible and Scheuer found inconsistent evidence for cardiac enlargement after exercise training [6]. Changes in cardiac dimension in the longitudinal studies were not nearly as great as the

Table 27.1 Classification of sports. From [12]

INTENSITY AND TYPE OF EXERCISE PERFORMED	
High-to-moderate intensity	Static with low dynamic demands (*contd*)
Dynamic and static demands	Field events (throwing)
Boxing	Gymnastics
Crew/rowing	Karate or judo
Cross-country skiing	Motorcycling
Cycling	Rodeoing
Downhill skiing	Sailing
Fencing	Ski jumping
Football	Water skiing
Ice hockey	Weight lifting
Rugby	
Running (sprint)	*Low intensity (low dynamic and low static demands)*
Speed skating	Bowling
Water polo	Cricket
Wrestling	Curling
	Golf
Dynamic with low static demands	Riflery
Badminton	
Baseball	DANGER OF BODY COLLISION
Basketball	Auto racing*
Field hockey	Bicycling*
Lacrosse	Boxing
Orienteering	Diving*
Ping-pong	Downhill skiing*
Race walking	Equestrian*
Racquetball	Football
Running (distance)	Gymnastics*
Soccer	Ice hockey
Squash	Karate or judo
Swimming	Lacrosse
Tennis	Motorcycling*
Volleyball	Polo*
	Rodeoing*
Static with low dynamic demands	Rugby
Archery	Ski jumping*
Auto racing	Soccer
Diving	Water polo*
Equestrian	Water skiing*
Field events (jumping)	Weight lifting*
	Wrestling

* Increased risk if syncope occurs.

morphologic differences between athletes and non-athletes. Factors which may have accounted for the inconsistency included: differences in pre-existing levels of fitness, differences in the duration and intensity of training, as well as sex and age factors.

The cardiac hypertrophy commonly observed in athletes has intrigued scientists because it represents a form of hypertrophy associated with normal or enhanced cardiac function. This contrasts with cardiac hypertrophy associated with chronic pathologic pressure overload as observed in hypertension and aortic stenosis. Both are frequently associated with impaired cardiac function. The morphologic response of the heart to static exercise mimics that of its response to chronic pressure overload, with the exception that left ventricular function in response to isometric stress is normal in the power athlete but depressed in patients with long-standing hypertension [6]. Furthermore, a more sensitive and earlier index of cardiac dysfunction may be abnormalities in diastolic function as measured by digitized echocardiography. In a study comparing top-class endurance swimmers with patients having nonmalignant hypertension of varying severity, diastolic function indices were abnormal in all of the hypertensive subjects, even in those with mild hypertension not associated with echocardiographic evidence of cardiac hypertrophy. On the other hand, athletes with degrees of cardiac hypertrophy equivalent to that in patients with moderate or severe hypertension had entirely normal diastolic function [17]. Another study comparing echocardiographic indices of left ventricular diastolic function in swimmers, power lifters, and age-matched normal control subjects demonstrated that cardiac hypertrophy associated with volume and pressure overload related to physical training resulted in enhanced diastolic function, in contrast to patients with pathologic conditions associated with these factors [18]. This suggested that the abnormalities in pathologic hypertrophy might be due to factors other than the cardiac hypertrophy itself. Chronic pressure overload is associated with eventual pathologic sequelae. However, in the power athlete, the intermittent nature of this overload results in hypertrophy which is a physiologic adaptation and probably without pathologic significance [6]. Studies of aerobically trained animals with chronic pathologic pressure overload (spontaneously hypertensive rats) have shown that cardiac hypertrophy intrinsic to the pathologic condition was exaggerated by training. But rather than being harmful, aerobic training reversed the contractile protein abnormalities associated with the pathologic stimulus [19,20].

EXERCISE TRAINING IN HYPERTENSION

Multiple studies have analyzed the relationship between physical activity and blood pressure, and many have implied that exercise training has been effective in lowering blood pressure at rest in both normotensive and hypertensive subjects. However, in a critique of cross-sectional and longitudinal studies supporting this effect, Seals and Hagberg [21] list numerous methodologic shortcomings and faults in study design that indicate that caution should be taken before accepting these conclusions. Problems which they identified included small sample size; limitations of age and sex of control and study groups; differences in stratification of blood pressure groups between studies; differences in the number of blood pressure measurements used to classify subjects as hypertensive; lack of nonexercising hypertensive control groups in some studies; lack of standardization of blood pressure recording technique (sitting,

supine); differences in the intensity, frequency, and duration of the exercise training program, and failure in some instances to control for changes in body weight. They concluded that the average blood pressure reduction reported from these studies (9 mmHg systolic and 7 mmHg diastolic) could have clinical implications for the hypertensive individual by lowering the risk of stroke and the development of cardiovascular disease [22]. However, the magnitude of these reductions would indicate that exercise training cannot replace pharmacologic therapy in persons with sustained moderate-to-severe hypertension. Exercise training thus may have a greater benefit to persons with borderline or mild hypertension, or in younger individuals in whom the pathologic process has not become fixed.

This conclusion contrasts with that of Fagard and colleagues [23], in a critical analysis of longitudinal studies in which a nonexercising hypertensive control group was incorporated. The analysis of the effect of dynamic exercise training on blood pressure in normotensive and hypertensive subjects found that only small decreases in pressure occurred with a pretraining systolic blood pressure of ≤140 mmHg. They suggested that dynamic exercise training was likely to be capable of a biologically significant reduction of a more elevated blood pressure level, with the important determinants of the pressure response being the pretraining blood pressure level and the magnitude of the increase in physical working capacity induced by training. On the other hand, Kiyonaga and co-workers [24] maintain that studies which failed to observe the effectiveness of exercise training on blood pressure tended to use too strenuous an exercise load, while those with optimal results employed milder degrees of exercise. Their study of 12 patients with essential hypertension trained on a cyclergometer (50% of maximum $\dot{V}o_2$) showed significant reductions in systolic and diastolic blood pressure. The effectiveness of training on resting blood pressure was dependent upon the patient's initial plasma renin activity. Exercise training was also found to be associated with a significant reduction in plasma catecholamine levels, an elevation of prostaglandin E levels, and increased urinary sodium excretion.

In addition to the evidence for a salutary effect of dynamic exercise on elevated blood pressure, the positive effect of isometric training on blood pressure control has been demonstrated. In 6 adolescents with essential hypertension, weight training alone maintained previous blood pressure reductions achieved by endurance training [25].

Two well documented responses to exercise have been cited as possible mechanisms by which a reduction in blood pressure might be mediated [21]. First, the vasodilating effect of an acute bout of exercise suggests the possibility that regular exercise could produce a state of chronic vasodilation with a resultant reduction of vascular resistance and blood pressure at rest. Second, the commonly reported reduction in heart rate at rest following exercise training has been postulated as a means of reducing the blood pressure of hypertensive individuals who exhibit a hyperkinetic circulation (increased heart rate and cardiac output at rest). Either or both of these mechanisms could be linked to the reduction in sympathetic tone known to occur in normotensive individuals with training. The increase in prostaglandin E levels after mild aerobic exercise training may reduce blood pressure by enhancement of sodium excretion by the kidney [24]. Prostaglandin E may also act as a local vasodilator after its liberation from skeletal muscle [26]. It may also inhibit norepinephrine release from nerve terminals which might result in a further reduction of sympathetic nerve activity [27].

HYPERTENSION IN ATHLETES

The current definition of hypertension in children and adolescents is a blood pressure exceeding the 95th percentile confirmed by three measurements on separate occasions. One-third of youths diagnosed by this criterion will have a return to normal blood pressure when followed over a 3–8-year period [28]. Therefore, to avoid undue prejudice against the competitive athlete with elevated blood pressure, caution is warranted in labeling one "hypertensive." Nevertheless, in terms of establishing guidelines for athletic participation, some stratification of blood pressure level is necessary. The majority of competitive athletes with hypertension will be adolescents. For this group, adult standards of hypertension, as listed by the Task Force on systemic arterial hypertension of the 16th Bethesda Conference on cardiovascular abnormalities in the athlete may be used [12] (Table 27.2).

In younger children and pre-adolescents, the issue may be more complicated since blood pressure is significantly related to height and weight. Certain sports emphasize size and maturity as positive attri-

Table 27.2 Classification of blood pressure in adults. From [29]

Classification

	Diastolic (mmHg)
Normal blood pressure	<85
High-normal blood pressure	85–89
Mild hypertension	90–104
Moderate hypertension	105–114
Severe hypertension	>115

	Systolic (when diastolic pressure is <90 mmHg)
Normal blood pressure	<140
Borderline isolated systolic hypertension	150–159
Isolated systolic hypertension	>160

Table 27.3 Pathogenetic mechanisms of chemically induced hypertension. From [31]

Predominant mechanism	Chemical agent
Expansion of extracellular fluid volume	Sodium
	Antacids
	Glycyrrhiza (licorice) and derivatives
	Mineralocorticoids
	Anabolic or androgenic steroids
	Oral contraceptives
	Nonsteroidal anti-inflammatory agents (aspirin, indomethacin, phenylbutazone)
Affecting autonomic nervous system	Direct or indirect sympathomimetic agents (amphetamines, phenylpropanolamine)
	Narcotics
	Ergot alkaloids

butes for optimal performance. These factors should not be overlooked in the evaluation of youths who may have higher blood pressures than their age group because of early maturity and growth of lean body mass [30]. To avoid misclassifying the young athlete as hypertensive, the blood pressure ranking percentile should be determined and compared to height and weight rankings, so that age is not the sole determining factor. The reader is referred to percentile rankings for age, height, weight, and sex given in Chapter 8. Another important factor is the use of blood pressure cuffs of an appropriate size (see Chapters 6 and 8), particularly for athletes whose arm girth may be exceedingly large because of resistance training. Additionally, a careful review of an athlete's drug regimen, including over-the-counter preparations, may assist in the diagnosis of chemically induced hypertension. The most common offenders in the athletic population include nonsteroidal anti-inflammatory drugs, anabolic and other steroidal agents, oral contraceptives, and nose drops containing sympathomimetic amines which act as nasal decongestants. Less common agents include amphetamines and narcotics [31] (Table 27.3).

Finally, the level of arterial blood pressure may not be the sole criterion for decision-making. The presence of other cardiovascular risk factors as well as target organ involvement may be helpful in making recommendations [12]. The target organ most likely affected in the young will be the heart, as manifested by echocardiographically assessed left ventricular hypertrophy.

The possibility that a subset of athletes with elevated blood pressure represent normal variants, as opposed to persons with underlying pathology, is found in a review of the features of the athletic heart and the hyperkinetic heart syndromes [32]. A significant number of well trained athletes have high resting systolic and normal diastolic blood pressures [4]. One should be wary of establishing the diagnosis of hypertension too early in this population.

Epidemiologic studies are sorely lacking in descriptive data for the prevalence and natural history of hypertension in the competitive athlete. However, a review of published reports suggests that high blood pressure is relatively common in football players [30,33] and possibly weight lifters [10], but this provides no clue to its etiology, since multiple factors could be involved. Training methods, lean body mass and maturity, or use of exogenous pharmacologic agents are all potential confounders. In this regard it is interesting to report the findings of a moderately exaggerated systolic blood pressure to exercise in a team of water polo players when compared to older control subjects [34].

In an attempt to establish the relative risk of hypertension in sports, it must be remembered that normal athletes may have extreme elevations of blood pressure during certain types of activity [3]. This may be related to their ability to increase their cardiac output. Furthermore, an elevated arterial pressure has not yet been observed to be related directly to sudden death during athletic participation. In reviews of pathologic series, hypertension *per se* has not been implicated

as a cause of acute morbidity or mortality [35,36]. Whether athletic participation affects hypertension positively or negatively over time has not been evaluated by appropriate longitudinal studies.

THERAPEUTIC CONCERNS

Exercise stress testing and evaluation of hypertensive individuals

There is currently a controversy about the value of exercise testing in the evaluation of athletes with elevated blood pressure [34,37,38]. Those who stress its value maintain that it can give a more accurate representation of blood pressure response to conditions simulating those which occur during competition. In addition, in this setting the contribution of resting anxiety to baseline blood pressure is abolished. Unfortunately, an exercise test is not the same as competitive athletics and direct comparisons cannot be made. Exercise testing has also been suggested to be able to detect the initial phases of cardiac involvement in hypertensive heart disease by the presence of abnormal ST changes, cardiac arrhythmias, or excessive blood pressure rise with exercise [13,37]. Nevertheless, a study by Spirito and colleagues of 75 isometrically trained athletes found a significant incidence (10%) of false-positive ST segment changes in maximal graded exercise stress testing with subsequent negative radionuclide exercise studies [39]. It was concluded that a high incidence of false-positive treadmill exercise tests was a major limitation in screening for underlying cardiovascular disease in athletes by this method.

Pharmacologic options

Indications for antihypertensive drug therapy for young athletes is also a controversial issue. In a prior publication, we suggested that pharmacologic therapy was probably not indicated for a blood pressure of less than 170/100 mmHg in an adolescent in the absence of a definable etiology [38]. At that time the following factors were considered in the rationale: elevated blood pressure in an adolescent had at least a one-third chance of returning to normal without any intervention; compliance with drug therapy would likely be low, and the side-effects of diuretics, the primary drugs used at that time, could reduce physical performance and also affect serum electrolyte and water homeostasis. Most importantly, data were beginning to appear that suggested that aerobic conditioning could reduce blood pressure and potentially reverse certain end-organ sequelae, especially the myocardial. Additionally, there have been few or no data to demonstrate the ill effects of athletic participation on hypertension and its complications. Therefore, we currently suggest that pharmacologic therapy should not be initiated in an athlete with mild hypertension without evidence of significant end-organ damage (e.g. retinal lesions). An exception to this recognized arbitrary recommendation would be the athlete whose blood pressure response to maximum exercise testing is greater than 240 mmHg systolic and 95 mmHg diastolic. A similar approach is taken in dealing with isolated systolic hypertension. Hygienic measures are initiated if the resting systolic blood pressure exceeds 160 mmHg. An exercise test is then performed. If the peak systolic blood pressure exceeds 240 mmHg we consider pharmacologic intervention earlier. The rationale for the level of 240 mmHg is that this pressure significantly exceeds the 95th percentile of blood pressure response to exercise in adolescents [40].

It is not the purpose of this chapter to outline the pharmacology of antihypertensive drugs since it has been described extensively elsewhere (see Chapters 12–15). Rather, it is appropriate when contemplating pharmacologic therapy in the competitive athlete to consider the interaction of the physiologic effects of therapy with athletic performance. An ideal antihypertensive drug would:

1 reduce systolic and diastolic blood pressure at rest and during exercise;
2 allow maximal performance in the athlete's sport;
3 produce no undesirable side-effects; and
4 have no short- or long-term harmful effects such as electrolyte imbalance or lipid changes [4].

Few, if any, currently available antihypertensive agents meet all of these criteria, but certain features of their action allow clear preferences to be made. In general, most cardiovascular drugs, with the exception of the β-blocking agents, permit a normal blood pressure response to dynamic exercise, with an increase in systolic blood pressure, a stable or mildly decreased diastolic blood pressure, and an increased heart rate, stroke volume, and cardiac index [41] (Tables 27.4 and 27.5).

Diuretic therapy has been used as a first step for many years [5]. The main drawbacks of diuretic therapy for athletic participation are volume contraction, hypokalemia, and failure to control exercise blood pressure. Additionally the negative effects of thiazides on serum lipoproteins and glucose tolerance are long-term considerations, in view of other cardiovascular risk factors. Furthermore, diuretic therapy in athletes requires knowledge of changes in the acclimatization to exercise workouts, especially during warm, humid seasons [4]. In the early phase of vigorous workouts, salt and water loss is excessive. This results in secondary aldosteronism with a reduction in further losses of sodium and chloride. However, potassium losses through sweat are constant and not affected by heat acclimatization. Diuretic therapy administered during the early training may thus exacerbate volume depletion and potassium loss. Some athletes may continue to lose large volumes of sweat, and those who persistently lose 3% or more of their body weight in the course of a

Table 27.4 Hemodynamic effects of antihypertensive agents. From [4]

Agent	Cardiac output		Total peripheral resistance		
Diuretics	→	↓	↓	↓	
Propranolol hydrochloride	↓	↓	↑		
Timolol maleate	↓	↓	↑		
Nadolol	↓	↓	↑		
Metoprolol tartrate	↓	↓	↑		
Atenolol	↓	↓	↑		
Pindolol	→	↓	↓		
Reserpine	↓		↓		
Guanethidine monosulfate	↓		↓	↓	↓
Methyldopa	→	↓	↓		
Clonidine hydrochloride	→	↓	↓		
Prazosin hydrochloride	→		↓	↓	
Hydralazine hydrochloride	↑		↓	↓	
Minoxidil	↑		↓	↓	
Captopril	→		↓	↓	
Nifedipine	→		↓	↓	
Verapamil hydrochloride	→		↓	↓	

→ Minimal or no change; ↓ decrease; ↑ increase.

Table 27.5 Antihypertensive agents that allow a normal cardiovascular response during dynamic exercise. From [41]

Clonidine	Prazosin
Methyldopa	Verapamil
Nifedipine	Captopril
	Diuretics

workout are probably not good candidates for diuretic therapy.

β-Blocking agents have become a cornerstone in the pharmacologic therapy of hypertension [5,42]. Most have significant disadvantages in the athlete (Table 27.6).

From these considerations, a modified stepped-care approach to the treatment of hypertension in an athlete can be constructed (Table 27.7). When hygienic measures have been attempted without an adequate hypotensive response, the first step would utilize drugs that lower peripheral vascular resistance but have minimal or no effect on resting or exercise cardiac output. Prazosin hydrochloride has many advantages in this regard. It acts like a vasodilator, thereby reducing peripheral vascular resistance. In addition it does not alter blood lipids, which enhances its long-term effectiveness in reducing coronary disease risk factors [22]. As with many of these agents, sexual dysfunction can occur. Prazosin seems to have the lowest incidence of this problem. Compliance may well be the most significant problem with the required dosing frequency of these agents.

Once initiated, the goal of therapy should be to achieve a resting systolic and diastolic blood pressure in the normal range. To attain this level may require the addition of a thiazide diuretic with potassium supplementation or a potassium-sparing agent, as noted above. Calcium channel blockers, such as nifedipine and verapamil, may also hold promise as therapy for the athlete with high blood pressure. Both have been shown to reduce resting blood pressure and the absolute response to static and dynamic exercise [43].

CONCLUSIONS AND RECOMMENDATIONS

1 Most young athletes should be allowed to participate in all competitive athletics in the presence of mild-to-moderate essential hypertension. This recommendation is based on several factors. First, reports are lacking describing sudden death or acute morbid events on the field, or shortly after athletic participation, that can be directly ascribed to hypertension. Second, in many young hypertensive athletes, hypertension may disappear with time. Finally, aerobic conditioning appears to be able to decrease resting blood pressure.

2 Those athletes with severe hypertension (by adult standards, greater than 115 mmHg diastolic blood

Table 27.6 Adverse effects of β-blockade during exercise. Adapted from [41] and [4]

Hyperkalemia
Inhibition of muscle and hepatic glycogenolysis (risk for hypoglycemia)
Inhibition of lipolysis
Muscle fatigue
Blunted heart rate response (especially cardiac output)
Reduction of FEV_1 and FEV_2

FEV_1 and FEV_2 = Forced expiratory volume in 1 and 2s, respectively

Table 27.7 Stepped-care approach to hypertension in the athlete. From [4]

Initial hygienic measures	Sodium restriction
	Caloric restriction
	Relaxation techniques
	Aerobic conditioning
Step 1	Prazosin
	Clonidine
	Methyldopa
Step 2	Low-dose diuretic with potassium chloride supplementation or potassium-sparing agent

pressure and/or target organ damage) must receive pharmacologic therapy. The type of competition allowed should be based on the response to therapy and the risk of causing further injury to target organs. The sport should be tailored to the young athlete, i.e. all athletes need not participate in strenuous or collision types of sport.

3 At the present time, there is inconclusive evidence to prohibit the isometric training of athletes with mild-to-moderate hypertension in the absence of target organ damage (especially cardiac). Early evidence suggests that this training may in fact aid in the control of both systolic and diastolic blood pressure.

4 Based on current evidence, the routine prescription of dynamic exercise for antihypertensive therapy seems appropriate for those athletes with mild-to-moderate hypertension. However, further information needs to be gained from controlled longitudinal studies.

5 When presented with a young athlete who manifests evidence of early maturity and increased lean

body mass, and whose blood pressure exceeds the 95th percentile for age, it is prudent to follow the blood pressure for a period of time in order to evaluate its trend.

6 When pharmacologic therapy is indicated, stepped-care is recommended with initial drug therapy consisting of a sympatholytic agent.

7 Drug therapy used for the treatment of hypertension should not exclude an individual from competition in athletic activities.

8 At present, our understanding of the effects of hypertension in this special group of patients is limited. The current recommendations are an attempt to balance practical considerations with scientific evidence. In this regard, directions for future investigation should aim to:

(a) define more clearly the role of exercise as therapy in controlling hypertension through well constructed and more closely controlled studies;

(b) expand the role of noninvasive investigation of the hypertensive patient in terms of early diagnosis and therapeutic monitoring (digitized echocardiography, peripheral renin activity screening, Doppler echocardiographic analysis);

(c) evaluate more precisely the risk of hypertension in the context of athletic competition;

(d) understand the special problem of isolated systolic hypertension and its short- and long-term ramifications; and

(e) evaluate new antihypertensive therapies in terms of their effects on athletic performance.

REFERENCES

1 Michener JA. *Sports in America*. New York: Random House, 1976.

2 Fixler DE, Laird WP, Fitzgerald V, Stead S, Adams R. Hypertension screening in schools; results of the Dallas study. *Pediatrics* 1979;63:32−6.

3 Bryan GT. Hypertension in the young athlete. *Texas Med* 1969;65:62−5.

4 Walther RJ, Tifft CP. High blood pressure in the competitive athlete: guidelines and recommendations. *Phys Sportsmed* 1985;13:93−114.

5 Strong WB, Steed D. Cardiovascular evaluation of the young athlete. *Pediatr Clin North Am* 1982;29:1334−7.

6 Schaible TF, Scheuer J. Cardiac adaptations to chronic exercise. *Prog Cardiovasc Dis* 1985;XXVII:297−324.

7 Asmussen E. Similarities and dissimilarities between static and dynamic exercise. *Circ Res* 1981;48(suppl 1):3−10.

8 Blomqvist CG, Saltin B. Cardiovascular adaptations to physical training. *Annu Rev Physiol* 1983;45:169−89.

9 Nutter DO, Schlant RC, Hurst JW. Isometric exercise and the cardiovascular system. *Mod Conc Cardiovasc Dis* 1972;41:11−15.

10 MacDougall JD, Tuxen D, Sale DG, Moroz JR, Sutton JR. Arterial blood pressure response to heavy resistance exercise. *J Appl Physiol* 1985;58:785−90.

11 Mitchell JH, Wildenthal K. Static (isometric) exercise and the heart: physiological and clinical considerations. *Annu Rev Med* 1974;25:369−81.

12 Mitchell JH, Blomqvist CG, Haskell WL *et al*. Classification of sports. Bethesda conference no. 16: cardiovascular abnormalities in the athlete: recommendations regarding eligibility for competition. *J Am Coll Cardiol* 1985;6:1198−9.

13 Fixler DE, Laird WP, Browne R, Fitzgerald V, Wilson S, Vance R. Response of hypertensive adolescents to dynamic and isometric exercise stress. *Pediatrics* 1979;64:579−83.

14 Sonnenblick EH, Ross J Jr, Braunwald E. Oxygen consumption of the heart: newer concepts of its multifactorial determination. *Am J Cardiol* 1968;22:328−40.

15 Mitchell JH, Hefner LL, Monroe RG. Performance of the left ventricle. *Am J Med* 1972;53:481−94.

16 Morganroth J, Maron BJ, Henry WL, Epstein SE. Comparative left ventricular dimensions in trained athletes. *Ann Int Med* 1975;82:521−4.

17 Shapiro LM, McKenna WJ. Left ventricular hypertrophy: relation of structure to diastolic function in hypertension. *Br Heart J* 1984;51:637−42.

18 Colan SD, Sanders SP, MacPherson D, Borow KM. Left ventricular diastolic function in elite athletes with physiologic cardiac hypertrophy. *J Am Coll Cardiol* 1985;6:545−9.

19 Rupp H, Jacob R. Response of blood pressure and cardiac myosin polymorphism to swimming training in the spontaneously hypertensive rat. *Can J Physiol Pharmacol* 1982;60:1098−103.

20 Scheuer J, Malhotra A, Hirsch C *et al*. Physiological cardiac hypertrophy corrects contractile protein abnormalities associated with pathological hypertrophy in rats. *J Clin Invest* 1982;70:1300−5.

21 Seals DR, Hagberg JM. The effect of exercise training on human hypertension: a review. *Med Sci Sports Exerc* 1984;16:207−15.

22 Kaplan NM. Therapy of mild hypertension: an overview. *Am J Cardiol* 1984;53:2A−3A.

23 Fagard R, M'Buyamba JR, Staessen J, Vanhees L, Amery A. Physical activity and blood pressure. In: Bulpitt CJ, ed. *Handbook of Hypertension*. New York: Elsevier Science, 1985:104−30.

24 Kiyonaga A, Arakawa K, Tanaka H, Shindo M. Blood pressure and hormonal responses to aerobic exercise. *Hypertension* 1985;7:125−31.

25 Hagberg JM, Ehsani AA, Goldring D, Hernandez A, Sinacore DR, Holloszy JO. Effect of weight training on blood pressure and hemodynamics in hypertensive adolescents. *J Pediatr* 1984;104:125−31.

26 Nowak J, Wennmalm A. Effect of exercise on human arterial and regional venous plasma concentrations of prostaglandin E. *Prostaglandins Med* 1978;1:489−97.

27 Hedqvist P. Studies on the effect of prostaglandin E_1 and E_2 on the sympathetic neuromuscular transmission in some animal tissues. *Acta Physiol Scand* 1970;(suppl 345):1−40.

28 Londe S, Bougoignie JJ, Robson AM *et al*. Hypertension in apparently normal children. *J Pediatr* 1971;78:569−73.

29 Frohlich ED, Lowenthal DT, Miller HS, Pickering T, Strong

WB. Systemic arterial hypertension. Bethesda conference no. 16: cardiovascular abnormalities in the athlete: recommendations regarding eligibility for competition. *J Am Coll Cardiol* 1985;6:1219.

30 Wilson SL, Gaffney FA, Laird WP, Fixler DE. Body size, composition, and fitness in adolescents with elevated blood pressure. *Hypertension* 1985;7:417−22.

31 Messerli FH, Frohlich E. High blood pressure: a side effect of drugs, poisons, and food. *Arch Intern Med* 1979;139: 682−6.

32 Huston TP, Puffer JC, Rodney WM. The athletic heart syndrome. *N Engl J Med* 1985;313:24−32.

33 Grossman M, Baker BE. Current cardiology problems in sports medicine. *Am J Sports Med* 1984;12:262−7.

34 Dlin RA, Dotan R, Inbar O, Rotstein A, Jacobs I, Karlson J. Exaggerated systolic blood pressure response to exercise in a water polo team. *Med Sci Sports Exerc* 1984;16:294−8.

35 Maron BJ, Roberts WC, McAllister HA, Rosing DR, Epstein SE. Sudden death in young athletes. *Circulation* 1980;62:218−29.

36 Virmani R, Robinowitz M, McAllister HA. Nontraumatic death in joggers. *Am J Med* 1982;72:784−8.

37 Wu SC, Secchi MB, Mancarella S *et al.* Usefulness of stress testing for the evaluation of hypertensive heart disease in young hypertensive subjects. *Cardiology* 1984;71:277−83.

38 Strong WB. Hypertension and sports. *Pediatrics* 1979;64:693−5.

39 Spirito P, Maron BJ, Bonow RO, Epstein SE. Prevalence and significance of an abnormal S−T segment response to exercise in a young athletic population. *Am J Cardiol* 1983;51:1663−6.

40 Alpert BS, Dover EV, Booker DL, Martin AM, Strong WB. Blood pressure response to dynamic exercise in healthy children − black vs. white. *J Pediatr* 1981;99:556−61.

41 Lowenthal DT, Stein D, Hare TW *et al.* The clinical pharmacology of cardiovascular drugs during exercise. *J Cardiac Rehabil* 1983;3:829−37.

42 Hull DH. Mild hypertension. *Aviat Space Environ Med* 1985;56:304−9.

43 Gould B, Hornung RS, Mann S, Balasubramanian V, Raftery EB. Slow channel inhibitors verapamil and nifedipine in the management of hypertension. *J Cardiovasc Pharmacol* 1982;4:S369−73.

28 Hypertension and Pregnancy: Maternal, Fetal, and Neonatal Manifestations

JANE E. BRAZY AND ALLEN P. KILLAM

The incidence of hypertension in pregnancy varies from 5% in healthy women in their 20s to over 20% in primigravidas whose sisters or mothers had severe pre-eclampsia as primigravidas, diabetics, and patients with chronic renal disease. Hypertension during pregnancy remains one of the three leading causes of maternal mortality, with death most often resulting from intracranial hemorrhage. Furthermore, medical intervention necessary to prevent possible maternal and fetal mortality often results in the birth of a preterm infant who requires intensive care. In this chapter we will first discuss hypertension in pregnancy and its treatment, then associated fetal and neonatal problems, and finally the effects of drugs used in the treatment of the maternal hypertension upon the fetus and nursing infant.

HYPERTENSION IN PREGNANCY

Hypertensive disorders of pregnancy may be divided into four categories:
1 coincidental chronic hypertension;
2 transient hypertension;
3 pre-eclampsia or pregnancy-induced hypertension; and
4 chronic hypertension with superimposed pre-eclampsia.

The importance of this type of classification is to distinguish patients who present different problems in pregnancy and benefit from different forms of management. The most severe problems in pregnancy occur with pre-eclampsia originating before the 34th week of pregnancy, and with pre-eclampsia superimposed upon chronic hypertension.

Pathogenesis

The causes of coincidental hypertension and pregnancy are those of hypertension in the general adult population. Like this population, usually no specific cause of hypertension is identified, and thus the label "essential hypertension" is applied. The specific etiology of pre-eclampsia is also unknown, but it is most likely related to a failure of vascular changes which should occur with placentation [1]. In a normal pregnancy, the fetal chorionic cytotrophoblast invades the walls of the branches of the uterine arteries that perfuse the placenta. With this invasion, the trophoblast erodes into the muscular layer converting the artery into a passive conduit which is relatively unresponsive to vasodilator influences. With pre-eclampsia this process is incomplete, and the arteries are more susceptible to vasoconstriction. There is considerable evidence that the invasion of the uterine arteries is enhanced by prior exposure to the fetal antigens [2]. This may explain why a prior pregnancy with the same father lowers the incidence of pre-eclampsia.

Placental hypoxia probably triggers the events which cause the elevated blood pressure and other manifestations of pre-eclampsia. For years researchers looked for a vasoconstrictor produced in excessive amounts by a hypoxic placenta. Rather than excessive production of a vasoconstrictor, there may be inadequate production of a vasodilator, such as prostacyclin or bradykinin [3,4]. Normally, the endothelial cells which line the blood vessels produce vasodilators that maintain the lower vascular resistance necessary to cope with the increase in blood volume and cardiac output which occurs during a normal pregnancy. With pre-eclampsia endothelial damage may occur, reducing vasodilator production. At other times the placental mass may be excessive, as in multifetal pregnancies, very large fetuses, or fetal hydrops. Intrauterine or, more specifically, placental hypoxia appears to be the common denominator for all of the conditions which predispose a patient to pre-eclampsia. Any factor that decreases placental perfusion, including well meaning attempts to lower a patient's blood pressure, tends to make pre-eclampsia worse.

Of particular importance to understanding the pathophysiology of severe hypertension in pregnancy is an appreciation of the vulnerability of the fetus to reduced placental perfusion and the unique features of pre-eclampsia. It appears that there are two pathophysiologic patterns in pre-eclampsia. The classic presentation of pre-eclampsia in a young primigravida is to have an apparently normal response to early pregnancy. The fetus and placenta grow well. Maternal blood volume expands normally and amniotic fluid volume is normal, as is maternal blood pressure. Before a woman develops signs of pre-eclampsia, she will have abnormal physiologic responses which accurately predict that she will later develop the overt signs and symptoms of pre-eclampsia. These responses include a greater sensitivity to the vasoconstrictors, angiotensin II and norepinephrine and altered intracellular calcium transport [5]. As the disease progresses, the patient develops a contracted blood volume, hypertension, proteinuria, and other sequelae of pre-eclampsia.

The second pattern, seen in women who are normotensive throughout the first 24 weeks of pregnancy, resembles the pattern more typical of the patient with known chronic hypertensive disease. These patients never have the normal expansion of blood volume. The fetus and placenta remain small and amniotic fluid volume may remain below normal throughout pregnancy.

Whether or not these two patterns represent two different disease processes is open to question. Much of the confusion about the nature of pre-eclampsia is due to the fact that it may present in many different ways depending on which organ is predominantly affected.

When the brain is affected, the patient may have severe headaches, visual disturbances, or convulsions and coma. When the liver is affected there may be epigastric pain, jaundice, or elevated liver enzymes. When the kidneys are affected proteinuria, oliguria, and azotemia are evident. Intrauterine growth retardation may be the predominant or first evidence of a hypertensive disorder in pregnancy. In other patients intrauterine growth retardation may be a late manifestation.

One of the most unique features of pre-eclampsia is the way it affects platelets, red blood cells, and intravascular coagulation. Thrombocytopenia, in-

creased red blood cell destruction, and the increased generation of fibrin set pre-eclampsia apart from chronic hypertension. Other typical features of pre-eclampsia include a markedly contracted plasma volume with hemoconcentration and low central venous pressure, pulmonary wedge pressures, and colloid osmotic pressures. Cardiac output is often high with normal total systemic vascular resistance. There is a strong tendency for capillaries in the lungs and other organs to become leaky. A relative excess of thromboxane production, especially if expressed as a ratio with prostacyclin productions, forms the rationale behind prophylactic treatment with low dose aspirin.

Diagnosis

The diagnosis of the hypertensive disorders during pregnancy is not difficult if the patient is seen early in pregnancy. When the woman is known to have hypertension before becoming pregnant or is found to be hypertensive prior to 20 weeks of gestation then she has coincidental chronic hypertension. A resting blood pressure of 140/90 mmHg on two occasions more than 6 h apart establishes the diagnosis of hypertension. Age must also be considered. A 14-year-old with a blood pressure of 130/86 mmHg or greater should be regarded as hypertensive for her age and followed accordingly. When the diagnosis of chronic hypertension is first established during pregnancy, evaluation for an underlying disorder may be indicated if the hypertension is severe or other abnormalities are appreciated on physical and laboratory examinations.

In contrast to underlying hypertension, pre-eclampsia has its onset after the 24th week. The cardinal features are hypertension, proteinuria, and edema. Edema is not specific for pre-eclampsia and does not correlate with pregnancy outcome. Hypertension defined as a pressure of 140/90 mmHg or a rise in pressure of 30 mmHg systolic or 15 mmHg diastolic is the keystone to the diagnosis of pre-eclampsia and the degree of hypertension correlates with the severity of the illness. This correlation, however, is not perfect; there are patients with minimal hypertension who have severe fetal growth retardation, liver or renal involvement, thrombocytopenia, hemolysis, and intravascular coagulation.

The diagnosis of pre-eclampsia without significant proteinuria must be suspect. Early in the course of the disease the patient may have only a trace of protein in her urine as measured by dipstick and less than 300 mg of protein in a 24-h specimen. Quantitative 24-h urine specimens and concomitant determination of creatinine clearance are very useful in following the course of pre-eclampsia and in deciding whether a patient with chronic hypertension is developing superimposed pre-eclampsia.

Symptoms frequently associated with pre-eclampsia include severe headaches, visual changes such as tiny, bright light spots and blurring, and swelling of the face and hands in the morning and the feet and legs in the afternoon. Epigastric or right subcostal pain with tenderness is often mistaken for a hiatal hernia, heartburn, gallbladder or renal disease when it actually represents swelling of the liver capsule from edema or hemorrhage. The hypertension may be labile at first and respond to brief periods of rest, then become more consistent and pronounced later. Deep tendon hyperreflexia, like edema, is very nonspecific but, when combined with other signs, may be useful in establishing the diagnosis. Edema of the retina and segmental constriction of the retinal arteries in the absence of signs of chronic hypertension such as thickening of the arterial walls, retinal hemorrhages, or exudates may help confirm the diagnosis of pre-eclampsia.

Laboratory tests in addition to proteinuria and creatinine clearance may help to establish the diagnosis of pre-eclampsia or to follow its course. Platelets may decrease and hematocrit and hemoglobin frequently increase with pre-eclampsia, but all three are usually unchanged in patients with chronic hypertension. Liver function tests may become elevated with pre-eclampsia. Rarely a patient becomes jaundiced and has liver enzyme levels similar to those seen in viral hepatitis. This is an ominous finding and, coupled with epigastric pain and evidence of disseminated intravascular coagulation, constitutes an urgent need to deliver the patient.

A number of tests have been found to serve as markers for pre-eclampsia. Most of these involve red blood cells, platelets, or factors involved in coagulation. Why increased red blood cell destruction, thrombocytopenia, and intravascular fibrin formation are specific for pre-eclampsia is unknown, but altered prostacyclin and thromboxane production is suspected. Serum iron, antithrombin III, fibronectin, D-D dimer, urinary calcium excretion and the nephelometric analysis of the urine proteins may be specific and sensitive markers of pre-eclampsia [6-8].

Diagnostic ultrasound is very useful in establishing the diagnosis and progression of intrauterine growth retardation and oligohydramnios. Doppler flowmeters can be used to follow flow patterns of the uterine and umbilical arteries. The resistance indices derived from peak systolic and diastolic flows in these arteries have been reported to be very predictive of pregnancy outcome as well as specific for pre-eclampsia [9,10].

Management

Management should include early detection, bedrest, close surveillance, and proper timing of delivery. Early entrance into the health care system is critical. First-trimester visits make the differential between chronic hypertension and pre-eclampsia infinitely easier. In addition, they facilitate more precise timing of conception through serial ultrasound studies. Hypertension during the first half of gestation is assumed to be chronic and coincidental to the pregnancy as long as the uterine size is appropriate and fetal heart tones are present. A baseline 24-h urine for total protein and creatinine clearance should be obtained. When there is significant proteinuria, a false-positive test for syphilis, arthralgias, or recurrent pregnancy losses, tests to screen for systemic lupus erythematosus and specific associated autoantibodies (lupus anticoagulant and anticardiolipin) are indicated.

Which patients require antihypertensive medication is a matter of judgment. If a patient is taking diuretics, they are generally stopped because diuretics tend to make the volume depletion associated with pre-eclampsia worse. There is also evidence that placental clearance is diminished and angiotensin II sensitivity is increased with diuretic usage. In addition to diuretics, powerful long-acting antihypertensive drugs are avoided to insure optimal placental perfusion. If the patient is on prazosin or propranolol and is doing well, it is generally reasonable to leave her on her current medication, particularly if she is beyond the first trimester when any teratogenesis would have already occurred. If the patient needs antihypertensive medication, α-methyldopa 1−2 g/day in divided doses two to four times a day can be used. Treatment is usually not begun unless the diastolic pressure is consistently over 95 mmHg. Although there is ample evidence of benefit in treating hypertension with antihypertensive medication if the diastolic pressure is over 110 mmHg blinded placebo-controlled studies have not indicated that there is any improvement in fetal or maternal outcome if methyldopa or any other drug is given to women whose diastolic pressure is 95 mmHg or below [11]. We aim to keep a patient with chronic hypertension at 90—95 mmHg diastolic and generally reduce her medication if her diastolic pressure stays below 80 mmHg for several visits.

A different plan of therapy is necessary for the pre-eclamptic patient. With pre-eclampsia, bedrest is the most effective way of reducing the patient's blood pressure without compromising placental perfusion. When a woman at high risk for developing pre-eclampsia has a slight increase in her pressure or some other indication that she is developing the disease, bedrest at home should be initiated. Once a patient has met the criteria for the diagnosis of pre-eclampsia she should remain in the hospital at bed-rest until she delivers.

Antihypertensive medications must be used with care. Whenever mean arterial pressure is reduced by more than 10 or 15% by any medication uterine perfusion is decreased consistently, indicating that the uterine arteries that perfuse the placenta are maintained at 90% of their maximum dilation and cannot dilate more than an additional 10% under any condition or with any known drug. For this reason medication to reduce the blood pressure of a patient with pre-eclampsia is withheld until her diastolic pressure is above 110 mmHg. The pressure is lowered cautiously with intravenous boluses of hydralazine 5 mg every 20 min until the diastolic pressure is between 100 and 105 mmHg.

Occasionally a patient's pressure cannot be controlled with hydralazine alone. Propranolol may be added or, if the patient is about to be delivered, short courses of intravenous nitroprusside or nitroglycerin may be given. Postpartum a whole range of newer drugs may be used, if necessary, to keep the diastolic pressure below 110 mmHg. Prazosin, an α-blocking agent, appears to be effective and safe.

The use of colloid solutions such as 5% albumin and invasive monitoring with the Swan—Gantz catheter have been controversial. It is tempting to try to expand plasma volume when it is known to be low in an effort to improve perfusion. We have used it briefly intrapartum under close, usually invasive, monitoring when we expect bleeding or anesthetics to precipitate a sharp drop in pressure. There is considerable risk of pulmonary edema and heart failure. The use of the Swan—Gantz catheter has resulted in some very valuable information about the pathophysiology of severe pre-eclampsia. Unexpectedly in most patients total peripheral resistance

is normal and cardiac output is high, especially if the patient has received vasodilators magnesium sulfate and intravenous fluids. A few patients have high total peripheral resistance and may have low cardiac output and evidence of heart failure. When the heart is on the verge of failure even a moderate amount of intravenous fluids may cause pulmonary edema. In this setting, colloid solutions are especially dangerous. Therefore, since it is impossible to tell if a woman with pre-eclampsia is at risk for heart failure by routine clinical parameters alone, one should avoid over-hydrating a patient with severe disease.

Patients with pre-eclampsia will often have enough endothelial damage that fluid easily leaks out into the lungs, causing pulmonary edema at pulmonary arterial pressures and colloid osmotic pressures that would not normally result in pulmonary edema. The central venous pressure does not correlate well with the pulmonary arterial wedge pressure. Thus, pushing intravenous fluids with only a central venous pressure catheter can be dangerous. It is possible for a patient to develop either pulmonary edema or left heart failure with relatively normal central venous pressures. Furosemide should be given for pulmonary edema and heart failure. Invasive monitoring should be used if there is intrinsic heart disease and the pre-eclampsia is especially severe and there is protracted oliguria or extensive blood loss.

Optimal timing of delivery should maximize perinatal survival and minimize morbidity. A woman who develops pre-eclampsia after the 37th week is promptly delivered since her infant is already near term. If the patient is remote from term when she develops pre-eclampsia then delivery may be delayed for several weeks. Factors which dictate prompt delivery regardless of prematurity include worsening hypertension, increasing proteinuria, deteriorating renal function, signs of fetal compromise, abnormal liver enzymes, thrombocytopenia, epigastric pain, convulsions, and signs of heart failure.

The route of delivery should be vaginal if it does not compromise the fetus. Cesarean birth is indicated when there is fetal distress or the mother's condition warrants an expedited delivery. Once the patient delivers, she should improve promptly and correct her physiologic parameters without much medication. If her diastolic blood pressure remains over 110 mmHg her blood pressure should be reduced to near 100 mmHg diastolic with antihypertensive medication.

There is mounting evidence from international

studies that low dose (60—80 mg/day) aspirin may prevent as much as 80% of clinical pre-eclampsia. Calcium supplementation has also shown promise. The National Institutes of Health have funded studies to confirm these studies and to determine which populations would benefit.

Conclusion

Patients found to be hypertensive during pregnancy may have coincidental chronic hypertension and/or a unique pregnancy-induced hypertension, usually referred to as pre-eclampsia. Early identification and prompt treatment with strict bedrest are important. If the disease does not respond to bedrest and becomes severe, delivery before term may be necessary.

INFANTS OF HYPERTENSIVE MOTHERS

Evidence is rapidly accumulating which suggests that, like infants of diabetic mothers, infants of hypertensive mothers (IHMs) have a specific constellation of problems which result from their abnormal intrauterine environment. Although they are often delivered before term, their problems are not simply those of prematurity. Likewise, not all are explainable by chronic asphyxia or growth retardation. Several papers have suggested that severe hypertension in pregnancy, particularly that beginning before the 37th week, may be a multisystem disease shared by the mother and fetus [12,13]. This section will first address fetal and neonatal mortality risks associated with hypertension in pregnancy and then elaborate on specific problems associated with this maternal disease.

Morbidity and mortality

Fetuses and infants of mothers with elevated blood pressure during pregnancy constitute a group at significantly increased risk for perinatal morbidity and mortality. Mortality rates in pregnancies complicated by hypertension are influenced predominantly by four factors:

1 the presence or absence of pre-existing hypertension;

2 the development of pre-eclampsia;

3 the gestational age when signs and symptoms begin; and

4 the severity of the maternal disease.

Perinatal mortality increases only slightly when pre-eclampsia develops after the 37th week or when mild essential hypertension is unchanged by pregnancy. But the development of severe pre-eclampsia before the 37th week markedly increases mortality. This increase is inversely related to gestational age, with rates as high as 100% reported for women with the onset of severe pre-eclampsia before the 28th week [14].

Long and colleagues [15] reported a mortality rate of 6.7 per thousand with onset of pre-eclampsia on or after the 37th week, but 133 per thousand in pregnancies with onset before the 37th week of gestation. Other studies support a perinatal mortality rate of 7—15% with onset of pre-eclampsia on or before 36 weeks of gestation [12,16]. Similarly, mortality is greatly influenced by the severity of the maternal disease, with the highest risk for fetal, neonatal, and maternal mortality in women with hemolysis, elevated liver enzymes, and thrombocytopenia [14]. Aggressive intervention with early delivery may significantly decrease the mortality rate in this group [13].

Like mortality, infant morbidity is influenced by gestational age at onset of hypertension and the

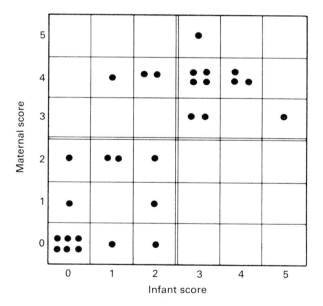

Fig. 28.1 Maternal score: 1 point for lactic dehydrogenase >350 iu, serum glutamic oxaloacetic transaminase >50 iu, platelet count <150 000, fibrin split products >32 μg/ml, and creatinine >1.5 mg/dl.

Infant score: 1 point for 1-min Apgar score <5, platelet count <150 000, weight <10%, head circumference <10%, neutrophils <2000/mm³.

severity of the maternal disease. Most studies addressing the acute morbidity risks to IHMs have concentrated on those infants in whom the severity of maternal disease gave rise to early delivery. With milder maternal disease and/or onset near term, the incidence and severity of all forms of neonatal disease decrease. In severe pre-eclampsia, however, the severity of the disease in the mother highly predicts the severity of disease in the infant (Fig. 28.1). It is not yet possible to establish if the different forms of neonatal morbidity are due to a shared fetal—maternal factor which is precipitating abnormalities in the infant as well as the mother, or if the state of hypertension in pregnancy exerts its fetal influence predominantly through reducing placental perfusion. If the latter is true, then we must assume that most, if not all, fetal and neonatal morbidity is the result of asphyxia, intrauterine malnutrition, and prematurity.

Another important confounding variable is the possibility of therapy-related morbidity. Nearly all mothers with severe disease receive antihypertensive and/or anti-epileptic therapy. Drugs used to treat these mothers cross the placenta, with most achieving a fetal:maternal ratio in plasma of nearly 1. Although they are used to reduce the potential risk for maternal hemorrhagic complications and seizures, each may have potentially deleterious side-effects upon the fetus and the infant in transition to extrauterine life.

FETAL AND NEONATAL PROBLEMS ASSOCIATED WITH MATERNAL HYPERTENSION

Growth

Hypertension commonly compromises growth of the fetus *in utero*. The noted incidence of intrauterine growth retardation, defined as a birthweight less than the 10th percentile for gestational age, varies with the definition of the population studied and the therapeutic approach applied to the mother, i.e. conservative therapy trying to extend the time *in utero*, or delivery of the infant. Long and colleagues [15] noted the incidence of growth retardation to be 5.6% in women with the onset of pre-eclampsia after the 37th week, but 18.2% in women with the onset before the 37th week. If severe hypertension (blood pressure ≥160/110 mmHg) occurs early in pregnancy (<36 weeks), the incidence of growth retardation is much higher—39%, as reported by Brazy and co-authors [12], with obstetric approach of stabilization

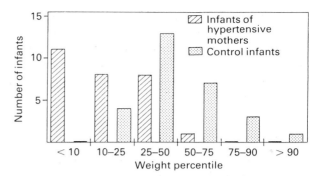

Fig. 28.2 Birth weight distribution of infants of hypertensive mothers (IHMs) and control infants using Colorado intrauterine growth curves.

and early delivery, and 56.5% in a similar population managed conservatively to extend the time *in utero* [17]. Data from Sibai and coworkers [14] revealed an 80% incidence of growth retardation in IHMs delivered at less than 28 weeks. Far more revealing, however, is the overall pattern of intrauterine fetal growth in women with severe early-onset disease. In a study of 28 infants of less than 36 weeks gestation, delivered because of severe maternal hypertension, only 1 had a birthweight above the 50th percentile [12]. A control group of gestationally matched infants without maternal hypertension demonstrated a normal distribution of birthweight (Fig. 28.2). Thus, although many infants did not fall below the 10th percentile at birth, the overall weight distribution was markedly skewed to the lower percentiles, indicating slowing of intrauterine weight accretion in almost all infants.

Few studies address the effect of maternal hypertension on fetal head growth. In the same preterm population, a plot of head growth demonstrated the same lowering of head circumference percentile distribution (Fig. 28.3). Only 2 of 28 infants retained head growth at the 50th percentile or above. Although the absolute effect of hypertension on fetal head growth is less than on weight (29 versus 39% falling below the 10th percentile), the impact is still appreciable and may be of greater importance for long-term outcome.

Asphyxia

Uteroplacental insufficiency associated with hypertensive disease in pregnancy renders the fetus at an increased risk for asphyxia both *in utero* and during the labor and delivery process. A study by

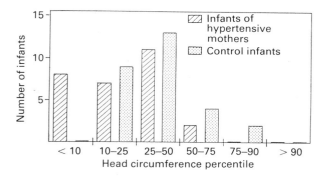

Fig. 28.3 Birth head circumference percentile distribution of infants of hypertensive mothers (IHMs) and control infants using Colorado intrauterine growth curves.

Rasmussen [18], using the pulsed Doppler technique with ultrasound, demonstrated decreased blood flow in the umbilical vein and aorta in fetuses of women with pre-eclampsia, suggesting that abnormalities in the fetal part of the placenta are a major cause of the increased total peripheral resistance in these fetuses. Regardless of the site of origin of placental insufficiency, most studies suggest IHMs are at increased risk for asphyxia as assessed by Apgar scores after birth. Lin and associates [19] reported a 37% incidence of 1-min Apgar scores of 6 or under in IHMs, compared to 18% in a high-risk normotensive population. Brazy and co-authors [12] demonstrated a significantly higher incidence of both 1- and 5-min Apgar scores of less than 5 in IHMs compared to gestational age-matched control subjects. In this study, the degree of asphyxia, as indicated by the Apgar score, highly correlated with the severity of the maternal disease as manifested by elevation in liver enzymes and thrombocytopenia.

Vital signs in transition to extrauterine life

If the fetus *in utero* shares the mother's vascular reactivity, then one might expect elevated blood pressure in IHMs. Results of studies relating the effect of maternal hypertension on neonatal blood pressure and heart rate initially appear in conflict, but discrepancies predominantly reflect differences in study design, population observed, and timing of data collection. Miller and colleagues [20] studied heart rate and aortic blood pressure during the first hour of life in 18 IHMs and 22 control subjects, all born at term. Mean arterial blood pressure was significantly higher in IHMs during the first 20 min of life, but fell to control levels between 30 and 60 min. Heart rate was

significantly lower for the first 50 min of life. Mausner and co-authors [21] assessed blood pressure on the third day of life using the Doppler technique and found no differences between IHMs and control infants born at term. A study of preterm infants born to severely hypertensive mothers did not find any significant differences in the incidence of abnormal blood pressures in IHMs and age-matched control babies [12].

Infants of hypertensive mothers may have difficulty in converting from the fetal to the postnatal circulatory pattern. Delay in this adaptation was noted in 32% of preterm IHMs during the first 24 h of life [12]. All of these infants responded to increased environmental oxygen and none displayed the more severe form of pulmonary hypertension of the newborn. In this same study, left-to-right shunting through the ductus arteriosus after 24 h of age was noted in 39% of IHMs.

Hematologic complications

The major hematologic complications of IHMs include neutropenia, thrombocytopenia, abnormal coagulation factors, and an elevated hematocrit. Although the occurrences of these abnormalities are well documented, the mechanisms by which they develop are still poorly defined.

Manroe and associates [22], while establishing normal values for neonatal neutrophil counts, documented maternal hypertension to be an important cause of neutropenia at birth. In a subsequent study, they noted that 50% of IHMs (mean gestational age 32.6 weeks) demonstrated neutrophil values below the lower limit of the normal range for chronologic age [23]. Others [12,13] have confirmed the incidence of neutropenia to be 42−50% in infants delivered of mothers with severe manifestations of hypertension. The degree of neutropenia correlates with the severity of the maternal disease, but the mothers do not similarly manifest neutrophil reduction [12]. Neutropenia of IHMs is unaccompanied by a left shift and persists for several days [12,23]. Gradually the counts rise to approach the lower limits of the normal range, usually after 72 h of age [23]. Although most neutropenic infants are evaluated for sepsis, cultures are negative.

Neonatal thrombocytopenia, defined as a platelet count <150 000, occurs frequently if maternal thrombocytopenia is present. The incidence of neonatal thrombocytopenia varies from 32 to 63% of thrombocytopenic mothers [12,24]; the depression of the platelet count correlates with the severity of the maternal abnormality [12]. Although hypertensive mothers rarely have coagulopathies consistent with disseminated intravascular coagulation, occasionally severely affected infants may have clinical and laboratory evidence of this condition [12]. Nielsen [25] studied coagulation parameters in IHMs. They noted a reduction in factor V, fibrinogen, and prothrombin-proconvertin as well as a prolonged partial thromboplastin time and thrombin time, indicating that some degree of intravascular coagulation may be present. Lox and coworkers [26] evaluated the effects of pre-eclampsia near term on cord blood clotting parameters and came to a somewhat different conclusion. They found elevated fibrinogen, decreased factors II, V, and VII activity and decreased factor II antigen in IHMs, suggesting impairment of liver function.

Hematocrits of IHMs are often elevated. Infants of mothers with early and severe hypertension have hematocrits that average 5 percentage points higher than those of age-matched control infants [12]. The highest values are from growth-retarded infants, but only a few of these reach hematocrits greater than 62–65% where hyperviscosity becomes a concern.

Respiratory problems

Because many IHMs must be delivered preterm, the possible development of respiratory distress syndrome (RDS) is of great concern. In a population study between 1968 and 1975, Yoon and co-authors [27] noted a decreased incidence of RDS in IHMs of all gestational ages. This difference was most significant in the infants who were 33 weeks' gestation or older. Other studies, however, specifically looking at the incidence of RDS in infants of mothers with early onset of severe hypertension, have failed to support a protective effect [12,16]. The role of β-methasone in altering the relative risk for RDS in IHMs is unknown. Thus, while mild hypertension may stimulate lung maturation and reduce the incidence of RDS, severe maternal hypertensive disease before term does not appear to confer any demonstrable pulmonary benefits.

Metabolic problems

Metabolic problems (hypoglycemia, hypocalcemia, hyperbilirubinemia) are commonly seen in preterm infants and infants who sustain growth impairment or asphyxia *in utero*. Thus, most infants delivered of mothers with severe disease should be considered at risk for these problems and monitored accordingly. In addition, specific abnormalities and increased risks result from being an IHM.

Neonatal hypoglycemia, defined as a blood glucose <20 mg/100 ml, occurred in 24% of 131 infants of toxemic mothers studied by Koivisto and Jouppila [28]. The incidence was highest when toxemia was severe (35%) and when fetal growth retardation was present (37%). Fifteen per cent of infants were symptomatic. Careful screening for hypoglycemia is therefore indicated for all IHMs.

Varner and associates [29] studied calcium metabolism in term pregnancies associated with essential hypertension. They demonstrated reduced levels of parathyroid hormone, reduced ionized calcium, and elevated levels of phosphorus in both the mother and the fetus. Treatment of women with pre-eclampsia with magnesium sulfate poses additional factors which alter calcium homeostasis. Cruikshank and coworkers [30] and Brazy and colleagues [12] both noted a lower cord blood calcium in infants of magnesium-treated mothers. In the postnatal adaptive period calcium values fell, as expected. The nadir of the calcium decline was no lower than that of age-matched controls, but the lowest value occurred a few hours earlier in postnatal life [12].

The incidence and severity of hyperbilirubinemia do not appear to be influenced by maternal hypertension. Its occurrence parallels that of age-matched control infants.

Adrenal function and fetal plasma lipoprotein cholesterol metabolism in IHMs have been studied by Parker and co-authors [31]. They divided their study groups into 30–33 weeks and 34–41 weeks and compared them to a normal control population. Umbilical cord plasma cortisol concentrations were similar in both groups at each gestational period. Fetal plasma dehydroisoandrosterone sulfate was similar before 34 weeks, but was significantly reduced in the more mature IHMs. At term, fetal plasma total cholesterol and low density lipoprotein cholesterol were higher in IHMs while high density lipoprotein cholesterol and very low density lipoprotein cholesterol were not different. They concluded that maternal hypertensive disease decreases the rate of steroidogenesis in the neocortical zone of the fetal adrenal and leads to hypercholesterolemia in the fetus as a consequence of reduced adrenal utilization of low density lipoprotein cholesterol.

Central nervous system complications

One might hypothesize that chronic stress *in utero* would give rise to accelerated maturation of vital organ systems including the brain. To investigate this possibility, Hadi [32] looked at anatomic brain maturation in autopsy material from 23 preterm IHMs. Cerebral maturation, of 2 or more weeks in advance of gestational age, was noted in 74%. Consistent with this observation of accelerated anatomic development is the failure to find an increased incidence of intraventricular hemorrhage in IHMs despite their high incidence of predisposing conditions such as asphyxia, thrombocytopenia, and lung disease [12,33].

Functional maturation, however, may not be so advanced. Shulte and co-authors [34,35] noted normal nerve conduction in small-for-gestational-age IHMs, but muscle tone, general excitability, and bioelectric brain activity were all delayed for age. Thus, evidence suggests that although the IHM may have accelerated anatomic maturation, functionally the IHM performs at or below the level appropriate for gestational age.

Other

Other problems have been noted to occur with increased frequency in IHMs, including delayed stooling (50%), ileus (25%), and hypotonia (18%) [12]. Since none of these correlate with the severity of the maternal disease, they are thought to be secondary to transplacental passage of drugs, particularly magnesium sulfate, used in treating the maternal disease.

Long-term outcome

Information regarding the long-term outcome of IHMs is sparse. Ounsted and colleagues [36,37] noted slight developmental delay in IHMs in the area of gross, fine, and visual motor skills, but not in language, comprehension, or global scores when compared to a matched control population. This delay was less apparent if the mother had received antihypertensive therapy during pregnancy. They noted no difference in outcome of children at school age between mothers with hypertension alone and those with pre-eclampsia superimposed upon hypertension.

Winer and coworkers [38] assessed intellectual and neurologic development at 4–7 years in two groups of small-for-gestational-age infants, IHMs, and non-IHMs: IHMs scored better than non-IHMs on almost all tests of intellectual development. In contrast to growth-retarded infants from other causes, there was an inverse relationship between gestational age (and birth-weight) and developmental scores in the IHMs, indicating that early delivery resulted in smaller infants but better outcomes.

Risk for subsequent hypertension

Like their mothers, IHMs are at greater risk for subsequent hypertension and this tendency toward increased pressure is evident from early childhood. When Mausner and co-authors [21] compared blood pressures of IHMs to control infants from normotensive pregnancies, no differences were seen at 9 months. However, by 24 months the systolic blood pressure of IHMs was significantly higher than that of control babies. Children 6–16 years of age, born of mothers with hypertension in pregnancy, were studied extensively by Svensson [39]. Both systolic and diastolic blood pressures of children from hypertensive pregnancies were significantly higher than those of matched control infants. These differences were apparent whether or not the mother's blood pressure had returned to normal after pregnancy; however, the highest pressures were in children of mothers who remained hypertensive after pregnancy. There were no indications of increased hemodynamic reactivity to stress as assessed by reaction to noise, video games, and physical exercise in either group. Erythrocyte studies performed on these children showed no difference in erythrocyte sodium concentration, but children with elevated blood pressures had reduced Na^+-K^+-ATPase activity in erythrocyte membranes. It is likely, therefore, that children born of hypertensive pregnancies represent a group at increased genetic risk for subsequent hypertension. Infants born of mothers with hypertension in pregnancy should be monitored frequently throughout childhood for the emergence of hypertension. Mild blood pressure elevations may be apparent by early childhood, especially if maternal hypertension has persisted after pregnancy.

FETAL/NEONATAL EFFECTS OF DRUGS USED TO TREAT HYPERTENSION IN PREGNANCY

Table 28.1 summarizes the fetal and neonatal effects

Table 28.1 Drugs used in the treatment of hypertension in pregnancy and lactation

Drug	Fetal: maternal ratio	Fetal effects	Neonatal effects	Excretion in milk	Breast-feeding comments
Magnesium sulfate	~1		Hypotension responsiveness Hypotonia Delayed neuromuscular transmission Respiratory depression Ileus/delayed stooling Low cord calcium Urinary retention	Yes $\dfrac{Milk}{Plasma} = \sim 2$	No additional adverse effects likely
Methyldopa	~1	Microcephaly if started at 16–20 weeks of gestation	Decrease in BP of 4–5 mmHg for 2 days	Yes $\dfrac{Milk}{Plasma} = 2$	Infant level, 0.09 mg/ml Insufficient information available
Hydralazine	~1	? ↑ Malformation with first-trimester use Deceleration of heart rate in a fetus with IUGR	Thrombocytopenia Bleeding Decrease in BP Hypothermia	Yes $\dfrac{Milk}{Plasma} = 0.05-1$	No adverse effects expected
Propranolol	0.2–1.2	? Premature labor ↓ Fetal heart rate in response to sound ? ↑ Fetal death IUGR	Hypoglycemia Respiratory depression Bradycardia ? Hyperbilirubinemia ? Polycythemia	Yes $\dfrac{Milk}{Plasma} = 0.2-0.7$	No adverse effects expected
Clonidine			Insufficient information	Yes $\dfrac{Milk}{Plasma} = 1.5$	Insufficient information available
Captopril		Embryocidal in some animals (↑ stillbirths) Unknown in humans	Insufficient information	Very low $\dfrac{Milk}{Plasma} = 0.01$	No adverse effects expected

Sodium nitroprusside	Fetal > maternal in animals	Transient fetal bradycardia; Low cyanide levels in fetal liver and cord blood	Insufficient information		Insufficient information available
Diazoxide	~1	Transient fetal bradycardia; Destruction of fetal islets in sheep and goats	Hyperglycemia (may last several days); ? Alopecia; ? Hypertrichosis lanuginosa; ? Decreased ossification of wrist		Insufficient information available
Reserpine	Crosses placenta	? Teratogen	↑ Nasal discharge; Nasal stuffiness and obstruction of nasal airway; Lethargy (all three of the above occur in 10%, lasting 1–5 days); Neonatal cold injury	Yes	Avoid if possible
Thiazide diuretics	0.1–0.8	↑ Risk of malformation early in pregnancy; ↓ Placental perfusion; ↑ Meconium staining; ? ↑ Perinatal mortality; Fetal bradycardia	Hypoglycemia; Thrombocytopenia; Hemolytic anemia; Hyponatremia; Hypokalemia	Yes; $\dfrac{\text{Milk}}{\text{Plasma}} = 0.05\text{–}0.43$	↓ Milk production (avoid use in first month)
Furosemide	1	↑ Postnatal diuresis; Hyponatremia; Hypokalemia		Yes	↓ Milk production (avoid use in first month)

BP = Blood pressure; IUGR = intrauterine growth retardation; ↑ = increase; ↓ = decrease.

of the drugs commonly used to treat hypertension in pregnancy [40–46]. In general, these medications cross the placenta readily, with most achieving a fetal:maternal ratio of 1. Therefore, in treating the neonate exposed *in utero*, one must assume a "therapeutic" drug concentration to be present at the time of delivery. The half-life of the drug within the infant will be prolonged whether the drug requires liver metabolism, renal excretion, or both. The younger the gestational age of the infant, the greater will be the time for clearance.

Magnesium sulfate is used frequently to prevent seizures in the toxemic patient. With increased use of the intravenous route and higher infusion rates, neonatal manifestations are more apparent. As expected, infants of treated mothers have elevated cord magnesium and lower cord calcium concentrations [12,30]. In addition, hypotension, respiratory depression, hypotonia, urinary retention, ileus, and delay in passage of meconium may occur [45,46]. Magnesium is completely dependent upon the kidney for excretion; therefore, gestational age, postnatal age, and asphyxial renal damage all influence the infant's ability to clear this drug.

Of all the antihypertensive agents, the most extensive studies have occurred with methyldopa [36,37]. Deleterious effects have not been seen when therapy was initiated after the 20th week of gestation. Microcephaly at birth was noted in children treated between the 16th and 20th weeks of gestation, but did not persist in later childhood and was not associated with long-term sequelae [36,37]. The only documented neonatal effect is a 4–5 mmHg decrease in blood pressure, lasting 2 days [47].

Hydralazine, another commonly used drug, is less well studied. There is a question of increase in malformations with first-trimester use and a few reports of neonatal thrombocytopenia and bleeding with use in later pregnancy. It too can cause a small decrease in the blood pressure of the newborn child.

The use of β-blocking agents in pregnancy appears to be increasing. Most neonatal information relates to propranolol. Propranolol has been reported to contribute to intrauterine growth retardation and may possibly cause fetal death [48]. Newborn infants may have problems with hypoglycemia, respiratory depression, and bradycardia. Other β-blockers, metoprolol, sotolol, and atenolol, all have maternal:fetal ratios of 1. Small trials of these agents in hypertensive pregnant women have not noted adverse fetal effects; however, infants of treated mothers merit careful monitoring for evidence of β-blockade.

Information on clonidine, captopril, sodium nitroprusside, and diazoxide is too sparse to draw definite conclusions on their safety to the fetus and newborn infant. Of concern is the possible risk for fetal cyanide toxicity [49] with the use of nitroprusside and pancreatic islet cell destruction [50] with the use of diazoxide.

In contrast, reserpine has well documented deleterious effects upon the neonate with 10% having nasal stuffiness, nasal airway obstruction, and lethargy. Increased susceptibility to cold injury is an additional potential problem. Therefore, reserpine is rarely, if ever, the drug of choice for use in pregnancy.

Diuretics are seldom indicated in pregnancy, and may have adverse effects upon placental perfusion and upon the newborn infant. If given near delivery, the baby will respond with diuresis, and must be monitored for the possible development of dehydration and electrolyte imbalance.

BLOOD PRESSURE THERAPY AND LACTATION

Most medications used to treat hypertension in the lactating woman appear in her breast milk (Table 28.1) [40,42,43,51]. Although milk:plasma ratios vary markedly, even for those with ratios >1, the total amount of drug presented to the nursing infant is small. Rarely are significant levels detected in the infant. One drug, captopril, appears to be unique in its extremely poor passage into breast milk and it may therefore offer a specific advantage to the nursing mother [52]. We suggest the avoidance of reserpine in lactation predominantly because of the known dangerous effects of transplacental drug acquisition. Even though the risks for toxicity should be markedly less with nursing, other drugs may be safer.

Use of diuretics may pose a significant problem to the lactating woman by decreasing milk production. For this reason, diuretic use should be avoided if possible during the first month postpartum when lactation is becoming established.

REFERENCES

1 Ramsey EM, Donner MW. *Placental Vasculature and Circulation*. Stuttgart: Thieme, 1980.
2 Feeney JG, Scott JS. Pre-eclampsia and changed paternity. *Eur J Obstet Gynaecol Reprod Biol* 1980;11:35–8.
3 Mikila UM, Viinikka L, Ylikorkala O. Evidence that prostacyclin deficiency is a specific feature in preeclampsia. *Am J*

Obstet Gynecol 1980;148:772−4.

4 Goodman RP, Killam AP, Biash AR, Branch RA. Prostacyclin production during pregnancy: comparison of production during normal and pregnancy complicated by hypertension. *Am J Obstet Gynecol* 1982;142:817−22.

5 Worley RJ, Gant NF, Everett RB, MacDonald PC. Vascular responsiveness to pressor agents during human pregnancy. *J Reprod Med* 1979;23:115−27.

6 Entman SS, Richardson LD, Killam AP. Elevated serum ferritin in the altered ferrokinetics of toxemia of pregnancy. *Am J Obstet Gynecol* 1982;144:418−22.

7 Stubbs TM, Lazarchick J, Harger EO. Plasma fibronectin levels in preeclampsia: a possible biochemical marker for vascular endothelial damage. *Am J Obstet Gynecol* 1984;150:885−7.

8 Eden RD, Wahbeh CJ, Barter JF, Williams AY, Killam AP, Gall SA. Serial nephelometric urinary protein profile as an index of renal involvement in severe pregnancy-induced hypertension: a case report. *Am J Obstet Gynecol* 1983;147:106−8.

9 Trudinger BJ, Gibs WB, Cook CM. Uteroplacental blood flow velocity−time waveforms in normal and complicated pregnancy. *Br J Obstet Gynaecol* 1985;92:39−45.

10 Giles WB, Trudinger BJ, Baird PJ. Fetal umbilical artery flow velocity waveforms and placental resistance: pathologic correlation. *Br J Obstet Gynaecol* 1985;92:31−8.

11 Pritchard JA, MacDonald PC, Gant NF. *Williams Obstetrics*. Norwalk: Appleton-Century-Crofts, 1985:527−60.

12 Brazy JE, Grimm JK, Little VA. Neonatal manifestations of severe maternal hypertension occurring before the 36th week of pregnancy. *J Pediatr* 1982;100:265−71.

13 Weinsten L. Syndrome of hemolysis, elevated liver enzymes, and low platelet count: a severe consequence of hypertension in pregnancy. *Am J Obstet Gynecol* 1982;142:159−67.

14 Sibai BM, Spinnato JA, Watson DL, Hill GA, Anderson GD. Pregnancy outcome in 303 cases with severe preeclampsia. *Obstet Gynecol* 1984;64:319−25.

15 Long PA, Abell DA, Beischer NA. Fetal growth retardation and pre-eclampsia. *Br J Obstet Gynaecol* 1980;87:13−18.

16 Benedetti TJ, Benedetti KJ, Stenchever MA. Severe preeclampsia−maternal and fetal outcome. *Clin Exp Hypertens* 1982;B1:401−16.

17 Martin TR, Tupper WRC. The management of severe toxemia in patients at less than 36 weeks' gestation. *Obstet Gynecol* 1979;54:602−5.

18 Rasmussen K. Fetal hemodynamics in pre-eclampsia. Changes during antihypertensive treatment. *Acta Med Scand* 1985;693[suppl]:11−14.

19 Lin CC, Lindheimer MD, River P, Moawad AH. Fetal outcome in hypertensive disorders of pregnancy. *Am J Obstet Gynecol* 1982;142:255−60.

20 Miller FC, Read JA, Cabel L, Siassi B. Heart rate and blood pressure in infants of preeclamptic mothers during the first hour of life. *Crit Care Med* 1983;11:532−5.

21 Mausner JS, Hiner LB, Hediger ML, Gabrielson MO, Levison SP. Blood pressure of infants of hypertensive mothers: a two-year follow-up. *Int J Pediatr Nephrol* 1983;4:255−61.

22 Manroe BL, Weinberg AG, Rosenfeld CR, Browne R. The neonatal blood count in health and disease. *J Pediatr*

1979;95:89−98.

23 Engle WD, Rosenfeld CR. Neutropenia in high-risk neonates. *J Pediatr* 1984;105:982−5.

24 Kleckner HB, Giles HR, Corrigan JJ. The association of maternal and neonatal thrombocytopenia in high-risk pregnancies. *Am J Obstet Gynecol* 1977;128:235−8.

25 Nielsen N. Influence of pre-eclampsia upon coagulation and fibrinolysis in women and their newborn infants immediately after delivery. *Acta Obstet Gynecol Scand* 1969;48:523−41.

26 Lox CD, Word RA, Corrigan JJ. Effects of pre-eclampsia on maternal and cord blood clotting activity. *Am J Perinatol* 1985;2:279−82.

27 Yoon JJ, Kohl S, Harper RG. The relationship between maternal hypertensive disease of pregnancy and the incidence of idiopathic respiratory distress syndrome. *Pediatrics* 1980;65:735−9.

28 Koivisto M, Jouppila P. Neonatal hypoglycemia and maternal toxemia. *Acta Paediatr Scand* 1974;63:743−9.

29 Varner MW, Cruikshank DP, Pitkin RM. Calcium metabolism in the hypertensive mother, fetus, and newborn infant. *Am J Obstet Gynecol* 1983;147:762−5.

30 Cruikshank DP, Pitkin RM, Reynolds WA, Williams GA, Hargis GK. Effects of magnesium sulfate treatment on perinatal calcium metabolism. I Maternal and fetal responses. *Am J Obstet Gynecol* 1979;134:243.

31 Parker CR, Hankins GD, Carr BP, Leveno KJ, Gant NF, MacDonald PC. The effect of hypertension in pregnant women on fetal adrenal function and fetal plasma lipoprotein-cholesterol metabolism. *Am J Obstet Gynecol* 1984;150:263−9.

32 Hadi HA. Fetal cerebral maturation in hypertensive disorders of pregnancy. *Obstet Gynecol* 1984;63:214−9.

33 Sibai BM, Watson DL, Hill GA, Spinnato JA, Anderson GD. Maternal fetal correlations in patients with severe preeclampsia/eclampsia. *Obstet Gynecol* 1983;62:745−50.

34 Shulte FJ, Schrempf G, Hinze G. Maternal toxemia, fetal malnutrition, and motor behavior of the newborn. *Pediatrics* 1971;48:871−81.

35 Shulte FJ, Hinze G, Schrempf G. Maternal toxemia, fetal malnutrition and bioelectric brain activity of the newborn. *Neuropadiatre* 1971;2:439−60.

36 Ounsted MK, Moar VA, Good FJ, Redman CWG. Hypertension during pregnancy with and without specific treatment; the development of the children at the age of four years. *Br J Obstet Gynaecol* 1980;87:19−24.

37 Ounsted MK, Cockburn J, Moar VA, Redman CW. Maternal hypertension with superimposed pre-eclampsia: effects on child development at $7\frac{1}{2}$ years. *Br J Obstet Gynaecol* 1983;90:644−9.

38 Winer EK, Tejani NA, Atluru VL, DiGiuseppe R, Borofsky LG. Four- to seven-year evaluation in two groups of small-for-gestational age infants. *Am J Obstet Gynecol* 1982;143:425−9.

39 Svensson A. Hypertension in pregnancy−long-term effects on blood pressure in mothers and children. *Acta Med Scand* 1985;695(suppl):1−50.

40 Briggs GG, Bodendorfer TW, Freeman RK, Yaffe SJ. *Drugs in Pregnancy and Lactation*. Baltimore: Williams & Wilkins, 1983.

41 Witter FR, King TM, Blake LDA. Adverse effects of cardio-vascular drug therapy on the fetus and neonate. *Obstet Gynecol* 1981;58:100S−105S.

42 Roberts RJ. *Drug Therapy in Infants*. Philadelphia: WB Saunders, 1984:346−72.

43 Marx CM. Effects of maternal drugs on the fetus. In: Cloherty JP, Stark AR, *Manual of Neonatal Care*. eds. Boston: Little, Brown, 1985;521−58.

44 Rasch DK, Huber PA, Richardson CJ, L'Hommedieu CS, Nelson TE, Reddi R. Neurobehavioral effects of neonatal hypermagnesemia. *J Pediatr* 1982;100:272−6.

45 Lipsitz PJ, English IC. Hypermagnesemia of newborn. *Pediatrics* 1967;40:856−62.

46 Sokal MM, Koeningsberger MR, Rose JS, Berdon WE, Santulli V. Neonatal hypermagnesemia and the meconium plug syndrome. *N Engl J Med* 1972;286:823−5.

47 Whitelaw A. Maternal methyldopa treatment and neonatal blood pressure. *Br Med J* 1981;283:471.

48 Lieberman BA, Stirrat GM, Cohen SL, Beard RW, Pinker GD. The possible adverse effect of propranolol on the fetus in pregnancies complicated by severe hypertension. *Br J Obstet Gynaecol* 1978;85:678−83.

49 Shoemaker CT, Meyers M. Sodium nitroprusside for control of severe hypertensive disease in pregnancy: a case report and discussion of potential toxicity. *Am J Obstet Gynecol* 1984;149:171−3.

50 Boulos BM, Davis LE, Almond CH, Jackson, RL. Placental transfer of diazoxide and its hazardous effects on the new-born. *J Clin Pharmacol* 1971;11:206−10.

51 White WV. Management of hypertension during lactation. *Hypertension* 1984;6:279−300.

52 Devlin RG, Fleiss PM. Captopril in human blood and breast milk. *J Clin Pharmacol* 1981;21:110−13.

29 Hypertension in Newborn Infants

JEFFREY M. PERLMAN

INTRODUCTION

During the past decade, advances in perinatal care have resulted in an improved neonatal survival rate. However, a concomitant increase in neonatal morbidity has also occurred. Hypertension is one such example of increased morbidity. Prior to 1970, hypertension was rarely reported in newborn babies, but recent evidence points to an increased occurrence in infants surviving in neonatal intensive care units. Thus, in two reports, 2.5% of such infants developed hypertension [1,2]. Whether this is only an apparent increase in incidence reflecting an improvement in blood pressure monitoring techniques, or whether it is a real increase consequent upon complications of the much more aggressive management of newborn infants is an important issue to resolve. This chapter reviews the problem of hypertension in newborn infants in terms of definition, etiology, complications, diagnosis, and treatment.

DEFINITION OF HYPERTENSION

Previously published reports have been limited by a lack of a consistent definition of hypertension. Thus, Adelman in a review of the subject defined neonatal hypertension as a systolic blood pressure >90 mmHg and a diastolic blood pressure >60 mmHg [1]. In other reports, a systolic blood pressure ranging from 70 mmHg [3] to 100 mmHg [4] has been used to define hypertension. Furthermore, it has become apparent that many variables may affect blood pressure measurement in the newborn baby. These variables include cuff size [5], the infant's state of arousal [5,6], and both the infant's gestational and postnatal ages [5–7].

With this as background, a review of normal blood pressure distribution in term and preterm infants is outlined below.

Term infant

Table 29.1 summarizes previous data concerning normal blood pressure values in the term infant. The systolic blood pressure at birth approximates 60 mmHg depending on the method used (transcutaneous Doppler versus direct intra-arterial). A progressive increase in blood pressure occurs during the first postnatal week. Thus, between the second and the fourth postnatal day, the blood pressure increases to approximately 75 mmHg with lower values obtained with the infant in quiet sleep, and higher values when the infant is awake and sucking. Thus, deSwiet and coworkers [5] did a longitudinal study of 1740 full-term babies and obtained a mean *systolic* blood pressure of 71 ± 8 mmHg in the sleep state versus 76 ± 10 mmHg in the awake state at the fourth postnatal day. The 95th percentile (regarded as the upper limit of normal) for the awake state in this study was a systolic blood pressure of 95 mmHg. In the same study the mean systolic blood pressure had increased to 96 ± 11 mmHg in the awake state at 6 weeks, was 93 ± 14 mmHg at 6 months, and 94 ± 11

Table 29.1 Postnatal changes in systolic blood pressure in healthy term infants

Blood pressure at birth (mmHg)		Blood pressure on second to fourth postnatal day (mmHg)				
		Asleep		Awake		
59.4 ± 8.7 [8]	D			69 ± 6	[8]	D
62 ± 6 [9]	SG			76 ± 8	[9]	SG
56 ± 8 [10]	D	73 ± 9.5 [6]	D	85.3 ± 9.5 [6]		D
70 [11]	A	71 ± 10 [5]	D	76.8 ± 8	[5]	D

D = Doppler method of determination; SG = strain gauge method of determination; A = intra-arterial method of determination.

All values are means ± SD.

mmHg at 1 year (Fig. 29.1). The 95th percentile at all later ages was 113 mmHg. The report of the Second Task Force on blood pressure control in children developed definitions and a classification of hypertension, based not upon risk data, but upon clinical experience and consensus [12]. Thus, for infants in the first postnatal week, significant hypertension was defined as a systolic blood pressure >96 mmHg; for infants beyond the first week but less than 1 month of age, hypertension was defined as a systolic blood pressure >104 mmHg, and for infants less than 2 years of age, hypertension was defined as a systolic blood pressure >112 mmHg.

Premature infant

There are limited data regarding blood pressure changes in the premature infant. Two studies have demonstrated a lower range of blood pressure at birth when compared to full-term infants. Thus, in infants weighing 750 g, the mean *systolic* arterial blood pressure was 44 mmHg (range 34–54 mmHg), reflecting average values over the first 12 h of life [13]. For infants of 1000 g birthweight in the same study, the mean systolic arterial blood pressure was 49 mmHg (range 39–59 mmHg), also reflecting average values over the first 12 h of life. Similarly, as in term infants, a progressive increase in blood pressure occurs during the first 48 h of life in the premature infant although exact limits are not clear from the published data [14]. Sheftel and colleagues [7] studied 99 premature infants at follow-up and found that the mean blood pressure at 14.7 ± 1.3 weeks was 93.3 ± 2 mmHg (mean ± SEM).

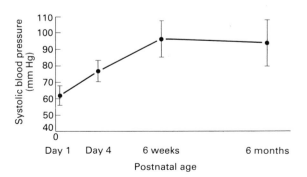

Fig. 29.1 Postnatal changes in systolic blood pressure in healthy awake term infants. Values are mean ± standard deviation. Adapted from [5,6,8,9,12].

ETIOLOGY

Hypertension in the newborn infant is usually secondary to known causes (Table 29.2). Our experience (Table 29.3) is similar to that reported in other series. Some of the more common causes are briefly reviewed below.

Vascular

Frequently neonatal hypertension is renovascular in nature secondary to thrombus or embolization of the renal vessels. This may in part reflect the widespread use of indwelling intra-arterial catheters [4,15]. The incidence of clinically inapparent thrombi is high; thrombotic lesions were detected by angiography in 21 (91%) infants studied (Table 29.4). Furthermore, in one clinical pathologic study, thrombi were more frequently noted at autopsy when compared to prior angiographic studies (Table 29.4). Additionally, severe, clinically evident thromboembolic complications requiring aggressive therapeutic intervention

Table 29.2 Causes of secondary hypertension in infancy

Vascular	Renal artery thrombus [4,15–17]
	Renal artery stenosis
	Renal artery hypoplasia
	Coarctation of the aorta [18]
	Aneurysm of the ductus arteriosus [17]
	Aortic thrombus [16,19,20]
Renal	Polycystic kidney
	Multicystic dysplastic kidney
	Hypoplastic kidney
	Obstructive uropathy [21]
Tumors	Neuroblastoma [22]
	Mesoblastoma [23]
	Pheochromocytoma [24]
Endocrine	Congenital adrenal hyperplasia
	Cushing's syndrome
	Neonatal thyrotoxicosis [25,26]
Central nervous system	Raised intracranial pressure
	Seizures [27]
	Meningitis
Respiratory	Bronchopulmonary dysplasia [28,29]
Miscellaneous	Drugs, e.g. phenylephrine [30], steroids
	Post surgery, e.g. closure of abdominal wall

Table 29.3 Causes of hypertension in newborn infants admitted between February 1984 and June 1985* at St Louis Children's Hospital, MO

Underlying cause		No. of infants
Bronchopulmonary dysplasia		9
Aortic and renal thrombi		5
Renal parenchymal lesions		3
Multicystic/dysplastic kidney with contralateral hydronephrosis	(2)	
Polycystic kidney	(1)	
Neurologic		2
Subdural hematoma	(1)	
Meningitis	(1)	
No etiology		3
Normal renin	(1)	
Elevated renin	(2)	
Total number of infants		22

* 22 of 881 infants (2.5%).

Table 29.4 Thrombus associated with umbilical artery catheters as determined at angiography and postmortem examination

Author	Aortic thrombi at angiography (%)	Aortic thrombi at autopsy (%)
Goetzman et al. [31]	23/98 (24)	9/42 (21)
Olinsky et al. [32]	9/30 (30)	5/8 (63)
Mokrohisky et al. [33]	21/23 (91)	
Tyson et al. [34]		33/56 (59)

occurred in 1% of newborn infants with umbilical artery catheters [35]. The incidence of renal arterial involvement in infants with umbilical artery catheters has been reported to range from 1 to 20% [34,36].

The ideal location of the catheter tip is still controversial. Thus, both high and low placement of umbilical artery catheters have been implicated in the genesis of thrombus formation in renal arteries [19,34,22]. Furthermore, whether the catheter alone or other additional factors are important in thrombus formation is unclear. Thus, aortic and renal artery thrombi have occurred in infants without umbilical artery catheter placement [16,19]. In one infant, antithrombin III deficiency was presumed to be the mechanism for the thrombus formation [16]. Furthermore, the association of renal artery thrombus in the presence of an aneurysm of the patent ductus arteriosus has been repeatedly identified [17]. In summary, while placement of an umbilical arterial cath-

eter increases the risk for thrombus formation, the additional role of other factors, such as the condition of the infant at birth (e.g. coagulation status) or the presence of a patent ductus arteriosus, should be considered in any infant with documented thrombus formation.

Other renovascular causes, such as renal artery stenosis and hypoplasia and cardiovascular causes, i.e. coarctation of the aorta [18], are less likely causes of hypertension, accounting for a small number of cases in our experience. Aortic thrombosis, clinically mimicking coarctation of the aorta, may complicate umbilical artery catheterization and present with hypertension [20] (see above).

Renal

Structural and parenchymal renal lesions may be associated with hypertension. Thus, renal cystic disease, such as infantile polycystic (recessive inheritance form) or multicystic dysplastic kidneys, has, in our experience, presented with both early and severe hypertension. Other developmental anomalies, such as hypoplasia of the kidney [21], are rare causes of hypertension in the neonatal period.

Involvement of the genitourinary tract from obstructive uropathy has also been associated with hypertension, and in our series 2 such infants (9%) presented with hypertension.

Tumors

Tumors associated with hypertension are extremely rare in the newborn period. However, neuroblastoma [22], renal mesoblastoma [23], and pheochromocytoma [24] have been associated with hypertension.

Endocrine

Congenital adrenal hyperplasia, specifically an 11-hydroxylase defect, can present with hypertension in infancy. Cushing's syndrome can rarely occur in infancy. More recently there have been two reports of several newborn infants with thyrotoxicosis and systolic hypertension [25,26].

Neurologic

Central nervous system injury, particularly when associated with elevations in intracranial pressure, is, in our experience, not an infrequent cause of hypertension. Thus, with continuous blood pressure monitoring, we have demonstrated a direct relationship between seizures (including subtle seizures) and hypertension in the newborn infant [27]. In animals, central hypertension appears to be sympathetically mediated since it can be abolished with ganglion-blocking agents. [37]. In our small series (Table 29.3), hypertension occurred in 1 infant with meningitis complicated by hydrocephalus. The hypertension only resolved after placement of a ventriculoperitoneal shunt. Another newborn infant admitted with hypertension was noted to have bilateral subdural hematomas on a computerized tomographic scan and clinically to have status epilepticus. The hypertension in this infant resolved only after resolution of the neurologic problems by control of seizure activity.

Respiratory

In our experience, the most common situation in which hypertension occurs in newborn infants is with bronchopulmonary dysplasia (BPD) [28] (Table 29.3) and this is discussed in detail below.

HYPERTENSION IN INFANTS WITH BRONCHOPULMONARY DYSPLASIA

In infants, the association of hypertension with BPD has been reported [28,29]. Briefly, BPD is a form of chronic lung disease which usually occurs in the premature infant in whom, following a course of hyaline membrane disease, chronic lung changes develop often necessitating prolonged oxygen and ventilator usage. Radiologically, in the more advanced cases (stage IV), cystic changes with lung overexpansion and right-sided cardiomegaly are frequently seen [38]. These infants often develop cor pulmonale; management includes treatment with fluid restriction and diuretics for this complication. We have reviewed the courses of 23 infants admitted to St Louis Children's Hospital, MO between July 1977 and March 1980 with severe BPD (stage IV). Each infant required hospitalization for at least 100 days [28]. Hypertension (defined as a systolic blood pressure >113 mmHg) [5,12] occurred in 39% of these infants. The onset of hypertension was late — 160 ± 15.84 postnatal days (mean ± SD) — and the duration averaged 65 ± 10.8 days (mean ± SD). However, this duration may be misleading since more than 80% of these hypertensive infants died.

Only 1 infant was treated with antihypertensive therapy, for a systolic blood pressure in excess of 150 mmHg. None of the infants demonstrated the cardiovascular, neurologic, or retinal complications described below. Abdman and colleagues also noted a low incidence of such complications in their series of infants with BPD [29].

The etiology for the hypertension in these infants is not clear. In our patients it could not be related to umbilical artery catheter placement or renal disease as these had a similar incidence in infants without hypertension. Renal scans also failed to demonstrate asymmetrical renal blood flow or abnormal renal excretory function in the infants studied. It is possible that microemboli to the kidneys with subsequent infarction were responsible for the hypertension. The late onset of an elevated blood pressure would, however, make this etiology less likely.

A striking association in the infants with hypertension was metabolic alkalosis (pH >7.45) and profound hypochloremia (chloride <90 mmol/l). Indeed, several of the infants manifested severe hypochloremia with serum chloride values below 80 mmol/l. We believe the hypochloremia may in part be explained via one of three mechanisms acting either singularly or in combination:

1 a compensatory response to the chronic hypercapnia;
2 the liberal use of diuretics; and
3 ineffective replacement of ongoing chloride losses. It is reasonable to postulate that the chloride deficiency reflects a volume depletion state. This would result in release of renin and subsequent hypertension. Support for this hypothesis is suggested by a lowering of blood pressure with correction of the chloride-deficient state in some of these infants.

The natural history of hypertension in the surviving infants with BPD is also of interest. In all but 1 patient seen in our institution between June 1977 and July 1985 (42 in total with hypertension), the blood pressure had returned to normal by the second year of life.

Miscellaneous

IATROGENIC

The administration of a variety of medications may cause transient blood pressure elevations. Thus, phenylephrine eyedrops have been noted to cause hypertension in infants. This occurred when a 10%

concentration was used [30]. Use of a lower concentration (2.5%) has resolved the problem. Other drugs, e.g. steroids, may also cause hypertension.

Adelman and Sherman noted hypertension following surgical closure of abdominal wall defects in infants [39]. It generally resolves within 48 h. The mechanism for the hypertension is not clear.

COMPLICATIONS

The signs and symptoms of hypertension in the newborn infant are often nonspecific. Most often the cardiovascular and neurologic systems are affected, although more recently retinal changes have been described too.

Cardiovascular system

Adelman [1] described frequent findings of tachycardia, apnea, and muffled heart sounds in 17 infants with hypertension. He attributed these findings to the hypertension. However, in his series, over half of the infants were premature; in addition, approximately 50% had a patent ductus arteriosus. Other medical problems, such as sepsis, apnea, and hypoxia, were also present, all of which could have contributed to the findings that were described. In our experience, cardiac failure is unusual and is most likely to occur in two clinical settings — in infants with either coarctation of the aorta or aortic thrombus.

Central nervous system

In the immediate perinatal period, acute elevations in blood pressure are thought to be important in the pathogenesis of intraventricular hemorrhage in the preterm infant [40]. Potential mechanisms for this association include: (a) vulnerable capillary beds, which are at risk to rupture, such as those within the germinal matrix adjacent to the lateral ventricles; and (b) cerebral blood flow which appears to be pressure-passive, as there is a lack of autoregulation in the stressed newborn infant. These mechanisms have been suggested by work in a beagle puppy model in which acute rises in blood pressure have been shown to provoke germinal matrix/intraventricular hemorrhage [41]. Beyond the immediate newborn period,

hypertension has been causally associated with neurologic symptoms, such as coma, lethargy, or seizures. Indeed, in some reports, resolution of the neurologic symptoms occurred only after control of the hypertension [42].

Retinal

A report by Skalina and colleagues in a group of hypertensive premature infants described a "hypertension-like" retinopathy in approximately 50% of the infants [3]. Some of the abnormalities included increased ratio of venous to arterial caliber vessels, vascular tortuosity, as well as superficial and deep exudates. The retinopathy appeared to resolve after control of the hypertension. The findings in this report should be interpreted with caution. First, the definition of hypertension used in the study — mean arterial blood pressure >70 mmHg — is lower than is currently accepted for such infants (see above). Second, other medical diagnoses, such as retinopathy of prematurity, were not completely excluded as a cause for the retinal changes. None the less, the data do stress the need for opthalmologic examination in newborn infants with hypertension.

MANAGEMENT

When managing an infant with hypertension, the clinician needs to consider the following:
1 What is the cause of the hypertension?
2 What are the risks of hypertension to the infant?
3 What intervention should be used?

What is the cause of the hypertension?

Table 29.5 illustrates the approach we adopt to find a cause for hypertension in the newborn infant. The method of determination of the blood pressure, including the cuff size used, is of primary importance. An expensive and unnecessary work-up can, on occasions, be avoided if it is found that an inappropriately small-sized cuff was used, since this may give a spuriously elevated blood pressure [5,12]. Further information to elicit includes the age at onset of hypertension, the names of recently used medications, whether there has been any recent surgery, and whether the infant has had an umbilical artery catheter. The clinical examination should focus on excluding obvious causes of hypertension, such as coarctation of the aorta, enlarged kidneys, evidence

Table 29.5 Clinical evaluation of the newborn infant with hypertension

History	Examination [System]	Examination Evaluation	Ancillary
Age at onset	Cardiovascular system	Four extremity blood pressure measurements (exclude coarctation), murmur of PDA	*Laboratory* BUN, creatinine, electrolytes, urinalysis, peripheral plasma renin activity, T4
UAC placement, recent surgery	Respiratory system	Evidence for bronchopulmonary dysplasia	*Sonography* Kidney evaluation, other abdominal organ evaluation
	Abdomen	Examine for masses; auscultate for bruit — may suggest aortic or renal artery stenosis	*Renal scan* Evaluate blood flow, excretory function
	Central nervous system	Examine for increased intracranial pressure	*Intravenous pyelogram* Rarely indicated
	Thyroid	Examine for a mass	*Arteriography and renal vein determination* Rarely indicated
	Genitalia	Examine for virilization	*Endocrine (17-ketosteroids, etc.)* Rarely indicated

UAC = Umbilical artery catheter; PDA = patent ductus arteriosus; BUN = blood urea nitrogen.

for raised intracranial pressure, seizures, evidence of virilization, or evidence for hyperthyroidism. The ancillary work-up should in part be guided by the clinical history and examination. Thus, for example, if coarctation of the aorta is suspected, the appropriate evaluation should be undertaken (Chapter 24).

Urinalysis should be performed. Serum urea nitrogen and creatinine determinations may be useful in the assessment of renal function. Serum electrolytes should be checked for evidence of adrenal abnormalities. For example, adrenal hyperplasia may be recognized by the presence of hyperkalemia with associated hyponatremia. We recommend that peripheral blood be obtained to measure venous plasma renin activity in all newborn infants who are hypertensive (see Table 29.6 for normal plasma renin activity). However, caution is necessary when interpreting the levels since they may be normal in the presence of renovascular hypertension [45], or elevated in infants with hyaline membrane disease or renal failure (43,44), and in the presence of a variety of drugs, such as diuretics. Furthermore, not all laboratories have adequate normal values for the newborn age group. A T4 level should be obtained to exclude hyperthyroidism, particularly with early-onset systolic hypertension.

Table 29.6 Plasma renin activity (ng/ml per h) in healthy infants

Day 1	Day 3–6	3–6 Weeks
8.24 ± 0.06*	5.39 ± 1.1*	
8.8 ± 2.8†	11.6 ± 2.8†	2.3 ± 0.6†

* [43] — Renin determined by radioimmunoassay, obtained in the supine position.
† [44] — Renin determined utilizing an immunoassay method with the infant in the supine position prior to a feeding.
All values are means ± SD

The use of real-time ultrasound in the assessment of renal parenchymal diseases has replaced the need for intravenous pyelography in newborn infants in the majority of patients. Furthermore, the role of sonography in the detection of aortic and renal thrombi (Fig. 29.2) has reduced the need for diagnostic angiography in the majority of infants. Thus, we recommend sonography in any infants with unexplained hypertension.

A radionuclide scan to determine blood flow and excretory function is an important and valuable diagnostic aid (Fig. 29.3). Because the technique is portable, it can be performed at the bedside, thus

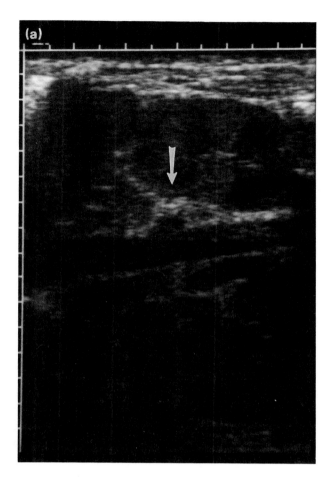

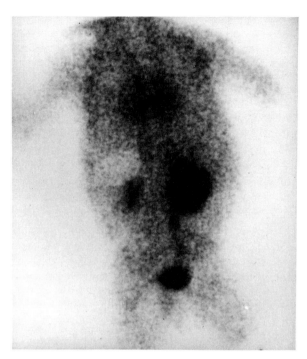

Fig. 29.3 Scintigram from the same patient obtained 6 min after injection of Tc-99m glucoheptonase demonstrates a small left kidney that concentrates the tracer poorly and contributes only 8% of total renal function. The right kidney shows normal accumulation and excretion of the radiopharmaceutic tracer. Decreased activity superior to the left kidney represents a distended stomach. (Courtesy of Dr Barry Siegel.)

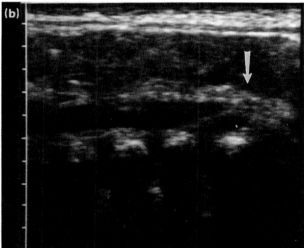

Fig. 29.2 (a) Abdominal ultrasound of the aorta (longitudinal view) in a hypertensive infant. The arrow demonstrates the presence of an echogenic structure (aortic thrombus) within the aorta at the bifurcation and extending proximally.

(b) Renal sonogram in the same patient. The arrow demonstrates an echogenic structure within the left renal artery (renal artery thrombus).

permitting repeated follow-up studies.

Endocrine causes of hypertension in newborn infants are rare; thus, unless strongly indicated, we do not recommend evaluation for these diseases on a routine basis.

What are the risks of hypertension to the infant?

The natural history of hypertension in newborn infants is unclear from available data. In our experience of 70 infants with hypertension, admitted between January 1980 and July 1985, only 4 (5%) developed complications that appeared to be directly and causally related to the hypertension, i.e. all 4 infants presented with congestive heart failure. In 3 infants, hypertension was secondary to an aortic thrombus and in the remaining infant secondary to a coarctation of the aorta. We were unable to detect neurologic or ophthalmologic complications directly attributable to hypertension beyond the immediate newborn period (see above), despite the fact that the majority of the infants were not treated with antihypertensive therapy. Conversely, in infants with hypertension secondary to a central nervous system disturbance, the hypertension is probably an adaptive response to maintain cerebral perfusion pressure (cerebral perfusion pressure is derived from the arterial blood pressure minus the intracranial pressure). It may thus be speculated that treating the hypertension in such infants might compromise cerebral blood flow.

The natural history of hypertension in the infants followed in our institution is as follows. If those with parenchymal renal disease or with obstructive uropathy are excluded, hypertension in all but 2 of the remaining infants resolved by the middle of the second year of life. One infant has BPD and the second renal artery thrombosis. This information raises the important questions: who to treat and when to treat? This is discussed below.

What intervention should be used?

Treatment should be directed toward correction of a primary disorder causing the hypertension, such as coarctation of the aorta, endocrine disorder, or a central nervous system disturbance. In infants without a surgically treatable disorder, such as those with structural renal disease or aortic thrombosis, antihypertensive medication should be implemented when blood pressure is *persistently* elevated above the 95th per-

centile corrected for weight and age (see definition above) [5,12].

There are increasing data regarding the use of antihypertensive medication in the neonatal period [46,47] (Table 29.7). Since pharmacokinetics differ between newborn infants and older children with regard to such variables as absorption, volume of distribution, metabolism, and excretion [47], the management of hypertension is often empiric. Furthermore, the preference for a particular antihypertensive agent will vary from one institution to another.

The choice of initial antihypertensive agent used currently in our institution is indicated below:
1 If the systolic blood pressure is markedly elevated, i.e. >160 mmHg, we use either diazoxide or nitroprusside [48] initially to lower the blood pressure rapidly. Following lowering and/or stabilization of the systolic blood pressure to <120 mmHg, additional antihypertensive medications are introduced to maintain blood pressure control. This facilitates the withdrawal of either the diazoxide or nitroprusside. The antihypertensive medication of our choice at this stage is hydralazine administered either intravenously or orally. However, the response to this drug is varied in our experience. Thus, in some infants it is effective alone in lowering blood pressure; in other infants a combination of other

Table 29.7 Recommended dosages of antihypertensive agents in newborn infants

Agent	Method of administration	Recommended dosage
Diazoxide*	i.v.	Starting dose: 1–2 mg/kg per dose administered either rapidly over 15–30 s or slowly over 15–30 min Maximum dose: 5 mg/kg per dose; repeat effective dose q. 2–6 h as required for control
Nitroprusside*	i.v.	Starting dose: 0.25–0.50 µg/kg per min, doubling q. 15–30 min
Hydralazine	i.v., p.o.	Starting dose: 0.1–0.5 mg/kg per dose q. 3–6 h Maximum dose: 2 mg/kg per dose q. 6 h —*Note*: p.o. dose is often twice the i.v. dose
Methyldopa	i.v., p.o.	Starting dose: 2–3 mg/kg per dose q. 6–8 h Maximum dose: 10–15 mg/kg per dose q. 6–8 h
Propranolol	i.v., p.o.	Starting dose: (p.o.) 0.25 mg/kg per dose q. 6–8 h Maximum dose: 1–4 mg/kg per dose q. 6–8 h i.v. starting dose: 0.01–0.15 mg/kg per dose q. 6 h i.v. maximum dose: 4 mg/kg q. dose q. 6 h
Captopril	p.o.	Starting dose: 0.1–0.15 mg/kg per dose q. 6 h Maximum dose: 0.1–1.0 mg/kg per dose q. 6 h

* Used for rapid lowering of blood pressure.
Adapted from our own experience [46–48].

antihypertensive agents, such as methyldopa, propranolol, or a diuretic, is required to lower the blood pressure. More recently, in infants with markedly elevated plasma renin activity who have failed to respond to hydralazine, captopril (an inhibitor of angiotensin converting enzyme) has been effective in lowering blood pressure [47,49−51]. However, we have observed unpredictable prolonged decreases in blood pressure on maintenance captopril therapy which, in several instances, were associated with oliguria [50].

2 When the *initial* systolic blood pressure is in the range of 120−150 mmHg, the treatment is as above except that we do not attempt to lower the blood pressure rapidly with diazoxide or nitroprusside but will initiate therapy with hydralazine.

The above approach is suggested for infants presenting with conditions such as structural renal disease or vascular thrombus. On the other hand, the most appropriate management of hypertension in infants with BPD is unclear. Our data [28] suggest that despite persistently elevated blood pressure, complications are surprisingly rare in these infants. Furthermore, correction of the chloride-deficient state appears to lower the blood pressure in some infants. Thus, our current approach in infants with BPD is to treat only those infants with a persistent systolic blood pressure >130 mmHg and in whom no electrolyte or acid−base disturbance is noted.

The majority of infants with hypertension will respond to one agent, and unless there is a primary renal parenchymal disease, medications are usually tapered and discontinued within 1 year after initiating therapy. The need for nephrectomy to control renovascular hypertension was suggested from earlier reports [4]. However, recent data suggest that aggressive medical management should obviate this need in the future [46,52]. We would concur with this latter approach.

CONCLUSIONS

Hypertension is not an insignificant problem in the neonatal period. We believe that there is a real increase in incidence and that the hypertension is often secondary to complications of the management of the sick newborn infant. Moreover, our data suggest that the hypertension in most infants will resolve within the first 2 years of life. The frequency of complications secondary to hypertension is unclear and needs to be better defined. Future studies should, in addition, be concerned with issues such as prevention and the need for appropriate intervention in infants with hypertension.

REFERENCES

1 Adelman RD. Neonatal hypertension. *Pediatr Clin North Am* 1978;25:99−110.

2 Leder ME, Kliegman RE, Fanaroff AA. Severe symptomatic hypertension in the newborn. *Pediatr Res* 1981;4:162.

3 Skalina ME, Annable WL, Kliegman RM, Fanaroff AA. Hypertensive retinopathy in the newborn infant. *J Pediatr* 1983;103:781−6.

4 Plummer LB, Kaplan EW, Mendoza SA. Hypertension in infants−a complication of umbilical arterial catheterization. *J Pediatr* 1976;89:802−5.

5 deSwiet M, Fayer P, Shinebourne EA. Systolic blood pressure in a population of infants in the first year of life: the Brompton study. *Pediatrics* 1980;65:1028−35.

6 Lee YH, Rosner B, Gould JB, Lowe EW, Kass EH. Familial aggregation of blood pressure of newborn infants and their mothers. *Pediatrics* 1976;58:722−9.

7 Sheftel DN, Hustead V, Friedman A. Hypertension screening in the follow-up of premature infants. *Pediatrics* 1983;71:763−6.

8 Kirkland RT, Kirkland JL. Systolic blood pressure measurement in the newborn with the transcutaneous Doppler method. *J Pediatr* 1972;80:52−6.

9 Levinson H, Kidd SL, Gemmell PA, Swyer PR. Blood pressure in normal full-term and premature infants. *Am J Dis Child* 1966;111:374−9.

10 Lagler U, Duc G. Systolic blood pressure in normal newborn infants during the first 6 hours of life: transcutaneous Doppler ultrasonic technique. *Biol Neonate* 1980;37:243−5.

11 Kitterman JA, Phibbs RH, Tooley WH. Aortic blood pressure in normal newborn infants during the first 12 hours of life. *Pediatrics* 1969;44:959−68.

12 Task Force on Blood Pressure Control in Children. Report of the Second Task Force on blood pressure control in children−1987. *Pediatrics* 1987;79:1−25.

13 Verswold HT, Kitterman JA, Phibbs GA, Gregory GA, Tooley WH. Aortic blood pressure during the first 12 hours of life in infants with birthweight 610 to 4220 grams. *Pediatrics* 1981;67:607−13.

14 Adams MA, Pasternak JF, Kupfer BM, Gardner TH. A computerized system for continuous physiologic data collection and analysis: initial report on mean arterial blood pressure in very low birthweight infants. *Pediatrics* 1983;71:23−30.

15 Ford KT, Teplick SK, Clark RE. Renal artery embolism causing neonatal hypertension. *Radiology* 1974;113:169−70.

16 Bjarke B, Herin P, Blomback M. Neonatal aortic thrombosis. A possible clinical manifestation of congenital antithrombin III deficiency. *Acta Ped Scand* 1974;63:297−301.

17 Dimmick JE, Patterson MWH, Wu HW. Systemic hypertension in a newborn infant. *J Pediatr* 1979;95:321−4.

18 Keith JD. Coarctation of the aorta. In: Keith JD, Vlad P, eds. *Heart Disease in Infancy and Childhood*. New York: Macmillan, 1978:736−57.

19 Knowlson GT, Marsden HB. Aortic thrombosis in the newborn period. *Arch Dis Child* 1978;53:164−6.

20 Henry CG, Gutierrez F, Lee JT et al. Aortic thrombosis presenting as congestive heart failure: an umbilical artery catheter complication. *J Pediatr* 1981;98:820−2.

21 Gilboa N, Bartoletti A, Unizar RE. Severe hypertension in a newborn associated with increased renin production by a hypoplastic kidney. *J Urol* 1982;128:570−1.

22 Weinblatt ME, Heisel MA, Siegel SE. Hypertension in children with neurogenic tumors. *Pediatrics* 1983;71:947−51.

23 Hendren WH, Kim SH, Herrin JT, Crawford JD. Surgically correctable hypertension of renal origin in childhood. *Am J Surg* 1982;143:432−42.

24 Greenberg RE, Gardner LI. Pheochromocytoma in father and son. Report of the eight affected kindred. *J Clin Endocrinol* 1959;19:351−3.

25 Eason E, Costom B, Papageorgiou AN. Hypertension in neonatal thyrotoxicosis. *J Pediatr* 1982;100:766−8.

26 Schonwetter BS, Libbes SM, Jones MD, Park KJ, Plotnick LP. Hypertension in neonatal hyperthyroidism. *Am J Dis Child* 1983;137:954−5.

27 Perlman JM, Volpe JJ. Seizures in the preterm infant. Effects on cerebral blood flow velocity, intracranial pressure and arterial blood pressure. *J Pediatr* 1983;102:288−93.

28 Perlman JM, Moore V, Siegel M, Dawson J. Is chloride deficiency an important contributing cause of death in infants with bronchopulmonary dysplasia? *Pediatrics* 1986;77:212−16.

29 Abdman SH, Marady BA, Lum GM et al. Systemic hypertension in infants with bronchopulmonary dysplasia. *J Pediatr* 1984;104:928−31.

30 Borromeo-McGrail V, Bordink JM, Keibel H. Systemic hypertension following ocular administration of 10% phenylephrine in the neonate. *Pediatrics* 1973;51:1032−6.

31 Goetzman BW, Stadalnik RC, Bogren HG, Blankenship WJ, Ikeda RM, Thayer J. Thrombotic complications of umbilical artery catheters: a clinical and radiographic study. *Pediatrics* 1975;56:374−9.

32 Olinsky A, Aitken FG, Isdale JM. Thrombus formation after umbilical arterial catheterization. An angiographic study. *South Afr Med J* 1975;49:1467−70.

33 Mokrohisky ST, Levene RT, Blumhagen JD, Wesenberg RL, Simmons MA. Low position of umbilical artery catheters increases associated complications in newborn infants. *N Engl J Med* 1978;299:561−3.

34 Tyson JE, DeSa DJ, Moore S. Thromboatheromatosis complications of umbilical arterial catheterization in the newborn period. *Arch Dis Child* 1976;51:744−54.

35 O'Neill JA, Neblett WW, Born ML. Management of major thromboembolic complications of umbilical artery catheters. *J Pediatr Surg* 1981;16:972−7.

36 Tooley W. What is the risk of umbilical artery catheters? *Pediatrics* 1972;50:1−2.

37 Plum F, Posner JB, Troy B. Cerebral metabolic and circulatory responses to induced convulsions in animals. *Arch Neurol* 1966;18:1−5.

38 Northway WH Jr, Rosan RC, Porter DY. Pulmonary disease following respiratory therapy of hyaline membrane disease: bronchopulmonary dysplasia. *N Engl J Med* 1967;276:357−62.

39 Adelman RD, Sherman MP. Hypertension in the neonate following closure of abdominal wall defects. *J Pediatr* 1980;97:642−4.

40 Perlman JM, McMenamin JB, Volpe JJ. Fluctuating cerebral blood flow velocity in respiratory distress syndrome: relation to the development of intraventricular hemorrhage. *N Engl J Med* 1983;309:204−8.

41 Goddard J, Lewis RM, Armstrong DL, Zeller RS. Moderately rapidly induced hypertension as a cause of intraventricular hemorrhage in the newborn beagle model. *J Pediatr* 1980;96:1057−60.

42 Mace S, Hirschfeld S. Hypertensive encephalopathy. A cause of neonatal seizures. *Am J Dis Child* 1983;137:32−3.

43 Marshall R, Bartlett C, Sheehan M, Mauer M. Plasma renin activity in healthy and sick newborns. *Pediatr Res* 1976;10:333.

44 Kotchen TA, Strickland AL, Rice MS, Walters DR. A study of the renin−angiotensin system in newborn infants. *J Pediatr* 1972;80:938−46.

45 Poutasse EF, Marks LS, Wisoff CP, Vinson AM, Wan AT. Renal vein renin determinations in hypertension: falsely negative tests. *J Urol* 1973;110:371−4.

46 Adelman RD, Merten D, Vogel J, Goetzman BW, Wennberg RP. Nonsurgical management of renovascular hypertension. *Pediatrics* 1978;62:71−6.

47 Roberts RJ. *Drug Therapy in Infants. Pharmacologic Principles and Clinical Experience.* Philadelphia: WB Saunders, 1984:173−205.

48 Benitz WE, Malachowski N, Cohen RS, Stevenson DK, Ariagno RL, Sunshine P. Use of sodium nitroprusside in neonates: efficacy and safety. *J Pediatr* 1985;106:102−10.

49 Hymes LC, Warshaw BL. Captopril: long term treatment of hypertension in a preterm infant and in older children. *Am J Dis Child* 1983;137:263−6.

50 Tack ED, Perlman JM. Renal failure in sick hypertensive premature infants receiving captopril therapy. *J Pediatr* 1988;112:805−10.

51 O'Dea RF, Mirkin BL, Alward CT, Sinaiko AR. Treatment of neonatal hypertension with captopril. *J Pediatr* 1988;113:403−6.

52 Strife JL, Ball WS, Towbin R, Keller MS, Dillon T. Arterial occlusions in neonates: use of fibrinolytic therapy. *Radiology* 1988;166:395−400.

30 Hypertension in the Black Population

JONATHAN D. HEILICZER AND EDDIE S. MOORE

Racial differences in blood pressure between black and white adult populations in the USA are now well documented. The differences that exist include those in average blood pressure, incidence of hypertension, prevalence of secondary relative to primary (essential) hypertension, and morbidity and mortality from hypertension. The reason for these racial differences is currently unknown; however, a number of factors including alterations in renal and endocrine physiology, the autonomic nervous system, and cardiac function may all play a role. In addition there are different genetic and environmental factors. Although the time of its precise onset is not known, essential hypertension is increasingly thought to begin during childhood and adolescence. Given that a racial effect on blood pressure is present in the adult population and that essential hypertension may begin in childhood, this review will focus on the above variables as presently reported in black and white children.

AVERAGE BLOOD PRESSURE

Newborn babies and infants

Early studies by Zinner and colleagues demonstrated a familial aggregation of blood pressure in young children with relatively higher values in those children whose parents also had high-normal values or overt hypertension [1]. To investigate whether or not this relationship was present shortly after birth, mean diastolic blood pressure was studied in black and white low-birthweight and premature infants during the first 8 days of life (Moore, personal observation). Mean diastolic pressure determined by multiple observations positively correlated with a parental history of hypertension; however, no racial differences were observed. In a study of systolic blood pressure during non-rapid eye movement sleep

in term newborn infants by Schachter and colleagues, no difference was noted between black and white babies [2]. These authors also referred to unpublished data that did not demonstrate a racial influence on average blood pressure during different behavioral states in 257 newborn babies. It appears that beginning shortly after birth, average blood pressure correlates with parental blood pressure; however no racial influence is present.

There may be racial differences in the effect of dietary sodium on blood pressure in infants. Schachter and colleagues [2] reported that white infants with increased dietary sodium intake had higher blood pressures than white infants receiving a lower sodium intake; a similar relationship was not found in black infants. Hofman and coworkers reported that dietary sodium intake beginning at birth had a small but significant effect on systolic blood pressure measured at 6 months of age in white infants in the Netherlands [3]. However, Whitten and Stewart [4] found no effect of dietary sodium on blood pressure in a study of black infants that started at birth and with follow-up at age 4 months, 2, and 8 years of age. Unfortunately, in these studies no mention was made of any possible relationship between blood pressure in the newborn period to that in the parent.

Infants and preschool age children

As stated previously, Zinner and co-authors [1] reported a close parent–child correlation for average blood pressure in young children; follow-up studies demonstrated that the level of blood pressure relative to peers tended to remain stable in later childhood [1,5]. Schachter and coworkers measured mean blood pressure in the same infants at birth and followed them up with repeat measurements until 5 years of age [6]. Diastolic blood pressure increased up to age

24 months with minimal change thereafter, and there was no apparent racial difference in either systolic or diastolic blood pressure. Zinner and colleagues reported no racial influence on systolic or diastolic blood pressure in children 2–14 years of age [7]. Additionally, Londe and co-authors [8], Levine and colleagues [9], and Londe and Goldring [10] investigated average blood pressure in young children and found no racial differences in either mean systolic or diastolic blood pressure. Thus, during the first 6 years of life, race has no effect on average blood pressure.

School-age children and adolescents

Most of the controversy regarding possible racial differences in blood pressure distribution during development is in adolescence. The disparate results may be related, at least in part, to differences in measurement techniques and in the definition of what constitutes elevated blood pressure. In many studies only a single blood pressure measurement has been reported. In other studies multiple measurements of blood pressure have been obtained. Therefore differences in methodology make it difficult to compare studies with different results.

In the Bogalusa (Louisiana) Heart Study, black children had significantly higher systolic and diastolic blood pressures beginning before 10 years of age compared to white children [11]. This apparent racial effect was greatest in the upper 5% of blood pressure rank. Similarly, Kotchen and co-authors [12], Haggerty and colleagues [13], and Kilcoyne and associates [14] all reported higher blood pressure in black children and adolescents compared to age-matched control white populations. More recently, Pratt and colleagues reported higher systolic and diastolic blood pressures in black children and adolescents studied in the midwestern USA [15].

In contrast to the above reports, Goldring and coworkers reported lower mean diastolic blood pressure in black boys 14–17 years of age compared to white boys of the same age [16]. Additionally, Dube and associates studied 1668 healthy children in Brooklyn, New York and found lower mean diastolic blood pressure in black children [17]. Rames and coworkers [18], Rose [19], and Fixler and co-authors [20] all reported no racial effect on mean systolic or diastolic blood pressure in children and adolescents. Furthermore the report of the Second Task Force on blood pressure control in children indicated that no

differences were found by race from birth to age 18 years in systolic or diastolic blood pressure when the results of several large studies were combined in a metaanalysis. If the above studies are considered in light of a report on adults in the Baltimore area, it seems likely that a racial effect on average blood pressure is not present during childhood or adolescence [21]. That study clearly showed that the incidence of essential hypertension in blacks was not significantly different from that in white adults until approximately the third to fourth decade of life, strongly suggesting that racial differences in average blood pressure are not present until early to mid adult life. Why then is there confusion regarding whether there is a racial effect on average blood pressure during adolescence? The specific explanation is unknown. Studies demonstrating a racial effect on mean blood pressure during development have been primarily from the southeastern USA, suggesting important environmental influences. These may include but are not limited to diet, stress, socioeconomic status, and availability of health care. Alternatively, but less likely, a difference in gene pool could be implicated. As stated above, another major explanation includes differences in investigative techniques. In any event, based on available data, there is no racial effect on mean blood pressure during childhood and adolescence in the USA.

Recently differences in ambulatory blood pressure have been found between black and white adults. Harshfield and coworkers [22] and Murphy and colleagues [23] reported that there is a smaller decline in sleeping blood pressure in blacks than in whites. In evaluating ambulatory blood pressure in 199 youngsters ranging in age from 9 to 18 years—107 of whom were black and 92 white—it has also been reported [24] that black boys had significantly higher systolic blood pressure while asleep than the three other sex/race groups studied. In addition, the black teenagers as a group had higher sleeping diastolic blood pressures than the whites. The investigators put forward the hypothesis that the additional cardiovascular strain imposed by the lack of a nocturnal decline in blood pressure in black children might be the cause of preventable cardiovascular damage.

PREVALENCE OF HYPERTENSION

An acceptable definition of hypertension is required to determine the prevalence of this condition and, until recently, the definition of what is high normal blood pressure and what is significant hypertension has been variable for American children [25]. Furthermore, differences in measurement techniques and the phenomenon of regression toward the mean, when multiple blood pressures are recorded, significantly influenced the reported prevalence of high blood pressure in children. In a recent report, Sinaiko and co-authors [26] have shown that the prevalence of systolic hypertension in school-age children decreased from 1.0% initially to 0.3% with subsequent readings. The prevalence of diastolic hypertension decreased from an initial 3.5% to 0.8% and the prevalence of combined systolic and diastolic hypertension decreased from 4.2% to 1.1%.

In earlier studies such as the Muscatine (Iowa) Study, initial recordings indicated a prevalence of childhood hypertension of 13%; this was reduced to approximately 1% with follow-up measurements [18]. Similar significant reductions in the initial prevalence of high blood pressure in children with use of multiple blood pressure determinations were reported in the Dallas Study, and in two studies from New York, [14,17,20]. This has led investigators to use persistent blood pressure elevation to define hypertension.

Londe and associates used systolic and diastolic blood pressures greater than the 90th percentile to define hypertension in children, observing a prevalence of 1.9 and 2.2% in white and black children, respectively; these prevalences were not significantly different statistically [8]. In a screening study of high school students 14–18 years of age, Goldring and co-authors [16] found blood pressures above the 95th percentile to be more frequent in white males than in black males only in 14-year-old subjects. In girls, the same was true for 14- and 18-year-old students. When all age groups were combined, the percentage of students with blood pressure exceeding the 95th percentile was greater in white boys. There was no racial difference in the 14–18-year-old girls [16].

One of the most striking studies relative to a racial effect on the prevalence of high blood pressure in childhood was that of Kotchen and coworkers who reported that more than 11% of black adolescents had systolic blood pressures greater than 140 mmHg compared to none for white children of the same age [12]. Similarly, the Bogalusa Heart Study reported striking racial differences in the upper 5% of mean blood pressures, with black children having higher levels than white children [27]. This may suggest that while the prevalence of blood pressure elevation is similar for black and white children, black children

with hypertension have higher blood pressures than white children with hypertension. Further study of this question is needed.

The report by Sinaiko and associates [26] and the review by Jesse [28] indicate that available data suggest a prevalence of high blood pressure from 1.1 to 4.5% in children from birth to 18 years of age with no apparent racial differences.

GENETIC FACTORS

Studies in various populations consistently have shown [29,30] that primary hypertension is an inherited disorder. Furthermore, an inherited factor has also been shown to be present in some laboratory animal models used to study human essential hypertension [31]. Therefore, during growth and development in black and white children, the predilection to develop essential hypertension may be related to genetic factors, as has been suggested for black and white adults. However, there is compelling evidence that environmental factors can and do affect the expression of these genetic factors. Environmental factors such as obesity, dietary sodium and calcium intake, and stress can precipitate as well as aggravate previously established hypertension [32–35].

In the USA, the original gene pool of blacks was principally from the West African coast. However, of interest is the study of Blankson and his coworkers who showed a lower mean blood pressure in West African children compared to American black children of a similar age [36]. This observation implies either a primary evolutionary change in the gene pool of American blacks, or supports the concept that environmental factors operate in concert with genetic factors to influence the ultimate level of blood pressure. Gleiberman [33] has proposed that during evolution, African blacks adapted physiologically so that the kidneys retained sodium in the face of a low dietary sodium intake and increased perspiration in the African heat. It can be further postulated that enforced relocation of these African blacks to America, as a result of the slave trade, exposed them to quite different environmental conditions. This may have resulted in selective mortality with those individuals with the greatest ability to retain salt and water being more likely to survive.

Further changes in diet and other environmental conditions are likely to have occurred as blacks began living in the USA. These factors, when combined with the prior evolutionary adaptation, may have resulted in a greater incidence of abnormally elevated blood pressure in American blacks. At present the polygenic inheritance of high blood pressure in both blacks and whites is not well characterized. However molecular geneticists are actively studying the problem and new information should be forthcoming within the next decade [37].

SECONDARY HYPERTENSION

In adults, hypertension due to renovascular disease is reported to be less common in blacks compared to whites [38,39]. However, adult blacks are reported to have a greater incidence of secondary high blood pressure due to diseases such as diabetes mellitus and parenchymal renal disease [40,41]. Assuming that genetic as well as socioeconomic and environmental factors may be associated with the incidence of diseases that may cause hypertension during childhood, such as glomerulonephritis and urinary tract infection, a racial effect on the occurrence of secondary hypertension in this age group could be postulated. However, in the Chicago area during an 11-year period, no racial difference in disease categories leading to end-stage renal failure in children 2–18 years of age was noted [42]. In the one disease particularly correlated with race, sickle cell anemia, hypertension has been rarely reported [43]. Sellers observed intermittent hypertension during sickle cell crisis in a 13-year-old black boy [44]. Of interest is the fact that Matustik and colleagues reported elevated plasma renin and aldosterone levels in 14 black patients with sickle cell anemia who had normal blood pressures [45]. Thus, there presently is insufficient clinical evidence to suggest a racial influence on the prevalence of secondary hypertension in childhood.

MORBIDITY AND MORTALITY

In general, the clinical manifestations of acute and chronic disease in infants and children are independent of race. For those rare instances where differences exist, host characteristics and environmental factors must be included in any possible explanation. Clinical manifestations of early essential hypertension in the young are no different from those in adults with mild and moderate hypertension. The majority of adolescents are asymptomatic; when symptomatology is present, according to an early

report by Lieberman, the manifestations are frontal headaches and palpitations [46]. There have been no reports of a racial influence on the clinical manifestations of hypertension in children.

An important question is whether or not essential hypertension during childhood will ultimately be shown to lead to target-organ disease in the affected individual, thereby having an impact on morbidity and mortality during subsequent adult life (see Chapter 33). The overwhelming clinical experience is that hypertension in adults has a significantly higher morbidity and mortality in blacks than in whites [21,47,48].

Lauer and co-authors [49] as well as Nora [50] have suggested formulas that may be useful for assessing the child at risk for developing coronary heart disease in adult life. The formula proposed by Nora involves family history, blood lipid levels, weight, somatotype, and level of blood pressure [50]. Recent studies have reported that plasma levels of cholesterol and high density lipoproteins are lower in black compared to white children. This leads us to speculate that a racial influence on Nora's proposed formula might be anticipated [50,51]. In the Chicago study of end-stage renal failure previously noted, only 1 child, (black) of a total of 296 children had end-stage renal failure due to hypertensive nephrosclerosis [42].

There are no literature references indicating a racial influence on mortality from high blood pressure during childhood. Clearly, long-term evaluation of black and white children with high blood pressure during childhood is needed to investigate adequately any possible racial effect on eventual outcome in subsequent adult life [52].

PHYSIOLOGIC RACIAL DIFFERENCES

Studies of the pathophysiology of elevated blood pressure in adult populations include those of the renal control of plasma volume, urinary sodium and electrolyte excretion, the renin–angiotensin system, renal vasodepressor substances, red cell sodium content, membrane electrolyte transport, and cardiovascular physiology [53–58]. In the majority of these studies, a racial influence on these determinants of blood pressure has been reported. As will be discussed, similar studies of the racial differences in the pathophysiology of elevated blood pressure have also been reported during childhood and adolescence.

Plasma volume and urine electrolyte excretion

Renal control of plasma volume via urinary sodium excretion is different in black and white adult hypertensive subjects [53,59]. For example, Luft and associates reported that adult black subjects excreted significantly less sodium following a salt load than adult white subjects [34]. In addition, several investigators have shown salt sensitivity in blacks [60–62]. Berenson and colleagues showed that in the Bogalusa Heart Study, 24-h urine sodium excretion was positively correlated with blood pressure level measured on the same day, particularly in the higher percentile ranks; this association was greater for black children [63]. Interestingly, however, there was no racial difference in the amount of urinary sodium excretion — a finding corroborated by Pratt and his coworkers [15]. The Evans County, Georgia Study also did not find a racial effect on urinary sodium excretion [64].

Studies in very low-birthweight newborn infants have shown that they can regulate plasma and extracellular volume by renal sodium excretion; however, an effect on blood pressure has not been reported [65]. In the studies of blood pressure in young infants by Schachter and colleagues [2] and by Hofman and coworkers [3] dietary sodium intake was shown to influence systolic blood pressure in white but not black infants, but urinary excretion of sodium was not measured. Thus, the racial differences in renal sodium excretion and subsequent regulation of plasma volume in adult populations are apparently not manifest during childhood.

Alterations in calcium homeostasis have been reported in essential hypertension and dietary calcium intake is being studied in the pathogenesis of essential hypertension [32,36]. The Bogalusa Heart Study addressed the possibility of a role for altered calcium homeostasis in blood pressure control during development [66]. In these studies, it was found that serum total calcium concentration correlated with blood pressure strata and, in addition, white children had higher rates of urinary calcium excretion than black children of comparable age. However, Perlman and coworkers reported that urinary calcium excretion in hypertensive adolescents did not differ from that of normotensive adolescents [67]. Additionally, urinary calcium excretion correlated with sodium excretion in the control but not in the hypertensive subjects. There was no mention of racial influences in this study.

In adult populations, increased potassium relative to sodium intake is thought to be protective against an elevation in blood pressure. The role of potassium homeostasis in blood pressure control has been reviewed by Parfrey and associates [68]. Black adults with or without hypertension excrete urinary potassium at lower rates than white adults [69,70] and this has been attributed to reduced dietary potassium intake [70]. At least two studies have been reported concerning potassium homeostasis and blood pressure control in children. In the Bogalusa Heart Study [66] and the Evans County, Georgia Study [64], urinary potassium excretion was lower in black children at any level of dietary potassium intake. In both black and white children, however, there was no correlation between urinary potassium excretion and blood pressure strata.

Finally, perturbations in uric acid homeostasis have been reported to occur with high blood pressure in adults [71]. Prebis and associates studied renal uric acid excretion in normotensive and hypertensive children and adolescents 3–18 years of age [72]. They reported that fractional uric acid excretion was inversely related to plasma uric acid concentration in both normotensive as well as hypertensive children. In this study of two groups of predominantly black children, Prebis and coworkers further reported plasma uric acid levels to be significantly higher in hypertensive compared to normotensive youths [72].

Hormonal systems

In the Bogalusa Heart Study, peripheral plasma renin activity was measured in free-living children. It was shown to be lower in black boys in the high blood pressure strata than in white boys and girls and black girls [63]. Moreover, racial differences in peripheral plasma renin activity were inversely correlated with blood pressure strata and with age. Low plasma renin activity is also found in black adults; it has been postulated that this is due to expanded plasma volume.

Recently Pratt and colleagues [15] studied 715 normotensive children aged 6–16 years, 249 of whom were black. No dietary interventions were prescribed prior to the measurement of urinary sodium, potassium, and aldosterone. The mean rate of sodium excretion was similar for blacks and whites but the rate of urinary potassium excretion was lower for blacks. In addition the rate of urinary aldosterone excretion was also lower in blacks than in whites. In a second study of 99 children between the ages of 6 and 14 years, blood pressure, plasma aldosterone, cortisol, and plasma renin activity were measured. Again, physical activity and diet were not controlled for in this study. It was found that the mean serum sodium and potassium concentrations, levels of plasma renin activity, and plasma cortisol were the same in the two races. The value for plasma aldosterone in black children was 58% of that in white children. This was the same percentage difference that had been found in the earlier study for urinary aldosterone excretion. This racial difference in aldosterone excretion could not be explained purely on the basis of differences in dietary potassium intake. However, it could be partially explained by a lower degree of responsiveness in black children since they excreted less aldosterone than white children at any level of potassium intake. The physiologic importance of these findings with regard to racial differences in blood pressure control is unknown.

Renal vasodepressor substances

Zinner and coworkers investigated the familial aggregation of urinary kallikrein excretion in childhood [73]. Familial aggregation was demonstrated for both black and white children; however, urine kallikrein excretion was significantly lower in black children, in whom it was positively correlated with potassium excretion and inversely correlated with sodium excretion. Families with the lowest urine kallikrein excretion tended to have higher blood pressure levels. In a more recent study, Hohn and colleagues confirmed that there is lower urine kallikrein excretion in black children [74].

It has been found that dopamine β-hydroxylase levels are higher in white children for all blood pressure strata. In addition Hohn and colleagues measured unstimulated circulating plasma catecholamine levels in normotensive children of parents with and without essential hypertension [74]. In both groups, plasma catecholamine levels were lower in black children.

Cardiovascular physiology

As already discussed, Schachter and co-authors [2] reported a racial difference in heart rate in newborn infants. In that study, 61 apparently unstressed, appropriate-for-gestational-age black infants had

significantly higher heart rates than comparable white infants. This difference was noted to disappear by 24 months of age [75]. However in older children Shekelle and co-authors reported lower mean heart rates in apparently unstimulated black children 6–11 years of age compared to age-matched white children [76]. Similarly, in the Bogalusa Heart Study lower resting heart rate was noted in black children [63].

Several studies investigating cardiovascular responses in stimulated or stressed children have also been reported. Strong and colleagues found no racial influence on the response of healthy and normotensive children undergoing isometric and dynamic exercise [77]. The Bogalusa Heart Study demonstrated an increase in resting heart rate over blood pressure strata in white but not in black boys [63]. However, black boys in the high blood pressure strata had higher resting supine and stressed systolic blood pressure levels than any other group, both black and white. Falkner and colleagues reported an exaggerated increase in blood pressure and pulse rate in predominantly black adolescents with mild elevations of blood pressure who had a family history of essential hypertension, compared to those who did not [78]. It also took longer for the elevated blood pressure to return to baseline levels in those adolescents with a positive family history of hypertension.

Red cell sodium fluxes (see also Chapter 16)

Canessa and co-authors [79] as well as Wedes [80] demonstrated a significant reduction in red cell sodium–lithium countertransport in black adults with essential hypertension compared to white subjects. Norling and coworkers studied red cell sodium–lithium countertransport in normotensive and hypertensive children and, similar to observations in the adult, found lower rates in black children in both groups [81]. In a study of young college students, Filer and associates also found lower red cell sodium–lithium countertransport in black compared to white subjects [82]. At variance with these reports, however, are the studies in normotensive children by Woods and colleagues, who found no racial difference in this countertransport system [83].

Red cell membrane sodium–potassium cotransport has been shown to be lower in both normotensive and hypertensive black adults compared to whites [84] but there is geographic variability of this system [85]. McCrory and associates investigated red cell sodium—potassium cotransport in normotensive black and white children with hypertensive parents and found lower mean values in black children [86]. Some black children had no detectable red cell membrane sodium—potassium cotransport.

Most studies have shown that erythrocytes from blacks have a higher sodium concentration than erythrocytes from whites. For example, Lasker and coworkers reported higher red cell free sodium concentrations in both normotensive and hypertensive black adults compared to white adults [87]. However, in a study of children 11—15 years of age, Trevisan and colleagues noted red cell free sodium concentration to be correlated with age, but there were no differences based on race [88]. Na^+-K^+-ATPase activity has also been studied in both black and white populations and has generally been lower in erythrocytes from blacks. However, at present there are no consistent correlations between Na^+-K^+-ATPase activity and blood pressure [89].

In summary, similar to adults, significant racial differences in the determinants of blood pressure have been found in children. The determinants measured have often been noted to be correlated with blood pressure strata or to show familial aggregation. However, during childhood, these determinants have not yet been associated with overt hypertension as they are in the adult black population in the USA.

ENVIRONMENTAL FACTORS AND PERSONAL CHARACTERISTICS

Various environmental factors in addition to diet have been considered important in the etiology of essential hypertension. These include social class, occupation, stress, level of education, domicile, weight, height, alcohol intake, and smoking [90] (see also Chapter 17). Some of these have been evaluated in children but not as extensively as in adults.

There is a great deal of evidence that in both adults and children body weight and blood pressure are positively correlated [91]. For example, in 1971 Londe and co-authors reported an association between obesity and elevated blood pressure in asymptomatic children [92]. In children in western cultures not only body weight but also height is related to blood pressure [93]. Lynds and associates correlated height and weight with blood pressure in black children 5—11 years of age [94]. In single observations of blood pressure, hypertension was three times more likely

to occur in obese black children than in the general black population.

In studies using multiple blood pressure measurements, Londe and Goldring showed a positive correlation between blood pressure and weight as well as with height in both black and white children [10]. However, in all blood pressure strata, the relationship was stronger in black children. In older adolescents, Johnson and coworkers reported that the correlation between weight and blood pressure was lower in black males [95]. When all of the data for children were analyzed the relationship of obesity to hypertension was found to be weakest for black females. Regardless of race, it is currently recommended that blood pressure measurements for a given child should be correlated with that individual's height and weight [52].

In a review of the pathophysiology of high blood pressure, Gillum noted that the black population is more frequently exposed to conditions of poverty, low occupational and educational status, and high levels of socioeconomic stress [96]. These factors are known to have an effect on the prevalence of hypertension in adult populations. Our experience with middle-class black children may represent an example of a result of stress of "upward mobility" in this high-risk group [97]. As mentioned previously, Falkner and coworkers showed an exaggerated cardiovascular response to verbal stress in black adolescents [78]. Light and colleagues have also demonstrated that young marginally hypertensive blacks have a greater systolic pressure response to competitive stress than do comparable whites [98].

Level of education is often used as a measure of socioeconomic status. Studies in adults have shown an inverse relationship between level of education and the incidence of high blood pressure [99]. In the study of heart rate and blood pressure in newborn infants described earlier, the higher heart rate in blacks was in infants of low socioeconomic status [75]. Similarly, reports from the southeastern USA showing a higher level of blood pressure in black children also found an inverse correlation of blood pressure with social class in the black children [11,27]. In contrast, Walter and Hofman did not find a relationship of social class with blood pressure [100]. Additionally, Londe and coworkers [8] and Goldring and colleagues [16] did not find a correlation between blood pressure and social class in the St Louis area. Neither in a study in New Jersey did Scholl and coworkers find a relationship between socioeconomic status and blood pressure in black school children [101]. We found hypertension in black children to occur more often in middle-class families [97]. The disparate results reported for the relationship of socioeconomic status to blood pressure in children may be related to different methodology for determining socioeconomic status and to selection of subjects. For example, some studies investigated patients seen at medical centers while others included people from private office practice.

In black adults, rural subjects have been shown to have a higher prevalence of hypertension than urban blacks [102]. Early studies in children suggest a similar relationship. As mentioned previously, our experience in the large metropolitan Chicago area indicated a greater prevalence of hypertension in black urban children [97]. A high prevalence of hypertension in urban black children was also reported by de Castro and colleagues [103].

Hypertension is reported to be more prevalent among adults who drink large amounts of alcohol than in those who do not [104]. Klatsky and co-authors reported that this relationship is independent of race [105]. Although smoking is associated with increased cardiovascular morbidity and mortality, blood pressure levels are said to be lower in smokers than in nonsmokers.

TREATMENT CONSIDERATIONS

Racial differences in response to different antihypertensive drugs have recently received considerable attention as discussed by Arradondo [106] and by Saunders [107]. It is presently unclear to what extent they correlate with the racial differences in the determinants of blood pressure which have been previously discussed.

Initial studies suggested that treatment with β-blocking agents was less effective in black adults than in white adults [108]. However, the combination of a diuretic with a β-blocking drug was found to enhance the effect of the β-blocker in the treatment of high blood pressure in blacks [107]. Presumably this is due to stimulation of the renin—angiotensin system by the diuretic. Shulman reported that monotherapy with angiotensin converting enzyme inhibitors for high blood pressure was also less effective in black subjects [109]. However similar to the response with β-blocking drugs, addition of a diuretic to therapy with angiotensin converting enzyme inhibitors improved the control of high blood pressure in blacks.

Finally, calcium channel blocking agents have been shown to be effective as monotherapy in the treatment of hypertension in black adults [110]. Diuretics, β- and calcium channel blocking agents, as well as angiotensin converting enzyme inhibitors, have been used with variable success for the treatment of high blood pressure in childhood; no racial influence has been reported [111]—however observations suggesting similar efficacy are quite limited.

SUMMARY

Systematic investigation of the effects of pathophysiologic and environmental factors on blood pressure control in childhood has lagged far behind studies in adults. Based on available data, certain differences demonstrating a racial influence on blood pressure in children and adolescents are known and are summarized in Table 30.1. These racial differences in blood pressure determinants are present in both normotensive and hypertensive black children. Falkner has questioned whether there is a distinctive "black hypertension" [112]. She stated that issues such as aging, genetics, and environment alter the biological interaction of determinants of blood pressure control. Subsequent development of hypertension would be consistent with Guyton's theory on the development of high blood pressure [113]. Thus race may be

Table 30.1 Summary of variables associated with blood pressure control in black children from birth to age 17 years compared to age-matched white children

Variable	Observation in black children
Average blood pressure	Not different or slightly higher
Incidence of hypertension	Not different
Resting heart rate	Lower
Dopamine β-hydroxylase	Lower
Plasma renin activity	Lower
Plasma catecholamine activity	Lower
Response to stress	Greater increase in systolic pressure
Response to exercise	Less increase in heart rate
Dietary potassium	Lower
Dietary calcium	Lower
24-h urine Na^+ excretion	Not different
24-h urine K^+ excretion	Lower
24-h urine Ca^{++} excretion	Lower
24-h urine kallikrein	Lower
Red cell Na^+ fluxes	Lower

merely a marker for other factors which are at present poorly understood.

As discussed above, a racial influence on variables related to blood pressure control is present throughout life. However, the prevalence of overt hypertension does not correlate with race until adult life. If we are to have an impact on the disproportionate morbidity and mortality of hypertension in adult blacks in the USA greater attention must be given to understanding blood pressure control in black children and adolescents. The observation of a different blood pressure distribution in West African blacks and the possible effect of westernization on blood pressure in American blacks should receive particular attention. Of related interest is the observed effect of western culture and dietary sodium intake on blood pressure in the inhabitants of the Solomon Islands and the Yanomamo Indians of Venezuela [114,115]. In these cultures prior to westernization, blood pressure was noted to remain relatively level throughout the life cycle. Following exposure to western civilization, blood pressure was found to increase with age, as is true in western culture. The explanation for this change is not known but several factors, such as stress and changes in diet with an increased sodium and caloric intake, have been suggested to play a role.

In recognition of the greater morbidity and mortality in adult blacks with hypertension, it is possible that the definition of elevated blood pressure in American black children should be lower than for American white children. This would result in earlier initiation of hygienic interventions as well as specific pharmacologic treatment in blacks. The ultimate objective would be to effect a reduction in hypertensive morbidity and mortality in blacks.

REFERENCES

1 Zinner SH, Levy PS, Kass EH. Familial aggregation of blood pressure in childhood. *N Engl J Med* 1971;284:401–4.

2 Schachter J, Lachin JM III, Kerr JL, Wimberly FC III, Ratey JJ. Heart rate and blood pressure in black newborns and in white newborns. *Pediatrics* 1976;58:283–7.

3 Hofman A, Hazebroek A, Volkenburg HA. A randomized trial of sodium intake and blood pressure in newborn infants. *JAMA* 1983;250:370–3.

4 Whitten CF, Stewart RA. The effect of dietary sodium in infancy on blood pressure and related factors. Studies of infants fed salted and unsalted diets for five months at eight months and eight years of age. *Acta Paediatr Scand* 1980;279(suppl):1–17.

5 Zinner SH, Rosner B, Oh W, Kass EH. Significance of blood pressure in infancy. Familial aggregation and predictive effect on later blood pressure. *Hypertension* 1985;7:411–16.

6 Schachter J, Kuller LH, Perfetti C. Blood pressure during the first five years of life: relation to ethnic group (black or white) and to parental hypertension. *Am J Epidemiol* 1984;119:541–53.

7 Zinner SH, Martin LF, Sacks F, Rosner B, Kass EH. A longitudinal study of blood pressure in childhood. *Am J Epidemiol* 1974;100:437–42.

8 Londe S, Gollub SW, Goldring D. Blood pressure in black and in white children. *J Pediatr* 1977;90:93–5.

9 Levine RS, Hennekens CH, Klein B et al. Tracking correlations of blood pressure levels in infancy. *Pediatrics* 1978;61:121–5.

10 Londe S, Goldring D. Hypertension in children. *Am Heart J* 1972;84:1–4.

11 Voors AW, Foster TA, Frerichs RR, Webber LS, Berenson GS. Studies of blood pressure in children, ages 5–14 years, in a total biracial community: the Bogalusa heart study. *Circulation* 1976;54:319–27.

12 Kotchen JM, Kotchen TA, Schwertman NC, Kuller LH. Blood pressure distributions of urban adolescents. *Am J Epidemiol* 1974;99:315–24.

13 Haggerty RJ, Maroney MS, Nadas AS. Essential hypertension in infancy and childhood. *Am J Dis Child* 1956;92:535–41.

14 Kilcoyne MM, Richter RW, Alsup PA. Adolescent hypertension. I. Detection and prevalence. *Circulation* 1974;40:758–64.

15 Pratt JH, Jones JJ, Miller JZ et al. Racial differences in aldosterone excretion and plasma aldosterone concentrations in children. *N Engl J Med* 1989;321:1152–7.

16 Goldring D, Londe S, Sivakoff M, Hernandez A, Britton C, Choi S. Blood pressure in a high school population. I. Standards for blood pressure and the relation of age, sex, weight, height, and race to blood pressure in children 14 to 18 years of age. *J Pediatr* 1977;91:884–9.

17 Dube SK, Kapoor S, Ratner H, Turnick FL. Blood pressure studies in black children. *Am J Dis Child* 1975;129:1177–80.

18 Rames LK, Clarke WR, Connor WE, Reiter MA, Lauer RM. Normal blood pressure and the evaluation of sustained blood pressure elevation in childhood: the Muscatine study. *Pediatrics* 1978;61:245–51.

19 Rose G. A study of blood pressure among negro school children. *J Chronic Dis* 1961;15:373–80.

20 Fixler DE, Laird WP, Fitzgerald V, Stead S, Adams R. Hypertension screening in schools: results of the Dallas study. *Pediatrics* 1979;63:32–6.

21 Saunders E. Hypertension in blacks. *Med Clin North Am* 1987;71:1013–29.

22 Harshfield GA, Hwang C, Grim CE. Circadian variation of blood pressure during a normal day in normotensive blacks. *Circulation* 1988;78(suppl II):II–188.

23 Murphy MB, Nelson KS, Elliott WJ. Racial differences in diurnal blood pressure profile. *Am J Hypertens* 1988;1:55A.

24 Harshfield GA, Alpert BS, Willey ES et al. Race and gender influence: ambulatory blood pressure patterns of adolescents. *Hypertension* 1989;14:598–603.

25 Blumenthal S, Epps RP, Heavenrich R et al. Report of the

Task Force on blood pressure control in children. *Pediatrics* 1977;59(suppl):797−820.

26 Sinaiko AR, Gomez-Marin O, Prineas RJ. Prevalence of "significant" hypertension in junior high school-aged children: the children and adolescent blood pressure program. *J Pediatr* 1989;114:664−9.

27 Voors AW, Webber LS, Berenson GS. Time course studies of blood pressure in children−the Bogalusa heart study. *Am J Epidemiol* 1979;109:320−34.

28 Jesse MJ. Essential hypertension in children. *Hosp Pract* 1982;17:81−8.

29 Murphy EA. Genetics in hypertension: a perspective. *Circ Res* 1973;32(suppl I):129−38.

30 Moll PP, Harburg E, Burns TL, Schork MA, Ozgoren F. Heredity, stress and blood pressure, a family set approach: the Detroit project revisited. *J Chronic Dis* 1983;36:317−28.

31 Okamoto K. Spontaneous hypertension in rats. *Int Rev Exp Pathol* 1969;7:227−70.

32 McCarron DA, Morris DA, Cole C. Dietary calcium in human hypertension. *Science* 1982;217:267−9.

33 Gleibermann L. Blood pressure and dietary salt in human populations. *Ecol Food Nutr* 1973;2:143−56.

34 Luft FC, Grim CE, Higgins JT Jr, Weinberger MH. Differences in response to sodium administration in normotensive white and black subjects. *J Lab Clin Med* 1977;90:555−62.

35 Weir MR, Saunders E. Pharmacologic management of systemic • hypertension in blacks. *Am J Cardiol* 1988;61:46H−52H.

36 Blankson JM, Larbi EB, Pobee JO. Blood pressure levels of African children. *J Chronic Dis* 1977;30:735−43.

37 Williams RR. Will gene markers predict hypertension? *Hypertension* 1989;14:610−13.

38 Simon N, Franklin SS, Bleifer KH, Maxwell MH. Clinical characteristics of renovascular hypertension. *JAMA* 1972;220:1209−18.

39 Hypertension Detection and Follow-up Program Cooperative Group. Five-year findings of the hypertension detection and follow-up program. II. Mortality by race, sex and age. *JAMA* 1979;242:2572−7.

40 Miller JM. Diabetes mellitus and hypertension in black and white populations. *South Med J* 1986;79:1229−34.

41 Persky V, Pan WH, Stamler J *et al*. Time trends in the US racial difference in hypertension. *Am J Epidemiol* 1986;124:724−37.

42 Moore ES, Cohn RA, John E *et al*. Race is a factor in end stage renal failure (ESRF) in children. *Pediatr Res* 1986;20:454A.

43 Konotey-Ahulu FI. The sickle cell diseases. Clinical manifestations including the "sickle crisis." *Arch Intern Med* 1974;133:611−9.

44 Sellers BB Jr. Intermittent hypertension during sickle cell crisis. *J Pediatr* 1978;94:941−3.

45 Matustik MC, Carpentieri U, Corn C, Meyer WJ III. Hyperreninemia and hyperaldosteronism in sickle cell anemia. *J Pediatr* 1979;95:206−9.

46 Lieberman E. Essential hypertension in children and youth: a pediatric perspective. *J Pediatr* 1974;85:1−11.

47 McClellan W, Tuttle E, Issa A. Racial differences in the incidence of hypertensive end-stage renal disease (ESRD) are not entirely explained by differences in the prevalence of hypertension. *Am J Kidney Dis* 1988;12:285−90.

48 Cook CA. Pathophysiologic and pharmacotherapy considerations in the management of the black hypertensive patient. *Am Heart J* 1988;116:288−95.

49 Lauer RM, Conner WE, Leaverton PE *et al*. Coronary heart disease risk factors in school children: the Muscatine study. *J Pediatr* 1975;86:697−704.

50 Nora JJ. Identifying the child at risk for coronary disease as an adult: a strategy for prevention. *J Pediatr* 1980;97:706−14.

51 Frerichs RR, Srinivasan SR, Webber LS, Berenson GR. Serum cholesterol and triglyceride levels in 3446 children from a biracial community: the Bogalusa heart study. *Circulation* 1976;54:302−9.

52 Report of the Second Task Force on blood pressure control in children−1987. *Pediatrics* 1987;79:1−25.

53 Trevisan M, Ostrow D, Cooper R *et al*. Abnormal red blood cell ion transport and hypertension. The People's Gas company study. *Hypertension* 1983;5:363−7.

54 Kaplan NM, ed. Primary (essential) hypertension: pathogenesis. *Clinical Hypertension*. Baltimore, MD: Williams & Wilkins, 1990:54−112.

55 Robinson BF. Altered calcium handling as a cause of primary hypertension. *J Hypertens* 1984;2:453−60.

56 Weder AB, Torretti BA, Julius S. Racial differences in erythrocyte cation transport. *Hypertension* 1984;6:115−23.

57 Dustan HP, Tarazi RC, Bravo EL, Dart RA. Plasma and extracellular fluid volume in hypertension. *Circ Res* 1973;32(suppl 1):73−83.

58 Dagnino J, Prys-Roberts C. Studies of anaesthesia in relation to hypertension. VI: Cardiovascular responses to extradural blockade of treated and untreated hypertensive patients. *Br J Anaesth* 1984;56:1065−73.

59 Folkow B. Physiological aspects of primary hypertension. *Physiol Rev* 1982;62:347−504.

60 Dustan HP, Valdes G, Bravo EL, Tarazi RC. Excessive sodium retention as a characteristic of salt sensitive hypertension. *Am J Med Sci* 1986;292:67−74.

61 Luft FC, Weinberger MH, Grim CE. Sodium sensitivity and resistance in normotensive humans. *Am J Med* 1982;72:726−32.

62 Weinberger MH, Luft FC, Block R *et al*. The blood pressure-raising effect of high dietary sodium intake: racial differences and the role of potassium. *J Am Coll Nutr* 1982;1:139−49.

63 Berenson GS, Voors AW, Webber LS, Dalferes ER Jr, Harsha DW. Racial differences of parameters associated with blood pressure levels in children−the Bogalusa heart study. *Metabolism* 1979;28:1218−28.

64 Heyden S, Bartel AG, Hames CG, McDonough JR. Elevated blood pressure levels in adolescents, Evans County, Georgia. Seven year follow-up of 30 patients and 30 controls. *JAMA* 1969;209:1683−9.

65 Shaffer SG, Meade VM. Sodium balance and extracellular volume regulation in very low birth weight infants. *J Pediatr* 1989;115:285−90.

66 Frank GC, Webber LS, Nicklas TA, Berenson GS. Sodium, potassium, calcium, magnesium, and phosphorous intakes of infants and children: Bogalusa heart study. *J Am Diet*

Assoc 1988;88:801—7.

67 Perlman SA, Gruskin AB, Prebis JW et al. Urinary calcium (Ca) excretion in adolescent essential hypertension. *Pediatr Res* 1975;10:91A.

68 Parfrey PS, Vandenburg MJ, Wright P et al. Blood pressure and hormonal changes following alteration in dietary sodium and potassium in mild essential hypertension. *Lancet* 1981;i:59—63.

69 Watson RL, Langford HG, Abernethy J et al. Urinary electrolytes, body weight, and blood pressure: pooled cross-sectional results among four groups of adolescent females. *Hypertension* 1980;2:93—8.

70 Grim CE, Luft FC, Miller JZ et al. Racial differences in blood pressure in Evans County, Georgia; relationship to sodium and potassium intake and plasma renin activity. *J Chronic Dis* 1980;33:87—94.

71 Breckenridge A. Hypertension and hyperuricemia. *Lancet* 1966;i:15—18.

72 Prebis JW, Gruskin AB, Polinsky MS, Baluarte HJ. Uric acid in childhood essential hypertension. *J Pediatr* 1981;98:702—7.

73 Zinner SH, Margolius HS, Rosner B, Keiser HR, Kass EH. Familial aggregation of urinary kallikrein concentration in childhood: relation to blood pressure, race and urinary electrolytes. *Am J Epidemiol* 1976;104:124—32.

74 Hohn A, Riopel DA, Keil JE et al. Childhood familial and racial differences in physiologic and biochemical factors related to hypertension. *Hypertension* 1983;5:56—70.

75 Schachter J, Kuller LH, Perkins JM, Radin ME. Infant blood pressure and heart rate: relation to ethnic group (black or white), nutrition and electrolyte intake. *Am J Epidemiol* 1979;110:205—18.

76 Shekelle RB, Liu S, Raynor WJ, Miller RA. Racial difference in mean pulse rate of children age 6 to 11 years. *Pediatrics* 1978;61:119—21.

77 Strong WB, Miller MD, Striplin M, Salehbhai M. Blood pressure response to isometric and dynamic exercise in healthy black children. *Am J Dis Child* 1978;132:587—91.

78 Falkner B, Onesti G, Angelakos ET, Fernandes M, Langman CB. Cardiovascular response to mental stress in normal adolescents with hypertensive parents. Hemodynamic and mental stress in adolescents. *Hypertension* 1979;1:23—30.

79 Canessa M, Adragna N, Solomon HS, Connolly TM, Tosteson DC. Increased sodium—lithium countertransport in red cells of patients with essential hypertension. *N Engl J Med* 1980;302:772—6.

80 Wedes AB. Red cell lithium—sodium countertransport and renal lithium clearance in hypertension. *N Engl J Med* 1986;314:198—201.

81 Norling LL, Landt M, Goldring D, Robson AM. Lithium—sodium (Li—Na) countertransport (CT) in erythrocytes of children with hypertension (HPT). *Pediatr Res* 1982;16:104A.

82 Filer LJ, Clarke WR, Lauer R, Burke GL. Blood pressure and sodium—lithium countertransport. In: Loggie JMH, Horan MJ, Gruskin AB et al. eds. *NHLBI Workshop on Juvenile Hypertension*. Bethesda, MD: Biomedical Information Corporation, 1983:173—9.

83 Woods JW, Falk RJ, Pittman AW, Klemmer PJ, Watson BS, Namboodiri K. Increased red-cell sodium—lithium countertransport in normotensive sons of hypertensive parents. *N Engl J Med* 1982;306:593—5.

84 Garay RP, Elghozi JL, Dagher G et al. Laboratory distinction between essential and secondary hypertension by measurement of erythrocyte cation fluxes. *N Engl J Med* 1982;302:772—6.

85 Aviv A, Gardner J. Racial differences in ion regulation and their possible links to hypertension in blacks. *Hypertension* 1989;14:584—9.

86 McCrory WW, Kelin AA, Fallo F. Predictors of blood pressure: humoral factors. In: Loggie JMH, Horan MJ, Gruskin AB et al., eds. *NHLBI Workshop on Juvenile Hypertension*. Bethesda, MD: Biomedical Information Corporation, 1983:181—202.

87 Lasker N, Hopp L, Grossman S, Bamforth R, Aviv A. Race and sex difference in erythrocyte Na^+-K^+-adenosine triphosphate. *J Clin Invest* 1985;75:1813—20.

88 Trevisan M, Cooper R, Ostrow D et al. Dietary sodium, erythrocyte sodium concentration, sodium-stimulated lithium efflux, and blood pressure. *Clin Sci* 1981;61:29s—32s.

89 Ives HE. Ion transport defects and hypertension. Where is the link? *Hypertension* 1989;14:590—7.

90 Ingelfinger JR. Epidemiology of hypertension. *Pediatric Hypertension*. Philadelphia: WB Saunders, 1982:79—92.

91 Mann GV. The influence of obesity on health. *N Engl J Med* 1974;291:178—85.

92 Londe S, Bourgoignie JJ, Robson AM, Goldring D. Hypertension in apparently normal children. *J Pediatr* 1971;78:569—77.

93 Frerichs RR, Webber LS, Voors AW, Srinivasan SR, Berenson GS. Cardiovascular disease risk factor variables in children at two successive years—the Bogalusa heart study. *J Chronic Dis* 1979;32:251—62.

94 Lynds BG, Seyler SK, Morgan BM. The relationship between elevated blood pressure and obesity in black children. *Am J Public Health* 1980;70:171—3.

95 Johnson AL, Cornoni JC, Cassel JC, Tyroler HA, Heyden S, Hames CG. Influence of race, sex and weight on blood pressure behavior in young adults. *Am J Cardiol* 1975;35:523—30.

96 Gillum RF. Pathophysiology of hypertension in blacks and whites: a review of the basis of racial blood pressure differences. *Hypertension* 1979;1:468—75.

97 McMann BJ, Moore ES, Cevallos EE et al. The relationship between obesity, anxiety and other risk factors to onset of essential hypertension in children. *Pediatr Res* 1976;10:441.

98 Light KC, Obrist PA, Sherwood A, James SA, Strogatz DS. Effects of race and marginally elevated blood pressure on responses to stress. *Hypertension* 1987;10:555—63.

99 Lee RE, Schneider RF. Hypertension and arteriosclerosis in executive and non-executive personnel. *JAMA* 1958;167:1447—50.

100 Walter HJ, Hofman A. Socioeconomic status, ethnic origin, and risk factors for coronary heart disease in children. *Am Heart J* 1987;113:812—18.

101 Scholl TO, Karp RJ, Theophano J, Decker E. Ethnic differences in growth and nutritional status: a study of poor schoolchildren in southern New Jersey. *Public Health Rep* 1987;102:278—83.

102 National Center for Health Statistics. *Hypertension and Hypertensive Heart Disease in Adults*. Vital and Health Statistics series II no. 13. Washington, DC: US Government Printing Office, 1966.

103 de Castro FJ, Biesbroeck R, Erickson C *et al*. Hypertension in adolescents. A significantly higher prevalence among students attending an inner city school. *Clin Pediatr* 1976; 15:24–6.

104 Mathew J. Alcohol use, hypertension and coronary heart disease. *Clin Sci Mol Med* 1976;51:661s–3s.

105 Klatsky AL, Friedman GD, Siegelaub AB, Gerard MJ. Alcohol consumption and blood pressure. Kaiser-Permanente multiphasic health examination data. *N Engl J Med* 1977;296:1194–200.

106 Arradondo J. Tailoring antihypertensive drug therapy for the black patient. *J Natl Med Assoc* 1987;79:149–54.

107 Saunders E. Drug treatment considerations for the hypertensive black patient. *J Fam Pract* 1988;26:659–64.

108 Veterans Administration cooperative study group on antihypertensive agents. Comparison of propranolol and hydrochlorothiazide for the initial treatment of hypertension. II. Results of long-term therapy. *JAMA* 1982;248: 2004–11.

109 Shulman NB. Treatment of hypertension in black patients with angiotensin-converting enzyme inhibitors. *J Natl Med Assoc* 1988;80:265–72.

110 Fadayomi MO, Akinroye KK, Ajao RO, Awosiki LA. Monotherapy with nifedipine for essential hypertension in adult blacks. *J Cardiovasc Pharmacol* 1986;8:466–9.

111 Ingelfinger JR. Antihypertensive therapy in childhood. *Pediatric Hypertension*. Philadelphia: WB Saunders, 1982:24–44.

112 Falkner B. Is there a black hypertension? *Hypertension* 1987;10:551–4.

113 Guyton AC. Personal views on mechanisms of hypertension. In: Genest J, Koiw E, Kuchel O, eds. *Hypertension*. New York: McGraw Hill, 1977:566–75.

114 Page LB, Moellering RC Jr, Lubin N, Rhoads J. Blood pressure, sodium intake and renin activity in two isolated Pacific Island populations. In: Thurm RH, ed. *Essential Hypertension*. Chicago: Yearbook, 1979:11–19.

115 Oliver WJ, Cohen EL, Neel JV. Blood pressure, sodium intake and sodium related hormones in the Yanomamo Indians, a no salt culture. *Circulation* 1975;52:146–55.

31 Management of Hypertensive Emergencies in Children

GERALD S. ARBUS AND MICHELLE FARINE

INTRODUCTION

A hypertensive emergency is one in which the blood pressure must be lowered within a few hours because the patient is experiencing or is about to experience a complication of severe hypertension, such as hypertensive encephalopathy, an intracranial hemorrhage, or acute left ventricular failure with pulmonary edema [1].

Hypertensive urgencies usually require the blood pressure to be lowered within 24 h. These situations involve patients who have accelerated or malignant hypertension without encephalopathy (see below), severe end-organ damage, a need for surgery, or perioperative hypertension. The terms hypertensive emergency and urgency may overlap and are often used interchangeably; in this chapter we have used the term hypertensive emergency to cover both. The general categories of emergencies seen in pediatrics are listed in Table 31.1 [2].

Children rarely develop accelerated or malignant hypertension [3], whereas adults can develop these conditions when the diastolic pressure remains above 130 mmHg. Malignant hypertension is accompanied by papilledema along with retinal striate hemorrhages and soft exudates, whereas in accelerated hypertension there is a retinopathy but not papil-

ledema. Malignant hypertension is usually associated with necrotizing arteriolitis. Microangiopathic hemolytic anemia or renal failure may also be associated with the vascular lesions of malignant hypertension. If left untreated, malignant hypertension has a mortality rate of 90% within 1 year. Each day that the blood pressure is not reduced, the greater is the risk of additional and potentially irreversible damage to vital organs.

ETIOLOGY OF HYPERTENSIVE EMERGENCIES

The most common cause of severe hypertension in children is intrinsic renal disease. In the series of Rance and coworkers, reflux nephropathy accounted for 40% of cases [4] and in the Still and Cottom series, which included only patients with severe sustained hypertension (diastolic blood pressure >120 mmHg with evidence of cardiac involvement), 64% of children had evidence of pyelonephritis [3]. In the latter series, children with acute nephritis in which hypertension was a temporary phenomenon were excluded. Both these series were reported from referral centers. Dillon reports that the most common cause (36% of cases) seen in his tertiary referral center was renal scarring from either reflux nephropathy or obstructive uropathy. Glomerulonephritis accounted for 23% of cases, renovascular disease for 10%, and coarctation of the aorta for 9% [5].

In our tertiary center, most pediatric emergencies occur in patients with end-stage renal disease who may be on dialysis or have renal transplants (Table 31.2).

Chronic hypertensive conditions can now be more effectively controlled with the newer, more powerful antihypertensive medications (captopril, nifedipine). When taken as prescribed, they not only reduce the incidence of hypertensive emergencies but, in some

Table 31.1 Hypertensive emergencies in pediatrics

Malignant or accelerated hypertension
Hypertensive encephalopathy
Hypertension complicated by intracranial hemorrhage
Hypertension associated with acute left ventricular failure
Hypertensive crises with pheochromocytoma
Uncontrolled hypertension in a patient needing emergency surgery
Blindness due to hypertension

Table 31.2 Possible causes of hypertension in renal transplant recipients [6]

Native kidneys
Transplant renal artery stenosis
Acute or chronic rejection
Fluid overload associated with renal failure
High-dose steroids
Cyclosporine
Obstructive uropathy

Table 31.3 Differential diagnosis of hypertensive encephalopathy

Intracranial hemorrhage
Cerebral thrombosis and infarction
Uremia with encephalopathy
Rapidly growing brain tumors
Anxiety of hysterical states
Encephalitis
Pseudotumor cerebri

cases, provide a reasonable alternative to such surgical interventions as nephrectomy or difficult reconstructive surgery in transplant recipients with renal artery stenosis.

SIGNS AND SYMPTOMS

The signs and symptoms of hypertensive emergencies are related either to the complications of the high blood pressure or to the etiology (e.g. pheochromocytoma) of the hypertension. The main target organs are the brain (hypertensive encephalopathy), eye (visual complications), heart (cardiac failure), and kidney (nephrosclerosis).

Neurologic complications

Severe childhood hypertension is associated with neurologic symptoms in 8.8–33% of patients [3]. Clinical features include headache, convulsions, nausea, vomiting, apraxia, hemiplegia, transverse myelopathy, visual disturbances, dizziness, coma, and personality changes (including irritability, hyperactivity, anxiety, and confusion).

Transient cerebral dysfunction associated with a rapid increase in blood pressure is referred to as hypertensive encephalopathy [7]. It is accompanied by decreased effective cerebral blood flow, and if left untreated can be fatal. The differential diagnosis of hypertensive encephalopathy in children is shown in Table 31.3.

The brain attempts to maintain a mean brain arterial blood pressure of 60–100 mmHg by a process called autoregulation. The cerebral arterial smooth muscles constrict against excessive filling pressure as systemic blood pressure rises, and dilate when the blood pressure is low.

At least two theories attempt to explain the pathogenesis of hypertensive encephalopathy, both based in part on the phenomenon of autoregulation [8,9].

The first claims that an overregulation of cerebral blood flow leads to severe vasospasm and a decrease in cerebral blood flow with ischemia to various parts of the brain. This results in capillary permeability, increasing capillary wall rupture, and hemorrhage. The second theory suggests that when the systemic blood pressure reaches an upper limit there is a breakthrough in autoregulation. A sudden increase in systemic pressure above this level leads to a lack of vasoconstriction, and as a result, an increase in cerebral venous pressure and transudation of plasma. This in turn leads to focal cerebral edema, compression of capillaries, and various central nervous system manifestations.

Damage to the cerebral arterioles appears to depend on the rapidity of onset, severity, and duration of hypertension, the extent of vasoconstriction; and the location of the affected vessels in the brain [10]. The vessels undergo necrotizing arteriolitis. At autopsy one finds fibrinoid necrosis with petechial hemorrhages, multiple small thrombi, and infarcts. There is an increase in brain weight from cerebral edema. The cerebrospinal fluid can show an increased amount of protein, elevated pressure, and xanthochromia.

Visual complications

Possible visual disturbances associated with hypertension are listed in Table 31.4 [11]. Clinically there may be absent pupillary responses to light, visual field defects, blurring of vision, and abnormalities of the optic disc leading to optic atrophy.

A spectrum of retinal abnormalities has been noted in 55% of newborn infants with acute hypertension who were examined ophthalmologically [12]. They consistently showed an increase in venous/arterial caliber, and some patients had arteriolar spasm or venous dilatation or both. Also noted were abnormal tortuosity and nicking of the retinal vessels. Although hemorrhages and exudates are a frequent finding in

Table 31.4 Possible ophthalmologic disturbances in malignant hypertension in children

Direct retinal disruption
  Retinal infarcts
  Hemorrhages
  Disc edema
Cortical blindness
Vitreous hemorrhage
Visual disturbances with increased intracranial pressure
Infarction of the anterior visual pathways

adults with hypertensive retinopathy, they are less common in newborn infants with hypertension. In all the infants studied, the retinopathy resolved when the blood pressure was corrected.

The classification of hypertensive retinopathy devised by Keith, Wagener, and Barker is adapted and reproduced in Table 31.5 [13]. Although grades III and IV rarely occur in children, hypertensive changes are graded according to this classification when they are present.

Cardiac complications

Cardiac failure may be a complication of hypertension. Unexplained congestive heart failure and respiratory distress may be the first signs of hypertension and may be the initial presentation of infants with coarctation of the aorta.

Renal complications

Many parenchymal lesions can cause hypertension, but sustained severe hypertension may also lead to abnormalities of the kidney, including hematuria, proteinuria, and the excretion of large volumes of urine. In newborn infants with renovascular hypertension, sodium loss may be a major finding. Sustained hypertension can lead to compromised renal function, which is usually reversible when the hypertension is controlled.

EVALUATION

When the blood pressure of a patient with known hypertension suddenly appears to be out of control, an evaluation is necessary (Table 31.6) [14]. If the patient is asymptomatic and has an unusually high blood pressure, the size of the cuff (the inflatable inner bladder, not its cloth covering) must be checked, as must the accuracy of the sphygmomanometer or electronic unit providing the reading. Automatic blood pressure devices need to be serviced regularly to provide accurate readings. They have been shown to provide accurate systolic blood pressure measurements; the Dynamap has also been shown to give accurate diastolic blood pressure readings [15]. The elevation in blood pressure may be transient, in which case it will settle down to previous levels if the usual medication is taken and/or the patient relaxes. However, when the elevated blood pressure is found to be true and persistent, the possibility of worsening of the underlying condition (e.g. the primary kidney disease) must be investigated. Noncompliance with medication as a cause of a rise in blood pressure must be considered in patients already being treated with antihypertensive drugs.

Clues that a patient and/or parent may not be complying with antihypertensive medication are listed in Table 31.7 [14]. Although checks such as pill counts are helpful in assessing compliance, the noncompliant patient may stop bringing the pill bottles to the physician for checking or remove the required

Table 31.5 Classification of hypertensive retinopathy

Degree of A/V dissociation	General narrowing of A/V ratio*	Focal arteriolar spasm[†]	Hemorrhages	Exudates	Papilledema
Normal	3/4	1/1	0	0	0
Grade I	1/2	1/1	0	0	0
Grade II	1/3	2/3	0	0	0
Grade III	1/4	1/3	+	+	0
Grade IV	Fine fibrous cords	Distal flow obliterated	+	+	+

A/V = Arteriolar/venous.
* Ratio of arteriolar/venous diameters.
[†] Ratio of diameters of region of spasm/proximal arteriole.

Table 31.6 Why is the blood pressure in a previously known hypertensive now out of control?

Wrong blood pressure recorded
Defective sphygmomanometer, cuff
Improper cuff size
Cuff not at heart level

Transient elevation/anxiety

Insufficient medications given
Too small a dose
Improper time schedule
Interfering factors
    Excess sodium consumption
    Drug interaction

Noncompliance
Has bad side-effects from medication
Is asymptomatic off medication
Finds treatment regime too complicated
Health beliefs preclude taking medication

Worsening of primary condition

Table 31.7 Possible indicators of noncompliance

Gives evasive answers
Does not keep appointments
Does not renew prescriptions
Complains about the cost of medication
Complains about side-effects of medication
Is unsure of name or description of medication
Does not know how often medication is taken

---

number of pills before the visit.

The newly identified symptomatic hypertensive patient constitutes a medical emergency. History and physical examination should be done as treatment is being initiated and should attempt to identify the etiology of the hypertension and the involved target organs.

Abdominal examination may indicate a bruit that suggests renal artery stenosis, while the absence of femoral pulses indicates coarctation of the aorta. A complete neurologic examination, paying particular attention to the pupillary reflex and visual acuity, must be done before initiating therapy; too aggressive therapy may itself cause deficits in the visual pathways. The presence or absence of heart failure should also be determined.

Blood should be drawn for laboratory investigations and intravenous lines started as soon as possible.

Blood tests should include urea and creatinine to identify renal disease, gases and electrolytes to detect renal disease or excessive mineralocorticoids, and hemoglobin to test for the presence of chronic renal disease. Although an elevation in plasma renin activity (PRA) may signify renal artery disease, PRA may be altered if antihypertensive medications have been given. Thus it is important to obtain a blood sample for renin determination before therapy is started. When the blood pressure is better controlled, chest X-ray and electrocardiogram may be done to try to determine the duration and severity of the hypertension. Echocardiography is a more sensitive test of cardiac status that can also be done later when the patient is stabilized. Invasive tests should not be undertaken during the acute period.

TREATMENT

Ideally the symptomatic patient should be managed in an intensive care setting where careful monitoring of the blood pressure and neurologic status are possible. Prompt therapy for severe hypertension is mandatory when the blood pressure affects the normal functioning of vital organs such as the brain, heart, eyes, and kidneys. Therapy may have to be initiated even though the etiology of the hypertension is unknown.

In the presence of long-standing hypertension, the autoregulation curve may shift to the right so that the patient has a lower cerebral blood flow for a given mean arteriolar pressure [16]. This shift may be due to an adaptive hypertrophy of the arteriolar walls and may explain why neurologic deficits develop in some patients when the blood pressure is rapidly decreased [10]. Although severe hypertension must be treated rapidly and efficiently to avoid complications, the blood pressure must not be reduced to levels below which the autoregulatory mechanisms cease to be effective.

In the severely hypertensive asymptomatic patient, Dillon has suggested that the blood pressure should be lowered by approximately one-third of the planned reduction during the first 6 h, by another third during the next 12−36 h, and by the final third over the next 48−96 h [5].

Drugs that allow the physician to control the rate of blood pressure decrease are preferable, especially for what appears to be long-standing severe hypertension. For example, sodium nitroprusside, diazoxide, and labetalol can be given through incremental infusions, thereby allowing better monitoring of the reduction in blood pressure. The second-line drugs listed below do not allow as careful control of the blood pressure drop and may subject the patient to relative hypotension. Their advantage is that they do not require continuous, stringent monitoring of the blood pressure once it has reached its lowest level.

Antihypertensive medication should not be given unless an intravenous line with normal saline or colloid solution is available to counteract the possible occurrence of relative hypotension. If the patient's neurologic status appears to deteriorate as the blood pressure is being reduced, intravenous saline boluses should be used to raise the pressure.

Maintenance antihypertensive medication must be started as soon as the blood pressure is brought down to the desired level. At this point, further investigation into the etiology of the hypertension is indicated and can be carried out in a rational way.

More experience is being gained with oral agents. New drugs are constantly being added or are replacing old ones. Consequently, a review of such drugs may be somewhat out of date by the time of publication.

PREFERRED DRUGS

A summary of the drugs considered most effective in treating hypertensive emergencies is presented in Table 31.8.

Sodium nitroprusside

It is the preferred drug for treating hypertensive crises in children [17] particularly when the etiology of the hypertension is unclear. In the past it has been used for periods of up to 28 days [18] but, with the current arsenal of drugs available to treat hypertension, this is no longer necessary. The drug is given as an intravenous infusion at a dose of 0.5−8 µg/Kg body weight per minute. It acts within seconds and is effective for only minutes after the infusion is discontinued. The risk of cyanide toxicity mandates that the drug be used at low infusion rates (<2 µg/Kg/min). Infusions of sodium nitroprusside at the maximum dose should not last for more than 10−15 minutes. Since nitroprusside causes venous dilatation, there is no increase in cardiac output or reflex tachycardia as is seen with other vasodilators. In patients not properly monitored, nitroprusside can cause precipitous falls in blood pressure.

Sodium nitroprusside is broken down into cyanide, which is in part detoxified by the liver to thiocyanate. Thiocyanate is then excreted by the kidneys. Blood thiocyanate and cyanide levels do not fully reflect the extent to which free cyanide limits oxygen utilization by the tissues. Reliable early indicators of cyanide poisoning are the presence of a metabolic acidosis, increased lactate levels, increased lactate:pyruvate ratio, and an increased, mixed venous oxygen content [19]. Suspected cyanide toxicity should be treated immediately without waiting for confirmatory tests.

Labetalol

Labetalol is a combined α- and β-receptor blocking agent [20]. When given as an intravenous infusion rather than orally, it allows more accurate control of the reduction in blood pressure. The initial dose is 1 mg/kg body weight per h, and this may be increased to a maximum of 3 mg/kg body weight per h. It may be administered diluted to a convenient volume with dextrose-containing intravenous fluids. The onset of action is within 5 min and the plasma half-life is 4.9 h after intravenous administration; the effect may last for up to 24 h. The side-effects of labetalol include hypotension (especially postural), dizziness, gastrointestinal upset, headaches, scalp tingling, and urinary retention.

Diazoxide

Diazoxide is considered one of the best drugs in the treatment of hypertensive emergencies. Its onset of action is prompt and it is easy to administer. A benzothiadiazine derivative, diazoxide is a powerful vasodilator with no diuretic activity. For a long time it was advocated that diazoxide should be given as a rapid bolus injection (5 mg/kg) in order to prevent it from binding to serum albumin and thus becoming pharmacologically inactive [21]. However, hypotension following bolus diazoxide therapy was reported to be associated with serious complications such as coma and renal failure. These are more likely to occur if diazoxide is combined with other antihypertensive medications, such as hydralazine [22].

An infusion regimen has been developed to try to avoid the complication of hypotension associated with a bolus injection [23]. The infusion rate is 0.25 mg/kg per min with a maximum dose of 5 mg/kg per min or 300 mg over 20 min.

Intravenous pulse diazoxide therapy has also been

Table 31.8 Drugs used in hypertensive emergencies

Preferred drugs	Dose	Mechanism of action	Onset of action	Duration of action	Side-effects and disadvantages
First-line drugs					
Nitroprusside	0.5–8 µg/kg per min i.v.	Direct arteriolar and venous vasodilator	Immediate	Only during infusion	Risk of cyanide and thiocyanate toxicity, chest pain, nausea, abdominal pain, headaches
Labetalol	1–3 mg/kg per h i.v.	α- and β-receptor blocker	Within minutes	Up to 24 h after end of infusion	Gastrointestinal upset, headaches, scalp tingling, dizziness
Diazoxide	1–2 mg/kg per dose i.v. over 30 s to be given q. 10–15 min until blood pressure is under control, or 0.25–5 mg/kg per min (max. 300 mg/20 min)	Direct arteriolar vasodilator	Within minutes	Up to 24 h	Hyperglycemia, hyperuricemia, salt and water retention, acute hypotension
Phentolamine	0.1–0.2 mg/kg i.v.	α-Blocker (used for hypertensive emergencies associated with pheochromocytoma)	Immediate	30–60 min	Tachycardia, abdominal pain, nausea, vomiting, hypotension
Second-line drugs					
Nifedipine	0.25–0.5 mg/kg p.o. bite and swallow capsule; maximum dose = 20 mg	Calcium channel blocker	Within 20–30 min	6 h	Dizziness, facial flushing
Hydralazine	0.1–0.5 mg/kg i.v., maximum dose = 25 mg	Direct arteriolar vasodilator	Within 30 min	4–12 h	Tachycardia, headaches, flushing, vomiting, acute hypotension
Captopril age <6 months age >6 months	0.05–0.5 mg/kg p.o. 0.3–2 mg/kg p.o.	Angiotensin converting enzyme inhibitor	Within 15 min	8–12 h	Neutropenia, proteinuria, reversible renal failure in renovascular disease, dysgeusia
Propranolol	0.01–0.05 mg/kg i.v. over 1 h; maximum dose = 10 mg	β-Receptor antagonist	Immediate for heart rate, 24 h for blood pressure	Up to 8 h	Bradycardia, bronchospasm in predisposed individuals
Furosemide	1–4 mg/kg i.v.	Loop diuretic	5 min	2–3 h	Electrolyte imbalance, hearing deficit, hyperglycemia

used in an attempt to avert hypotension [24,25]. This consists of repeated small doses of diazoxide (1−2 mg/kg body weight), as opposed to the usual bolus of 5 mg/kg, given over a 30-s period at 10−15 minute intervals until the desired diastolic pressure is reached.

In addition to hypotension, the side-effects of diazoxide include hyperglycemia, retention of salt and water, hyperuricemia, hypertrichosis, nausea, and vomiting.

Phentolamine

Phentolamine, an intravenous α-receptor antagonist, is used in the hypertensive emergencies of pheochromocytoma. It is an α-adrenergic blocking agent with immediate onset but short duration of action.

SECOND-LINE DRUGS

Nifedipine

Nifedipine, a calcium channel blocking agent that reduces peripheral resistance, has lowered blood pressure safely and effectively in both adults and children [26]. In children, it has been used sublingually at a dose of 0.25−0.5 mg/kg body weight. The maximal effect is achieved after 30 min and continues for at least 6 h. It has been shown that peak levels higher than those achieved through sublingual use, and quicker onset of action, are attained through biting and then swallowing the capsules [27]. In adults, nifedipine is given orally in a dose of 20 mg two to four times a day to treat chronic hypertension. When it was used as acute antihypertensive therapy, 4 of 5 patients had an increase in cerebral blood flow [28].

Hydralazine

Hydralazine is an arteriolar vasodilator that can be given either orally or parenterally. It causes reflex tachycardia and increased cardiac output. Its plasma half-life varies from 1.5 to 8 h. However, its duration of action is longer because it is retained in the vascular walls. Hydralazine has been demonstrated to be effective when given twice daily in adults with chronic hypertension, but it is usually given more frequently. When given intravenously, it is started at 0.2 mg/kg body weight per dose and increased to 0.5 mg/kg body weight per dose; the maximum intravenous dose is 25 mg.

Captopril

Captopril, an angiotensin converting enzyme inhibitor given orally, has been used to treat adults with hypertensive crises [29]. The onset of hypotensive action occurs within 15 min of ingesting the drug. The initial single dose is 0.3 mg/kg body weight. Patients who show no significant change in blood pressure 2−3 h after a dose can have the previous dose doubled. Thus the dose can be increased in a steplike manner, each time doubling the previous dose to a maximum of 2 mg/kg body weight per dose. The recommended dose of captopril in infants less than 6 months old is 0.05−0.5 mg/kg. The nadir of its effect is reached at 90 min. Captopril is given twice or three times a day when used as a maintenance antihypertensive drug. Usually the blood pressure returns to previous levels 6−10 h after the dose. Captopril does not cause reflex tachycardia or affect the central nervous system.

Propranolol

Propranolol, a β-receptor antagonist, is not useful in hypertensive emergencies except to counteract the reflex tachycardia from other drugs. When given intravenously it has an immediate effect on heart rate but no hypotensive effect for approximately 24 h because of the reflex vasoconstriction that occurs.

Furosemide

Furosemide is a loop diuretic that may be helpful in treating fluid overload in nephritic patients. It may also be necessary if fluid retention becomes evident as a result of the salt retention seen when vasodilator antihypertensive medication is used.

Diuretics should be avoided in the acute treatment of hypertensive emergencies because many patients are already salt-depleted [14].

MANAGEMENT OF SPECIFIC HYPERTENSIVE EMERGENCIES

Hypertensive encephalopathy

Acute hypertensive encephalopathy may result from almost any cause of acute or chronic hypertension.

Often it occurs at lower blood pressure levels in patients who develop acute hypertension than in those with long-standing hypertension.

The therapy of hypertensive convulsions consists of stopping the seizure with anticonvulsant medication and lowering the blood pressure with antihypertensive medications. Intravenous diazepam 0.1–0.3 mg/kg body weight or intravenous phenytoin up to a total of 20 mg/kg body weight can be used as the blood pressure is being decreased. If the seizure is short with no sequelae, anticonvulsants should be tapered quickly. If the seizure is prolonged or associated with sequelae such as a hemiparesis or if there are electroencephalogram changes, the anticonvulsants should be maintained for 6 months and then their use re-evaluated.

The agents of choice for treating this emergency are drugs that act rapidly and those that allow control of the blood pressure as it is lowered [30]. Obviously, drugs that do not affect the level of consciousness are preferable.

Intracerebral hemorrhage

Intracerebral hemorrhage must be treated rapidly with a controlled decrease in blood pressure, using drugs that will not interfere with the neurologic evaluation of the patient. Nitroprusside and labetalol are particularly useful. Nifedipine, which increases cerebral blood flow, is contraindicated when this diagnosis is suspected.

Acute left ventricular failure

Acute left ventricular failure requires rapid reduction of arterial blood pressure and left ventricular afterload. Drugs that do not increase cardiac workload, such as sodium nitroprusside and labetalol, are preferred.

ACKNOWLEDGMENT

This chapter was prepared with the assistance of the Medical Publications Department, The Hospital for Sick Children, Toronto.

REFERENCES

1 The Joint National Committee on detection, evaluation, and treatment of high blood pressure. The 1984 report of the joint national committee on detection, evaluation, and treatment of high blood pressure. *Arch Intern Med* 1984;144:1045–57.

2 Koch-Weser J. Hypertensive emergencies. *N Engl J Med* 1974;290:211–14.

3 Still JL, Cottom D. Severe hypertension in childhood. *Arch Dis Child* 1967;42:34–9.

4 Rance CP, Arbus GS, Balfe JW, Kooh SW. Persistent systemic hypertension in infants and children. *Pediatr Clin North Am* 1974;21:801–24.

5 Dillon MJ. Modern management of hypertension. In: Meadow R, ed. *Recent Advances in Paediatrics*. Edinburgh: Churchill Livingstone, 1984;35–55.

6 Luke RG, Curtis JJ, Jones P, Whelchel JD, Diethelm AG. Mechanisms of posttransplant hypertension. Hypertension and the kidney. *Am J Kidney Dis* 1985;5:479–84.

7 van Vught AJ, Troost J, Willemse J. Hypertensive encephalopathy in childhood diagnostic problems. *Neuropädiatrie* 1976;7:92–100.

8 Gifford RW Jr, Westbrook E. Hypertensive encephalopathy: mechanisms, clinical features, and treatment. *Prog Cardiovasc Dis* 1974;17:115–24.

9 Kirkendall WM. *Hypertensive Emergencies. Dialogues in Hypertension, Hypertension Update.* Vol. II. Bloomfield, NJ: Health Learning Systems, 1980:8–23.

10 Ledingham JGG, Rajagopalan B. Cerebral complications in the treatment of accelerated hypertension. *Q J Med* 1979;48:25–41.

11 Hulse JA, Taylor DSI, Dillon MJ. Blindness and paraplegia in severe childhood hypertension. *Lancet* 1979;ii:553–6.

12 Skalina MEL, Annable WL, Kliegman RM, Panaroff AA. Hypertensive retinopathy in the newborn infant. *J Pediatr* 1983;103:781–6.

13 Williams GH. Hypertensive vascular disease. In: Wilson JD, Braunwald E, Isselbacher KJ, Petersdorf RG, Martin JB, Fauci AS, Root RK, eds. *Harrison's Principles of Internal Medicine.* 12th edn, New York: McGraw-Hill, 1991;1006.

14 Gifford RW Jr, Tarazi C. Resistant hypertension: diagnosis and management. *Ann Intern Med* 1978;88:661–5.

15 Task Force on blood pressure control in children. Report of the second task force on blood pressure control in children. *Pediatrics* 1987;79:1–25.

16 Strandgaard S, Olesen J, Skinhøj E, Lassen NA. Autoregulation of brain circulation in severe arterial hypertension. *Br Med J* 1973;1:507–10.

17 Palmer RF, Lasseter KC. Sodium nitroprusside. *N Engl J Med* 1975;292:294–7.

18 Luderer JR, Hayes AH Jr, Dubynsky O, Berlin CM. Long-term administration of sodium nitroprusside in childhood. *J Pediatr* 1977;91:490–1.

19 Tinker JH, Michenfelder JD. Sodium nitroprusside: pharmacology, toxicology and therapeutics. *Anesthesiology* 1976;45:340–54.

20 Wallin JD, O'Neill WM Jr. Labetalol: current research and therapeutic status. *Arch Intern Med* 1983;143:485–90.

21 McCrory WW, Kohaut EC, Lewy JE, Lieberman E, Travis LB. Safety of intravenous diazoxide in children with severe hypertension. *Clin Pediatr* 1979;18:661–71.

22 Henrich WL, Cronin R, Miller PD, Anderson RJ. Hypotensive sequelae of diazoxide and hydralazine therapy. *JAMA* 1977;237:264–5.

23 Thien TA, Huysmans FTM, Gerlag PGG, Koene RAP, Wijdeveld PGAB. Diazoxide infusion in severe hypertension and hypertensive crisis. *Clin Pharmacol Ther* 1979;25:795−9.

24 Ram CVS, Kaplan NM. Individual titration of diazoxide dosage in the treatment of severe hypertension. *Am J Cardiol* 1979;43:627−9.

25 Wilson DJ, Lewis RC, Vidt DG. Control of severe hypertension with pulse diazoxide. *Cardiovasc Ther* 1981;12:79−91.

26 Dilmen U, Cağlar MK, Senses A, Kinik E. Nifedipine in hypertensive emergencies of children. *Am J Dis Child* 1983;137:1162−5.

27 McAllister RG Jr. Kinetics and dynamics of nifedipine after oral and sublingual doses. *Am J Med* 1986;81(suppl 6A):2−5.

28 Bertel O, Conen D, Radü EW, Müller J, Lang C, Dubach UC. Nifedipine in hypertensive emergencies. *Br Med J* 1983;286:19−21.

29 Biollaz J, Waeber B, Brunner HR. Hypertensive crisis treated with orally administered captopril. *Eur J Clin Pharmacol* 1983;25:145−9.

30 Romankiewicz JA. Pharmacology and clinical use of drugs in hypertensive emergencies. *Am J Hosp Pharm* 1977;34:185−93.

32 Vascular Pathology in Hypertensive Children

WILL R. BLACKBURN AND NELSON REEDE COOLEY JR

INTRODUCTION

Hypertension (HBP) in adults is often idiopathic (primary) while the disorder in children is frequently associated with an identifiable etiology [1,2]. Renal vascular and parenchymal diseases account for many cases of HBP in pediatric medicine. Other causes of HBP in this age group (coarctation, endocrine abnormalities, neurofibromatosis, neoplasms) are far less common [3]. Recently physicians have begun to appreciate the fact that idiopathic HBP is not a rarity in children and adolescents [4–6]. In our hospital, preeclampsia and gestational HBP are the most frequent causes of HBP in teenage girls. Many of these girls are at high risk for the subsequent development of idiopathic HBP.

In spite of our increasing awareness of the incidence, etiology, and treatment of HBP in pediatric medicine, relatively little is known of the attending vascular pathology. Pediatric and perinatal pathologists have remained conspicuously quiet on the subject of the cellular and molecular lesions developing in arteries of children with HBP. In not one of the recent symposia on pediatric hypertension were there detailed discussions of the structural or compositional nature of the vascular lesions [2–4,6,7]. This chapter describes the arterial lesions accompanying HBP in children. The differences between these lesions as they appear in children and young animals and those observed in the arteries of adults and older animals are emphasized.

For purposes of presentation, the arterial lesions in hypertensive states in children will be considered in two general categories: arterial lesions *producing* HBP and lesions developing in the arteries of children as a *result* of HBP of nonvascular origin (e.g. endocrine, central nervous system disease, essential HBP).

ANATOMIC CONSIDERATIONS

The mean arterial pressure is the product of cardiac output and the total peripheral resistance. In hypertensive children, the blood pressure elevation is abnormal in repeated examinations (at least above the 90th percentile rank for age–sex comparable peers) if not associated at the time of initial examination with signs and/or symptoms commonly found with hypertensive cardiovascular disease [7]. The pathologic changes developing in the arteries of a child with HBP depend on several factors:
1 age of onset;
2 degree and duration of pressure elevation;
3 alterations in pulse pressure;
4 the vascular circuit involved; and
5 the caliber of artery examined.

The vascular bed is a continuum composed of vessels of different size and structure. The arterial component of this system consists of large elastic arteries (aorta, pulmonary artery); large, medium, and small muscular arteries (e.g. brachiocephalic, internal carotid, and radial artery); arterioles, and arterial capillaries. Only the response of the arterial component of the vascular bed to HBP will be considered in this paper. The uniqueness of the pulmonary and renal arterial circuits in HBP will be emphasized when appropriate.

The reactivity of the arterial wall to HBP (or any other insult) is dependent upon its cellular composition, extracellular matrix-fiber system (elastin, collagen), and structural organization. Because of these structural and compositional variables, large elastic arteries, muscular arteries, arterioles, and capillaries respond differently to HBP.

The basic structure of all vessels is similar throughout the cardiovascular system (including the heart).

The walls of arteries are organized into layers or tunics: the innermost tunica intima (intima), the middle tunica media (media), and the outer tunica adventitia (adventitia). The thickness of each tunic varies in different arteries; however, their composition and structural organization are relatively similar since the tunics are continuous.

The intima consists of an inner layer of endothelial cells (ECs), overlying a basement membrane (BM) and a thin layer of subendothelial connective tissue. In the fetus and infant, the subendothelial connective tissue is quite thin but with aging this tissue becomes progressively thickened due to an accumulation of both fibers and cells. By 14 years of age, smooth muscle cells (SMCs) begin to appear within the subendothelial connective tissue.

The media is characterized by SMCs in all vessels except capillaries; in the latter vessels, a modified SMC (the pericyte) acts as the entire media. In all other arteries, the SMC is the only cell normally present in the media; the orientation of the SMC and its internal organelles varies considerably with age [8]. The SMC is a multipotential cell capable of synthesizing elastin, collagen, myosin, actin, and certain constituents of the extracellular ground substance [9]. In the muscular arteries where the media is most conspicuous, the SMCs are arranged circumferentially in concentric layers separated by a thick envelope of collagen and elastic fibers. At the inner and outer boundaries of the media are bands of elastin-rich tissue which comprise the internal and external elastic lamellae, respectively. The media of the aorta is unique in that it contains as many as 70 fenestrated lamellae dispersed throughout the media. The orientation of the elastic fibers is in one direction (clockwise or counterclockwise) which alternates with each lamella.

The adventitia is the outermost tunic and is composed of a matrix of loose connective tissue containing macrophages, nerves, and vasa vasorum. The connective tissue fibers are arranged parallel and tangential to the lumen and are anchored in a complex manner to similar fibers within the tunica media. Three types of nerve fibers are present within the adventitia (sensory, sympathetic, and parasympathetic). The vasa vasorum are present in all vessels of a size greater than about 200 μm.

The vascular bed is lined by ECs. If one visualizes the entire endothelial barrier as a single flat sheet one cell thick, it would be possible to detect specific anatomic regions. These specialized regions correspond to the structurally modified ECs in different types of specialty arteries (aorta, muscular arteries, cerebral arteries) and capillary beds (glomerular, liver sinusoids, brain, muscle). These modified areas of endothelium correspond to areas of functional specialization and account for the four general types of capillaries described by Rhodin [10] and others. Since the endothelium acts as a living antithrombotic barrier between the tissues of blood and those of the arterial wall and since these cells are known to secrete BM components and various trophic substances, the response of the endothelial cell to HBP is of major importance.

Smooth muscle cells maintain arterial wall compliance, contractibility, and, in turn, blood pressure. The surface of the SMC is in direct structural continuity with the extracellular fibrous matrix system and with the cell membranes of other SMCs and/or ECs. SMCs are now known to secrete and maintain much of the fibrous-matrix complex of the media. The latter complex plays a fundamental role in normal vascular compliance and in the adaptation to HBP.

ARTERIAL LESIONS PRODUCING HYPERTENSION IN CHILDREN

It is important to consider lesions arising within arteries which produce HBP. In general, these lesions produce HBP by either modifying vascular flow, compliance, and tone, or by indirectly bringing about the release of pressor substances (e.g. renin) which in turn alter vascular tone and compliance. In pediatric medicine the most important arterial lesions producing HBP are those associated with persistent fetal circulation, coarctation, renal artery stenosis, and pre-eclampsia.

Coarctation

Coarctation of the aorta is a frequent cause of HBP in infants. The lesion is most commonly congenital and involves the thoracic aorta at or near the junction with the ductus arteriosus [11]. Stenoses of this sort are interesting in that many of the lesions are associated with chromosomal abnormalities (Turner's syndrome, trisomy 9 syndrome), single mutant gene syndromes (e.g. Apert syndrome), inborn errors of metabolism (Hurler syndrome) [12], maternal diabetes mellitus, and fetal infection (rubella) [13]. A few cases are known to be familial [14]. Males are much more often affected than females. Some 25–50% of coarctations are associated with other congenital anomalies (e.g. endocardial fibroelastosis, bicuspid aortic valve, patent ductus arteriosus).

Recently it has been suggested that aortic coarctation associated with Turner's syndrome is due to lymphatic abnormalities which lead to lymphedema in the area of the developing aortic arch [15,16]. Other studies [17] suggest that although the coarctation lesion may be resected surgically, the patients are at extreme risk for premature cardiovascular disease [18] and a high (12%) premature death rate (average age 34 years) due primarily to rupture of a major artery (e.g. aorta, cerebral artery). Necropsy and other studies reveal an increased incidence of aortic root dilatation and aneurysms of the cerebral and internal carotid arteries [19]. These lesions are thought to be secondary to HBP which is present in 80% of Turner's syndrome patients [19]. Similar aneurysmal lesions are noted in children with HBP due to other causes (e.g. pheochromocytoma, renal artery stenosis, and polycystic kidney disease). Collectively these findings suggest that the fetus with coarctation of the aorta develops widespread vascular disease early in life and that the disease process in patients with HBP is progressive in spite of surgical treatment. Clearly this is an area for continued investigation.

Histologic studies of the stenotic aorta segment in infants indicate a lesion of the media composed of both smooth muscle and fibroelastic tissues. Intimal lesions develop at the site of narrowing as well as proximal and distal to the stenotic site. Proximal to the area of stenosis, the ECs develop "stress fibers" (modifications of the cytoskeletal system composed of bundles of actin filaments) and apparently undergo increased turnover rates [20]. At the site of stenosis, the intima often becomes thick and fibrous; distally the intima undergoes severe thickening due to increased numbers of cells and the quantity of fiber-rich matrix. With time, atheromas develop in the poststenotic dilated region. This area is known to be exposed to considerable flow turbulence.

In many patients with coarctation and HBP, death at an early age occurs as a result of arterial rupture [16,19]. In addition to the histologic changes described above, signs of widespread cystic medial arterial necrosis are detected. This is particularly true

of patients with Turner's syndrome. The lesions are quite similar to those seen in Marfan syndrome, a similarity that leads one to suspect an intrinsic mesenchymal defect in such patients [16,21].

Coarctation of the abdominal aorta is relatively rare with only about 70 cases having been reported to date. The lesion may produce HBP in a manner identical to that seen in coarctation of the thoracic aorta. If the lesion involves the renal arteries, however, renin-mediated HBP may develop. Most coarctations of the abdominal aorta appear to represent regional areas of hypoplasia. The usual aortic tissue layers are present but the overall mural region is thin and the lumen is reduced. Intimal lesions develop both at the site of narrowing and distally, as discussed above.

A significant number of children with coarctation of the abdominal aorta actually suffer from vascular neurofibromatosis (VNF) [22–26]. Such children may show café-au-lait spots but do not usually show the other stigmas of neurofibromatosis (e.g. hemangiomas and neurofibromas). Narrowing of the aortic lumen in neurofibromatosis may result from extrinsic compression by an adjacent neurofibroma or other neoplasm common to von Recklinghausen's disease. Most often, however, the narrowing of the lumen is the result of intrinsic, intramural, vascular disease (e.g. "true" VNF). While VNF is strongly associated with coarctation of the abdominal aorta, the disease most commonly involves medium-size muscular arteries where it produces vascular insufficiency. Vascular neurofibromatosis produces a progressive obliteration of the internal carotid artery and is a common cause of stroke in children (Moyamoya disease) [27]. Vascular neurofibromatosis of the mesenteric artery may produce malabsorption and sprue-like symptoms [28]. It is now known that VNF is a frequent cause of renal artery stenosis, a lesion triggering renal hypertension. These lesions will be described in the following discussion of renal artery stenosis.

Renal artery stenosis

Although there are several diseases which produce renal artery stenosis and lead to renal–renin-mediated HBP, only a few morphologically characteristic arterial lesions are recognized and only a few of the diseases are common to children (Table 32.1). The nomenclature used to reference the different types of renal artery stenoses was in a confusing state until

Table 32.1 Renal artery stenoses in children

Atherosclerosis
Progeroid syndromes
Inborn error of lipid metabolism

Fibrous and fibromuscular dysplasia
Intima
    Intimal fibroplasia
Media
    Fibromuscular dysplasia (with or without aneurysms)
    Medial fibroplasia
    Medial hyperplasia
    Perimedial fibroplasia
    Medial dissection
Adventitia
    Periarterial fibroplasia

Genetic disorders
Vascular neurofibromatosis
Williams syndrome
Klippel−Trenaunay−Weber syndrome
Feuerstein−Mimms syndrome

Thromboembolization
Postcatheterization

Inflammatory stenoses
Takayasu's arteritis
Aortitis
Sarcoidosis

Harrison and McCormack and their associates developed a classification based on vascular tunic involvement [29,30]. This classification, with recognized limitations, provides a framework for the evaluation of renal artery stenoses in pediatric pathology.

Atherosclerotic narrowing of the renal artery is a rare cause of HBP in pediatric pathology. The lesion is identical to that seen in adults and almost always is associated with either an inborn error in lipid metabolism [31] or a progeroid syndrome [32,33]. In the latter conditions, elevated blood levels of cholesterol and low density lipoproteins (LDLs) are almost always present. Elevated cholesterol is known to reduce the EC glycocalyx coat, enhance the rate of both EC death and mitosis, as well as promote the accumulation of lipid within intimal phagocytes (foam cells) [34].

Thromboembolic occlusion of the renal artery is a common cause of acute HBP in premature newborn infants; the lesion is rare in older infants and children [35]. Umbilical artery catheterization with subsequent thrombotic occlusion of a renal artery is the most common cause of HBP in the newborn child

[36]. The pathophysiologic process involves trauma to the endothelium with subsequent platelet adhesion and aggregation followed by clot formation and subsequent propagation of this clot into the renal artery or with embolization into the renal artery lumen. Renin-mediated renal hypertension follows shortly thereafter. Inflammatory processes involving the renal as well as other arteries are uncommon except in certain geographic areas: Takayasu's arteritis in Asia [37,38] and African arteritis [39]. Granulomatous arteritis may involve systemically the medium-size arteries and may produce renal artery stenosis. In this category belong the lesions of sarcoidosis and familial granulomatous arteritis. Some authors believe that the latter two disorders are one and the same [40,41].

In pediatric medicine, intimal fibroplasia, fibromuscular dysplasia, and VNF are the most frequent causes of renovascular HBP. Intimal fibroplasia is occasionally seen in fetuses, infants, and children. The lesion consists of a circumferential, often eccentric, accumulation of a relatively loose fibrous matrix tissue containing a moderate number of cells. There are no signs of inflammatory change or of lipid accumulation. The internal elastic lamellae may show duplications but are often intact and normal. The arterial lesions produced by congenital rubella most likely belong in this category. Congenital rubella produces intimal lesions which lead to stenoses in many arteries (pulmonary, aorta, renal, and others). Esterly and Oppenheimer [42] and others [43] have referred to these changes as "intimal fibromuscular proliferation" and/or "hyperplasia." Similar lesions have been seen in children without mention of congenital rubella [44−47] and in children with Williams syndrome [48,49].

Fibromuscular dysplasia with or without aneurysms is a frequent cause of renal artery stenosis in children. The disorder produces a segmental narrowing of the renal artery. The lesion involves the main renal artery, the segmental branches, or both. The arterial wall shows focal areas of thickening alternating with areas of extreme thinning with or without aneurysmal dilatation. The lesions resemble a string of beads when seen by arteriography [30]. The thick ridge-like zones of the media are partly or completely replaced by a collagenous fibrous matrix. These matrix deposits replace areas of degenerated elastic fibers within the media and displace and disorient the SMCs. In the thin wall regions, the smooth muscle tissue has been completely replaced and the elastic lamellae are deficient. In the adventitial regions, the longitudinally oriented SMCs appear hypertrophic. The lesions of fibromuscular dysplasia do not dissect, thrombose, or hemorrhage, and rarely cause progressive arterial obstruction.

Adventitial periarterial fibroplasia is a relatively rare lesion characterized by fibroplasia and the deposition of collagen within the adventitial and surrounding connective tissues. The lesion is accompanied by signs of chronic inflammation (plasma cells, lymphocytes) within the surrounding connective tissues of the renal arteries; the small vessels and capillaries within the connective tissues may also be cuffed by inflammatory cells. The latter aspects of the lesion are somewhat similar to those seen in idiopathic retroperitoneal fibrosis. Although it is a rare condition, it is more common in teenage girls [30].

Neurofibromatosis

Neurofibromatosis is a congenital hereditary dysplasia of mesodermal and ectodermal tissues and represents one of the neurocristopathies. Most, if not all, children with neurofibromatosis develop vascular lesions [26,50]. These lesions have been described in virtually all arteries but are most common in the aorta (coarctation), renal arteries (stenosis), internal carotid, and vertebral arteries (progressive obliterative stenosis) [51,52]. Feyrter [53] has described the lesions of VNF in arterioles and capillaries. Vascular lesions have been described in the kidneys, endocrine glands, heart, gastrointestinal tract, and brain [26,54]. VNF involving the renal arteries is one of the most common causes of renovascular HBP [23–25,54–58].

In extremely careful studies, Feyrter [53] described five different types of arterial lesions if VNF:

1 pure intimal lesions;
2 an advanced intimal lesion with medial changes;
3 nodular aneurysmal lesions with loss of medial elements and the formation of aneurysm-like nodules;
4 periarterial nodular lesions; and
5 an epithelioid lesion with marked cellular proliferation.
Reubi [50] more or less proposed a similar classification.

In our studies of VNF [25,26] the arterial lesions were found to be unusual and diagnostic. In the past we causally had interpreted the lesions of VNF in resected renal arteries as being part of the fibromuscular dysplasia group. In a review of renal artery

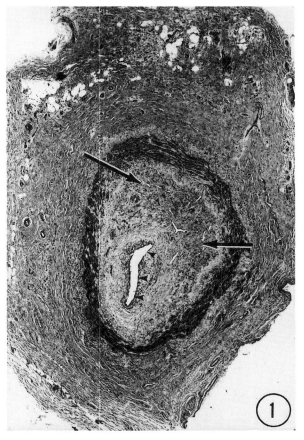

Fig. 32.1 Cross-section of artery with vascular neurofibromatosis showing severe stenosis of the lumen (arrow-heads) due to a fibrous thickening of the intima (arrows). The internal elastic membrane is also thickened. (Masson's trichome, × 38.)

stenoses in children, most of the lesions we once termed fibromuscular dysplasia were found to be those of VNF. The most conspicuous lesion in VNF is a fibrous thickening of the intima (Fig. 32.1) within which small blood vessels (vasa vasorum) may be seen with slit-like lumens (Fig. 32.2). The internal elastic membranes are often duplicated and fragmented. Often nodular aggregates of cells are noted within the junctional zones between the intima and the muscularis (Fig. 32.3) These nodules are thought to represent SMCs [51], or nodules of neural origin [53]. Our studies suggest that nodules of both neural and vascular etiology occur in VNF (Figs 32.3 and 32.4). The polar arrangement of SMCs within the arterial media is often disorganized in VNF. In many areas, the layers of smooth muscle in the media are thinner than normal while the matrix connective tissues are increased. The histopathologic lesions in

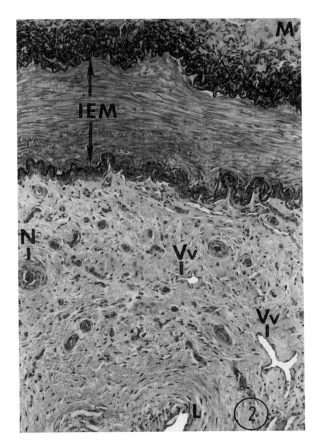

Fig. 32.2 An enlargement of the artery wall in Figure 32.1 showing the lumen (L) and tiny vasa vasoral-like vessels (Vv) within the thickened intima. The internal elastic membrane (IEM) is greatly thickened. M = Media; N = nodule. (Verhoeff Van Giesson × 150.)

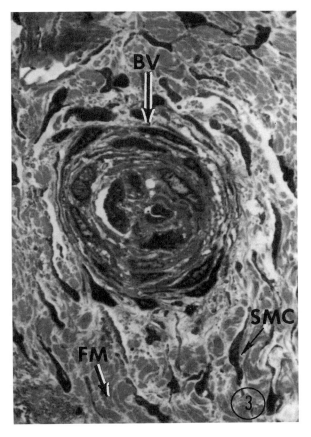

Fig. 32.3 Portion of vascular neurofibromatosis lesion showing nodule of smooth muscle cells (SMC). The structural arrangement suggests a vasa vasoral blood vessel (BV). FM = Fibrous matrix. (Epon, Paragon stain × 432.)

the intima and in the vasa vasora in VNF are quite similar to those seen in the intracranial arteries of children with vascular complications associated with sickle cell disease [59] and tuberous sclerosis [60].

Pre-eclampsia and gestational hypertension

Although many physicians may not consider pre-eclampsia a proper subject in a symposium on pediatric HBP, in my hospital this disorder is the most common acute hypertensive disorder seen in teenage girls. Secondly, many physicians may object to a consideration of pre-eclampsia in a discussion of arterial lesions *producing* HBP; however, there are many current data to support this concept. It should be pointed out that there are both similarities and differences between pre-eclampsia, gestational HBP,

and essential HBP [61−63]. The frequency of eclampsia and pre-eclampsia in families suggests that a single recessive gene may be responsible for the disorder. Mild pre-eclampsia (gestational hypertension) is often a sign of latent HBP unmasked by pregnancy [63]. Adolescents with gestational HBP ultimately have a high prevalence of idiopathic HBP whereas those pregnancies which are normotensive ultimately have a low prevalence of idiopathic HBP.

The pathogenesis of pre-eclampsia is unknown; however, there are many data to suggest that utero-placental hypoperfusion plays a triggering role in the development of this syndrome and that this phenomenon is mediated by the subplacental decidual vascular bed [64]. Studies [65−68] have indicated that abnormalities develop within the endometrial spiral arteries during the first trimester of pregnancy *prior*

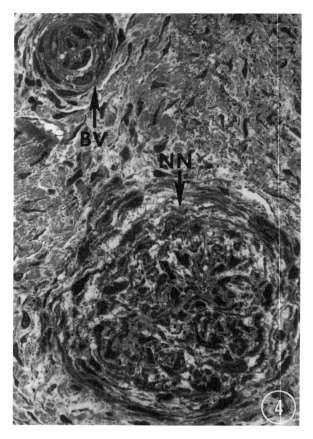

Fig. 32.4 Section of intimal lesion in vascular neurofibromatosis showing a nodule composed of neural elements (NN) and a small vasa vasoral blood vessel (BV). (Epon, Paragon stain × 432.)

to the development of HBP. During this period, cells derived from the cytotrophoblast (intermediate trophoblast) invade and modify the maternal spiral arteries and arterioles in both humans and primates [65,69,70]. There is a growing mass of data to suggest that the invading intermediate cytotrophoblast acts as an antigenic trigger for the maternal immunologic vascular reaction and that lesions develop within the spiral arteries and arterioles early in pregnancy [66,67]. These lesions act to constrict uteroplacental blood flow which, in turn, brings about a release of uterine renin and ultimately an increase in angiotensin II and the hypertensive state.

An alternative explanation for the pathobiology of pre-eclampsia involves intermediate trophoblast. Intermediate trophoblast cells are derived from cytotrophoblast, as is the syncytiotrophoblast. The intermediate trophoblast cells are most unique. Intermediate trophoblast cells invade the implantation

site, infiltrating the decidua and myometrium and ultimately the maternal spiral arteries. Within the spiral arteries, intermediate trophoblast cells replace the smooth muscle (forming the fibrin matrix) and the endothelium. In this process the distal segments of the spiral arteries are converted to flaccid tubes incapable of constriction. The physiologic effect is a conversion of the spiral artery blood pressure to the low-pressure system characteristic of the uteroplacental circulation. It has been suggested that certain maternal vascular abnormalities (e.g. pre-eclampsia, diabetes mellitus, lupus erythematosus) are the result of defective invasion of the implantation site by intermediate trophoblast cells. The result is inadequate development of the fibrin matrix in the myometrial and distal portion of the spiral arteries [71,72].

Histologic studies of the spiral arteries before [66,67] as well as after the development of pre-eclampsia [69] indicate a rather unique lesion in the arteries of teenage girls. These changes reduce the arterial lumen and consist of endothelial swelling, intimal hypercellularity, and the appearance of lipid-laden foam cells. The intimal lesions have been referred to as "acute atheroma" [68]. The lesions of the media include SMC hypertrophy, intramural fibrosis, and degenerative changes in elastic fibers and ground substances. The latter changes resemble fibrinoid necrosis [65,67]. A unique component of the arterial lesion is the frequent presence of mononuclear cells within the adventitial zones. The addition of the latter reaction makes the overall appearance of the arterial lesions in pre-eclampsia very similar to those seen in homograft rejection [69,73,74]. Electron microscopic studies of these lesions have added a more detailed description to the literature [75].

Most evidence suggests that the endometrial arterial lesions *precede* the development of acute HBP in pre-eclampsia. Once the acute hypertensive state has been established, the arterial, arteriolar, and capillary lesions appear secondarily within the kidney. In the afferent arteriole and the glomerular capillary tuft, these lesions consist of endothelial and mesangial cell swelling, EC denudation with fibrin deposition and platelet adhesion, electron-dense granular deposits between the endothelium and the BM and the mesangium, and, occasionally, fibrin depositions within the capillary wall. The lesions may progress to eclampsia—acute arteriolar necrosis with disseminated microembolization.

Experimental models of pre-eclampsia, utilizing the uteroplacental hypoperfusion concept as a triggering event, have been developed. These studies strongly support the aforegoing pathophysiologic chain of events in a variety of pregnant animals (rabbits, dogs, monkeys, and baboons) [76—79].

ARTERIAL LESIONS IN HYPERTENSION

There is general agreement that the final common path in the etiology of HBP is the arterial wall. The mechanism by which increased peripheral resistance is established in HBP is unknown. It is known that the response of arteries to increased hydrostatic pressure is dependent upon age, caliber of artery, as well as the degree and duration of HBP. The lesions associated with acute and chronic HBP are morphologically distinct and will be considered separately.

Acute hypertension

In acute malignant HBP there is a sudden, severe increase in blood pressure superimposed on an arterial wall with or without previous adaptation to HBP. The lesions of acute HBP are characterized by EC swelling (endotheliosis), EC disruption and denudation, platelet adhesion and degranulation, fibrin deposition, and arterionecrosis. The last two components are collectively referred to as "fibrinoid necrosis." The lesions are most prominent in the renal, pulmonary, and cerebral arterial circuits. In the brain, fibrinoid necrosis of the small arteries and arterioles leads to aneurysm formation (Charcot—Buchard aneurysms) with associated rupture and hemorrhage. Once the arterioles are overstretched and autoregulation is lost, the postresistance arterial capillaries are exposed to extreme pressures; EC disruption occurs and paracellular transport is markedly increased [80,81]. During healing, the areas of arterionecrosis become angioblastic nodules composed of fibrin, modified migrating endothelial cells [82], and loose connective tissue. Nodular lesions of this sort have been referred to as "plexiform," "glomoid," and "angiomatoid" [83].

The lesions of acute (malignant) HBP are seen in children with renal-mediated HBP; in these cases, the lesions are usually superimposed upon arteries undergoing adaptation to progressive HBP. In adolescent girls, pre-eclampsia and toxemia are the most common causes of malignant HBP. In this group, the lesions are particularly severe in the renal arterioles and glomerular capillaries. Neoplasms are relatively uncommon causes of acute HBP in pediatric medicine.

Chronic hypertension

It is known that the arterial vasculature undergoes considerable structural development during the fetal period and that growth continues in both the infant and child. During adolescence the arterial tunics become structurally mature. In the aorta, for example, the elastic lamellae are fully developed by about 12 years of age. The number of aortic elastic lamellae does not change thereafter, even though HBP may become clinically manifest [84]. It should also be pointed out that the growth and development of arteries are closely related to pulse pressure. For example, if there is little or no pulse pressure during fetal development, the elastic lamellae do not develop in the aorta (e.g. acardiac twin). The influence of a widening pulse pressure on the developing aorta is not known. Finally, it should be pointed out that the arterial tunics continue to change in the normotensive individual throughout life and that during this time period we cease to refer to *growth* and begin to refer to this process as *aging*. The structural expressions of arterial growth, aging, and the influences of HBP are overlapping phenomena which infinitely complicate our discussion.

HBP accelerates the growth process (and probably the aging process) in arteries of infants and children. These changes include a narrowing of the arterial lumen, thickening of the arterial wall, and increased vessel stiffness or tone [85,86]. Arteries from hypertensive children show thickening of the intima and the media early in the process (Fig. 32.5). Initially, the large elastic arteries appear relatively resistant to these structural changes. Light microscopy reveals an increase in both subendothelial connective tissue and cellularity. The increase in intimal cellularity is due to cells derived from blood and media (SMCs). Blood-derived cells enter the subendothelial space either at EC junctions or by actually passing through the EC wall. SMCs accumulate within the subendothelial space in HBP by migration from the media, entering through the fenestration in the elastic laminae. The accumulation of lipids within the intima occurs earlier than was initially thought. These lipid accumulations are mostly intracellular and consist of modified LDLs. If the hypertensive state continues, atheromas develop within the arteries of children in a manner identical to that seen in the adult. Severe

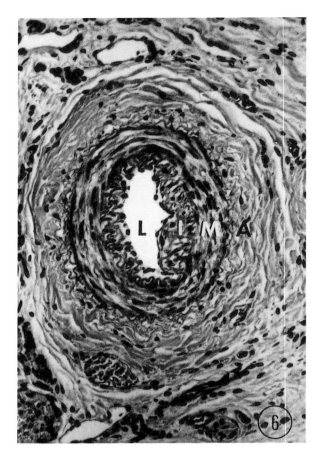

Fig. 32.5 Artery from hypertensive child showing reduced lumen (L), intimal thickening (I), and early smooth muscle cell hypertrophy in the media (M). (Hematoxylin and eosin × 256.)

obliterative atherosclerosis has been noted in the arteries of children with prolonged HBP. These lesions are particularly prominent in the coronary and systemic muscular arteries [31].

The arterial media is thickened in HBP [87]. The SMCs appear hypertrophic (enlarged) and excess extra-cellular fibrous tissue matrix is present. Initially, the elastic laminae do not show significant changes, but in time, signs of reduplication and even fragmentation appear. Studies have suggested that SMCs do not undergo hyperplasia (proliferation) but respond to increased wall tension by undergoing hypertrophy and increasing the synthesis of precursors of elastin, collagen, and extracellular ground substance [9,88]. These studies further emphasize the multipotential nature of vascular SMCs. The increase in the arterial wall content of both elastin and collagen is quantitatively similar and suggests that these two fibrous protein complexes act in concert at both normal and pathologic levels of tension [86].

A prominent but poorly appreciated lesion accompanying chronic HBP is *microvascular rarefaction*. This process appears in two stages: the first is functional rarefaction followed by anatomic rarefaction [89]. The process results in a quantitative reduction in parallel conductance microvascular channels due to rarefaction of arterioles and capillaries. This process accounts, at least in part, for the maintenance of chronic HBP. In a variety of studies in humans [90,91] and in experimental animals [89,92], prolonged HBP is noted to be associated with a decrease in the number of small arterioles and capillaries within a specific vascular bed (e.g. skeletal muscle, mesentery, skin, conjunctivae). *In vivo* microscopy, stereologic, and low-viscosity latex cast studies of the microvascular system subjected to HBP suggest that early in the process, functional capillary density is reduced. This is followed a few weeks later by a reduction in the density of both functioning arterioles and capillaries (functional rarefaction). Finally, an anatomic decrease in the density of both capillaries and arterioles (anatomic rarefaction) is noted. The latter process is apparently irreversible. Microvascular rarefaction is also noted in association with HBP in certain specialized vascular circuits. It is, for example, a serious anatomic complication of a variety of lung diseases characterized by pulmonary hypertension [93,94].

Compositional studies of the arterial wall of the human during growth [87,88,95] and during the adaptation to HBP [87,88,96] are few in number and the results are discordant. Most of the data suggests that in HBP there is an increase in the absolute amounts of water, collagen, elastin, sodium, and certain components of the media matrix (e.g. chondroitin sulfate). Alterations in the media matrix give rise to certain lesions which resemble cystic medial necrosis; such lesions are associated with chronic HBP and most often are found in cerebral and systemic medium-size arteries.

Relatively few changes have been described in the adventitia in human HBP. There is evidence that changes do occur and that there is an increase in the number of vasa vasorum accompanying the structural adaptation to HBP. Fibrosis and condensation of the adventitial tissues have also been described. It is not known whether or not this latter change is related to age or the duration of HBP.

Hypertension and atherogenesis

It is well established that HBP predisposes to atherosclerosis, particularly in coronary and cerebral arteries. Hypertension is an established major risk factor predisposing to the accumulation of lipid and ultimately fibrous connective tissue within the arterial intima at sites of high flow stress in both adults and children. In children the initial, and apparently reversible, lesions are confined to the intima and are referred to as "fatty streaks." In children, atheromas may develop in the absence of HBP, as in diseases with abnormal lipid metabolism (inborn errors, nephrotic syndrome) [31]. Studies by Moon [97] clearly indicate the presence of arteriosclerotic lesions in the coronary arteries of infants and children, a process most prominent in males and one thought to be related initially to rupture and degeneration of the internal elastic membrane. These lesions are accelerated by HBP, as demonstrated in the hypertensive circuit of congenital aortic coarctation [98].

The lesions of atherogenesis and hypertension share three basic vascular cell phenomena: proliferation of intimal SMCs; the accumulation of lipids within the extracellular matrix and SMCs, and the formation of new connective tissue elements (collagen, elastic fibers, and proteoglycans) [84]. The current basic concept regarding the relationship between HBP and atherogenesis is repeated EC injury (flow stress), EC death, and the establishment of a constant state of regeneration of the endothelial layer [34]. Under these conditions, the production of prostacyclin by ECs is thought to be reduced. Prostacyclin is a known antithrombotic agent and suppressor (through its inhibitory effects on platelet aggregation) of atherosclerotic lesions. With suppressed prostacyclin production, platelet aggregation is enhanced and SMC mitogens are released during the platelet degranulation phenomenon [99–101]. SMCs appear within the intima and, in time, modified forms of LDLs accumulate in the subendothelial region both extracellularly and within cells of either monocyte [34] or SMC origin. When these lesions are attended by increased fibrous matrix, the fibrous plaque (the hallmark of atherosclerosis) is established (Fig. 32.6).

EXPERIMENTAL HYPERTENSION

Animal models

A variety of models for experimental HBP have been developed [103–105]. Perhaps the greatest information has been derived from models involving experimental coarctation [106,107], renal artery stenosis and the Goldblatt kidney [104,108], genetic strains of rats [105,109,110], and certain drug and diet models [105,111–113]. Only a few of these models will be considered here and only in so far as they shed light on the vascular lesions in HBP, particularly in young animals.

TERATOGENESIS: HYPERTENSION IN THE FETUS AND EMBRYO

In 1932, Bremer [114] advanced the idea that spiral streams of blood flow within the developing heart played an important role in determining the location of developing cardiac septa. Conditions which altered blood pressure in the embryo would in turn alter these spiral streams and abnormally influence septation in the developing heart. Yoshida and associates [115] studied intracardiac flow patterns and observed changes, and did not support the traditional flow-molding hypothesis of Bremer. Most recently Stewart and coworkers [116] and Kirby [117] studied the effects of neural crest ablation on the developing chick heart; these studies revealed that neural crest ablation led to hemodynamic changes which *preceded* the appearance of heart defects (e.g. aortic arch anomalies, persistent truncus arteriosus, ventricular septal defect, and double outlet right ventricle). Ethyl alcohol induces similar cardiac anomalies in chick and mouse embryos [118] and in these species, anomalous neural crest migration with associated hemodynamic effects is suspected.

Methods are available in which the blood pressure in developing embryos and fetuses may be measured [119,120]. Although the number of studies are few, the available data indicate that HBP in the embryo or fetus plays a fundamental role in the initiation of teratogenic processes. Grabowski and colleagues [119] have shown that hypoxia in the embryo or fetus leads to hypervolemia and, after a time, HBP, vascular rupture, hemorrhage, and ultimately developmental anomalies. Ruckman and co-workers [121] have reviewed the role of HBP in the teratogenesis of hypoxia in the embryonic chick heart. The nature of the anomalies produced depended upon the stage of development at the time of the HBP insult.

In other experimental models, the teratogenic nature of HBP has been emphasized. Hyperthermia, for example, has been shown to increase heart rate, cardiac output, and arterial blood pressure in chick embryos; these hemodynamic effects are thought to be directly related to the teratogenic effects noted in the developing cardiovascular system [122]. A variety

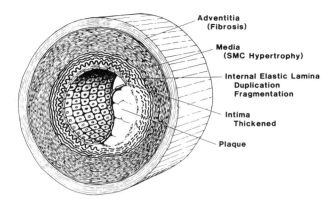

Fig. 32.6 Schematic depiction of the relationship between hypertension and atherogenesis within the vascular tunics. Modified from [102].

of drugs and chemicals, many of which are teratogens (e.g. trypan blue, cocaine, caffeine, xanthines, ethanol, dopamine, dextroamphetamine), are known to induce HBP in the embryo and fetus [123–127]. The most common abnormalities associated with exposure to these agents early in development are aortic anomalies and septation defects in the heart [124,128,129]. If agent exposure occurs after cardiac development is complete, the nature of the induced anomaly is altered. Rajala and Kaplan [113] have reported that late chick embryos treated with trypan blue developed severe HBP and dilatation and rupture of the caudal dorsal aortae; caudal hematomas were formed and the chicks were hatched with anomalous development of the tail regions.

Although the mechanisms are not fully delineated at this time, much of the evidence suggests that HBP plays a fundamental role in certain forms of teratogenesis. Early in development, HBP appears significantly to affect cardiac development while exposure late in development leads to distal end-organ abnormalities (hypoplasia, atresia, or agenesis). Collectively these data strongly suggest that the hypertensive state in the embryo or fetus is teratogenic and that the end-result is an array of birth defects, of which the nature and pattern depend upon both the duration and timing of the hypertensive insult.

HYPERTENSION IN GENETIC STRAINS OF RATS

Dahl and colleagues [109] have developed genetic strains of rats both highly sensitive (S) and highly

resistant (R) to the hypertensive effects of salt. The inheritance of blood pressure control in both S and R strains is polygenic, involving approximately two of four autosomal loci. One of these loci has been identified and involves the mutation of a cytochrome P-450 involved in adrenal steroid hydroxylation at positions 18 and 11 β. This locus has two alleles inherited by mendelian codominance and results in increased secretion and increased blood levels of the weak mineralocorticoid 18-hydroxy-11-deoxycorticosterone.

The spontaneously hypertensive rats (SHRs) of Okamoto and Aoki [110] and the Milan hypertensive strain (MHS) of Bianchi and coworkers [130] become hypertensive shortly after weaning. In the New Zealand genetically hypertensive rats, the blood pressure is elevated even at 2 days of age.

The arterial lesions in SHRs have been studied in some detail. Ichijima [131] was the first to demonstrate artery abnormalities in SHRs as compared to control rats. These lesions consisted of increased tortuosity and a decrease in the lumen size of mesenteric arterioles. Mulvany and colleagues [132] demonstrated in the small resistance arteries of SHRs a thickening of the media which was reflected by an increase in the number of layers of SMCs within the media. Gattone and co-authors [133] have suggested that a primary vascular abnormality is present in SHRs and that these lesions are present *before* the detection of clinical HBP. The lesions appear as an abnormally small renal afferent arteriole in SHRs as compared to controls (Fig. 32.7). Morkrid and associates [134] noted small afferent renal arterioles in rats with deoxycorticosterone acetate salt-induced HBP. Mulvany and colleagues [132] reported abnormally small mesenteric arteries in SHRs at all ages. There is also evidence that cardiomegaly (heart weight:body weight ratio) is present in SHRs at the time of birth [135].

While anatomic studies of the vessels in SHRs are few, the findings at this time suggest that:

1 vascular lesions may be present at or shortly after birth and before the appearance of HBP;

2 the growth of resistant arteries and arterioles may be inhibited, leading to hypoplastic or small-caliber vessels;

3 when HBP appears, signs of SMC hypertrophy (and possibly hyperplasia) develop along with increased tortuosity of the small arteries;

4 in adult animals with long-term HBP, the vascular lesions are virtually the same as those seen in other animals with other nongenetic forms of HBP.

Cell and molecular pathobiology

Most of the investigations of the effects of HBP on the components of the arterial wall have been limited to changes in ECs and SMCs. Changes in the intercellular matrix appear concomitantly with alterations in the EC barrier and with the response of the SMC to HBP. Each of these elements will be considered separately.

ENDOTHELIUM

The endothelium, being a living tissue barrier between the blood and vascular wall, quite naturally has been of great interest in studies of the pathobiology of HBP. A few studies have considered the effects of age on the endothelial lesions in HBP; these studies will be highlighted as we progress. The effect of injury on endothelium as it relates to atherogenesis and HBP is an elaborate construct based on a variety of investigative approaches [84,99,136].

In young animals, EC turnover is greater than in older animals. With aging, the cells undergo fewer and fewer mitoses [137]. ECs apparently die *in situ* and appear as dark cells which do not stain with vital dyes [135]. The fate of dead ECs is not known; possibly such cells are simply shed into the blood stream and subsequently are cleared by the reticuloendothelial system or within vascular circuits of certain organs (e.g. lung). Possibly such cells migrate into the subendothelial intima and are subsequently lysed and phagocytosed. Evidence indicates that ECs are capable of migrating through the underlying BM during angioblastic stimulus [82,138]. It is possible that a migration of this sort may also occur in the EC dying process. Most researchers believe that although ECs die *in situ* and that mitoses appear *in situ*, these are relatively "slow-rate" processes. Sites of single cell denudation are not seen in scanning electron microscopy studies of the endothelial surface. Schwartz [136] has studied the kinetics of EC repair and has noted that although numerous ECs are injured (e.g. after endotoxin), actual sites of denudation are not seen. It should also be pointed out that EC turnover varies within the vascular bed, some areas being much more rapid than others. Indirect evidence suggests that these foci of rapid turnover are those associated with increased shear injury (i.e. artery bifurcation sites); with age, these shear injury sites are unusually prone to the development of atherogenesis with or without HBP.

Hypertension is known to increase EC turnover

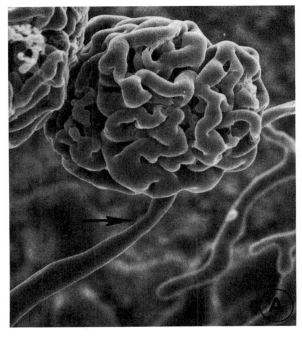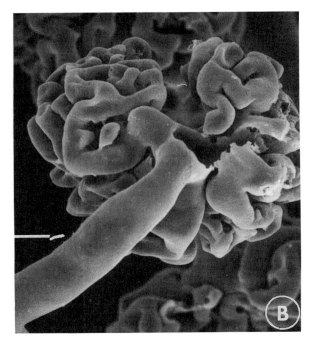

Fig. 32.7 Vascular casts of afferent renal arterioles showing abnormally small vessel in the spontaneously hypertensive rat (A), as compared to normotensive control (B); × 450. From Gattone and colleagues [133], with permission.

[139]; sites of actual denudation do appear and are the sites of subendothelial connective tissue exposure, platelet adhesion, degranulation, and release of a SMC mitogen [99]. The latter phenomenon is a key concept in the current Ross and Glomset hypothesis of atherogenesis [84]. Endothelial cell replication *in vitro* is altered by both age and hypertension. Aortic ECs from children have a greater *in vitro* replication potential than those from adults.

Scanning electron microscopy of arterial endothelium clearly delineates a specific orientation pattern in which the long axis of the EC is in the direction of blood flow [20]. The flow orientation pattern observed in ECs is most likely dictated by the cytoskeletal system and cell anchoring organelles. The EC surface is regionally specialized both structurally [10,137] and functionally (transport domains) [140,141]. The EC surface is marked by small cytoplasmic projections, caveolar pits, and tiny ridges near the cell junctions. In HBP, a variety of cell surface changes are noted. The number of cytoplasmic projections greatly increase, as do the number of caveolae (pinocytotic pits) [142]. The EC cytoskeletal system develops stress fibers (bundles of actin filaments) which further modify the surface of the cell and probably increase its anchoring [20]. In acute HBP the ECs become less firmly anchored and loose cytoplasmic flaps appear near the cell junctions [143]. Blood leukocytes adhere to the EC surface in great numbers (Fig. 32.8) and by transmission electron microscopy are noted to enter the subendothelial intima, particularly at EC junctions. As cells from the blood enter the subendothelial zone of the intima and as SMCs migrate into the intima, the overall endothelial surface lining becomes more irregular forming lumps and bumps [142,144]. Although there are conflicting reports, large areas of EC denudation are noted in HBP; these areas are quickly covered over by platelets, fibrin, and possibly other blood components.

The influence of HBP on macromolecular transport across the EC barrier is also a complicated and controversial issue. Most data suggest that if the increase in hydrostatic pressure is small and gradual, the ECs adapt by *decreasing* macromolecular transport in both the intracellular (pinocytotic) and pericellular (cell junction) routes. Hypertension alters transport in ECs with glycocalyx surface coats by increasing macromolecular trapping. This leads to tightening of the glycocalyx sieve-like meshwork and ultimately a reduction in further macromolecular transport [145].

In the small vessels of hypertensive SHRs, a rapid rise in pressure is not associated with an increase in peroxidase-labeled vesicles, nor is the amount of extravasation of peroxidase increased [135]. Most studies of EC transport in HBP appear to represent a sudden insult in unadapted vessels and hence the report of *increased* transport [80,81].

When arterioles are overstretched, as in acute HBP, they lose their ability to autoregulate. The postresistance vessels (arterial capillaries, venules) are then exposed to higher pressures than normal and a marked increase in permeability appears [80]. During this process, blood-derived macromolecules (fibrinogen) accumulate within the mural regions and account for the fibrinoid lesions described in the past [144].

Aside from a variety of other functions, ECs are known to be responsible for the synthesis of both BM materials and collagenase [82]. Little information is known as to the influences of HBP on the rates of these syntheses; most data seem to suggest, however, that BM materials (collagen IV and V, glycoproteins, and proteoglycans) are produced in increased quantity in HBP while collagenase production is reduced.

SMOOTH MUSCLE CELL

Relatively little is known of the biology of vascular SMC as it relates to the normal progression of blood pressure during human maturation. It is known that intimal SMC proliferation occurs at specific sites within the arterial bed; these sites are those which in time develop atherogenesis and correspond to sites of increased shear force activity [100]. Smooth muscle cells from different sites within the vascular tree show different replicative potentials *in vitro* [146].

Following intimal injury, SMC growth kinetics vary from site to site within the aorta; after intimal injury, SMC growth (replication) is much greater in the abdominal aorta than in the thoracic aorta. These regional differences in injury response by SMCs may account for some of the differences in pathologic lesions developing within an individual artery subjected to HBP [100].

In infants with coarctation, SMCs from the proximal hypertensive side of the stenosis will not replicate *in vitro* for as long as those harvested from the distal hypotensive side of the stenosis [147]. The implications of these observations as they relate to aging and to HBP are very provocative. Is it possible then, that SMCs from the arteries of children having a

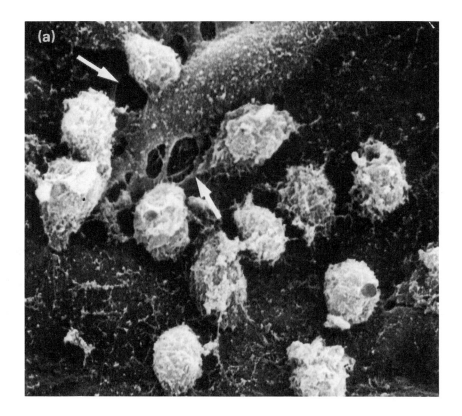

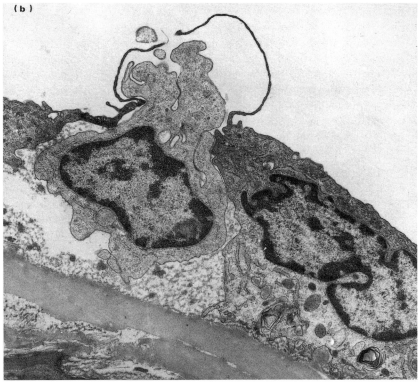

Fig. 32.8 (a) Scanning electron microscopy of aortic intima of hypertensive rat showing blood-derived leukocytes adhering in the vicinity of an endothelial cell surrounded by small gaps (arrows) (× 1500). (b) Transmission electron microscopy showing leukocyte within a small gap between two endothelial cells (× 9800). From Haudenschild and colleagues [137], with permission.

genetic predisposition for idiopathic HBP might not replicate *in vitro* as long as arterial SMCs from children without this risk factor? Such a phenomenon might provide a rapid and early screening test (using SMCs harvested at birth from the umbilical arteries) for children at risk for the subsequent development of HBP.

A basic component of the adaptation of arteries to HBP is mediated through SMCs. The mass of experimental data suggests that, concomitant with the alterations in the endothelial barrier cells (see above), SMCs increase in number, show signs of hypertrophy, increase the synthesis of fiber precursors, and undergo migrations within the vascular tunics. These changes appear within both the intima and the media. These SMC responses reduce the lumen area and alter the vascular wall contractility, and extensibility. The overall effect is thick-walled arteries with increased flow resistance. There is evidence to suggest that many of these changes are reversible during the early stages of HBP [137]; in time, however, certain changes become irreversible [148].

SMOOTH MUSCLE CELL HYPERPLASIA AND MIGRATION

It is known that the cellularity of the intima increases with aging in normotensive animals [149] and that some of these cells are of mural origin (SMCs) while others are of blood origin. In HBP this process is accelerated; increased numbers of SMCs appear within the intima and are derived from local mitoses and from SMCs migrating through the internal elastic membranes from the surrounding muscularis [137,150]. A current concept is that platelet degranulation releases a SMC mitogen (platelet-derived growth factor) which in turn induces SMC mitoses within both the intima and media [101]. There is evidence that HBP in infancy leads to a greater degree of vascular wall thickening (a SMC-mediated response) than when HBP develops during adulthood [87]. Haworth and Reid [74] have described an increase in the number of SMCs in the pulmonary arteries of infants with pulmonary hypertension. The authors describe the migration of SMCs distally in the arterial bed during HBP and the conversion of capillaries to arterioles. The authors imply that in children these alterations may be permanent. In HBP developing in the adult pulmonary arterial bed, SMC mitoses and migrations are either less severe or do not occur [151]. Clearly this concept needs further study.

It has been shown that platelet derived growth factor (PDGF) localizes in sites of SMC proliferation (e.g. atherosclerosis, hypertrophic pregnant uteri). Recent studies of the cardiovascular lesions in children with Williams syndrome (and associated supravalvular aortic stenosis with HBP) revealed quantitative signs of localized SMC proliferation. These localized areas of SMC proliferation within the aortic media grew progressively over time and produced stenosis. Immunohistochemical studies of these localized SMC proliferations revealed increased quantities of PDGF within SMCs. These data suggest that aortic supravalvular stenosis in Williams syndrome results from abnormally localized SMC proliferations stimulated by PDGF.

Perhaps the single most provocative study of SMC behavior in HBP is the report by Owens and coworkers [148] in which the SMCs were studied in hypertensive SHRs and normotensive rats. These data clearly indicated that the increased SMC mass in HBP arteries was due to *hypertrophy* rather than hyperplasia. Accompanying SMC hypertrophy was an increase in nuclear ploidy. The increase in nuclear ploidy (DNA/nucleus) attending HBP is most likely an irreversible change. Somewhat similar changes in heart muscle cells during hypertrophy and resolution are noted; the DNA remains elevated while other parameters (protein, RNA) revert to normal [103].

Electron microscopy studies of the SMC in HBP have further supported the concept of hypertrophy rather than hyperplasia. These studies have described cellular enlargement, nuclear enlargement with increased nuclear folding, increased concentrations of organelles including mitochondria, and contractile filaments. Abnormalities of the SMC surface have been described by scanning electron microscopy; these alterations have been described above, utilizing human tissues. Apparently, scanning electron microscopy studies of the SMC in experimental HBP have not been reported.

OTHER VASCULAR WALL COMPONENTS

In addition to the alterations in ECs and SMCs in HBP, the experimental data clearly indicate that other blood and vascular wall-derived cells participate. Blood-derived mononuclear cells have been shown to enter the intima in HBP [137]. These cells may play a role in the phagocytic clearing of dead cells (ECs), blood-derived proteins (fibrin, lipids, LDLs), and in the formation of fatty streaks and atheromas. In both human and experimental HBP, there is an increase in certain components of the intercellular fibrous matrix complex (BM-collagens, elastin) [88,95]. Much of the extracellular fibrous matrix accumulation in the arterial wall in long-term HBP is later described as "hyaline" by pathologists. The fine structure of this material is unexciting, consisting of granular materials with occasional filaments. Hyaline is thought to represent a condensation of altered BM as well as transudated plasma proteins [144].

Alteration in the biochemical composition of arteries in HBP is a controversial subject because of conflicting data and variations in information-gathering techniques. When these data are summarized, it is indicated that HBP is associated with an absolute increase in arterial wall collagen, elastin, water, sodium, and potassium [152,153]. Unfortunately, detailed biochemical studies of the influences of normal growth and HBP in the arteries of infants, children, and animals have not as yet appeared.

SUMMARY AND CONCLUSIONS

There is a serious shortage of information concerning the biology of blood vessels during normal growth, development, and aging. The thinness of this database and that relating to the effects of HBP on the blood vessels of infants and children seriously compromises our ability to prevent the morbidity and mortality of the disease in adults. It is now apparent that hypertension produces arterial lesions in the fetus and infant; it is also apparent from studies of genetic strains of SHR that arterial lesions are present at birth or shortly thereafter. These lesions are present *before* the development of hypertension. It is now important to determine if such lesions are present in infants with a genetic predisposition to essential hypertension. Experimental studies have also indicated that alterations in the biology of both EC and SMC may be present before the development of hypertension. Future research should investigate the activities of these cell lines in the arteries of the placenta and umbilical cord of infants with and without high genetic risk for hypertension. Similar studies should be carried out in controlled studies of arteries harvested from perinatal and neonatal necropsy materials.

Studies such as those proposed above may possibly provide a simple, effective screening test for idiopathic HBP at an age when therapy might prevent the serious arterial lesions that account for the morbidity and mortality of HBP.

Abnormalities in the capacity for *in vitro* replication of ECs harvested from aged and hypertensive individuals are now established. Future inquiries should determine whether or not these changes are present in ECs harvested from the arteries of fetuses at risk for essential hypertension. Finally, future research should include evaluations of the structural and biochemical composition of human and experimental arteries throughout the growth and aging periods of life. These data would then be available for comparative studies using similarly aged tissues from humans and animals with low and high risk potential for essential hypertension.

ACKNOWLEDGMENTS

The extraordinary support and contributions of my associates, Nelson Reede Cooley Jr (photographs) and Susan Dickinson and Betty Warren (editing), are recognized.

REFERENCES

1 Gill DG, Mendes da Costa B, Cameron JS, Joseph MC, Ogg CS, Chantler C. Analysis of 100 children with severe and persistent hypertension. *Arch Dis Child* 1976;51:951−6.

2 Kaplan MR, Hernandez LG. The pathogenesis and diagnosis of hypertension in children. *Pediatr Ann* 1982;11:592−602.

3 Lieberman E. Hypertension in childhood and adolescence. *Clin Symp* 1978;30:1−43.

4 Blaufox MD. Systemic arterial hypertension in pediatric practice. *Pediatr Clin North Am* 1971;18:577−93.

5 Kotchen T, Havlik RJ eds. High blood pressure in the young symposium. *Hypertension* 1980;2(suppl I):I-1−135.

6 Loggie JMH. Hypertension in children and adolescents. In: Davis JO, Laragh JH, Selwyn A, eds. *Hypertension Mechanisms, Diagnosis, and Management*. New York: HP Publishing, 1977:221−32.

7 McCrory WW. Finding an elevated blood pressure — what does it mean? *Pediatr Ann* 1982;11:581−4.

8 Cliff WJ. The aortic tunica media in growing rats studied with the electron microscope. *Lab Invest* 1967;17:599−615.

9 Jarmolych J, Daoud AS, Landau J, Fritz KE, McElvene E. Aortic media explants: cell proliferation and production of mucopolysaccharides, collagen, and elastic tissue. *Exp Mol Pathol* 1968;9:171−88.

10 Rhodin JAG. Fine structure of capillaries. In: Kramer A, ed. *Topics in the Study of Life: The Bioscience Book*. New York: Harper & Row, 1971:214−24.

11 Blackburn W, Wheeler VR, Cooley NR Jr, Manci EA. Studies of normal and abnormal aortic arch development in the fetus. *Proc Greenwood Genet Center* 1987;6:112.

12 Taylor J, Thorner P, Geary DF, Baumal R, Balfe JW. Nephrotic syndrome and hypertension in two children with Hurler syndrome. *J Pediatr* 1986;108:726−9.

13 Hastreiter AR, Joorabchi B, Pujatti G, van der Horst RL, Patacsil G, Sever JL. Cardiovascular lesions associated with

congenital rubella. *J Pediatr* 1967;71:59−65.

14 Gough JH. Coarctation of the aorta in father and son. *Br J Radiol* 1961;34:670−2.

15 Lacro RV, Jones KL, Benirschke K. Coarctation of the aorta in Turner syndrome: a pathologic study of fetuses with nuchal cystic hygromas, hydrops fetalis, and female genitalia. *Pediatrics* 1988;81:445−51.

16 Lin AE, Lippe BM, Geffner ME *et al.* Aortic dilation, dissection, and rupture in patients with Turner's syndrome. *J Pediatr* 1986;109:820−6.

17 Moss AJ. Coarctation of the aorta: current status. *J Pediatr* 1983;102:253−5.

18 Maron BJ, Humphries JO, Rowe RD, Mellits ED. Prognosis of surgically corrected coarctation of the aorta: a 20 year postoperative appraisal. *Circulation* 1973;47:119−26.

19 Allen DB, Hendricks SA, Levy JM. Aortic dilatation in Turner's syndrome. *J Pediatr* 1986;109:302−5.

20 Herman IM, Pollard TD, Wong AJ. Contractile proteins in endothelial cells. *Ann NY Acad Sci* 1982;401:50−60.

21 Kostich ND, Opitz JM. Ullrich−Turner syndrome associated with cystic medial necrosis of the aorta and great vessels: case report and review of the literature. *Am J Med* 1965;38:943−50.

22 Baird RJ, Evans JR, Labrosse CL. Coarctation of the abdominal aorta. *Arch Surg* 1964;89:466−74.

23 Glenn F, Keefer EBC, Speer DS, Dotter CT. Coarctation of the lower thoracic and abdominal aorta immediately proximal to celiac axis. *Surg Gynecol Obstet* 1952;94:561−9.

24 Senning A, Johansson L. Coarctation of the abdominal aorta. *J Thorac Cardiovasc Surg* 1960;40:517−23.

25 Superneau DW, Wertelecki W, Blackburn WR, Riddick L. The occurrence of vascular occlusion in neurofibromatosis. In: Saul RA, ed. *Proceedings of the Greenwood Genetics Center*. Clinton, SC: Jacobs Press, 1983:112−13.

26 Wertelecki W, Superneau DW, Blackburn WR, Varakis JN. Neurofibromatosis, skin hemangiomas, and arterial disease. In: Nyhan WL, Jones KL, eds. *Birth Defects: Original Article Series*. New York: Alan R. Liss, 1982:29−41.

27 Harvey FH, Alvord EC Jr. Juvenile cerebral arterosclerosis and other cerebral arteriopathies of childhood: six autopsied cases. *Acta Neurol Scand* 1972;48:479−509.

28 Brunner H, Stacher G, Bankl H, Grabner G. Chronic mesenteric arterial insufficiency caused by vascular neurofibromatosis. *Am J Gastroenterol* 1974;62:442−7.

29 Harrison EG Jr, McCormack LJ. Pathologic classification of renal arterial disease in renovascular hypertension. *Mayo Clin Proc* 1971;46:161−7.

30 McCormack LJ, Dustan HP, Meaney TF. Selected pathology of the renal artery. *Semin Roentgenol* 1967;2:126−38.

31 Oppenheimer EH, Esterly JR. Cardiac lesions in hypertensive infants and children. *Arch Pathol* 1967;84:318−25.

32 Higginbottom MC, Griswold WR, Jones KL, Vasquez MD, Mendoza SA, Wilson CB. The Cockayne syndrome: an evaluation of hypertension and studies of renal pathology. *Pediatrics* 1979;64:929−34.

33 Neill CA, Dingwall MM. A syndrome resembling progeria: a review of two cases. *Arch Dis Child* 1950;25:213−23.

34 Henriksen T, Mahoney EM, Steinberg D. Interactions of plasma lipoproteins with endothelial cells. *Ann NY Acad Sci* 1982;401:102−16.

35 Fischbach H, Riemenschneider T, Mentzel H. Morphologic aspects of Goldblatt hypertension in a newborn infant. *Clin Nephrol* 1982;17:41−5.

36 Vailas GN, Brouillette RT, Scott JP, Shkolnik A, Conway J, Wiringa K. Neonatal aortic thrombosis: recent experience. *J Pediatr* 1986;109:101−8.

37 Danaraj TJ, Ong WH. Primary arteritis of abdominal aorta in children causing bilateral stenosis of renal arteries and hypertension. *Circulation* 1959;20:856−63.

38 Vinijchaikul K, Blackburn WR. Takayasu's arteriopathy. *Int Pathol Bull* 1969;10:3−8.

39 Isaacson C. An idiopathic aortitis in young Africans. *J Pathol Bacteriol* 1961;81:69−79.

40 Gross KR, Malleson PN, Culham G, Lirenman DS, McCormick AQ, Petty RE. Vasculopathy with renal artery stenosis in a child with sarcoidosis. *J Pediatr* 1986;108:724−6.

41 Miller JJ. Early-onset "sarcoidosis" and "familial granulomatous arthritis (arteritis)": the same disease. *J Pediatr* 1986;109:387−8.

42 Esterly JR, Oppenheimer EH. Vascular lesions in infants with congenital rubella. *Circulation* 1967;36:544−54.

43 Menser MA, Dorman DC, Reye RDK, Reid RR. Renal artery stenosis in the rubella syndrome. *Lancet* 1966;i:790−2.

44 Formby D, Emery JL. Intimal hyperplasia of the aorta and renal vessels in an infant with hypertension. *J Pathol* 1969;98:205−8.

45 Hughes FWT, Perry CB. Senile arterial changes in a child aged 7 weeks. *Bristol Med Chir J* 1929;46:219−22.

46 Robertson JH. The significance of intimal thickening in the arteries of the newborn. *Arch Dis Child* 1960;35:588−90.

47 Schmidt DM, Rambo ON Jr. Segmental intimal hyperplasia of the abdominal aorta and renal arteries producing hypertension in an infant. *Am J Clin Pathol* 1965;44:546−55.

48 Daniels SR, Loggie JMH, Schwartz DC, Strife JL, Kaplan S. Systemic hypertension secondary to peripheral vascular anomalies in patients with Williams syndrome. *J Pediatr* 1985;106:249−51.

49 Ino T, Nishimoto K, Iwahara M *et al.* Progressive vascular lesions in Williams syndrome. *J Pediatr* 1985;107:826.

50 Reubi F. Les vaisseaux et les glandes endocrines dans la neurofibromatose. *Pathol Bakteriol* 1944;7:168−236.

51 Greene JF Jr, Fitzwater JE, Burgess J. Arterial lesions associated with neurofibromatosis. *Am J Clin Pathol* 1974;62:481−7.

52 Halonen H, Halonen V, Donner M, Iivanainen M, Vuolio M, Makinen J. Occlusive disease of intracranial main arteries with collateral networks in children. *Neuropaediatrie* 1973;4:187−206.

53 Feyrter F. Uber die vasculare Neurofibromatose, nach Untersuchungen am menschlichen Magen-Darmschlauch. *Virchows Arch Pathol Anat Physiol Klin Med* 1949;317:221−65.

54 Halpern M, Currarino G. Vascular lesions causing hypertension in neurofibromatosis. *N Engl J Med* 1965;273:248−52.

55 Bourke E, Gatenby PBB. Renal artery dysplasia with hypertension in neurofibromatosis. *Br Med J* 1971;3:681−2.

56 Fienman NL, Yakovac WC. Neurofibromatosis in childhood. *J Pediatr* 1970;76:339−46.

57 Grad E, Rance CP. Bilateral renal artery stenosis in association with neurofibromatosis (Recklinghausen's disease):

report of two cases. *J Pediatr* 1972;80:804−8.

58 Itzchak Y, Katznelson D, Boichis H, Jonas A, Deutsch V. Angiographic features of arterial lesions in neurofibromatosis. *Am J Roentgenol* 1974;122:643−7.

59 Van Hoff J, Ritchey AK, Shaywitz BA. Intracranial hemorrhage in children with sickle cell disease. *Am J Dis Child* 1985;139:1120−3.

60 Rolfes DB, Towbin R, Bove KE. Vascular dysplasia in a child with tuberous sclerosis. *Pediatr Pathol* 1985;3:359−73.

61 Adams EM, Finlayson A. Familial aspects of pre-eclampsia and hypertension in pregnancy. *Lancet* 1961;ii:1375−9.

62 Chesley LC, Annitto JE, Cosgrove RA. The familial factor in toxemia of pregnancy. *Obstet Gynecol* 1968;32:303−11.

63 Chesley LC. Hypertension in pregnancy: definitions, familial factor, and remote prognosis. *Kidney Int* 1980;18:234−40.

64 Swartz SL, Moore TJ, Schoenbaum SC. Theories of pathogenesis of preeclampsia. In: Brenner BM, Stein JH, eds. *Contemporary Issues in Nephrology, Hypertension.* New York: Churchill Livingstone, 1981:210−16.

65 Brosens IA. Morphological changes in the utero-placental bed in pregnancy hypertension. *Clin Obstet Gynecol* 1977;4:573−93.

66 Lichtig C, Brandes JM. Vascular changes of endometrium in early pregnancy, a possible marker for eclampsia. *Adv Pathol Anat Clin* 1982;2:427.

67 Nadji P, Sommers SC. Lesions of toxemia in first trimester pregnancies. *Am J Clin Pathol* 1973;59:344−9.

68 Zeek PM, Assali NS. Vascular changes in the decidua associated with eclamptogenic toxemia of pregnancy. *Am J Clin Pathol* 1950;20:1099−1109.

69 Kitzmiller JL, Benirschke K. Immunofluorescent study of placental bed vessels in pre-eclampsia of pregnancy. *Am J Obstet Gynecol* 1973;115:248−51.

70 Yeh IT, Kurman RJ. Functional and morphologic expressions of trophoblast. *Lab Invest* 1989;61:1−4.

71 Brosens IA, Robertson WB, Dixon HG. The role of the spiral arteries in the pathogenesis of pre-eclampsia. *Obstet Gynecol Ann* 1972;1:177.

72 Khong TY, De Wolf F, Robertson WB, Brosens I. Inadequate maternal vascular response to placentation in pregnancies complicated by pre-eclampsia and by small-for-gestational age infants. *Br J Obstet Gynaecol* 1986;93:1049−59.

73 Glassock RJ, Feldman D, Reynolds ES, Dammin GJ, Merrill JP. Human renal isografts: a clinical and pathologic analysis. *Medicine* 1968;47:411−54.

74 Haworth SG, Reid L. A morphometric study of regional variation in lung structure in infants with pulmonary hypertension and congenital cardiac defect: a justification of lung biopsy. *Br Heart J* 1978;40:825−31.

75 De Wolf F, Robertson WB, Brosens I. The ultrastructure of acute atherosis in hypertensive pregnancy. *Am J Obstet Gynecol* 1975;123:164−74.

76 Abitbol MM, Gallo GR, Pirani CL, Ober WB. Production of experimental toxemia in the pregnant rabbit. *Am J Obstet Gynecol* 1976;124:460−70.

77 Abitbol MM, Ober WB, Gallo GR, Driscoll SG, Pirani CL. Experimental toxemia of pregnancy in the monkey, with a preliminary report on renin and aldosterone. *Am J Pathol* 1977;86:573−83.

78 Abitbol MM, Pirani CL, Ober WB, Driscoll SG, Cohen MW. Production of experimental toxemia in the pregnant dog. *Obstet Gynecol* 1976;48:537−48.

79 Cavanagh D, Rao PS, Tsai CC, O'Connor TC. Experimental toxemia in the pregnant primate. *Am J Obstet Gynecol* 1977;128:75−85.

80 Haggendal E, Johansson B. On the pathophysiology of the increased cerebrovascular permeability in acute arterial hypertension in cats. *Acta Neurol Scand* 1972;48:265−70.

81 Nagy Z, Mathieson G, Huttner I. Blood−brain barrier opening to horseradish peroxidase in acute arterial hypertension. *Acta Neuropathol (Berl)* 1979;48:45−53.

82 Kalebic T, Garbisa S, Glaser B, Liotta LA. Basement membrane collagen: degradation by migrating endothelial cells. *Science* 1983;221:281−3.

83 Hughson MD, Harley RA, Henninger GR. Cellular arteriolar nodules: their presence in heart, pancreas, and kidneys of patients with malignant nephrosclerosis. *Arch Pathol Lab Med* 1982;106:71−4.

84 Ross R, Glomset JA. The pathogenesis of atherosclerosis. *N Engl J Med* 1976;295:369−77.

85 Feigl EO, Peterson LH, Jones AW. Mechanical and chemical properties of arteries in experimental hypertension. *J Clin Invest* 1963;42:1640−7.

86 Wolinsky H. Response of the rat aortic media to hypertension: morphological and chemical studies. *Circ Res* 1970;26:507−22.

87 Karsner HT. Thickness of aortic media in hypertension. *Trans Assoc Am Phys* 1938;53:54−9.

88 Faber M, Moller-Hou G. The human aorta: V. Collagen and elastin in the normal and hypertensive aorta. *Acta Pathol Microbiol Scand* 1952;31:377−82.

89 Alson RL, Dusseau JW, Hutchins PM. Arteriolar and systemic autoregulatory responses during the development of hypertension in the spontaneously hypertensive rat. *Proc Soc Exp Biol Med* 1985;180:62−71.

90 Harper RN, Moore MA, Marr MC, Watts LE, Hutchins PM. Arteriolar rarefaction in the conjunctiva of human essential hypertensives. *Microvasc Res* 1978;16:369−72.

91 Short DS. Arteries of intestinal wall in systemic hypertension. *Lancet* 1958;ii:1261−3.

92 Prewitt RL, Chen IIH, Dowell R. Development of microvascular rarefaction in the spontaneously hypertensive rat. *Am J Physiol* 1982;243:H243−51.

93 Khorsand J, Tennant R, Gillies C. Congenital alveolar capillary dysplasia: a developmental vascular anomaly causing persistent pulmonary hypertension of the newborn. *Pediatr Pathol* 1985;3:299−306.

94 Shaffer SG, O'Neill D, Bradt SK, Thibeault DW. Chronic vascular pulmonary dysplasia associated with neonatal hyperoxia exposure in the rat. *Pediatr Res* 1987;21:14−20.

95 Wolinsky H, Glagov S. Nature of species differences in the medial distribution of aortic vasa vasorum in mammals. *Circ Res* 1967;20:409−21.

96 Karnbaum S. Elastizitat und Morphologie des Aortenwindkessels beim Blutchochdruck. *Arch Kreislaufforsch* 1961;34:18−74.

97 Moon HD. Coronary arteries in fetuses, infants, and juveniles. *Circulation* 1957;16:263−7.

98 Nadas AS, Fyler DC. Valvular and vascular lesions with a right to left shunt or no shunt. In: *Pediatric Cardiology*, 3rd edn. Philadelphia: WB Saunders, 1972:452−607.

99 Goldberg ID, Stemerman MB, Handin RI. Vascular permeation of platelet factor 4 after endothelial injury. *Science* 1980;209:611−12.

100 Goldberg ID, Stemerman MB, Ransil BJ, Fuhro RL. *In vivo* aortic muscle cell growth kinetics: differences between thoracic and abdominal segments after intimal injury in the rabbit. *Circ Res* 1980;47:182−9.

101 Schwartz SM, Gajdusek CM, Reidy MA, Selden SC III, Haudenschild CC. Maintenance of integrity of aortic endothelium. *Fed Proc* 1980;39:2618−25.

102 Ginsberg R. Coronary artery spasm: clinical experience and implications. *Hospital practice* 1983;18:165−76.

103 Beznak M, Korecky B, Thomas G. Regression of cardiac hypertrophies of various origins. *Can J Physiol Pharmacol* 1969;47:579−86.

104 Page IH. The production of persistent arterial hypertension by cellophane perinephritis. *JAMA* 1939;113:2046−8.

105 Rapp JP. Hypertension in the young rat. In: New MI, Levine LS, eds. *Juvenile Hypertension*. New York: Raven Press, 1977:79−87.

106 Hollander W, Kramsch DM, Farmelant M, Madoff IM. Arterial wall metabolism in experimental hypertension of coarctation of the aorta of short duration. *J Clin Invest* 1968;47:1221−9.

107 Pamnani MB, Overbeck HW. Abnormal ion and water composition of veins and normotensive arteries in coarctation hypertension in rats. *Circ Res* 1976;38:375−8.

108 Goldblatt H, Lynch J, Hanzal RF, Summerville WW. Studies on experimental hypertension; production of persistent elevation of systolic blood pressure by means of renal ischemia. *J Exp Med* 1934;59:347−79.

109 Dahl LK, Heine M, Tassinari L. Effects of chronic excess salt ingestion. Evidence that genetic factors play an important role in susceptibility to experimental hypertension. *J Exp Med* 1962;115:1173−90.

110 Okamoto K, Aoki K. Development of a strain of spontaneously hypertensive rats. *Jpn Circ J* 1963;27:282−93.

111 Grollman A, Grollman EF. The teratogenic induction of hypertension. *J Clin Invest* 1962;41:710−14.

112 Grollman A, White FH. Induction of renal hypertension in rats and dogs by potassium or choline deficiency. *Am J Physiol* 1958;193:144−6.

113 Rajala GM, Kaplan S. Abnormally elevated blood pressure in the trypan blue-treated chick embryo during early morphogenesis. *Teratology* 1980;21:247−51.

114 Bremer JL. The presence and influence of two spiral streams in the heart of the chick embryo. *Am J Anat* 1932;49:409−40.

115 Yoshida H, Manasek F, Arcilla RA. Intracardiac flow patterns in early embryonic life: a reexamination. *Circ Res* 1983;53:363−71.

116 Stewart DE, Kirby ML, Sulik KK. Hemodynamic changes in chick embryos precede heart defects after cardiac neural crest ablation. *Circ Res* 1986;59:545−50.

117 Kirby ML. Cardiac morphogenesis − recent research advances. *Pediatr Res* 1987;21:219−24.

118 Fang TT, Bruyere HJ Jr, Kargas SA, Nishikawa T, Takagi Y, Gilbert EF. Ethyl alcohol-induced cardiovascular malformations in the chick embryo. *Teratology* 1987;35:95−103.

119 Grabowski CT, Tsai ENC, Toben HR. The effects of teratogenic doses of hypoxia on the blood pressure of chick embryos. *Teratology* 1969;2:67−76.

120 Paff GH, Boucek RJ, Gutten GS. Ventricular blood pressures and competency of valves in early embryonic chick heart. *Anat Rec* 1965;151:119−24.

121 Ruckman RN, Rosenquist GC, Rademaker DA, Morse DE, Getson PR. The effects of graded hypoxia on the embryonic chick heart. *Teratology* 1985;32:463−72.

122 Nakazawa M, Miyagama S, Takao A, Clark EB, Hu N. Hemodynamic effects of environmental hyperthermia in stage 18, 21, and 24 chick embryos. *Pediatr Res* 1986;20:1213−15.

123 Bingol N, Fuchs M, Diaz V, Stone RK, Gromisch DS. Teratogenicity of cocaine in humans. *J Pediatr* 1987;110:93−6.

124 Hodach RJ, Gilbert EF, Fallon JF. Aortic arch anomalies associated with the administration of epinephrine in chick embryos. *Teratology* 1974;9:203−10.

125 Kolesari GL, Schnitzler HJ. The differential effects of a teratogenic dose of epinephrine or dopamine on EKG patterns in the chick embryo. *Teratology* 1986;33:64C.

126 Lafond JS, Fouron JC, Bard H, Ducharme G. Effects of maternal alcohol intoxication on fetal circulation and myocardial function: an experimental study in the ovine fetus. *J Pediatr* 1985;107:947−50.

127 Temples TE, Geoffray DJ, Nakamoto T, Hartman AD, Miller HI. Effects of chronic caffeine ingestion on growth and myocardial function. *Proc Soc Exp Biol Med* 1985;179:388−95.

128 Cameron RH, Kolesari GL, Kalbfleisch JH. Pharmacology of dextroamphetamine-induced cardiovascular malformations in the chick embryo. *Teratology* 1983;27:253−9.

129 Nora JJ, Vargo TA, Nora AH, Love KE, McNamara DG. Dexamphetamine: a possible environmental trigger in cardiovascular malformations. *Lancet* 1970;i:1290.

130 Bianchi G, Fox U, Imbasciati E. The development of a new strain of spontaneously hypertensive rats. *Life Sci* 1974;14:339−47.

131 Ichijima K. Morphological studies on the peripheral small arteries of spontaneously hypertensive rats. *Jpn Circ J* 1969;33:785−813.

132 Mulvany MJ, Hansen PK, Aalkjaer C. Direct evidence that the greater contractility of resistance vessels in spontaneously hypertensive rats is associated with a narrowed lumen, a thickened media, and an increased number of smooth muscle cell layers. *Circ Res* 1978;43:854−64.

133 Gattone VH II, Evan AP, Willis LR, Luft FC. Renal afferent arteriole in the spontaneously hypertensive rat. *Hypertension* 1983;5:8−16.

134 Morkrid L, Iverson BM, Ofstad J. Afferent arteriolar diameter in DOCA-hypertensive and post-DOCA hypertensive rats estimated by means of microspheres. *Acta Med Scand* 1979;625(suppl):107−10.

135 Johansson BB, Nordborg C. Cerebral vessels in spontaneously hypertensive rats. In: Cervos-Navarro J *et al.*, eds. *Advances in Neurology*. New York: Raven Press, 1978:349−57.

136 Schwartz SM. Disturbances in endothelial integrity. *Ann NY Acad Sci* 1982;401:228−33.

137 Haudenschild CC, Prescott MF, Chobanian AV. Aortic endothelial and subendothelial cells in experimental hypertension and aging. *Hypertension* 1981;3(suppl I):148−53.

138 Ausprunk DH, Folkman J. Migration and proliferation of endothelial cells in preformed and newly formed blood vessels during tumor angiogenesis. *Microvasc Res* 1977;14:53−65.

139 Schwartz SM, Benditt EP. Aortic endothelial cell replication I. Effects of age and hypertension in the rat. *Circ Res* 1977;41:248−55.

140 Simionescu M, Simionescu N, Palade GE. Biochemically differentiated microdomains of the cell surface of capillary endothelium. *Ann NY Acad Sci* 1982;401:9−24.

141 Stalcup SA, Davidson D, Mellins RB. Endothelial cell functions in the hemodynamic responses to stress. *Ann NY Acad Sci* 1982;401:117−31.

142 Still WJS, Dennison S. The arterial endothelium of the hypertensive rat: a scanning and transmission electron microscopical study. *Arch Pathol* 1974;97:337−42.

143 Nagy Z, Mathieson G, Huttner I. Opening of tight junctions in cerebral endothelium.II. Effect of pressure-pulse induced acute arterial hypertension. *J Comp Neurol* 1979;185: 579−85.

144 Esterly JA, Glagov S. Altered permeability of the renal artery of the hypertensive rat: an electron microscopic study. *Am J Pathol* 1963;43:619−38.

145 Curry FE, Michel CC. A fiber matrix model of capillary permeability. *Microvasc Res* 1980;20:96−9.

146 Martin GM, Sprague CA. Symposium on *in vitro* studies related to atherogenesis: life histories of hyperplastoid cell lines from aorta and skin. *Exp Mol Pathol* 1973;18:125−41.

147 Bierman EL, Brewer C, Baum C. Hypertension decreases replication potential of arterial smooth muscle cells: aortic coarctation in humans as a model. *Proc Soc Exp Biol Med* 1981;166:335−8.

148 Owens GK, Rabinovitch PS, Schwartz SM. Smooth muscle cell hypertrophy versus hyperplasia in hypertension. *Proc Natl Acad Sci* 1981;78:7759−63.

149 Karrer HE. An electron microscope study of the aorta in young and in aging mice. *J Ultrastruct Res* 1961;5:1−27.

150 Greditzer HG III, Fisher VW. A sequential ultrastructural study of different arteries in the hypertensive rat. *Exp Mol Pathol* 1978;29:12−28.

151 Hoffmeister HM, Apitz J, Hoffmeister HE, Fischbach H. The correlation between blood pressure and morphometric findings in children with congenital heart disease and pulmonary hypertension. *Basic Res Cardiol* 1981;76:647−56.

152 Koletsky S, Resnick H, Behrin D. Mesenteric artery electrolytes in experimental hypertension. *Proc Soc Exp Biol Med* 1959;102:12−15.

153 Tobian L, Binion J. Artery wall electrolytes in renal and DCA hypertension. *J Clin Invest* 1954;33:1407−14.

33 Prognosis for Children with Primary and Secondary Hypertension

STEPHEN R. DANIELS

Blood pressure elevation represents the middle link in a pathophysiologic causal chain (Fig. 33.1) and is the result of a number of known and unknown processes. Hypertension is, in turn, the most important etiologic factor in many cardiovascular diseases observed in Western cultures. Some, such as intracranial hemorrhage, renal failure, and congestive heart failure, have been shown to be directly related to blood pressure elevation, while others, such as myocardial infarction, cerebral infarction, and peripheral vascular insufficiency, occur when elevated blood pressure acts in concert with other cardiovascular risk factors to cause accelerated arteriosclerosis [1].

Essential (primary) hypertension is one of the leading causes of morbidity and mortality among adults in the USA [2]. It is likely that its role as a cause of mortality may be underestimated in studies that rely on death certificate data. It has been shown that elevated blood pressure is recorded as a cause of death on fewer than 20% of death certificates, despite awareness of the attending physician that hypertension was present and may have been involved in the pathophysiologic process leading to death [3]. Death is often attributed solely to stroke or myocardial infarction with no consideration given to underlying blood pressure elevation.

Over the past 20 years, significant decreases in cardiovascular mortality have occurred in the USA [4]. This decline is probably related to a number of factors which include decreasing the population's overall cardiovascular risk status by changes in lifestyle, improved intensive care techniques, and, perhaps most importantly, by improved diagnosis and treatment of hypertension [5,6]. A number of studies have conclusively shown that the effective treatment of elevated blood pressure significantly reduces the risk of suffering cardiovascular morbidity and mortality. Furthermore, the beneficial effect

of treatment has been demonstrated for progressively lower levels of hypertension in adults. Studies suggest that therapy may even diminish morbidity and mortality for patients with diastolic blood pressures as low as 90–95 mmHg [7–9].

It has long been recognized that marked elevation of blood pressure may have sudden adverse consequences, such as hypertensive encephalopathy and stroke, in both adults and children [10–13]. Still and Cottom found that 18% of children presenting with severe hypertension had neurologic complications including convulsions, facial palsy, and hemiplegia [12]. Gill and colleagues [14] found that 11% of the children in their series had seizures as a result of hypertension. Nevertheless, Trompeter and co-workers [13] have reported that the prognosis for children who had had a single episode of hypertensive encephalopathy was good. Long-term follow-up showed no permanent neurologic sequelae and no significant differences in cognitive assessment between children who had had an episode of hypertensive encephalopathy and a control group with chronic renal disease [13].

It has become clear in adults that lesser elevations of blood pressure are predictive of various cardiovascular endpoints [15]. The association between blood pressure levels and outcome has been demonstrated for both systolic and diastolic pressure, with

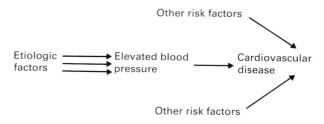

Fig. 33.1 The role of elevated blood pressure in the development of cardiovascular disease.

systolic levels having a closer relationship to risk than diastolic pressure levels [16]. These relationships have been established by longitudinal studies in which adults with varying levels of blood pressure are followed over time with respect to outcome. Studies of this type have not been performed beginning with a childhood population. Therefore, the relationship between blood pressure elevation in childhood and target-organ complications occurring in adulthood remains largely unknown.

OUTCOMES

The five major organ systems that may be affected by elevated blood pressure are:

1 blood vessels;
2 brain;
3 optic fundus;
4 kidneys; and
5 heart.

Blood vessels

Vascular disease of both proximal and peripheral arteries is increased in adults with hypertension and forms the basis for many hypertensive complications [17]. Vascular disease may be caused in a number of different ways. For example, an elevated blood pressure causes increased arterial wall tension which leads to arterial smooth muscle hyperplasia and hypertrophy. This process involves the increased synthesis of DNA, RNA, protein, collagen, elastin, and mucopolysaccharides, and leads to fibromuscular thickening of the intima and media of small and large arteries [18,19]. Other factors may be involved in this process including the tissue and plasma mediators of vascular injury which increase endothelial permeability to plasma, vasoactive substances, and the aggregation of platelets [18]. Hypertensive vascular disease may lead to a vicious cycle in which diseased vessels have decreased lumen size and reactivity leading to an increase in peripheral vascular resistance and further elevation of blood pressure (Fig. 33.2).

There is a shortage of information on the normal development of the vasculature as well as on the changes that take place with hypertension in children. The available evidence indicates that elevated blood pressure accelerates the growth and aging process leading to narrowing of the arterial lumen, thickening of the arterial wall, and increased vessel

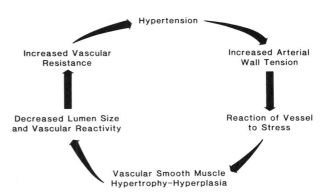

Fig. 33.2 The potential cyclic relationship between systemic hypertension and vascular abnormalities.

stiffness [19]. These vascular changes may be seen early in the development of hypertension in children and adolescents [19,20]. The acceleration of the atherosclerotic process caused by hypertension is increased in the presence of dyslipoproteinemia [18]. The relative importance of elevated systolic pressure, diastolic pressure, and widened pulse pressure in the pathophysiology of hypertensive vascular disease is not known.

Clinical evidence of hypertensive vascular disease is uncommon in children. Severe obliterative atherosclerosis and dissecting aneurysms of the aorta have been observed in children with hypertension, but they are extremely rare [20]. The lack of clinical signs suggests that overt manifestations of hypertensive vascular disease may be due to the combination of hypertension with other risk factors and changes related to aging.

Brain

Vascular diseases of the brain are the third leading cause of death in the USA [21]. The major cerebral complication of hypertension is that of cerebrovascular accident. Strokes can best be classified into two major categories, ischemic and hemorrhagic. Although there can be clinical problems with accurate differentiation, it appears that ischemic strokes are more common, while hemorrhagic strokes have a higher case-fatality ratio [18].

The mechanisms by which blood pressure elevation causes stroke are not completely understood. The pathologic characteristics and locations of the lesions produced suggest that mechanical distension plays a major role. Vessel wall integrity may be interrupted eventually leading to occlusion or rupture

[18,22,23]. Ischemic strokes are more likely to result from hypertension in combination with other risk factors. Hemorrhagic stroke is more directly related to the increased level of blood pressure alone [1]. Nevertheless, hypertension is the most important risk factor for both ischemic and hemorrhagic stroke [24]. In the Framingham study, brain infarcts occurred 5–30 times more commonly in hypertensive than in normotensive subjects [25]. In adults even moderate elevation of blood pressure, when untreated, predisposes to an incidence of stroke up to four times that of normotensive persons [26]. Systolic blood pressure is even more predictive of stroke than is the level of diastolic pressure [27].

In children, stroke can occur when the elevation of blood pressure is severe, as may be present in some secondary forms of hypertension [12]. Both the incidence of stroke and its mortality have been shown to increase markedly with age [28].

Transient ischemic attacks are brief episodes of focal cerebral dysfunction thought to result from periods of a relative decrease in cerebral perfusion. Although only about 10% of strokes are preceded by transient ischemic attacks, patients who suffer one or more of these have a 17 times greater risk of stroke during the following year [29]. When hypertensive adults are compared to normotensive control subjects, those with elevated blood pressure have a higher prevalence of transient ischemic attacks [30]. However, children very rarely have such episodes.

Subtle abnormalities of cerebral function have also been reported to accompany hypertension in adults. Boller and colleagues found that reaction time was slower and attention span was decreased in men with newly diagnosed hypertension and diastolic blood pressure greater than 105 mmHg when they were compared to normotensive control subjects matched for age, sex, education, and occupation [31]. Similar studies have not been performed in children and young adults. Trompeter and co-authors [13] did find reading skills which were behind for chronological age and an average IQ of 90 in a group of children presenting with severe arterial hypertension and identified as having neurologic complications. However, these findings were not significantly different than those of a control group of children with chronic renal disease.

Optic fundus

Changes in the retinal vessels have long been known to accompany both acute severe elevations of blood pressure as well as chronic lesser elevations. Changes in the optic fundi reflect both hypertensive retinopathy and arteriosclerotic retinopathy. Keith and coworkers divided these vascular changes into four grades [32]. Grade 1 includes narrowing of the arteriolar lumen. Grade 2 is arteriovenous nicking which is caused by sclerosis of the adventitia and/or thickening of the arteriolar wall. This may progress so that the vein becomes invisible below the arteriole and is obstructed. Grade 3 includes hemorrhages and exudates secondary to rupture of small vessels. Grade 4 is when papilledema is present. Fluorescein angiography may permit the investigation of the permeability of the vascular bed and identify leakage from vessels which would not otherwise be visible [33].

In adults, the grade of abnormality in the optic fundus has been found to be predictive of subsequent mortality from stroke and other arteriosclerotic diseases [34]. Retinal vascular changes have not been extensively investigated in children and adolescents. Skalina and associates found 11 of 21 hypertensive newborn infants to have ophthalmologic changes similar to those seen in hypertensive adults, including a decreased ratio of the arterial to venous calibers, vascular tortuosity, hemorrhage, and exudate [35]. Hemorrhages were present in 6, and exudates were present in 2 of the 11 infants. Seven infants had repeat examination at 1–6 months after the initial examination; 5 of them had complete clearing of the hypertensive changes with resolution or treatment of their hypertension [35]. Further studies are needed to investigate the retinal vasculature of older children and adolescents with hypertension and the potentially beneficial effect that treatment may have on those abnormalities.

Kidneys

Renal impairment may occur in both acute and longstanding hypertension. Elevated blood pressure is the most common cause of progressive renal insufficiency in adults in the USA. In accelerated hypertension, decreased glomerular filtration rate (GFR] and proteinuria are common [36]. With detailed study, functional and/or structural abnormalities can be found in adults with even apparently early and mild hypertension [37,38]. In them, there may be decreased renal plasma flow [39], while with longstanding hypertension most people develop nephrosclerosis [40].

Elevation of the serum uric acid level in adults

with hypertension constitutes evidence of early nephrosclerosis [41]. This abnormality is found in 33% of untreated adults with high blood pressure. It may also be true for juveniles with hypertension, but this has not been systematically studied in this age group. It is important to remember that diuretics used as therapy for hypertension quite often cause an elevation of serum uric acid. Thus, the usefulness of an elevated serum uric acid as evidence for the longevity of hypertension may be limited in patients taking these agents.

Schmieder and co-authors [42] have asserted that glomerular hyperfiltration is an indicator of early nephrosclerosis and incipient target-organ damage. Increased GFR may be a marker for loss of renal autoregulation. They found that GFR determined by creatinine clearance calculated from 24-h urine collection data was elevated in a subset of adult patients with primary hypertension. The patients with elevated GFR also had increased left ventricular mass index compared to those patients with normal GFR.

Renal dysfunction may also contribute to the etiology of both secondary and essential hypertension. In some cases this may make it difficult to determine which is the antecedent and which the consequence. The interrelationship may lead to a vicious cycle in which the target-organ damage causes an increased elevation of blood pressure, which in turn worsens the target-organ disease. In adults it has been shown that aggressive antihypertensive therapy protects the kidneys from further damage [43]. In children it is not common for elevated blood pressure to be the etiology of renal failure. Therefore, while it is important to treat hypertension in children with renal failure, this may not prevent progression of the primary cause of the renal insufficiency.

Heart

Hypertension increases left ventricular wall tension. This leads to structural, biochemical, and physiologic changes in the myocardium. Hypertension combined with dyslipoproteinemia and other cardiovascular risk factors leads to atherosclerosis of the coronary arteries. These pathophysiologic processes then lead to the two major cardiac consequences of elevated blood pressure: congestive heart failure and myocardial infarction [18].

The relationship between hypertension and congestive heart failure has been clearly established. The Framingham study has shown that hypertension

precedes clinically significant heart failure in 75% of cases [44]. The risk of developing heart failure was approximately six times greater for hypertensive than for normotensive adults [45]. Moreover, the incidence of congestive heart failure increased in both men and women of all ages as systolic or diastolic blood pressure increased [44].

The pathophysiologic evolution of left ventricular failure in hypertensive individuals is thought to occur when elevated blood pressure causes increasing afterload of the left ventricle. This results in ventricular hypertrophy which initially reduces wall stress. However, after a point, the hypertrophy does not significantly improve ventricular function, but does increase the oxygen demand of the myocardium. Continuing hypertrophy may lead to decreased ventricular function with a decreased ejection rate, a prolonged tension-time index, and ultimately congestive heart failure [44,46,47]. In the Framingham study, adults with long-standing hypertension and electrocardiographic evidence of left ventricular hypertrophy had a 10 times greater risk of developing congestive heart failure than those without evidence of hypertrophy [48].

Although the end-stages of hypertensive congestive heart failure have been well described, the early stages are not understood. Studies of both adults and children have clearly shown the epidemiologic association between hypertension and left ventricular hypertrophy. Laird and Fixler [49] studied a group of adolescents with elevated blood pressure and compared them to an age, race, sex, and body size matched group of normotensive subjects. Of the hypertensive subjects, 18% had left ventricular hypertrophy by echocardiography. They were unable to demonstrate a dose–response relationship between the level of blood pressure and the left ventricular wall thickness [49]. Schieken and colleagues found similar results when they investigated children in the Muscatine study [50], and other investigators have had similar findings in other childhood populations [51,52]. All of these studies have used echocardiography to measure left ventricular free wall and septal thickness. However, as Culpepper [53] has pointed out, each of the studies used somewhat different echocardiographic methods for measuring left ventricular dimensions and for calculating left ventricular mass. Therefore, while echocardiography has been demonstrated to be the most sensitive and specific noninvasive method for measuring cardiac chamber size and wall thickness [49,50,54], there is a need for agreement on one accurate method for making measurements and calculating left ventricular mass in children.

Daniels and co-authors [55] have reported a correlation of $r = 0.89$ between left ventricular mass calculated using the modified American Society of Echocardiography cube formula and the true left ventricular mass measured in children at necropsy. They also determined normal values for left ventricular mass indexed by body surface area and by height. The investigators found significant differences in indexed left ventricular mass by sex, but racial differences were not observed. Sex-specific criteria for left ventricular hypertrophy based on the 95th percentile of the left ventricular mass index distributions (Table 33.1) were presented. Use of these normal values in the future may make the echocardiogram a more useful clinical and research instrument for the evaluation of hypertension.

Ischemic heart disease is caused by coronary atherosclerosis. Hypertension and other coronary artery risk factors contribute to this. The Manitoba heart study showed that an increase in systolic blood pressure over time is even more strongly associated with the incidence of ischemic heart disease than an initially high level [56]. On the other hand, in individuals with other risk factors for ischemic heart disease, blood pressure control may not have the same dramatic effect on the incidence of myocardial infarction that it has on other cardiovascular endpoints [1,18]. Survival after myocardial infarction may be inversely related to the preinfarction level of blood pressure [57]. Newman and coworkers [58] report that young adults, found to have coronary artery fibrous plaques at autopsy, had significantly higher systolic blood pressure than other young adults who did not have plaques at autopsy. However, diastolic pressure did not differ between the two groups. The findings persisted even after the possible confounding effects of race, sex, and age were controlled. These results document the importance of risk factor levels to early arteriosclerotic changes in the coronary arteries at a young age.

PROGNOSIS

The prognosis for children with elevated blood pressure is variable and depends to some extent on the etiology of their high blood pressure. Secondary forms of hypertension usually present with marked elevations in pressure, but may be curable by specific treatment aimed at ameliorating the underlying

Table 33.1 Sex-specific criteria for increased left ventricular mass index

| | 95th Percentile | |
	Males	Females
Left ventricular mass/height (g/m)	99.8	81.0
Left ventricular mass/body surface area (g/m²)	103.0	84.2

cause. Primary hypertension has at present no known etiology. It has been suggested that it may represent a syndrome rather than a single disease entity [57]. This means that a number of separate, currently unknown, pathophysiologic processes which lead to the same outward manifestation (hypertension) may be involved in different individuals. Therefore, it may be that different children with primary hypertension have very different prognoses depending on the category of essential hypertension into which they fit. Unfortunately, at present it is not possible to categorize patients in this way. The next sections review what is known about the prognosis of children with secondary and primary hypertension.

SECONDARY HYPERTENSION

Renovascular hypertension

Renovascular hypertension may be the result of several different disease processes which cause abnormalities of the renal arteries. In 1938, Leadbetter and Burkland documented cure of renovascular hypertension by nephrectomy [59]. Since that time, surgical management has improved and techniques have been developed which provide cure of hypertension without loss of renal parenchyma [60]. Subsequently, nonsurgical transluminal balloon angioplastic techniques have been developed and used in selected children with renovascular hypertension [61].

The reports of surgical management of renovascular hypertension in children have shown this therapy to be successful when patients are properly selected and when the surgeon is experienced with renovascular surgery in this age group. However, poor selection of patients for surgery or performance of the operation by an inexperienced surgeon will adversely affect the results [62]. Stanley and Fry have reported that out of 40 young patients, 34 (85%) were cured, 5 (12.5%) were improved, and only 1 patient was unchanged after surgery for renovascular hypertension [60]. In this series 6 secondary operations, including 4 secondary nephrectomies, had to be performed when the initial procedure proved to be inadequate. No patients in their series died [60].

Defining a broad clinical spectrum of juvenile renovascular hypertension, Daniels and associates reported on 20 years of experience with this disorder at a single institution [63]. Target-organ damage at the time of presentation was common. In all, 23 of 27 patients (85%) presented with evidence of damage to the heart, kidneys, cerebral and/or retinal vasculature. Three patients (11%) presented with hypertensive encephalopathy, including 1 patient who also had a cerebrovascular accident. Eighteen patients (66%) had evidence of left ventricular hypertrophy, 2 of whom had clinically overt congestive heart failure. Sixteen patients (59%) had retinal vascular abnormalities at presentation [63].

Thirteen (48%) of the 27 patients were treated medically and 14 surgically. Four of the 13 patients treated medically are considered candidates for future surgery. For the remaining 9, surgery was considered either inadvisable or not possible. Four of the patients managed medically now have normal blood pressure without medication. Three had arteritis which subsequently resolved and the fourth had blunt abdominal trauma that resulted in renal artery thrombosis that eventually resolved. Of the remaining 5 patients treated medically, 1 now has normal blood pressure without antihypertensive medication, but after balloon angioplasty of an intrarenal lesion. One underwent nephrectomy of her one viable kidney and renal transplantation after failure of medical management to control her blood pressure. One patient died of causes unrelated to hypertension and 2 were lost to follow-up. Five (36%) of the surgically treated patients have normal blood pressure without medication; 5 are improved but still require antihypertensive drugs; 1 had two attempts at revascularization that failed but his blood pressure is now controlled following balloon angioplasty. Three patients died [63].

In summary, juvenile renovascular hypertension often presents with severe hypertension and evidence of target-organ damage. Its management must be individualized to give each patient the best prognosis; however, cure of the hypertension is by no means assured.

Coarctation of the aorta

Corrective surgery for coarctation of the aorta has been successfully performed since 1945 [64]. An analysis of the natural history of patients with coarctation has shown that without surgery 50% of those patients who survived the first 2 years of life died before age 32, 75% died before age 46, and by age 58, 98% had died [65]. A total of 75% of the deaths were a result of complications directly related to hypertension.

Maron and colleagues [66] published the results of 20 years of follow-up of patients who had undergone corrective surgery for coarctation of the aorta. They found that, of the 12% of patients who had died during the follow-up period, survival was not significantly longer than that of unoperated patients. In this group, hypertensive cardiovascular disease was the cause of death in 22 of 23 patients. The major difference between survivors and nonsurvivors was that survivors were operated on at a significantly younger age. Among the survivors, 33% had late postoperative systemic hypertension. One potential cause for this hypertension is residual coarctation or restenosis at the site of repair, but only 18% of the survivors with hypertension had clinical evidence of this [66]. The average age at operation in the series of Maron and colleagues was 20 years; however, even in series where surgery was performed at an earlier age, an increased incidence of hypertension and premature cardiovascular morbidity and mortality was found [67]. It has also been shown by James and Kaplan that the systolic blood pressure response to exercise is abnormal in patients who have had surgical correction of coarctation of the aorta [68]. This was found in 9 of 14 patients who had exercise testing after repair of coarctation. The finding offers further evidence that operative repair may not be a complete cure for this disease.

In a multivariable analysis, Daniels and coworkers investigated factors which may be associated with the level of late postoperative systolic blood pressure both at rest and during maximal exercise [69]. They found that the combination of variables that best explained the variance of these two dependent variables were:

1 height at the time of exercise testing;
2 the highest level of resting systolic blood pressure during the preoperative period; and
3 the residual postoperative gradient across the site of repair.

Increases in the three independent variables were associated with increased resting and maximal exercise systolic blood pressure in the late postoperative period. Other variables including age at surgery, age at the exercise test, and the time interval between the operation and the exercise tests were investigated, but were not associated with late postoperative levels of systolic blood pressure at rest or during maximal exercise [69]. These findings suggest that the preoperative level of systolic blood pressure should be the most important determinant for the timing of surgery. This means that it may be possible to delay surgery in a patient with no systolic hypertension until an age when repair is less likely to result in restenosis. However, systolic blood pressure that is tracking into higher percentiles for the patient's age and sex, or blood pressure above the normal range at presentation should be an indication for surgery. If the timing of surgery is optimized, it may be that the incidence of late postoperative cardiovascular complications can be decreased.

Pheochromocytoma

Pheochromocytoma is another potentially curable cause of hypertension. Children with this tumor usually present with sustained high blood pressure which can be quite elevated and accompanied by hypertensive encephalopathy [70]. The accelerated hypertension may also give rise to renal abnormalities manifested by proteinuria and hematuria [71,72]. Pheochromocytoma may also present with paroxysmal elevations of blood pressure and other symptoms more related to periodic release of catecholamines into the circulation [71]. Sometimes, because they can be similar, it may be difficult to distinguish if the symptoms in these patients are due to elevated blood pressure, catecholamine release, or both.

Pheochromocytomas in children are usually small and benign; however, there is a higher incidence of multiple and extra-adrenal tumors than in adults [71]. Malignant tumors have been reported that are locally invasive and that metastasize to bone and liver. The metastatic lesions may secrete catecholamines [73]. These characteristics sometimes make the management of pheochromocytoma difficult and the outcome uncertain. Familial pheochromocytoma may be complicated by other endocrine abnormalities (See Chapter 25).

Untreated pheochromocytoma carries a high risk of fatality [70,71]. Surgical removal is indicated, but may be difficult due to fluctuating blood pressure and cardiac arrhythmias that may occur during the procedure. Hypotension may complicate the postoperative course. Operative mortality has been reported to be as high as 13% in the most recent pediatric series, published over 20 years ago [70]. The authors found that the most important cause of death during the operative and immediate postoperative period was the presence of an undiscovered tumor leading to uncontrolled hypertension [70]. Anesthesia and operative intervention have been made safer with preoperative treatment with adrenergic blocking agents and/or tyrosine hydroxylase inhibitors. However, the use of these agents may interfere with tumor localization and they are not universally used. With benign tumors, blood pressure should return to normal after successful surgery and the prognosis should be good. It is important, however, to follow these children for a prolonged period in order to detect a possible recurrence. Patients with metastatic pheochromocytoma ultimately have a poor prognosis [73], but may live for many years unless they develop uncontrollable hypertension or arrhythmias. To date, chemotherapy has generally been unrewarding and radiation only palliative for pain.

Hypertension with renal parenchymal disease (see Chapters 19—21)

Renal parenchymal diseases are the most common cause of secondary hypertension in children. Some of these can be treated successfully, thereby improving the hypertension and the overall prognosis. In some instances, the elevation of blood pressure accompanies the progressive renal failure. In others—for example, infantile polycystic kidney disease—the hypertension actually precedes the renal insufficiency [74]. As with other secondary forms of hypertension, the prognosis for children with renal parenchymal disease depends on the underlying cause and course of the primary lesion. However, irrespective of the specific etiology, if hypertension secondary to renal parenchymal disease is treated, the prognosis for individual patients can be improved and renal function may also improve [12].

Renal transplantation has improved the prognosis for many children with renal parenchymal diseases which result in progressive renal failure. Unfortunately, some of the drugs used in the treatment of posttransplant rejection, such as corticosteroids and cyclosporine, can also cause elevated blood pressure [75]. Therefore, despite improved renal function, hypertension may continue to be a long-term problem for these patients. Ingelfinger and co-workers report that virtually every patient with a renal transplant has hypertension in the immediate posttransplant period [76]. These patients also can have higher elevations of blood pressure during periods of acute rejection [77]. Persistent hypertension may also occur in patients with chronic rejection [78] or with stenosis of the artery anastomosed at transplant (see Chapter 21).

The long-term effects of posttransplant hypertension are not known. In addition to causing the complications usually associated with elevated blood pressure, hypertension may also cause vascular injury which may lead to graft failure and further hypertension.

PRIMARY HYPERTENSION

In most cases of essential hypertension in childhood and adolescence, blood pressure levels are not severely elevated. For this reason, the consequences of childhood essential hypertension are likely to be the result of slow pathophysiologic processes occurring over time. Whether or not the outcomes for younger individuals with essential hypertension are the same as those for adults remains unknown. No long-term data about the persistence and sequelae of elevated blood pressure in childhood exist, and at present the long-term effects of childhood hypertension must be inferred from studies of adult populations.

Three target-organ systems are amenable to study in children with essential hypertension: the heart, the kidney, and the retinal vasculature. Daniels and colleagues studied the prevalence of left ventricular hypertrophy, glomerular hyperfiltration, and retinal vascular abnormality in 88 children aged 6–23 years with blood pressure persistently greater than the 90th percentile for age and sex [79]. Left ventricular hypertrophy was defined as echocardiographically determined left ventricular mass index greater than the 95th percentile compared to previously reported sex-specific standards [55]. Glomerular hyperfiltration was defined as creatinine clearance greater than 120 ml/min per 1.73 m^2 [42]. This was studied using creatinine clearance data from 24-h urine collections obtained during hospitalization in the Clini-

cal Research Center. Retinal vascular abnormality was determined from photographs of the optic fundus. These photographs were rated by two ophthalmologists for the presence of arteriolar narrowing, tortuosity, and arteriovenous nicking.

The prevalence of left ventricular hypertrophy was 36%, while 49% of the patients had glomerular hyperfiltration, and 50% had one or more retinal vascular abnormalities. It can be seen in Table 33.2 that these abnormalities were not all clustered in a single group of patients. Also, there was no clustering of abnormality by race or sex.

This study demonstrates that the early stages of target-organ disease are relatively common in children with essential hypertension. It also suggests that particular subgroups of patients may be at risk for certain end-organ problems. Further research will be necessary to elucidate the pathophysiology of these processes and to confirm the relationship between these early stages of target-organ abnormality and morbidity and mortality later in life.

The study of the consequences of blood pressure elevation in childhood should be a major area of investigation in the future. In order for clinicians rationally to manage children with hypertension, they need to know what the prognosis for them is and how treatment can affect the progression of target-organ complications in this population. It is hoped that in the not too distant future pediatricians will be able to predict which children are destined to maintain high blood pressure over a long period of

Table 33.2 Distribution of target-organ abnormalities in children with essential hypertension

Abnormality	Cases
LVH	11
GH	13
RVA	10
Total with one abnormality	34
LVH + GH	5
LVH + RVA	9
GH + RVA	18
Total with two abnormalities	32
LVH + GH + RVA	15
No abnormalities	15

GH = glomerular hyperfiltration; LVH = Left ventricular hypertrophy; RVA = retinal vascular abnormality.

time. It may also be possible to predict which among those children are likely to develop specific complications of hypertension. When this is known, physicians will be able to test specific therapeutic regimens to determine which therapies are effective in slowing the different pathophysiologic processes that lead to target-organ disease.

REFERENCES

1 Smith WM. Treatment of mild hypertension. Results of a ten-year intervention trial. *Circ Res* 1977;40(Suppl I):98–105.

2 Roberts WC. The hypertensive diseases. Evidence that systemic hypertension is a greater risk factor to the development of other cardiovascular diseases than previously suspected. *Am J Med* 1975;59:523–32.

3 Schweitzer MD, Gearing FR, Perera GA. The epidemiology of primary hypertension. Present status. *J Chronic Dis* 1965; 18:847–57.

4 Havlik RJ. Understanding the decline in coronary heart disease mortality. *JAMA* 1982;247:1605–6.

5 Kannel WB. Meaning of the downward trend in cardiovascular mortality. *JAMA* 1982;247:877–80.

6 Kaplan NM. *Clinical Hypertension*. 3rd edn. Baltimore: Williams & Wilkins, 1982.

7 Veterans Administration cooperative study group on antihypertensive agents. Effects of treatment on morbidity in hypertension. Results in patients with diastolic blood pressures averaging 115 through 129 mmHg. *JAMA* 1967;202(II): 116–22.

8 Veterans Administration cooperative study group on antihypertensive agents. Effects of treatment on morbidity in hypertension II. Results in patients with diastolic blood pressure averaging 90 through 114 mmHg. *JAMA* 1970;213: 1143–52.

9 Hypertension Detection and Follow-up Program cooperative group. Five year findings of the Hypertension Detection and Follow-up Program I. Reduction in mortality of persons with high blood pressure, including mild hypertension. *JAMA* 1979;242:2562–71.

10 Perera GA. Hypertensive vascular disease: description and natural history. *J Chronic Dis* 1955;1:33–42.

11 Heyden S, Bartel AG, Hames CG, McDonough JR. Elevated blood pressure levels in adolescents, Evans County, Georgia. Seven year follow-up of 30 patients and 30 controls. *JAMA* 1969;209:1683–9.

12 Still JL, Cottom DG. Severe hypertension in childhood. *Arch Dis Child* 1967;42:34–9.

13 Trompeter RS, Smith RL, Hoare RD, Neville BGR, Chantler C. Neurological complications of arterial hypertension. *Arch Dis Child* 1982;57:913–17.

14 Gill DG, Mendes da Costa B, Cameron JS, Joseph MC, Ogg CS, Chantler C. Analysis of 100 children with severe and persistent hypertension. *Arch Dis Child* 1976;51:951–6.

15 Hypertension Detection and Follow-up Program cooperative group. The Hypertension Detection and Follow-up Program. A progress report. *Circ Res* 1977;40:I 106–109.

16 Dawber TR. *The Framingham Study. The Epidemiology of Atherosclerotic Disease*. Cambridge, MA: Harvard University Press, 1980.

17 Robertson WB, Strong JP. Atherosclerosis in persons with hypertension and diabetes mellitus. *Lab Invest* 1968;18: 538–51.

18 Hollander W. Role of hypertension in atherosclerosis and cardiovascular disease. *Am J Cardiol* 1976;38:786–800.

19 Blackburn WR. Vascular pathology in hypertensive children. In: Loggie JMH, Horan MJ, Gruskin AB, Hohn AR, Dunbar JB, Havlik RJ, eds. *NHLBI Workshop on Juvenile Hypertension*. New York, NY: Biomedical Information, 1984.

20 Oppenheimer EH, Esterly JR. Cardiac lesions in hypertensive infants and children. *Arch Pathol* 1967;84:318–25.

21 Soltero I, Kiang L, Cooper R, Stamler J, Garside D. Trends in mortality from cerebrovascular diseases in the United States, 1960 to 1975. *Stroke* 1978;9:549–55.

22 Barnes KL, Brosnihan KB, Ferrario CM. Animal models, hypertension and central nervous system mechanisms. *Mayo Clin Proc* 1977;52:387–90.

23 Russel RWR. How does blood pressure cause stroke? *Lancet* 1975; ii:1283–8.

24 Kannel WB, Wolf PA, Vertes J, McNamara PM. Epidemiologic assessment of the role of blood pressure in stroke. *JAMA* 1970;214:301–10.

25 Kannel WB, Dawber TR, Sorlie P, Wolf PA. Components of blood pressure and risk of atherothrombotic brain infarction: the Framingham study. *Stroke* 1976;7:327–31.

26 Kannel WB, Wolf PA, McGee DL, Dawber TR, McNamara P, Castelli WP. Systolic blood pressure, arterial rigidity and risk of stroke. The Framingham study. *JAMA* 1981;245: 1225–9.

27 Rabkin SW, Mathewson FAL, Tate RB. Predicting risk of ischemic heart disease and cerebrovascular disease from systolic and diastolic blood pressures. *Ann Intern Med* 1978; 88:342–5.

28 Kurtzke JF. *Epidemiology of Cerebrovascular Disease*. Berlin: Springer-Verlag, 1969.

29 Cartlidge NEF, Whisnant JP, Elveback LR. Carotid and vertebral-basilar transient ischemic attacks: a community study, Rochester, Minnesota. *Mayo Clin Proc* 1977;52: 117–20.

30 Dyken JL, Conneally M, Haerer AF *et al.* Cooperative study of hospital frequency and character of transient ischemic attacks. I. Background organization and clinical survey. *JAMA* 1977;237:822–86.

31 Boller F, Vrtunski PB, Mack JL, Kim Y. Neuropsychological correlates of hypertension. *Arch Neurol* 1977;34:701–5.

32 Keith NM, Wagener HP, Barker NW. Some different types of essential hypertension, their course and prognosis. *Am J Med Sci* 1939;197:332–43.

33 Novotny HR, Alvis DL. A method of photographing fluorescence in circulating blood in the human retina. *Circulation* 1961;24:82–6.

34 Svardsudd K, Wedel H, Aurell E, Tibblin G. Hypertensive eye ground changes. *Acta Med Scand* 1978;204:159–67.

35 Skalina MEL, Annable WL, Kleigman RM, Fanaroff AA. Hypertensive retinopathy in the newborn infant. *J Pediatr* 1983;103:781–6.

36 Breckenridge A. Prognosis of treated hypertension. *Br Heart J* 1971; 33(suppl):127–8.

37 Hollenberg NK, Adams DF. The renal circulation in hypertensive disease. *Am J Med* 1976;60:773–84.

38 Wollam GL, Gifford RW. The kidney as a target organ in hypertension. *Geriatrics* 1976;31:71–9.

39 Goldring W, Chasis H. *Hypertension and Hypertensive Disease*. New York: NY Commonwealth Fund, 1944.

40 Fishberg AM. The arteriolar lesions of glomerulonephritis. *Arch Intern Med* 1927;40:80−97.

41 Messerli FH, Frohlich ED, Dreslinski GR, Svarez DH, Aristimuno GG. Serum uric acid in essential hypertension: an indicator of renovascular involvement. *Ann Intern Med* 1980; 93:817−21.

42 Schmieder RE, Messerli FH, Garavaglia GE, Nunez BD. Glomerular hyperfiltration indicates target organ disease in essential hypertension. *Circulation* 1987;76:III-273.

43 Woods JW, Blythe WB, Huffines WD. Management of malignant hypertension complicated by renal insufficiency. *N Engl J Med* 1974;291:10−14.

44 McKee PA, Castelli WP, McNamara PM, Kannel WB. The natural history of congestive heart failure. The Framingham study. *N Engl J Med* 1971;285:1441−6.

45 Tarazi RC. The heart in hypertension: its load and its role. *Hosp Pract* 1975;10:31−40.

46 Cohn JN. Blood pressure and cardiac performance. *Am J Med* 1973;55:351−61.

47 Tarazi RC, Levy MN. Cardiac responses to increased afterload. *Hypertension* 1982;4(suppl II):II 8−18.

48 Kannel WB, Castelli WP, McNamara PM, McKee P, Feinleib M. Role of blood pressure in the development of congestive heart failure: the Framingham study. *N Engl J Med* 1972;287: 781−7.

49 Laird WP, Fixler DE. Left ventricular hypertrophy in adolescents with elevated blood pressure: assessment by chest roentgenography, electrocardiography and echocardiography. *Pediatrics* 1981;67:255−9.

50 Schieken RM, Clarke WR, Lauer RM. Left ventricular hypertrophy in children with blood pressures in the upper quintile of the distribution: the Muscatine study. *Hypertension* 1981;3:669−75.

51 Culpepper WS, Sodt PC, Messerli FH, Ruschhaupt DG, Arcilla PA. Cardiac status in juvenile borderline hypertension. *Ann Intern Med* 1983;98:1−7.

52 Zahka KG, Neill CA, Kidd L, Cutilletta AF. Cardiac involvement in adolescent hypertension. *Hypertension* 1981;3: 664−8.

53 Culpepper WS. Cardiac anatomy and function in juvenile hypertension, current understanding and future concerns. *Am J Med* 1983;75(suppl): 57−61.

54 Murray JA, Johnson WE, Reid JM. Echocardiographic determination of left ventricular dimensions, volumes and performance. *Am J Cardiol* 1972;30:252−7.

55 Daniels SR, Meyer RA, Liang YC, Bove K. Echocardiographically determined left ventricular mass in normal children, adolescents and young adults. *J Am Coll Cardiol* 1988; 12:703−8.

56 Rabkin SW, Matthewson FAL, Tate RB. Longitudinal blood pressure measurements during a 26 year observation period and the risk of ischemic heart disease. *Am J Epidemiol* 1979;109:650−62.

57 Rabkin SW, Matthewson FAL, Tate RB. Prognosis after acute myocardial infarction: relation to blood pressure values before infarction in a prospective cardiovascular study. *Am J Cardiol* 1977;40:604−10.

58 Newman WP, Freedman DS, Voors AW et al. Relation of serum lipoprotein levels and systolic blood pressure to early atherosclerosis: the Bogalusa heart study. *N Engl J Med* 1986;314:138−44.

59 Leadbetter WF, Burkland CE. Hypertension in unilateral renal disease. *J Urol* 1938;39:611−26.

60 Stanley JC, Fry WJ. Pediatric renal artery occlusive disease and renovascular hypertension. Etiology, diagnosis and operative treatment. *Arch Surg* 1981;116:669−76.

61 McCook TA, Mills SR, Kirks DR. et al. Percutaneous transluminal renal artery angioplasty in a $3\frac{1}{2}$ year old hypertensive girl. *J Pediatr* 1980;97:958−60.

62 Ernst CB. Childhood renovascular hypertension. In: Kotchen TA, Kotchen JM, eds. *Clinical Approach to High Blood Pressure in the Young*. London: John Wright, 1983.

63 Daniels SR, Loggie JMH, Towbin RB, McEnery PT. The clinical spectrum of juvenile renovascular hypertension. *Pediatrics* 1987;80:698−704.

64 Crafoord C, Nylin G. Congenital coarctation of the aorta and its surgical treatment. *J Thorac Cardiovasc Surg* 1945;14: 347−52.

65 Campbell M. Natural history of coarctation of the aorta. *Br Heart J* 1970;32:633−40.

66 Maron BJ, Humphries JO, Rowe RD, Mellits ED. Prognosis of surgically corrected coarctation of the aorta: a 20 year post operative appraisal. *Circulation* 1973;47:119−26.

67 Simon AB, Zioto A. Coarctation of the aorta: longitudinal assessment of operated patients. *Circulation* 1974;50:456−64.

68 James FW, Kaplan S. Systolic hypertension during submaximal exercise after correction of coarctation of the aorta. *Circulation* 1974;49−50(suppl II):II 27−34.

69 Daniels SR, James FW, Loggie JMH, Kaplan S. Correlates of resting and maximal exercise systolic blood pressure after repair of coarctation of the aorta: a multivariable analysis. *Am Heart J* 1987;113:349−53.

70 Stackpole RH, Melicow MM, Uson AC. Pheochromocytoma in children. *J Pediatr* 1963;63:315−30.

71 Hume DM. Pheochromocytoma in the adult and in the child. *Am J Surg* 1960;99:458−96.

72 Alvestrand A, Bergstrom J, Wehle B. Pheochromocytoma and renovascular hypertension. *Acta Med Scand* 1977;202: 231−6.

73 Phillips AF, McMustry RJ, Taubman J. Malignant pheochromocytoma in childhood. *Am J Dis Child* 1976;130:1252−5.

74 Ingelfinger JR. *Pediatric Hypertension*. Philadelphia: WB Saunders, 1982.

75 Gartner C, Zitelli B, Malatack JJ, Shaw BW, Iwatsuki S, Starzi TE. Orthotopic liver transplantation in children. Two year experience with 47 patients. *Pediatrics* 1984;74:140−5.

76 Ingelfinger JR, Grupe WE, Levey RH. Post-transplant hypertension in the absence of rejection or recurrent disease. *Clin Nephrol* 1981;15:236−9.

77 Gunnells JG, Stickel DL, Robinson RR. Episodic hypertension associated with positive renin assays after renal transplantation. *N Engl J Med* 1966;274:543−7.

78 Malekzadeh MH, Brennen LP, Payne VC, Fine RN. Hypertension after renal transplantation in children. *J Pediatr* 1975;86:370−5.

79 Daniels SR, Loggie JMH, Strife CF, Lipman M, Meyer RA. Distribution of target-organ abnormalities by race and sex in children with essential hypertension. *J Human Hypertension* (in press).

Index